ATLAS OF
HUMAN
ANATOMY

F. Netter
M.D.

ATLAS

HUMAN

OF
ANATOMY

by FRANK H. NETTER, M.D.

Sharon Colacino, Ph.D., *Consulting Editor*

CIBA–GEIGY CORPORATION

SUMMIT, NEW JERSEY

Copies of *Atlas of Human Anatomy, The CIBA Collection of Medical
Illustrations, Clinical Symposia* reprints and color slides of all
illustrations are available from CIBA–GEIGY Medical Education,
14 Henderson Drive, West Caldwell, NJ 07006

Library of Congress Cataloging-in-Publication Data

Netter, Frank H. (Frank Henry), 1906–
      Atlas of human anatomy / by Frank H. Netter: Sharon Colacino,
   consulting editor.
         p.   cm,
      Includes bibliographies and index.
      ISBN 0-914168-18-5: $86.50.—ISBN 0-914168-19-3 (pbk.): $39.95
      1. Anatomy, Human—Atlases. I. Colacino, Sharon. II. Title.
      [DNLM: 1. Anatomy—atlases. QS 17 N474a]
   QM25. N46 1989
   611: 0022—dc20
   DNLM/DLC
      for Library of Congress   89-60477
                                                                 CIP

First Printing, 1989
Second Printing, 1990
Third Printing, 1990

ISBN 0-914168-19-3
Library of Congress Catalog No: 89-060477

Printed in Japan

Design and production by Philip Grushkin
Color separations, printing and binding by Daiichi Seihan
Composition by U.S. Lithograph, typographers

To my dear wife, Vera

INTRODUCTION

I have often said that my career as a medical artist for almost 50 years has been a sort of "command performance" in the sense that it has grown in response to the desires and requests of the medical profession. Over these many years, I have produced almost 4,000 illustrations, mostly for *The CIBA Collection of Medical Illustrations* but also for *Clinical Symposia*. These pictures have been concerned with the varied subdivisions of medical knowledge such as gross anatomy, histology, embryology, physiology, pathology, diagnostic modalities, surgical and therapeutic techniques and clinical manifestations of a multitude of diseases. As the years went by, however, there were more and more requests from physicians and students for me to produce an atlas purely of gross anatomy. Thus, this atlas has come about, not through any inspiration on my part but rather, like most of my previous works, as a fulfillment of the desires of the medical profession. I was, however, so occupied with other commitments that it took me a long time to get around to undertaking it. And then when I finally did, I found it to require much more work and time than I had anticipated. It involved going back over all the illustrations I had made over so many years, selecting those pertinent to gross anatomy, classifying them and organizing them by system and region, adapting them to page size and space and arranging them in logical sequence. Anatomy of course does not change, but our understanding of anatomy and its clinical significance does change as do anatomical terminology and nomenclature. This therefore required much updating of many of the older pictures and even revision of a number of them in order to make them more pertinent to today's ever-expanding scope of medical and surgical practice. In addition I found that there were gaps in the portrayal of medical knowledge as pictorialized in the illustrations I had previously done, and this necessitated my making a number of new pictures that are included in this volume.

In creating an atlas such as this, it is important to achieve a happy medium between complexity and simplification. If the pictures are too complex, they may be difficult and confusing to read; if oversimplified, they may not be adequately definitive or may even be misleading. I have therefore striven for a middle course of realism without the clutter of confusing minutiae. I hope that the students and members of the medical and allied professions will find the illustrations readily understandable, yet instructive and useful.

At one point Mr. Flagler, the publisher, and I thought it might be nice to include a foreword by a truly outstanding and renowned anatomist, but there are so many in that category, a considerable number of whom have collaborated with me in the past and who are listed elsewhere in this volume, that we could not make a choice. We did think of men like Vesalius, Leonardo da Vinci, William Hunter and Henry Gray, who of course are unfortunately unavailable, but I do wonder what their comments might have been about this atlas.

Frank H. Netter, M.D.

ACKNOWLEDGMENTS

I have not been alone in this entire venture of medical pictorialization. There has been first and foremost the CIBA Pharmaceutical Company (now the CIBA–GEIGY Corporation) that has sponsored the creation of *The CIBA Collection of Medical Illustrations* as well as of this *Atlas of Human Anatomy*, which has grown out of it. Ours has been a long, happy and productive association. Very significant in this connection was a very special person and good friend, Mr. Paul Roder, then a CIBA executive, who early recognized the artistic and educational value of my pictures, and who was a major influence in CIBA's undertaking their sponsorship, as well as in encouraging me to do more. Another person who was most important in these respects was the late Dr. Ernst Oppenheimer, then chief pharmacologist at CIBA, who edited the first three volumes of *The CIBA Collection*.

In the creation of this specific *Atlas of Human Anatomy*, Dr. Sharon Colacino, assistant professor of anatomy at the College of Physicians and Surgeons, Columbia University, and consulting editor of this volume, played so vital and diversified a role that I cannot find words to adequately describe it. I can only express my heartfelt thanks for her help in many, many ways such as in organization of the atlas, in proposing modification of many of the old plates, in suggesting additional new ones, in checking on anatomical details and nomenclature, in planning sectional and subsectional divisions of the book and, in general, for her tireless and dedicated devotion to the project.

I furthermore express herewith my admiration for the artistry and skill of Mr. Philip Grushkin, who did the overall and typographic design, made the mechanicals and oversaw the entire production and printing of this atlas. Its visual appeal, readability and fine quality of pictorial reproduction are largely attributable to him, and his efficiency of operation greatly expedited its production.

I thank also dear Ms. Jeffie Lemons, who kept track of the over 500 illustrations with numerous type overlays for each, and the multitude of typographic and organizational changes as we went along, and who made up the preliminary and revised dummies that were necessary. Her pleasantness and efficiency in handling these almost overwhelming detailed responsibilities were a delight to me.

Thanks as well to Ms. Sally Chichester without whose editorial expertise this book would not have been possible.

Finally I must give great credit to Mr. Philip Flagler, who kept the whole project moving along and the entire team working together, and on whom it befell to make many production and financial decisions; to Dr. Milton Donin and Dr. Roy A. Ellis, who both did much in initiating this undertaking; and to a great many others of the CIBA organization for their supporting roles.

Many of the illustrations in this atlas have been published previously in various volumes of *The CIBA Collection of Medical Illustrations* or *Clinical Symposia*. In creating those illustrations, I had the pleasure and benefit of collaborating with a number of outstanding anatomists from various parts of the world, some of whom are now deceased. Many of these knowledgeable people are listed below, but there were also many others who gave to me of their advice and criticism and I thank them all very much.

Frank H. Netter, M.D.

Jay B. Angevine, Jr., Ph.D.

Louis L. Bergmann, M.D.

Hyun Taik Cho, M.D.

Eugene Cliffton, M.D.

Edmund S. Crelin, Ph.D., D.Sc.

Calvin Ezrin, M.D.

Joseph A. Gaines, M.D.

Charles F. Geschickter, M.D.

Rudolph V. Gorsch, M.D.

Brian F. Hoffman, M.D.

John Franklin Huber, M.D., Ph.D.

W.R. Ingram, Ph.D.

Abraham Kaplan, M.D.

Albert Kuntz, Ph.D, M.D.

Nicholas A. Michels, M.A., D.Sc.

G.A.G. Mitchell, Ch.M., D.Sc., F.R.C.S.

Barry W. Peterson, Ph.D.

Hans Popper, M.D.

Lynne M. Reid, M.D.

Johannes A.G. Rhodin, M.D., Ph.D.

I.C. Rubin, M.D.

Jerome J. Sheldon, M.D.

Max L. Som, M.D.

F. Mason Sones, Jr., M.D.

Somers H. Sturgis, M.D.

Lodewyk H.S. Van Mierop, M.D.

Samuel A. Vest, M.D.

Gerhardt von Bonin, M.D.

Bernard S. Wolf, M.D.

Gerhard Wolf-Heidegger, M.D., Ph.D.

Russell T. Woodburne, M.A., Ph.D.

PUBLISHER'S NOTE

Completion of a project as large and complex as this atlas requires the work of many people with diverse skills, a wealth of talent and single-minded dedication to see their tasks through to the end. We have been most fortunate to have just such a group working together with Dr. Netter to publish this book, and they have done it with enthusiasm, tenacity and great care. I extend to them my personal thanks as well as those of CIBA–GEIGY.

Dr. Netter has worked primarily with his collaborators, our consultants and the editorial staff, all of whom he has thanked in his own acknowledgments. I am delighted to second that thanks. Many others were involved in important ways, however, and their contributions must also be acknowledged.

Between the editorial and production functions lies a land of unsung heroes, several of whom should be recognized by name. Proofreaders Jo Sacher and Robin Snowden provided invaluable assistance, as anyone who looks at the legends on the pictures will agree. Designer Clark Carroll assisted Philip Grushkin in the preparation of mechanicals, brackets, special figures and many of the leader lines. Editorial Assistant Nicole Friedman, though not officially assigned to the project, became involved frequently—and willingly.

I would be remiss not to mention an important attribute of this atlas, which along with so many other jobs, was taken on as a special project by Dr. Colacino, Sally Chichester and Jeffie Lemons. I think you will find that every legend on every painting in the book has been called out in the index—and in a very usable way too. An index of 36 pages is a book in itself, and it took many late nights with the exercise of infinite patience to prepare.

The paintings are reproduced with a clarity and accuracy never before possible, and this is due to the work of two companies whose people became full partners with us in this project. Don Sigovich and his staff at Gamma One Conversions in New York City photographed all of the paintings, both old and new, using a process that captures on film the colors, densities, shapes and textures of Dr. Netter's originals. These transparencies, color corrected by hand to precisely match the art, became the starting point in the reproduction process.

The transparencies, in turn, were handed over to Daiichi Seihan, who produced the color separations from which the printing plates were made and who also printed and bound the finished work. Tomeji Maruyama personally oversaw each step in the difficult process of color separation both here in the United States and in Japan where the films were physically prepared. His application of time, talent, patience, organization and hard work was extraordinary. Tomeji was assisted in these steps by Bill Bianco, also of Daiichi Seihan, and the company's staff in Japan (who at this writing I have not met, but who certainly will become colleagues and friends before the ink is dry and the covers are attached).

Finally, of course, we at CIBA–GEIGY thank Frank H. Netter, M.D., our friend, our colleague and our inspiration. We hope he has found as much satisfaction and pleasure in preparing this atlas as each of us has found in working with him. At 83, he is still the master artist, the master teacher and the master physician, and he can still outwork all of us. As we go to press with this atlas, he is ready with all the paintings for the next addition to *The CIBA Collection of Medical Illustrations, Musculoskeletal System*, Part II (tentative publishing date, September 1990), as well as many of the paintings for *Musculoskeletal System*, Part III. Perhaps we should say he is the master of productivity as well!

Again, many thanks to all who have had a hand in bringing this very special book to life. It is our hope it will help countless generations of students learn the complexities of human anatomy and find a place as a reference wherever the intricacies of the human body are studied and discussed.

Philip Flagler
Director
Medical Education

CONTENTS

NOMENCLATURE

The *Atlas of Human Anatomy* follows the nomenclature
adopted by the Eleventh International Congress of Anatomists
in 1980. In accordance with the recommendation of the
International Anatomical Nomenclature Committee, the
terminology in this book departs from the strict Latin in many
cases by either anglicizing names or by using direct English
translations. If the adopted *Nomina Anatomica* terms differ
substantially from the older terms or if eponyms and older
terms are still in common use by the medical community,
these alternate terms are given in parentheses.

Section I

HEAD AND NECK

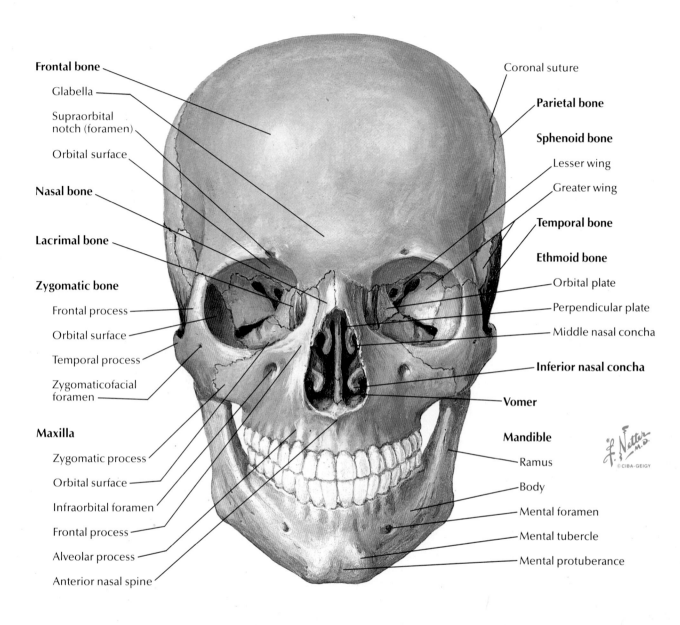

Frontal bone

Glabella

Supraorbital notch (foramen)

Orbital surface

Nasal bone

Lacrimal bone

Zygomatic bone

Frontal process

Orbital surface

Temporal process

Zygomaticofacial foramen

Maxilla

Zygomatic process

Orbital surface

Infraorbital foramen

Frontal process

Alveolar process

Anterior nasal spine

Coronal suture

Parietal bone

Sphenoid bone

Lesser wing

Greater wing

Temporal bone

Ethmoid bone

Orbital plate

Perpendicular plate

Middle nasal concha

Inferior nasal concha

Vomer

Mandible

Ramus

Body

Mental foramen

Mental tubercle

Mental protuberance

Right orbit: frontal and slightly lateral view

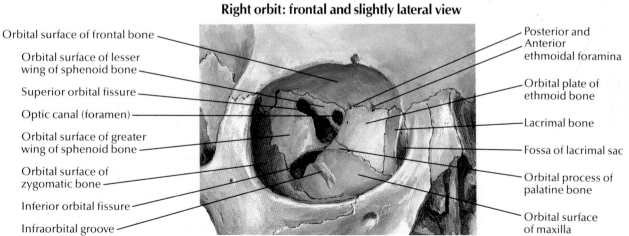

Orbital surface of frontal bone

Orbital surface of lesser wing of sphenoid bone

Superior orbital fissure

Optic canal (foramen)

Orbital surface of greater wing of sphenoid bone

Orbital surface of zygomatic bone

Inferior orbital fissure

Infraorbital groove

Posterior and Anterior ethmoidal foramina

Orbital plate of ethmoid bone

Lacrimal bone

Fossa of lacrimal sac

Orbital process of palatine bone

Orbital surface of maxilla

Skull: Lateral View

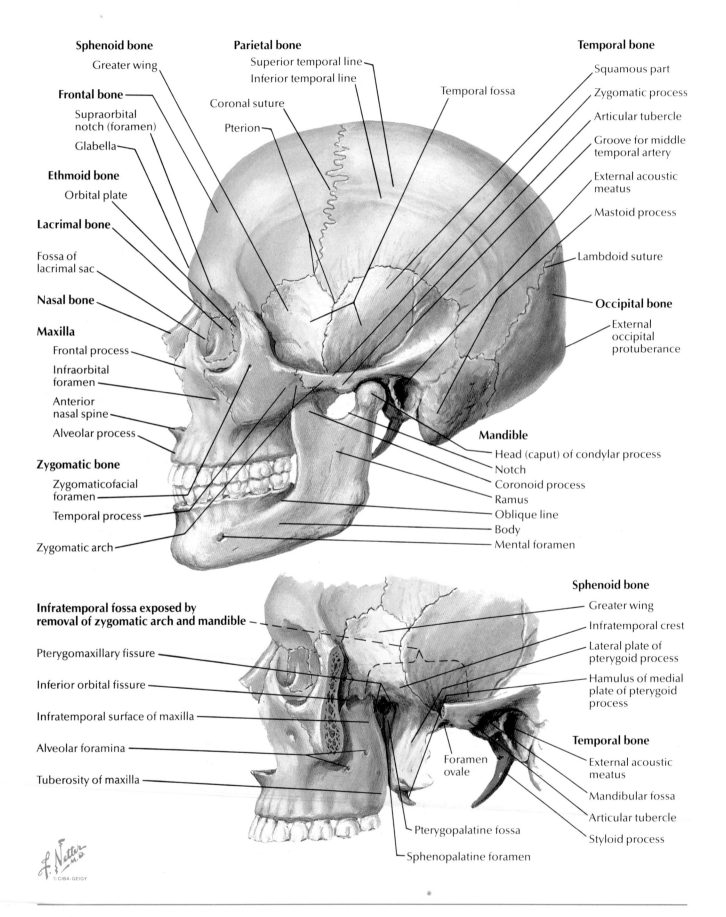

Sphenoid bone
Greater wing

Frontal bone
Supraorbital notch (foramen)
Glabella

Ethmoid bone
Orbital plate

Lacrimal bone
Fossa of lacrimal sac

Nasal bone

Maxilla
Frontal process
Infraorbital foramen
Anterior nasal spine
Alveolar process

Zygomatic bone
Zygomaticofacial foramen
Temporal process
Zygomatic arch

Parietal bone
Superior temporal line
Inferior temporal line
Coronal suture
Pterion

Temporal fossa

Temporal bone
Squamous part
Zygomatic process
Articular tubercle
Groove for middle temporal artery
External acoustic meatus
Mastoid process
Lambdoid suture

Occipital bone
External occipital protuberance

Mandible
Head (caput) of condylar process
Notch
Coronoid process
Ramus
Oblique line
Body
Mental foramen

Infratemporal fossa exposed by removal of zygomatic arch and mandible

Pterygomaxillary fissure

Inferior orbital fissure

Infratemporal surface of maxilla

Alveolar foramina

Tuberosity of maxilla

Foramen ovale

Pterygopalatine fossa

Sphenopalatine foramen

Sphenoid bone
Greater wing
Infratemporal crest
Lateral plate of pterygoid process
Hamulus of medial plate of pterygoid process

Temporal bone
External acoustic meatus
Mandibular fossa
Articular tubercle
Styloid process

PLATE 2

HEAD AND NECK

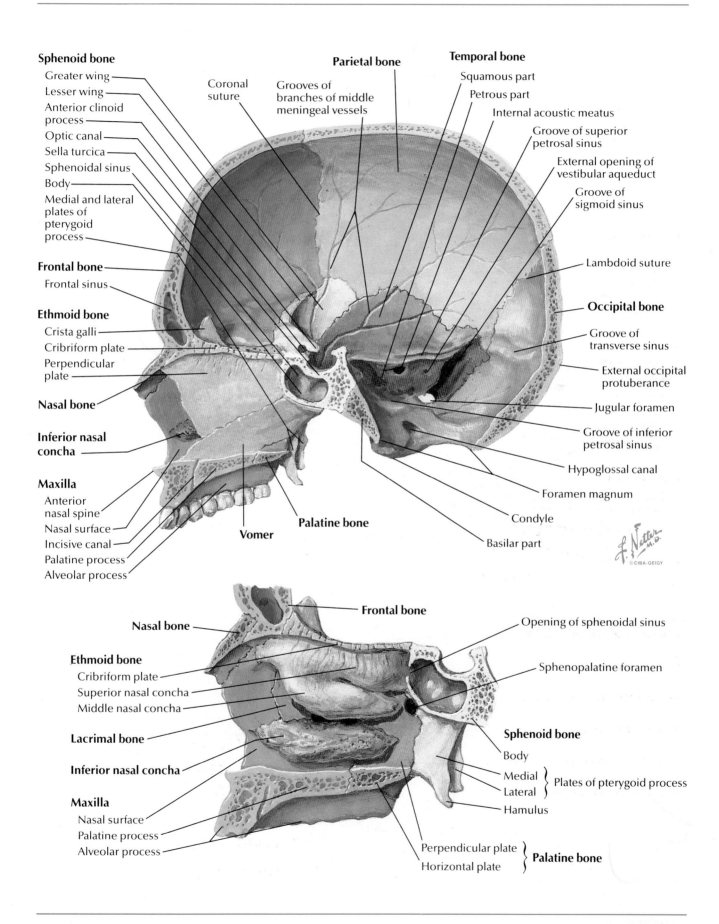

Sphenoid bone
Greater wing
Lesser wing
Anterior clinoid process
Optic canal
Sella turcica
Sphenoidal sinus
Body
Medial and lateral plates of pterygoid process

Frontal bone
Frontal sinus

Ethmoid bone
Crista galli
Cribriform plate
Perpendicular plate

Nasal bone

Inferior nasal concha

Maxilla
Anterior nasal spine
Nasal surface
Incisive canal
Palatine process
Alveolar process

Coronal suture

Grooves of branches of middle meningeal vessels

Parietal bone

Temporal bone
Squamous part
Petrous part
Internal acoustic meatus
Groove of superior petrosal sinus
External opening of vestibular aqueduct
Groove of sigmoid sinus

Lambdoid suture

Occipital bone
Groove of transverse sinus
External occipital protuberance
Jugular foramen
Groove of inferior petrosal sinus
Hypoglossal canal
Foramen magnum
Condyle
Basilar part

Vomer

Palatine bone

Nasal bone

Frontal bone

Opening of sphenoidal sinus

Sphenopalatine foramen

Ethmoid bone
Cribriform plate
Superior nasal concha
Middle nasal concha

Lacrimal bone

Inferior nasal concha

Maxilla
Nasal surface
Palatine process
Alveolar process

Sphenoid bone
Body
Medial ⎫
Lateral ⎬ Plates of pterygoid process
Hamulus

Perpendicular plate ⎫
Horizontal plate ⎬ **Palatine bone**

Calvaria

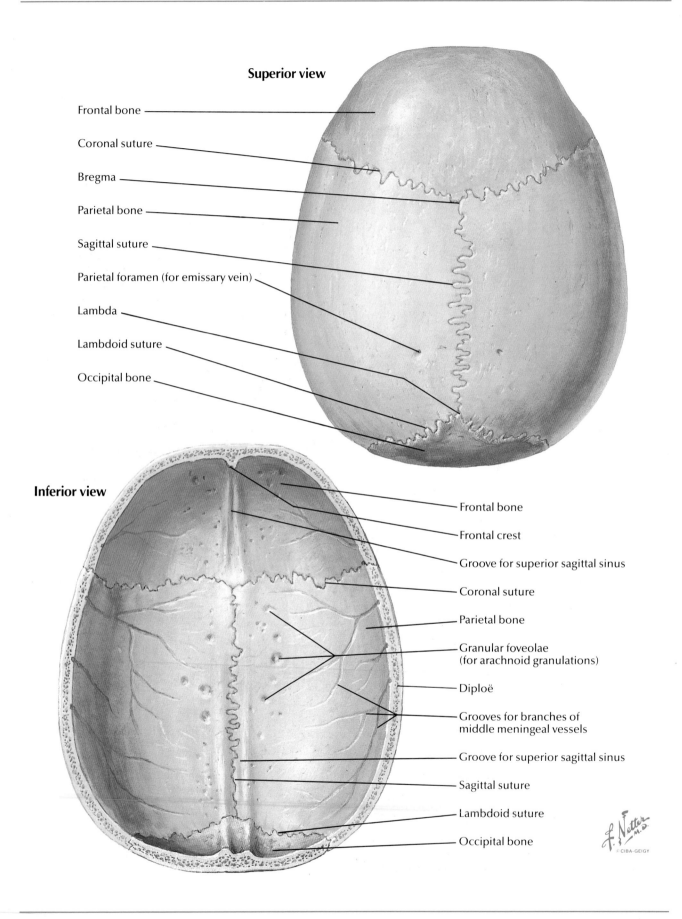

Superior view

Frontal bone

Coronal suture

Bregma

Parietal bone

Sagittal suture

Parietal foramen (for emissary vein)

Lambda

Lambdoid suture

Occipital bone

Inferior view

Frontal bone

Frontal crest

Groove for superior sagittal sinus

Coronal suture

Parietal bone

Granular foveolae
(for arachnoid granulations)

Diploë

Grooves for branches of
middle meningeal vessels

Groove for superior sagittal sinus

Sagittal suture

Lambdoid suture

Occipital bone

PLATE 4

HEAD AND NECK

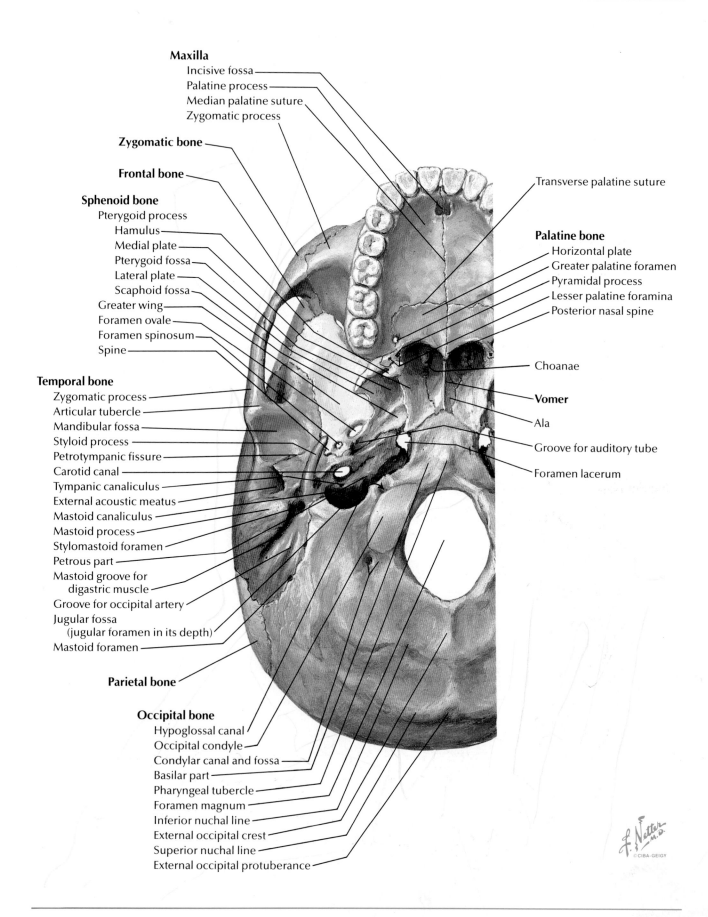

Maxilla
Incisive fossa
Palatine process
Median palatine suture
Zygomatic process

Zygomatic bone

Frontal bone

Sphenoid bone
Pterygoid process
Hamulus
Medial plate
Pterygoid fossa
Lateral plate
Scaphoid fossa
Greater wing
Foramen ovale
Foramen spinosum
Spine

Temporal bone
Zygomatic process
Articular tubercle
Mandibular fossa
Styloid process
Petrotympanic fissure
Carotid canal
Tympanic canaliculus
External acoustic meatus
Mastoid canaliculus
Mastoid process
Stylomastoid foramen
Petrous part
Mastoid groove for
    digastric muscle
Groove for occipital artery
Jugular fossa
    (jugular foramen in its depth)
Mastoid foramen

Parietal bone

Occipital bone
Hypoglossal canal
Occipital condyle
Condylar canal and fossa
Basilar part
Pharyngeal tubercle
Foramen magnum
Inferior nuchal line
External occipital crest
Superior nuchal line
External occipital protuberance

Transverse palatine suture

Palatine bone
Horizontal plate
Greater palatine foramen
Pyramidal process
Lesser palatine foramina
Posterior nasal spine

Choanae

Vomer

Ala

Groove for auditory tube

Foramen lacerum

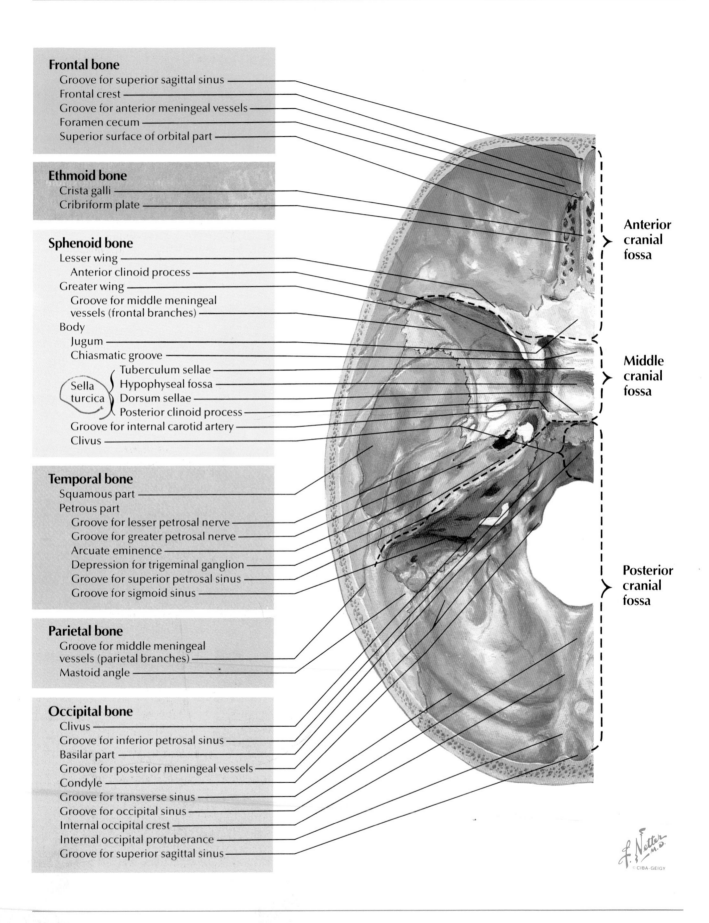

Frontal bone
Groove for superior sagittal sinus
Frontal crest
Groove for anterior meningeal vessels
Foramen cecum
Superior surface of orbital part

Ethmoid bone
Crista galli
Cribriform plate

Sphenoid bone
Lesser wing
Anterior clinoid process
Greater wing
Groove for middle meningeal
vessels (frontal branches)
Body
Jugum
Chiasmatic groove
Sella turcica {
Tuberculum sellae
Hypophyseal fossa
Dorsum sellae
Posterior clinoid process
Groove for internal carotid artery
Clivus

Temporal bone
Squamous part
Petrous part
Groove for lesser petrosal nerve
Groove for greater petrosal nerve
Arcuate eminence
Depression for trigeminal ganglion
Groove for superior petrosal sinus
Groove for sigmoid sinus

Parietal bone
Groove for middle meningeal
vessels (parietal branches)
Mastoid angle

Occipital bone
Clivus
Groove for inferior petrosal sinus
Basilar part
Groove for posterior meningeal vessels
Condyle
Groove for transverse sinus
Groove for occipital sinus
Internal occipital crest
Internal occipital protuberance
Groove for superior sagittal sinus

Anterior
cranial
fossa

Middle
cranial
fossa

Posterior
cranial
fossa

PLATE 6   **HEAD AND NECK**

Foramina of Cranial Base: Superior View

Foramen cecum ------------ Emissary vein to superior sagittal sinus

Nasal slit --------------- } {Anterior ethmoidal artery, vein
Anterior ethmoidal foramen } {   and nerve

Foramina of cribriform plate ----- Olfactory nerve bundles

Posterior ethmoidal foramen ---- Posterior ethmoidal artery, vein
and nerve

Optic canal --------------- { Optic nerve (II)
{ Ophthalmic artery

Superior orbital fissure ------ { Oculomotor nerve (III)
{ Trochlear nerve (IV)
{ Lacrimal, frontal and nasociliary
{   branches of ophthalmic nerve (V₁)
{ Abducens nerve (VI)
{ Superior ophthalmic vein

Foramen rotundum --------- Maxillary nerve (V₂)

Foramen ovale ----------- { Mandibular nerve (V₃)
{ Accessory meningeal artery
{ Lesser petrosal nerve (occasionally)

Foramen spinosum -------- { Middle meningeal artery and vein
{ Meningeal branch of mandibular nerve

Foramen of Vesalius (inconstant) – Small emissary vein

Foramen lacerum ---------- { Internal carotid artery
{ Internal carotid nerve plexus

Hiatus of canal of ----------- Lesser petrosal nerve

Hiatus of canal of ---------- Greater petrosal nerve

Internal acoustic meatus ------ { Facial nerve (VII)
{ Vestibulocochlear nerve (VIII)
{ Labyrinthine artery

External opening of
vestibular aqueduct --------- Endolymphatic duct

Mastoid foramen (inconstant) --- Emissary vein (branch of
occipital artery)

Jugular foramen ---------- { Inferior petrosal sinus
{ Glossopharyngeal nerve (IX)
{ Vagus nerve (X)
{ Accessory nerve (XI)
{ Sigmoid sinus
{ Posterior meningeal artery

Condylar canal (inconstant) ----{ Emissary vein and meningeal branch
{   of ascending pharyngeal artery

Hypoglossal canal ----------- Hypoglossal nerve (XII)

Foramen magnum -------- { Medulla oblongata
{ Meninges
{ Vertebral arteries
{ Meningeal branches of vertebral
{   arteries
{ Spinal roots of accessory nerves

Turbinate

f. Netter
©CIBA-GEIGY

BONES AND LIGAMENTS

PLATE 7

Skull of Newborn

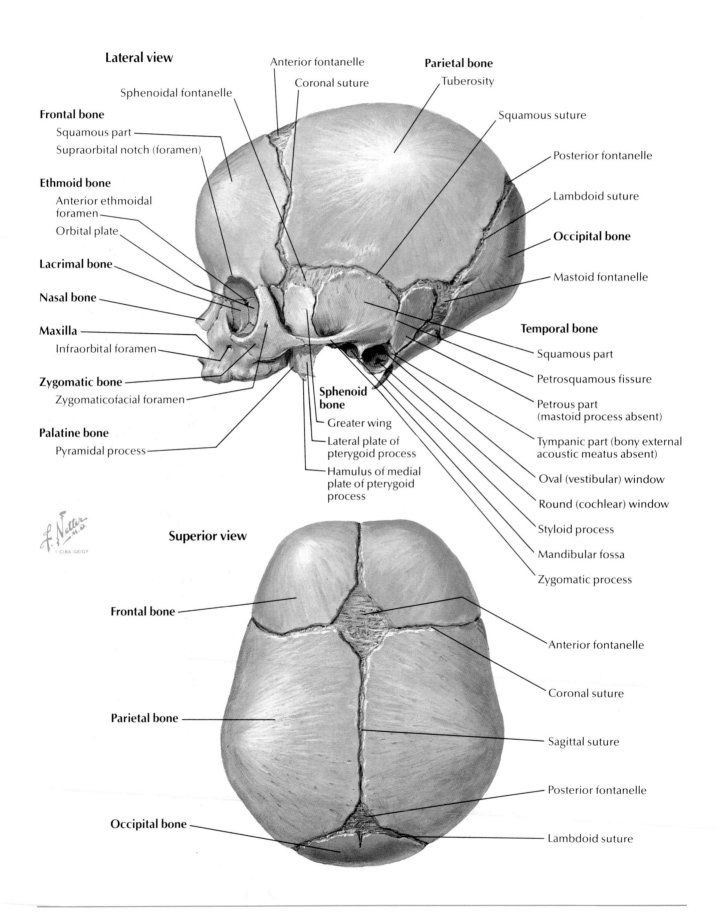

Lateral view

Anterior fontanelle

Coronal suture

Parietal bone

Tuberosity

Sphenoidal fontanelle

Frontal bone

Squamous part

Supraorbital notch (foramen)

Squamous suture

Posterior fontanelle

Ethmoid bone

Anterior ethmoidal foramen

Orbital plate

Lambdoid suture

Occipital bone

Lacrimal bone

Mastoid fontanelle

Nasal bone

Maxilla

Infraorbital foramen

Temporal bone

Squamous part

Petrosquamous fissure

Zygomatic bone

Zygomaticofacial foramen

Petrous part (mastoid process absent)

Sphenoid bone

Greater wing

Tympanic part (bony external acoustic meatus absent)

Palatine bone

Pyramidal process

Lateral plate of pterygoid process

Oval (vestibular) window

Round (cochlear) window

Hamulus of medial plate of pterygoid process

Styloid process

Mandibular fossa

Zygomatic process

Superior view

Frontal bone

Anterior fontanelle

Coronal suture

Parietal bone

Sagittal suture

Posterior fontanelle

Occipital bone

Lambdoid suture

PLATE 8

HEAD AND NECK

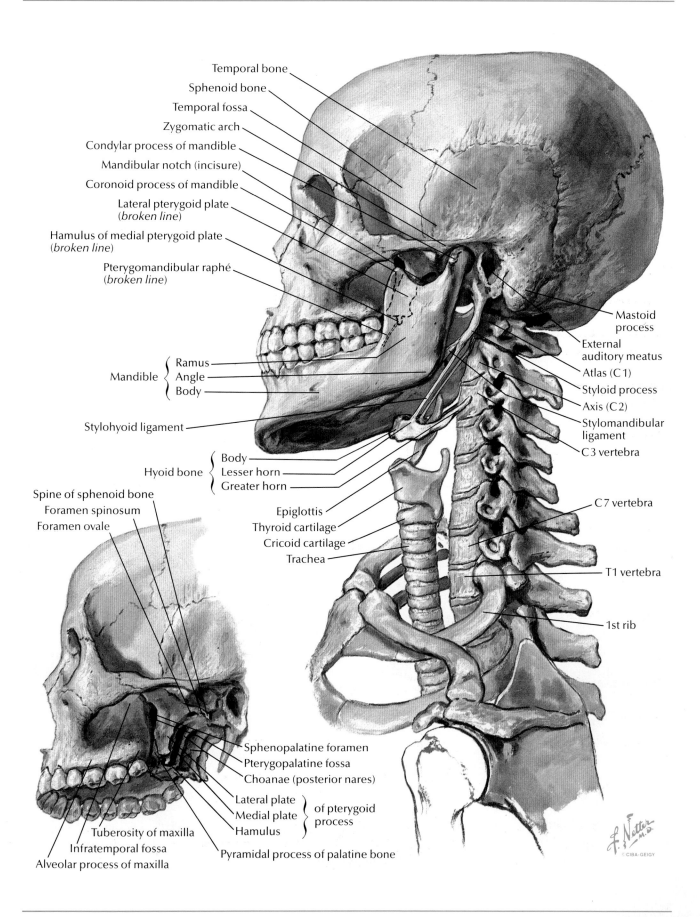

Temporal bone
Sphenoid bone
Temporal fossa
Zygomatic arch
Condylar process of mandible
Mandibular notch (incisure)
Coronoid process of mandible
Lateral pterygoid plate (*broken line*)
Hamulus of medial pterygoid plate (*broken line*)
Pterygomandibular raphé (*broken line*)

Mandible { Ramus / Angle / Body

Stylohyoid ligament

Spine of sphenoid bone
Foramen spinosum
Foramen ovale

Hyoid bone { Body / Lesser horn / Greater horn

Epiglottis
Thyroid cartilage
Cricoid cartilage
Trachea

Mastoid process
External auditory meatus
Atlas (C 1)
Styloid process
Axis (C 2)
Stylomandibular ligament
C 3 vertebra

C 7 vertebra

T1 vertebra

1st rib

Sphenopalatine foramen
Pterygopalatine fossa
Choanae (posterior nares)
Lateral plate }
Medial plate } of pterygoid process
Hamulus }
Tuberosity of maxilla
Infratemporal fossa
Pyramidal process of palatine bone
Alveolar process of maxilla

f. Netter
©CIBA-GEIGY

Mandible

Mandible of infant

Condylar process
Coronoid process
Head (caput)
Pterygoid fossa
Neck
Notch (incisure)
Mylohyoid groove
Lingula
Oblique line
Mandibular foramen
Submandibular fossa
Mylohyoid line
Sublingual fossa
Interalveolar septa
Ramus
Alveolar part (crest)
Mental foramen
Mental protuberance
Angle
Mental tubercle
Base of mandible
Body

**Mandible of adult:
anterolateral superior view**

Coronoid process
Head (caput)
Neck
Notch (incisure)
Pterygoid fossa
Condylar process
Lingula
Mandibular foramen
Mylohyoid groove
Mylohyoid line
Ramus
Angle
Body
Submandibular fossa
Sublingual fossa
Digastric fossa
Mental spines

**Mandible of adult:
left posterior view**

**Mandible of aged
person (edentulous)**

PLATE 10

HEAD AND NECK

Temporomandibular Joint

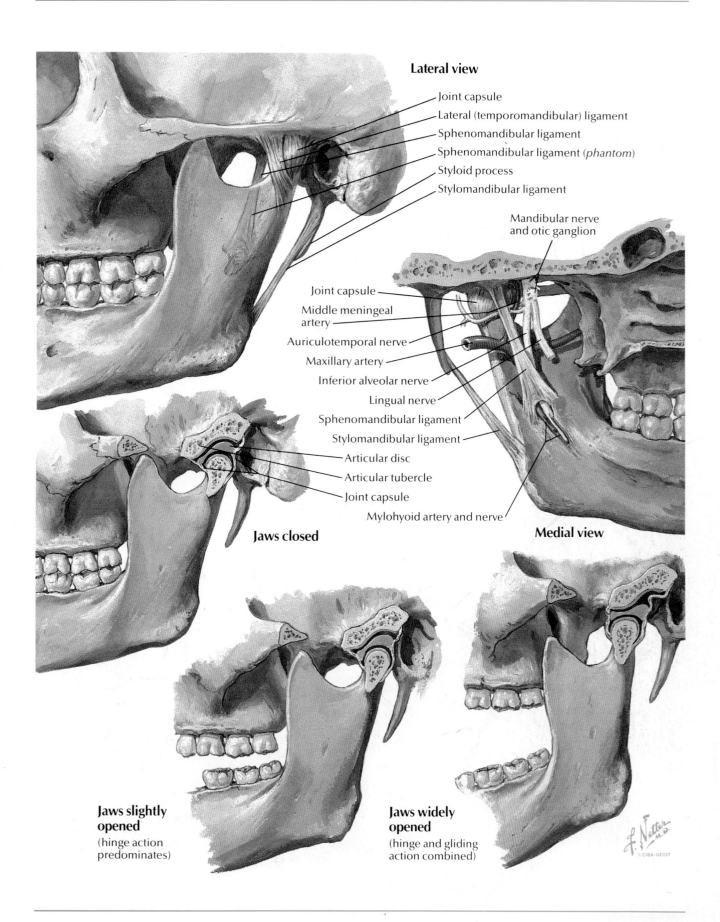

Lateral view

- Joint capsule
- Lateral (temporomandibular) ligament
- Sphenomandibular ligament
- Sphenomandibular ligament (*phantom*)
- Styloid process
- Stylomandibular ligament

Mandibular nerve and otic ganglion

- Joint capsule
- Middle meningeal artery
- Auriculotemporal nerve
- Maxillary artery
- Inferior alveolar nerve
- Lingual nerve
- Sphenomandibular ligament
- Stylomandibular ligament
- Articular disc
- Articular tubercle
- Joint capsule
- Mylohyoid artery and nerve

Jaws closed

Medial view

Jaws slightly opened
(hinge action predominates)

Jaws widely opened
(hinge and gliding action combined)

Cervical Vertebrae: Atlas and Axis

SEE ALSO PLATES 9, 142

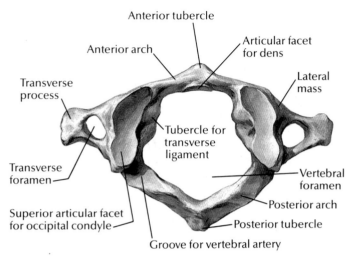

Anterior tubercle

Anterior arch

Articular facet for dens

Transverse process

Lateral mass

Tubercle for transverse ligament

Transverse foramen

Vertebral foramen

Superior articular facet for occipital condyle

Posterior arch

Posterior tubercle

Groove for vertebral artery

Atlas (C 1): superior view

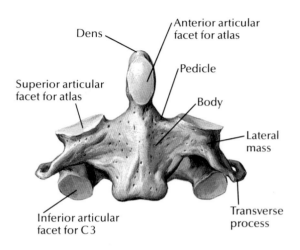

Dens

Anterior articular facet for atlas

Superior articular facet for atlas

Pedicle

Body

Lateral mass

Inferior articular facet for C 3

Transverse process

Axis (C 2): anterior view

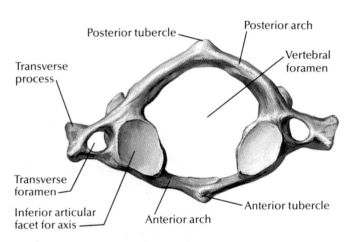

Posterior tubercle

Posterior arch

Transverse process

Vertebral foramen

Transverse foramen

Inferior articular facet for axis

Anterior tubercle

Anterior arch

Atlas (C 1): inferior view

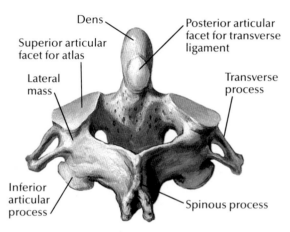

Dens

Posterior articular facet for transverse ligament

Superior articular facet for atlas

Lateral mass

Transverse process

Inferior articular process

Spinous process

Axis (C 2): posterosuperior view

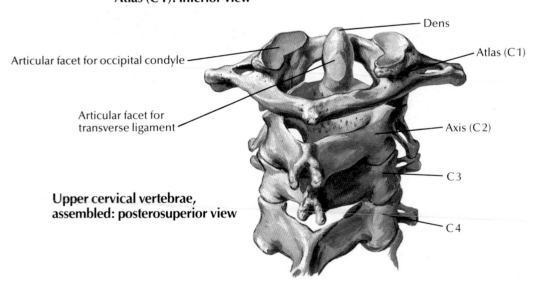

Dens

Atlas (C 1)

Articular facet for occipital condyle

Articular facet for transverse ligament

Axis (C 2)

C 3

C 4

Upper cervical vertebrae, assembled: posterosuperior view

PLATE 12

Anterior tubercle

Body

Transverse process

Groove for spinal nerve

Transverse foramen

Pedicle

Superior articular facet

Inferior articular process

Vertebral foramen (vertebral canal)

Spinous process

Posterior tubercle

Lamina

4th cervical vertebra: superior view

Body

Anterior tubercle

Posterior tubercle

Lamina

7th cervical vertebra: superior view

Dens

Cervical curvature

Intervertebral foramina for spinal nerves

Spinous processes

Lateral masses

C2

C3

C4

C5

C6

C7

T1

Zygapophyseal (lateral) articulation

Vertebral body (medial) articulation (*disc removed*)

Articular facets for 1st rib

2nd cervical to 1st thoracic vertebrae: right lateral view

Lateral mass

Zygapophyseal (lateral) articulation

Intervertebral foramen for spinal nerve

C3

C4

C5

3rd, 4th and 5th cervical vertebrae: anterior view

External Craniocervical Ligaments

Anterior view

Basilar part of occipital bone

Pharyngeal tubercle

Anterior atlantooccipital membrane

Capsule of atlantooccipital joint

Posterior atlantooccipital membrane

Lateral atlantoaxial joint (*opened up*)

Anterior longitudinal ligament

Atlas (C 1)

Capsule of lateral atlantoaxial joint

Axis (C 2)

Capsule of zygapophyseal (lateral) joint (C 3–4)

Posterior view

Posterior atlantooccipital membrane

Skull

Capsule of atlantooccipital joint

Atlas (C 1)

Capsule of lateral atlantoaxial joint

Axis (C 2)

Ligamentum flavum

Vertebral artery

Suboccipital nerve (dorsal ramus of C1)

Anterior atlantooccipital membrane

Capsule of atlantooccipital joint

Posterior atlantooccipital membrane

Atlas

Ligamenta flava

Ligamentum nuchae

Body of axis (C 2)

Intervertebral discs (C 2–3 and C 3–4)

Zygapophyseal (lateral) joints (C 4–5 and C 5–6)

Anterior tubercle of C6 vertebra (carotid tubercle)

Spinous process of C 7 vertebra (vertebra prominens)

Vertebral artery

T1 vertebra

Right lateral view

PLATE 14

HEAD AND NECK

Basilar part of occipital bone (clivus)

Upper part of vertebral canal with spinous processes and parts of vertebral arches removed to expose ligaments on posterior vertebral bodies: posterior view

Capsule of atlantooccipital joint

Atlas (C1)

Capsule of atlantoaxial joint

Axis (C2)

Capsule of zygapophyseal joint (C2–3)

Tectorial membrane

Deeper (accessory) part of tectorial membrane

Posterior longitudinal ligament

Alar ligaments

Cruciform ligament {
Superior longitudinal fibers

Transverse ligament of atlas

Inferior longitudinal fibers
}

Deeper (accessory) part of tectorial membrane

Atlas (C1)

Axis (C2)

Principal part of tectorial membrane removed to expose deeper ligaments: posterior view

Atlas (C1)

Axis (C2)

Apical ligament of dens

Alar ligament

Articular facet of dens for transverse ligament of atlas

Alar ligament

Anterior tubercle of atlas

Synovial cavities

Dens

Transverse ligament of atlas

Cruciform ligament removed to show deepest ligaments: posterior view

Median atlantoaxial joint: superior view

Atlantooccipital Junction

Vertebral artery

Posterior margin of foramen magnum

Posterior atlanto-occipital membrane

Posterior tubercle of atlas (C 1)

Ligamentum nuchae

Posterior atlantoaxial membrane

Spinous process of axis (C 2)

Ligamentum flavum

Hypoglossal canal

Tectorial membrane

Apical ligament of dens

Superior longitudinal fibers of cruciate ligament of atlas

Anterior atlantooccipital membrane

Anterior tubercle of atlas (C 1)

Articular cavity

Dens (odontoid process) of axis (C 2)

Transverse (cruciate) ligament of atlas

Inferior atlantooccipital fibers of cruciate ligament of atlas

Anterior longitudinal ligament

Posterior longitudinal ligament

Posterior tip of hard palate

Lowest level of occipital bone

McGregor's line, from posterior tip of hard palate to lowest point of occipital bone. Average normal position of odontoid tip is 1.32 mm above this line with standard deviation of ± 2.6 mm as measured on standard lateral radiograph. Tip > 4.5 mm above line is considered to indicate basilar impression

Odontoid abnormalities, most often associated with skeletal dysplasias such as Klippel-Feil, Down's or Morquio's syndromes

Hypoplastic dens (odontoid process)

Os odontoideum with fibrous union and narrowing of vertebral canal with head in extension

PLATE 16

HEAD AND NECK

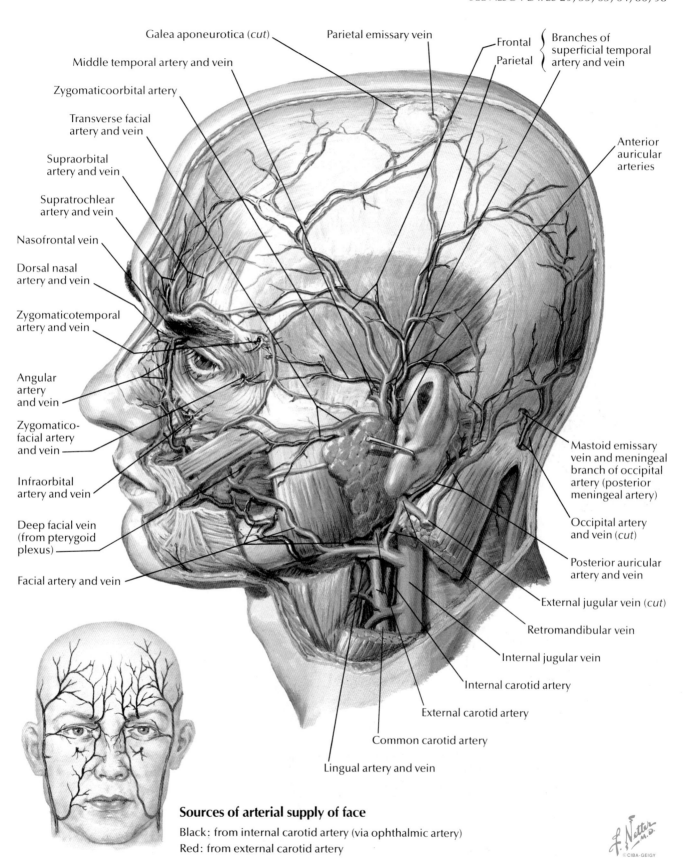

Galea aponeurotica (*cut*)

Middle temporal artery and vein

Zygomaticoorbital artery

Transverse facial artery and vein

Supraorbital artery and vein

Supratrochlear artery and vein

Nasofrontal vein

Dorsal nasal artery and vein

Zygomaticotemporal artery and vein

Angular artery and vein

Zygomatico-facial artery and vein

Infraorbital artery and vein

Deep facial vein (from pterygoid plexus)

Facial artery and vein

Parietal emissary vein

Frontal { Parietal { Branches of superficial temporal artery and vein

Anterior auricular arteries

Mastoid emissary vein and meningeal branch of occipital artery (posterior meningeal artery)

Occipital artery and vein (*cut*)

Posterior auricular artery and vein

External jugular vein (*cut*)

Retromandibular vein

Internal jugular vein

Internal carotid artery

External carotid artery

Common carotid artery

Lingual artery and vein

Sources of arterial supply of face

Black: from internal carotid artery (via ophthalmic artery)
Red: from external carotid artery

Cutaneous Nerves of Head and Neck

SEE ALSO PLATES 27, 31, 40, 41, 116

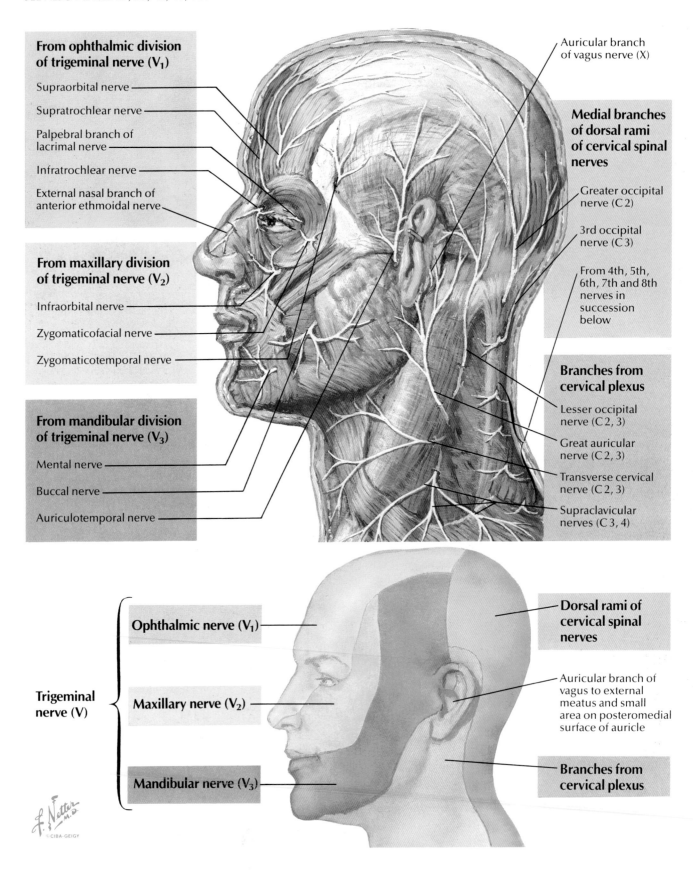

From ophthalmic division of trigeminal nerve (V₁)

Supraorbital nerve

Supratrochlear nerve

Palpebral branch of lacrimal nerve

Infratrochlear nerve

External nasal branch of anterior ethmoidal nerve

From maxillary division of trigeminal nerve (V₂)

Infraorbital nerve

Zygomaticofacial nerve

Zygomaticotemporal nerve

From mandibular division of trigeminal nerve (V₃)

Mental nerve

Buccal nerve

Auriculotemporal nerve

Auricular branch of vagus nerve (X)

Medial branches of dorsal rami of cervical spinal nerves

Greater occipital nerve (C 2)

3rd occipital nerve (C 3)

From 4th, 5th, 6th, 7th and 8th nerves in succession below

Branches from cervical plexus

Lesser occipital nerve (C 2, 3)

Great auricular nerve (C 2, 3)

Transverse cervical nerve (C 2, 3)

Supraclavicular nerves (C 3, 4)

Trigeminal nerve (V)

Ophthalmic nerve (V₁)

Maxillary nerve (V₂)

Mandibular nerve (V₃)

Dorsal rami of cervical spinal nerves

Auricular branch of vagus to external meatus and small area on posteromedial surface of auricle

Branches from cervical plexus

PLATE 18

HEAD AND NECK

Facial Nerve Branches and Parotid Gland

SEE ALSO PLATE 117

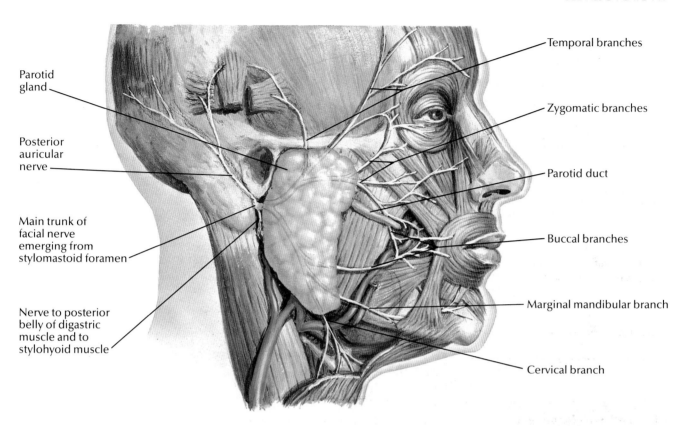

Parotid gland

Posterior auricular nerve

Main trunk of facial nerve emerging from stylomastoid foramen

Nerve to posterior belly of digastric muscle and to stylohyoid muscle

Temporal branches

Zygomatic branches

Parotid duct

Buccal branches

Marginal mandibular branch

Cervical branch

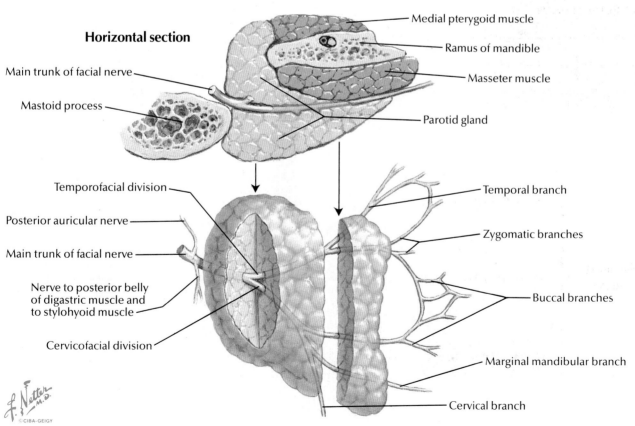

Horizontal section

Main trunk of facial nerve

Mastoid process

Medial pterygoid muscle

Ramus of mandible

Masseter muscle

Parotid gland

Temporofacial division

Posterior auricular nerve

Main trunk of facial nerve

Nerve to posterior belly of digastric muscle and to stylohyoid muscle

Cervicofacial division

Temporal branch

Zygomatic branches

Buccal branches

Marginal mandibular branch

Cervical branch

SUPERFICIAL FACE

PLATE 19

Muscles of Facial Expression: Anterior View

SEE ALSO PLATE 48

Galea aponeurotica

Frontal belly (frontalis) of epicranius muscle

Procerus muscle

Corrugator supercilii muscle

Orbital part
Palpebral part } of orbicularis oculi muscle

Levator labii superioris alaeque nasi muscle

Transverse part } of nasalis muscle
Alar part

Levator labii superioris muscle

Auricularis anterior muscle

Zygomaticus minor muscle

Zygomaticus major muscle

Levator anguli oris muscle

Depressor septi nasi muscle

Buccinator muscle

Risorius muscle

Orbicularis oris muscle

Depressor anguli oris muscle

Depressor labii inferioris muscle

Mentalis muscle

Platysma muscle

Course of wrinkle lines of skin is transverse to fiber direction of facial muscles. Elliptical incisions for removal of skin tumors conform to direction of wrinkle lines

PLATE 20

HEAD AND NECK

Galea aponeurotica

Temporalis fascia

Auricularis anterior muscle

Auricularis superior muscle

Auricularis posterior muscle

Occipital belly of epicranius (occipitalis) muscle

Orbicularis oculi muscle { Orbital part / Palpebral part

Frontal belly (frontalis) of epicranius muscle

Corrugator supercilii muscle (frontalis and orbicularis oculi, *partially cut away*)

Procerus muscle

Levator labii superioris muscle

Levator labii superioris alaeque nasi muscle (*partially cut away*)

Nasalis muscle { Transverse part / Alar part

Depressor septi nasi muscle

Orbicularis oris muscle

Zygomaticus minor muscle

Zygomaticus major muscle

Orbicularis oris muscle

Mentalis muscle

Depressor labii inferioris muscle

Depressor anguli oris muscle

Buccinator muscle

Risorius muscle

Platysma muscle

Sternum

Clavicle

Pectoralis major fascia

Parotid fascia

Masseteric fascia

Sternocleidomastoid fascia

Superficial cervical fascia of posterior (lateral) triangle over levator scapulae and splenius capitis muscles

Trapezius fascia

Deltoid fascia

Muscles of Neck: Lateral View

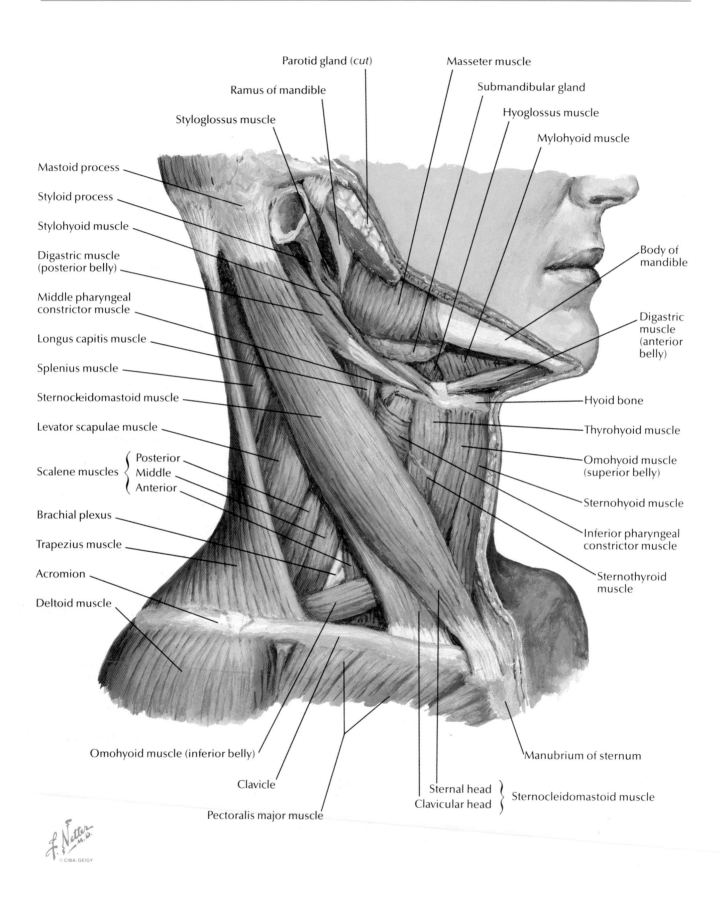

Parotid gland (*cut*)

Ramus of mandible

Styloglossus muscle

Masseter muscle

Submandibular gland

Hyoglossus muscle

Mylohyoid muscle

Mastoid process

Styloid process

Stylohyoid muscle

Digastric muscle
(posterior belly)

Middle pharyngeal
constrictor muscle

Longus capitis muscle

Splenius muscle

Sternocleidomastoid muscle

Levator scapulae muscle

Scalene muscles { Posterior / Middle / Anterior

Brachial plexus

Trapezius muscle

Acromion

Deltoid muscle

Body of
mandible

Digastric
muscle
(anterior
belly)

Hyoid bone

Thyrohyoid muscle

Omohyoid muscle
(superior belly)

Sternohyoid muscle

Inferior pharyngeal
constrictor muscle

Sternothyroid
muscle

Omohyoid muscle (inferior belly)

Clavicle

Pectoralis major muscle

Sternal head } Sternocleidomastoid muscle
Clavicular head }

Manubrium of sternum

PLATE 22

HEAD AND NECK

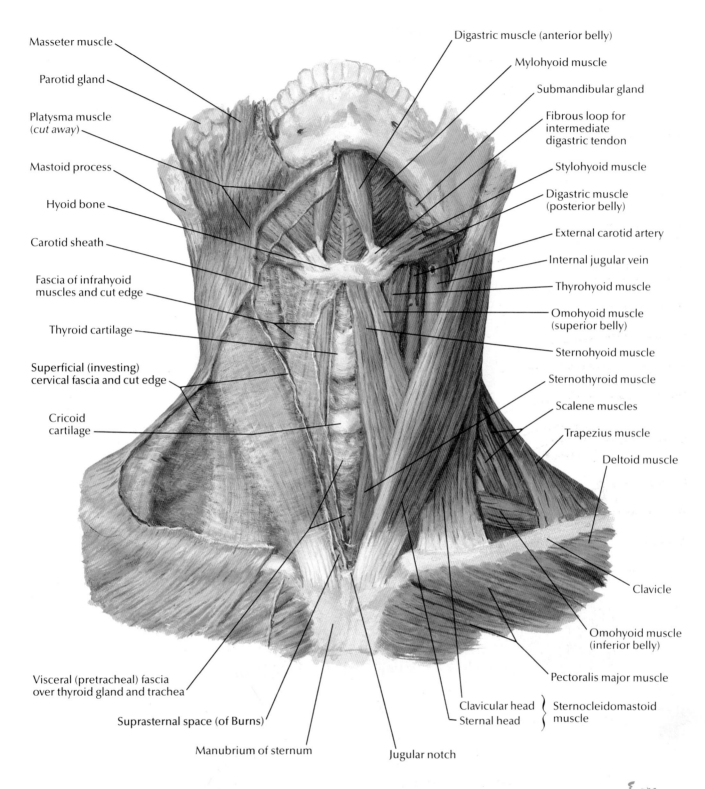

Masseter muscle

Parotid gland

Platysma muscle
(*cut away*)

Mastoid process

Hyoid bone

Carotid sheath

Fascia of infrahyoid
muscles and cut edge

Thyroid cartilage

Superficial (investing)
cervical fascia and cut edge

Cricoid
cartilage

Visceral (pretracheal) fascia
over thyroid gland and trachea

Suprasternal space (of Burns)

Manubrium of sternum

Digastric muscle (anterior belly)

Mylohyoid muscle

Submandibular gland

Fibrous loop for
intermediate
digastric tendon

Stylohyoid muscle

Digastric muscle
(posterior belly)

External carotid artery

Internal jugular vein

Thyrohyoid muscle

Omohyoid muscle
(superior belly)

Sternohyoid muscle

Sternothyroid muscle

Scalene muscles

Trapezius muscle

Deltoid muscle

Clavicle

Omohyoid muscle
(inferior belly)

Pectoralis major muscle

Clavicular head } Sternocleidomastoid
Sternal head   } muscle

Jugular notch

Infrahyoid and Suprahyoid Muscles

SEE ALSO PLATE 47

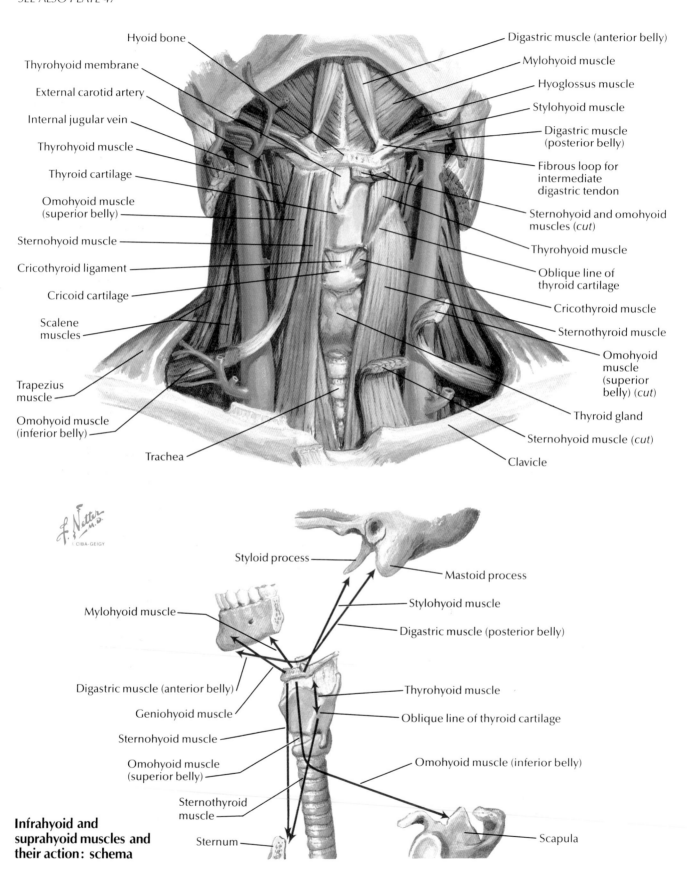

Hyoid bone

Thyrohyoid membrane

External carotid artery

Internal jugular vein

Thyrohyoid muscle

Thyroid cartilage

Omohyoid muscle (superior belly)

Sternohyoid muscle

Cricothyroid ligament

Cricoid cartilage

Scalene muscles

Trapezius muscle

Omohyoid muscle (inferior belly)

Trachea

Digastric muscle (anterior belly)

Mylohyoid muscle

Hyoglossus muscle

Stylohyoid muscle

Digastric muscle (posterior belly)

Fibrous loop for intermediate digastric tendon

Sternohyoid and omohyoid muscles (*cut*)

Thyrohyoid muscle

Oblique line of thyroid cartilage

Cricothyroid muscle

Sternothyroid muscle

Omohyoid muscle (superior belly) (*cut*)

Thyroid gland

Sternohyoid muscle (*cut*)

Clavicle

Styloid process

Mastoid process

Stylohyoid muscle

Digastric muscle (posterior belly)

Mylohyoid muscle

Digastric muscle (anterior belly)

Geniohyoid muscle

Sternohyoid muscle

Omohyoid muscle (superior belly)

Sternothyroid muscle

Sternum

Thyrohyoid muscle

Oblique line of thyroid cartilage

Omohyoid muscle (inferior belly)

Scapula

Infrahyoid and suprahyoid muscles and their action: schema

PLATE 24

HEAD AND NECK

Basilar part of
occipital bone

Longus capitis muscle (*cut*)

Occipital condyle

Rectus capitis
anterior muscle

Rectus capitis
lateralis muscle

Jugular process of
occipital bone

Mastoid process

Styloid process

Transverse process of atlas (C 1)

Longus capitis muscle

Anterior
Posterior } Tubercles of transverse
process of C3 vertebra

Posterior tubercle of
transverse process of axis (C 2)

Slips of origin of anterior
scalene muscle (*cut*)

Longus colli muscle

Slips of origin of posterior
scalene muscle

Scalene
muscles } Anterior
Middle
Posterior

Middle
Posterior } Scalene
muscles

Anterior scalene
muscle (*cut*)

Phrenic nerve

Brachial plexus

1st rib

Subclavian artery

Subclavian vein

Internal jugular vein

Common carotid artery

Posterior tubercle of transverse
process of C 7 vertebra

Superficial Veins and Cutaneous Nerves of Neck

FOR DEEP VEINS OF NECK SEE PLATE 64

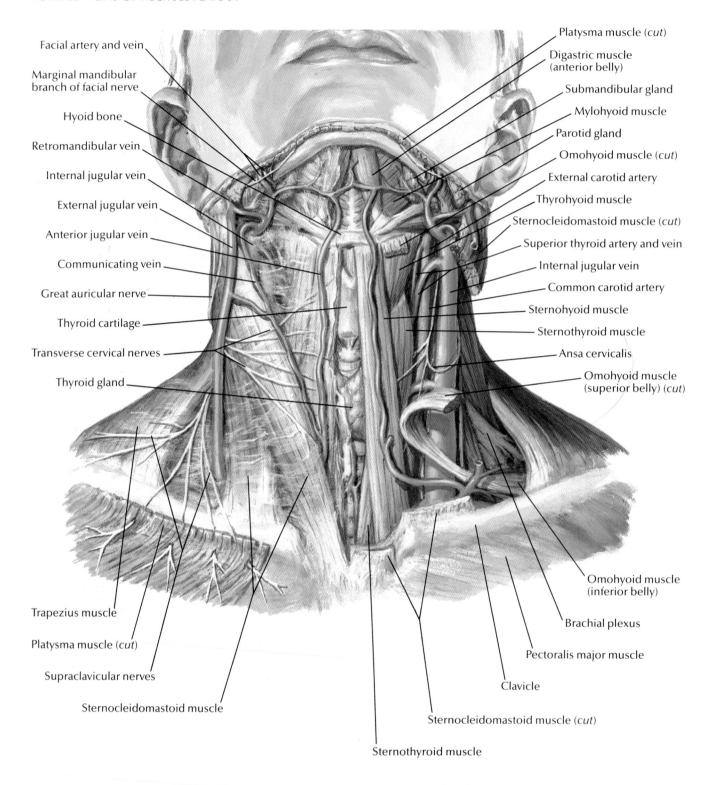

Facial artery and vein

Marginal mandibular branch of facial nerve

Hyoid bone

Retromandibular vein

Internal jugular vein

External jugular vein

Anterior jugular vein

Communicating vein

Great auricular nerve

Thyroid cartilage

Transverse cervical nerves

Thyroid gland

Trapezius muscle

Platysma muscle (*cut*)

Supraclavicular nerves

Sternocleidomastoid muscle

Sternothyroid muscle

Platysma muscle (*cut*)

Digastric muscle (anterior belly)

Submandibular gland

Mylohyoid muscle

Parotid gland

Omohyoid muscle (*cut*)

External carotid artery

Thyrohyoid muscle

Sternocleidomastoid muscle (*cut*)

Superior thyroid artery and vein

Internal jugular vein

Common carotid artery

Sternohyoid muscle

Sternothyroid muscle

Ansa cervicalis

Omohyoid muscle (superior belly) (*cut*)

Omohyoid muscle (inferior belly)

Brachial plexus

Pectoralis major muscle

Clavicle

Sternocleidomastoid muscle (*cut*)

PLATE 26

HEAD AND NECK

Parotid gland
Facial artery and vein
Submandibular gland
Mylohyoid muscle
Hypoglossal nerve (XII)
Digastric muscle (anterior belly)
Lingual artery
External carotid artery
Internal carotid artery
Thyrohyoid muscle
Superior thyroid artery
Omohyoid muscle (superior belly) (*cut*)
Ansa cervicalis { Superior root / Inferior root
Sternohyoid muscle
Sternothyroid muscle
Internal jugular vein
Common carotid artery
Inferior thyroid artery
Vagus nerve (X)
Vertebral artery
Thyrocervical trunk
Subclavian artery and vein

Great auricular nerve
Lesser occipital nerve
Sternocleidomastoid muscle (*cut, turned up*)
Stylohyoid muscle
Digastric muscle (posterior belly)
2nd cervical nerve (ventral ramus)
Accessory nerve (XI)
3rd cervical nerve (ventral ramus)
Levator scapulae muscle
Middle scalene muscle
Anterior scalene muscle
5th cervical nerve (ventral ramus)
Transverse cervical artery
Phrenic nerve
Omohyoid muscle (inferior belly) (*cut*)
Brachial plexus
Costocervical trunk
Suprascapular artery

Cervical plexus: schema
(S = gray ramus to superior sympathetic ganglion)

Hypoglossal nerve (XII)
Accessory nerve (XI)
Great auricular nerve
Lesser occipital nerve
To rectus capitis lateralis, longus capitis and rectus capitis anterior muscles

To geniohyoid muscle
To thyrohyoid muscle
Communication to vagus nerve

Transverse cervical nerves

To omohyoid muscle (superior belly)

Ansa cervicalis { Superior root / Inferior root

To sternothyroid muscle
To sternohyoid muscle
To omohyoid muscle (inferior belly)

To longus capitis and longus colli muscles

To scalene and levator scapulae muscles

Supraclavicular nerves
Phrenic nerve

S
C1
S C2
S C3
S C4

Subclavian Artery

SEE ALSO PLATE 402

Right anterior dissection

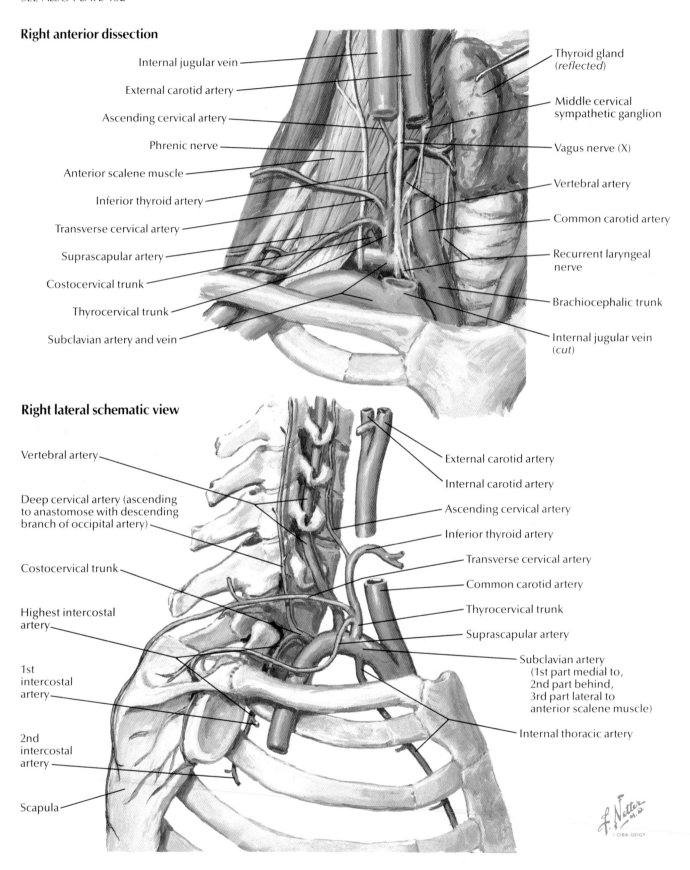

Internal jugular vein

External carotid artery

Ascending cervical artery

Phrenic nerve

Anterior scalene muscle

Inferior thyroid artery

Transverse cervical artery

Suprascapular artery

Costocervical trunk

Thyrocervical trunk

Subclavian artery and vein

Thyroid gland (*reflected*)

Middle cervical sympathetic ganglion

Vagus nerve (X)

Vertebral artery

Common carotid artery

Recurrent laryngeal nerve

Brachiocephalic trunk

Internal jugular vein (*cut*)

Right lateral schematic view

Vertebral artery

Deep cervical artery (ascending to anastomose with descending branch of occipital artery)

Costocervical trunk

Highest intercostal artery

1st intercostal artery

2nd intercostal artery

Scapula

External carotid artery

Internal carotid artery

Ascending cervical artery

Inferior thyroid artery

Transverse cervical artery

Common carotid artery

Thyrocervical trunk

Suprascapular artery

Subclavian artery (1st part medial to, 2nd part behind, 3rd part lateral to anterior scalene muscle)

Internal thoracic artery

PLATE 28   **HEAD AND NECK**

Parotid fossa: right lateral dissection

Mastoid process

Styloid process

Facial nerve (VII) (*cut*)

Sternocleidomastoid muscle (*cut*)

Digastric muscle (posterior belly) (*cut*)

Occipital artery and sternocleidomastoid branch

Accessory nerve (XI)

Ansa cervicalis { Superior root / Inferior root }

Vagus nerve (X)

Ascending pharyngeal artery

Carotid sinus nerve (IX) and carotid body

Internal carotid artery

Internal jugular vein

Superficial temporal artery

Transverse facial artery

Maxillary artery

External carotid artery

Posterior auricular artery

Glossopharyngeal nerve (IX)

Stylohyoid muscle

Hypoglossal nerve (XII)

Facial artery

Lingual artery

Mylohyoid muscle

Hyoglossus muscle

Digastric muscle (anterior belly)

Hyoid bone

Branch to thyrohyoid muscle (from ansa cervicalis)

Superior laryngeal artery

Superior thyroid artery

External carotid artery

Common carotid artery

Superficial temporal artery

Digastric muscle (*phantom*)

Occipital artery with sternocleidomastoid and descending branches

Internal carotid artery

External carotid artery

Common carotid artery

Thyrocervical trunk

Transverse facial artery

Maxillary artery

Posterior auricular artery

Facial artery

Lingual artery

Ascending pharyngeal artery

Superior thyroid artery and superior laryngeal branch

Omohyoid muscle (*phantom*)

External carotid branches: schema

Fascial Layers of Neck

FOR CONTENTS OF CAROTID SHEATH SEE PLATES 63, 64, 65

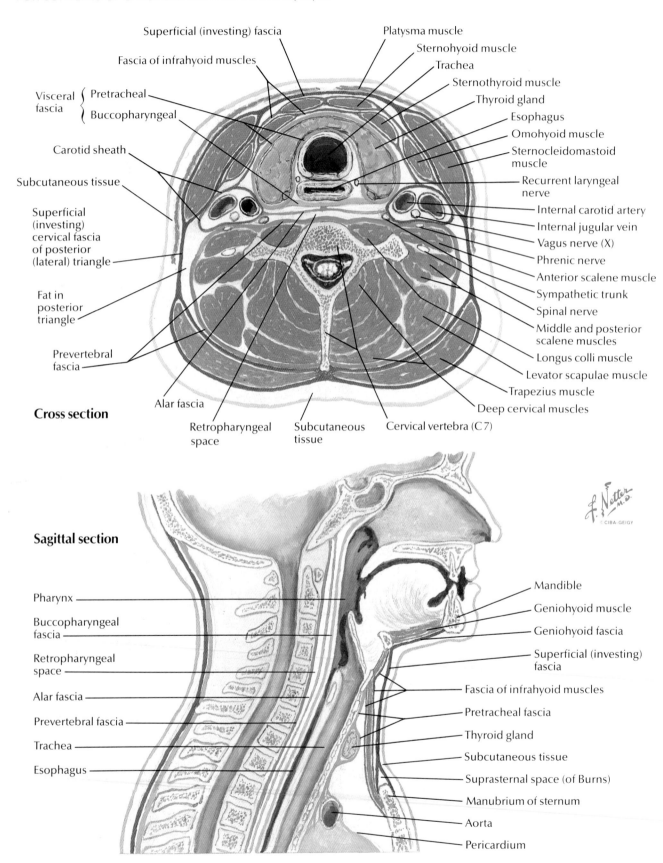

Superficial (investing) fascia

Fascia of infrahyoid muscles

Platysma muscle

Sternohyoid muscle

Trachea

Sternothyroid muscle

Thyroid gland

Visceral fascia { Pretracheal / Buccopharyngeal }

Esophagus

Omohyoid muscle

Carotid sheath

Sternocleidomastoid muscle

Subcutaneous tissue

Recurrent laryngeal nerve

Superficial (investing) cervical fascia of posterior (lateral) triangle

Internal carotid artery

Internal jugular vein

Vagus nerve (X)

Phrenic nerve

Fat in posterior triangle

Anterior scalene muscle

Sympathetic trunk

Spinal nerve

Prevertebral fascia

Middle and posterior scalene muscles

Longus colli muscle

Levator scapulae muscle

Cross section

Alar fascia

Retropharyngeal space

Subcutaneous tissue

Cervical vertebra (C 7)

Trapezius muscle

Deep cervical muscles

Sagittal section

Pharynx

Buccopharyngeal fascia

Retropharyngeal space

Alar fascia

Prevertebral fascia

Trachea

Esophagus

Mandible

Geniohyoid muscle

Geniohyoid fascia

Superficial (investing) fascia

Fascia of infrahyoid muscles

Pretracheal fascia

Thyroid gland

Subcutaneous tissue

Suprasternal space (of Burns)

Manubrium of sternum

Aorta

Pericardium

PLATE 30

HEAD AND NECK

Frontal bone

Nasal bones

Frontal process of maxilla

Lateral nasal cartilages

Septal cartilage

Lesser alar cartilage

Accessory alar (sesamoid) cartilage

Greater alar cartilage
Lateral crus
Medial crus

Septal cartilage

Anterior nasal spine of maxilla

Alar fibrofatty tissue

Infraorbital foramen

Greater alar cartilage
Lateral crus
Medial crus

Alar fibrofatty tissue

Septal cartilage

Anterior nasal spine of maxilla

Intermaxillary suture

Frontalis muscle

Supraorbital artery and nerve

Supratrochlear artery and nerve

Procerus muscle

Corrugator supercilii muscle

Dorsal nasal artery

Infratrochlear nerve

Angular artery

External nasal artery and nerve

Nasalis muscle (transverse part)

Infraorbital artery and nerve

Lateral nasal artery

Transverse facial artery

Nasalis muscle (alar part)

Depressor septi nasi muscle

Orbicularis oris muscle

Facial artery

Lateral Nasal Wall

Frontal sinus

Superior nasal concha (turbinate)

Superior nasal meatus

Middle nasal concha (turbinate)

Agger nasi

Atrium of middle nasal meatus

Middle nasal meatus

Inferior nasal concha (turbinate)

Limen

Vestibule

Inferior nasal meatus

Palatine process of maxilla

Incisive canal

Tongue

Sphenoethmoidal recess

Opening of sphenoidal sinus

Hypophysis (pituitary gland) in sella turcica

Sphenoidal sinus

Pharyngeal tonsil (adenoid if enlarged)

Basilar part of occipital bone

Pharyngobasilar fascia

Nasopharyngeal opening

Torus tubarius

Opening of auditory (Eustachian) tube

Pharyngeal recess

Horizontal plate of palatine bone

Soft palate

Middle nasal concha (turbinate)

Middle nasal meatus

Bulging septum

Airway to nasopharynx

Inferior nasal concha (turbinate)

Inferior nasal meatus

Floor of nasal cavity

Speculum view

Frontal sinus

Probe in nasofrontal duct from middle nasal meatus and semi-lunar hiatus via infundibulum

Middle nasal concha (*cut surface*)

Ethmoidal bulla

Openings of middle ethmoidal cells

Semilunar hiatus with openings of anterior ethmoidal cells

Uncinate process

Middle nasal concha (*cut surface*)

Opening of nasolacrimal duct

Inferior nasal meatus

Cribriform plate of ethmoid bone

Probe in opening of sphenoidal sinus

Sphenoidal sinus

Superior nasal meatus with openings of posterior ethmoidal cells

Basilar part of occipital bone

Torus tubarius

Opening of auditory (Eustachian) tube

Anterior tubercle of atlas (C1 vertebra)

Dens of axis (C2 vertebra)

Opening of maxillary sinus

PLATE 32

HEAD AND NECK

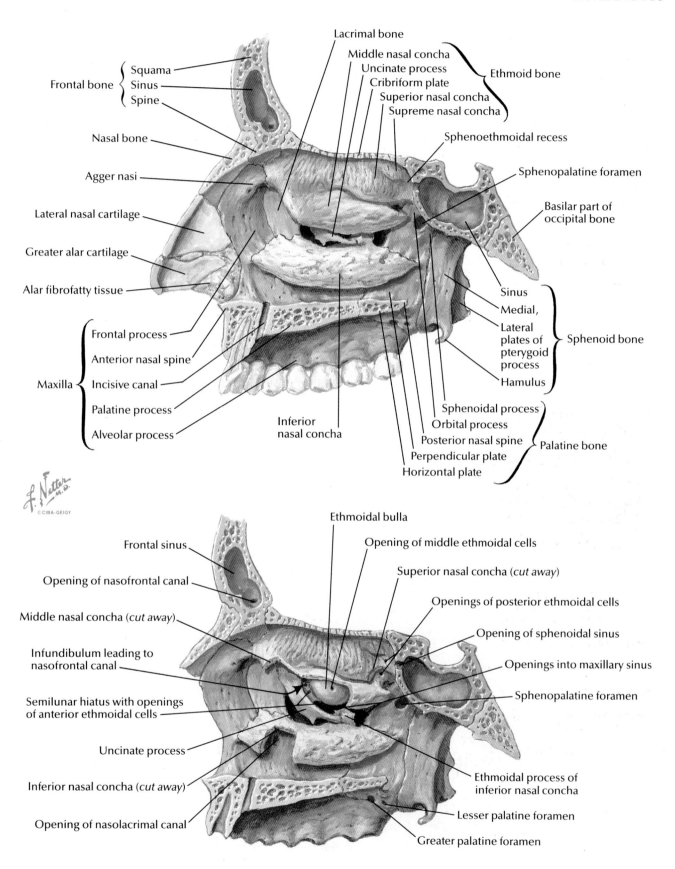

Lacrimal bone
Middle nasal concha
Uncinate process
Cribriform plate
Superior nasal concha
Supreme nasal concha
Ethmoid bone
Sphenoethmoidal recess
Sphenopalatine foramen
Basilar part of occipital bone

Frontal bone
  Squama
  Sinus
  Spine
Nasal bone
Agger nasi
Lateral nasal cartilage
Greater alar cartilage
Alar fibrofatty tissue

Maxilla
  Frontal process
  Anterior nasal spine
  Incisive canal
  Palatine process
  Alveolar process

Inferior nasal concha

Sinus
Medial,
Lateral plates of pterygoid process
Hamulus
Sphenoid bone

Sphenoidal process
Orbital process
Posterior nasal spine
Perpendicular plate
Horizontal plate
Palatine bone

Ethmoidal bulla
Opening of middle ethmoidal cells
Superior nasal concha (*cut away*)
Openings of posterior ethmoidal cells
Opening of sphenoidal sinus
Openings into maxillary sinus
Sphenopalatine foramen

Frontal sinus
Opening of nasofrontal canal
Middle nasal concha (*cut away*)
Infundibulum leading to nasofrontal canal
Semilunar hiatus with openings of anterior ethmoidal cells
Uncinate process
Inferior nasal concha (*cut away*)
Opening of nasolacrimal canal

Ethmoidal process of inferior nasal concha
Lesser palatine foramen
Greater palatine foramen

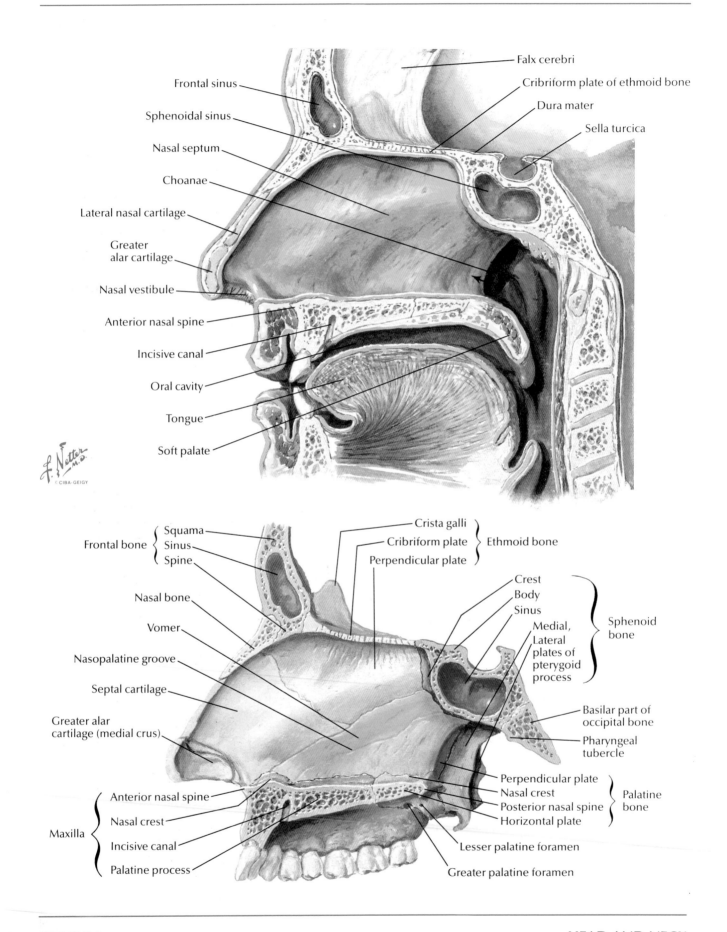

Falx cerebri

Frontal sinus

Cribriform plate of ethmoid bone

Sphenoidal sinus

Dura mater

Nasal septum

Sella turcica

Choanae

Lateral nasal cartilage

Greater alar cartilage

Nasal vestibule

Anterior nasal spine

Incisive canal

Oral cavity

Tongue

Soft palate

Squama

Crista galli

Frontal bone { Sinus

Cribriform plate } Ethmoid bone

Spine

Perpendicular plate

Nasal bone

Crest

Vomer

Body

Nasopalatine groove

Sinus

Septal cartilage

Medial, Lateral plates of pterygoid process } Sphenoid bone

Greater alar cartilage (medial crus)

Basilar part of occipital bone

Pharyngeal tubercle

Anterior nasal spine

Perpendicular plate

Nasal crest } Palatine bone

Nasal crest

Posterior nasal spine

Maxilla {

Incisive canal

Horizontal plate

Palatine process

Lesser palatine foramen

Greater palatine foramen

PLATE 34

HEAD AND NECK

Lateral pterygoid artery and muscle
Supraorbital artery
Supratrochlear artery
Ophthalmic artery
Dorsal nasal artery
Angular artery
Infraorbital artery
Superior alveolar arteries { Posterior / Middle / Anterior }
Buccal artery and nerve
Medial pterygoid artery and muscle
Pterygomandibular raphé
Lingual nerve
Facial artery
Mental artery
Submental artery

Anterior } Deep temporal arteries and nerves
Posterior }
Masseteric artery and nerve
Lateral ligament of temporomandibular joint
Middle meningeal artery
Auriculotemporal nerve
Maxillary artery
Superficial temporal artery
Posterior auricular artery
Facial nerve
Inferior alveolar artery and nerve
Sphenomandibular ligament
Mylohyoid artery and nerve
Digastric muscle (posterior belly)
Stylohyoid muscle
External carotid artery
Facial artery
Lingual artery

Sphenopalatine artery
Posterior lateral nasal artery
Infraorbital artery
Posterior superior alveolar artery
Sphenopalatine artery
Posterior septal branches
Descending palatine artery in pterygo-palatine fossa
Buccal artery
Anastomosis in incisive canal
Left and right greater palatine arteries
Left and right lesser palatine arteries

Artery of pterygoid canal
Pharyngeal artery
Sphenopalatine foramen

Anterior } Deep temporal arteries
Posterior } and nerves
Accessory meningeal artery
Middle meningeal artery
Anterior tympanic artery
Deep auricular artery
Auriculo-temporal nerve
Superficial temporal artery
Ascending pharyngeal artery
Ascending palatine artery
Tonsillar branches
Tonsillar artery
External carotid artery
Facial artery

Pterygoid arteries
Masseteric artery
Inferior alveolar artery
Superior pharyngeal constrictor muscle
Styloglossus muscle

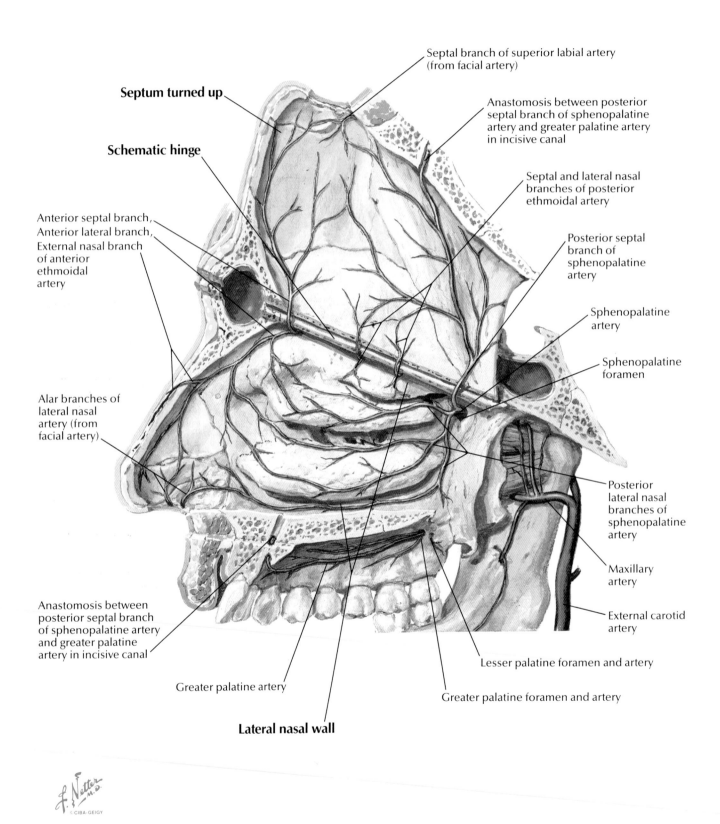

Septum turned up

Schematic hinge

Anterior septal branch,
Anterior lateral branch,
External nasal branch
of anterior
ethmoidal
artery

Alar branches of
lateral nasal
artery (from
facial artery)

Anastomosis between
posterior septal branch
of sphenopalatine artery
and greater palatine
artery in incisive
canal

Greater palatine artery

Lateral nasal wall

Septal branch of superior labial artery
(from facial artery)

Anastomosis between posterior
septal branch of sphenopalatine
artery and greater palatine artery
in incisive canal

Septal and lateral nasal
branches of posterior
ethmoidal artery

Posterior septal
branch of
sphenopalatine
artery

Sphenopalatine
artery

Sphenopalatine
foramen

Posterior
lateral nasal
branches of
sphenopalatine
artery

Maxillary
artery

External carotid
artery

Lesser palatine foramen and artery

Greater palatine foramen and artery

PLATE 36   **HEAD AND NECK**

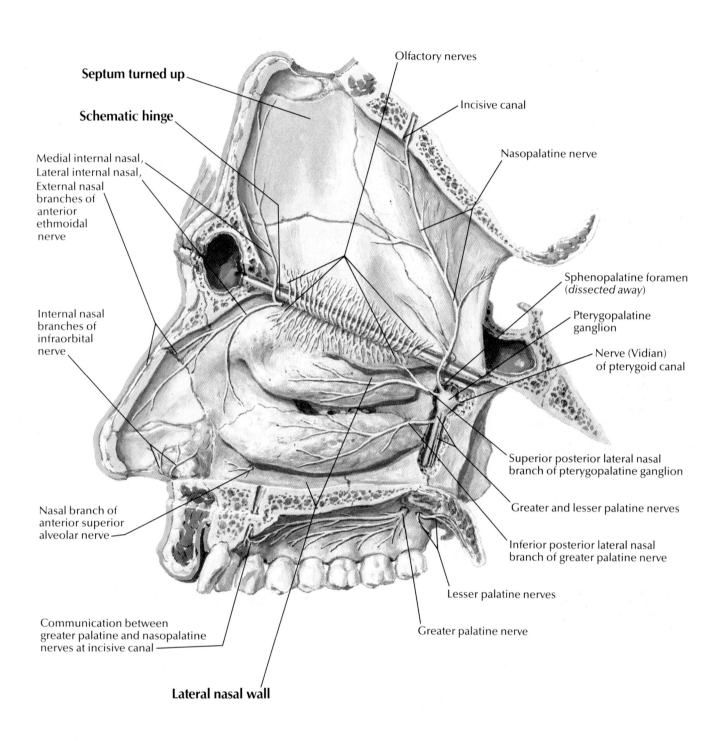

Septum turned up

Schematic hinge

Medial internal nasal,
Lateral internal nasal,
External nasal
branches of
anterior
ethmoidal
nerve

Internal nasal
branches of
infraorbital
nerve

Nasal branch of
anterior superior
alveolar nerve

Communication between
greater palatine and nasopalatine
nerves at incisive canal

Lateral nasal wall

Olfactory nerves

Incisive canal

Nasopalatine nerve

Sphenopalatine foramen
(*dissected away*)

Pterygopalatine
ganglion

Nerve (Vidian)
of pterygoid canal

Superior posterior lateral nasal
branch of pterygopalatine ganglion

Greater and lesser palatine nerves

Inferior posterior lateral nasal
branch of greater palatine nerve

Lesser palatine nerves

Greater palatine nerve

NASAL REGION

PLATE 37

Nerves of Nasal Cavity (continued)

SEE ALSO PLATE 113

Distribution of olfactory mucosa (*shaded blue*)

Lateral nasal wall

Nasal septum

External nasal branch of anterior ethmoidal nerve

Lateral internal nasal branch of anterior ethmoidal nerve

Olfactory bulb

Cribriform plate of ethmoid bone

Olfactory tract

Superior posterior lateral nasal branches from pterygopalatine ganglion

Maxillary nerve (sphenopalatine foramen dissected away)

Pterygopalatine ganglion

Greater petrosal nerve

Deep petrosal nerve

Nerve (Vidian) of pterygoid canal

Pharyngeal branch of pterygopalatine ganglion

Nasopalatine nerve passing to septum (*cut*)

Inferior posterior lateral nasal branch from greater palatine nerve

Lateral nasal wall

Olfactory nerves

Palatine nerves { Greater
Lesser

Olfactory bulb

Cribriform plate

Olfactory tract

Medial internal nasal branch of anterior ethmoidal nerve

Olfactory nerves

Nasopalatine nerve

Incisive foramen

Nasal septum

PLATE 38   **HEAD AND NECK**

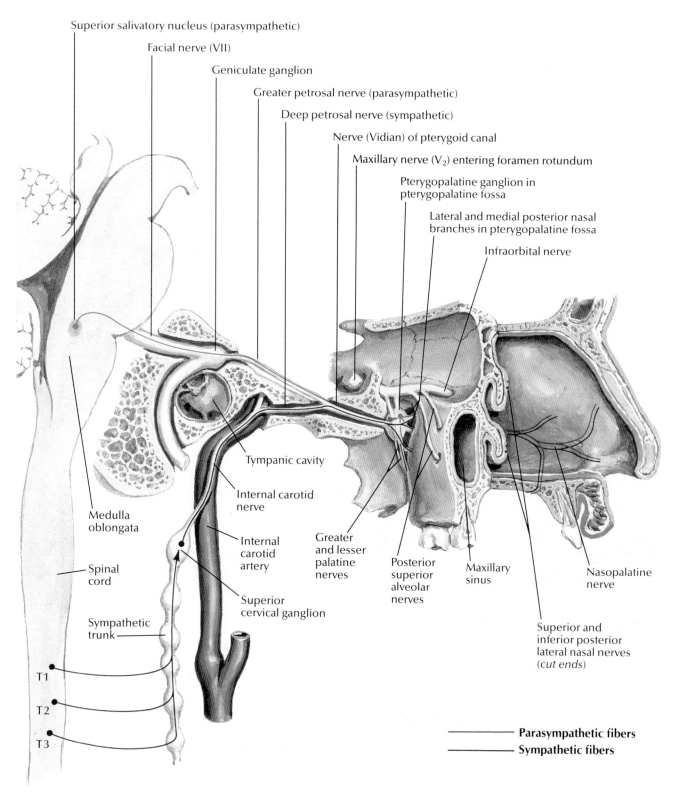

Superior salivatory nucleus (parasympathetic)

Facial nerve (VII)

Geniculate ganglion

Greater petrosal nerve (parasympathetic)

Deep petrosal nerve (sympathetic)

Nerve (Vidian) of pterygoid canal

Maxillary nerve (V_2) entering foramen rotundum

Pterygopalatine ganglion in pterygopalatine fossa

Lateral and medial posterior nasal branches in pterygopalatine fossa

Infraorbital nerve

Tympanic cavity

Internal carotid nerve

Medulla oblongata

Internal carotid artery

Spinal cord

Greater and lesser palatine nerves

Posterior superior alveolar nerves

Maxillary sinus

Nasopalatine nerve

Superior cervical ganglion

Sympathetic trunk

Superior and inferior posterior lateral nasal nerves (*cut ends*)

T1

T2

T3

———— Parasympathetic fibers
———— Sympathetic fibers

Ophthalmic and Maxillary Nerves

SEE ALSO PLATE 116

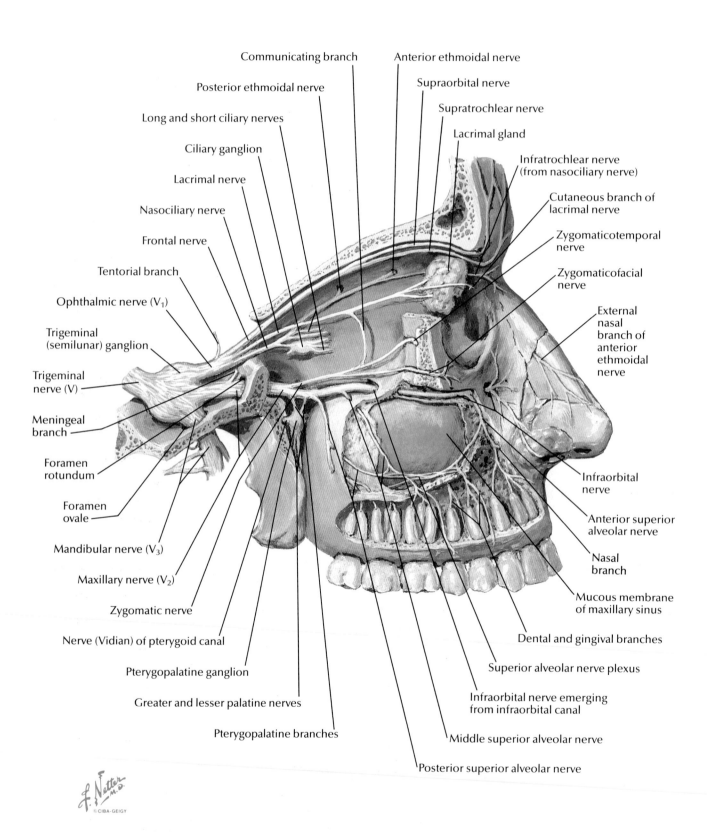

Communicating branch

Posterior ethmoidal nerve

Long and short ciliary nerves

Ciliary ganglion

Lacrimal nerve

Nasociliary nerve

Frontal nerve

Tentorial branch

Ophthalmic nerve (V₁)

Trigeminal (semilunar) ganglion

Trigeminal nerve (V)

Meningeal branch

Foramen rotundum

Foramen ovale

Mandibular nerve (V₃)

Maxillary nerve (V₂)

Zygomatic nerve

Nerve (Vidian) of pterygoid canal

Pterygopalatine ganglion

Greater and lesser palatine nerves

Pterygopalatine branches

Anterior ethmoidal nerve

Supraorbital nerve

Supratrochlear nerve

Lacrimal gland

Infratrochlear nerve (from nasociliary nerve)

Cutaneous branch of lacrimal nerve

Zygomaticotemporal nerve

Zygomaticofacial nerve

External nasal branch of anterior ethmoidal nerve

Infraorbital nerve

Anterior superior alveolar nerve

Nasal branch

Mucous membrane of maxillary sinus

Dental and gingival branches

Superior alveolar nerve plexus

Infraorbital nerve emerging from infraorbital canal

Middle superior alveolar nerve

Posterior superior alveolar nerve

PLATE 40

Lateral view

Anterior division
Posterior division
Temporalis fascia and muscle
Posterior
Anterior } Deep temporal nerves
Foramen ovale
Masseteric nerve
Meningeal branch
Lateral pterygoid nerve and muscle
Foramen spinosum
Middle meningeal artery
Auriculotemporal nerve
Posterior auricular nerve
Facial nerve (VII)
Buccal nerve and buccinator muscle (*cut*)
Chorda tympani nerve
Lingual nerve
Submandibular ganglion
Inferior alveolar nerve (*cut*)
Sublingual gland
Mylohyoid nerve
Medial pterygoid muscle (*cut*)
Mylohyoid muscle (*cut*)
Digastric muscle (posterior belly)
Mental nerve
Stylohyoid muscle
Hypoglossal nerve
Inferior alveolar nerve (*cut*)
Submandibular gland
Digastric muscle (anterior belly)
Sublingual nerve

Medial view

Trigeminal (semilunar) ganglion
Motor root
Sensory root
Geniculate ganglion
Ophthalmic nerve (V₁)
Maxillary nerve (V₂)
Tympanic cavity
Mandibular nerve (V₃)
Chorda tympani nerve
Anterior division
Facial nerve (VII)
Tensor veli palatini nerve and muscle
Tensor tympani muscle and nerve
Otic ganglion
Lesser petrosal nerve
Chorda tympani nerve
Auriculotemporal nerve
Medial pterygoid nerve and muscle (*cut*)
Maxillary artery
Pterygoid hamulus
Mylohyoid nerve
Lingual nerve
Inferior alveolar nerve emerging from mandibular foramen

Paranasal Sinuses

Coronal section

Brain

Nasal cavities

Nasal septum

Middle nasal concha

Middle nasal meatus

Maxillary sinus

Inferior nasal meatus

Inferior nasal concha

Hard palate

Oral cavity

Frontal sinus

Orbital fat

Ethmoidal cells

Opening of maxillary sinus

Infraorbital ⎫
Zygomatic ⎬ Recesses of maxillary sinus
Alveolar ⎭

Buccinator muscle

Alveolar process of maxilla

Body of tongue

Eyeball

Ethmoidal cells

Orbital fat and muscles

Sphenoidal sinuses

Nasal cavities

Nasal septum

Medial wall of orbit

Optic nerve (II)

Brain

Horizontal section

PLATE 42

HEAD AND NECK

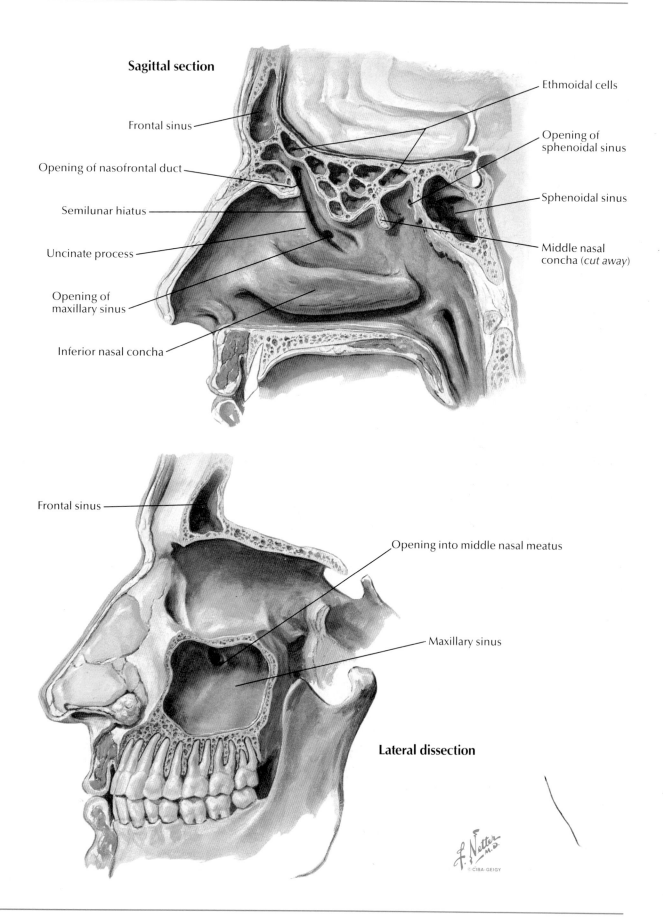

Sagittal section

Frontal sinus

Opening of nasofrontal duct

Semilunar hiatus

Uncinate process

Opening of maxillary sinus

Inferior nasal concha

Ethmoidal cells

Opening of sphenoidal sinus

Sphenoidal sinus

Middle nasal concha (*cut away*)

Frontal sinus

Opening into middle nasal meatus

Maxillary sinus

Lateral dissection

Paranasal Sinuses: Changes With Age

Bones of nasal cavity and paranasal sinuses at birth

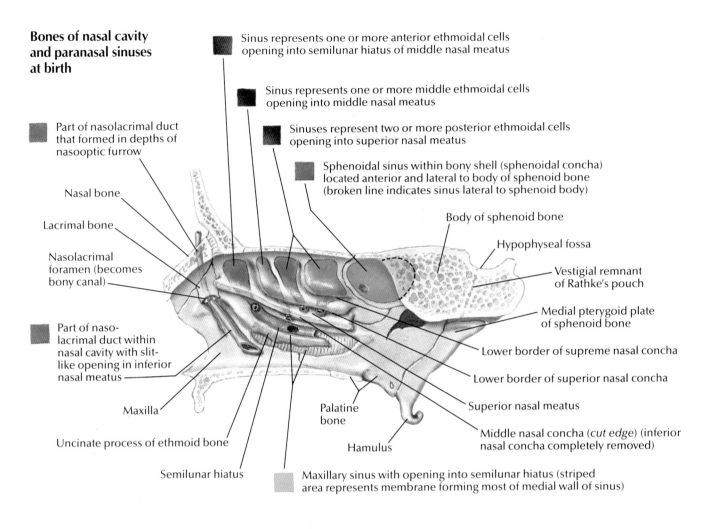

Sinus represents one or more anterior ethmoidal cells opening into semilunar hiatus of middle nasal meatus

Sinus represents one or more middle ethmoidal cells opening into middle nasal meatus

Sinuses represent two or more posterior ethmoidal cells opening into superior nasal meatus

Sphenoidal sinus within bony shell (sphenoidal concha) located anterior and lateral to body of sphenoid bone (broken line indicates sinus lateral to sphenoid body)

Part of nasolacrimal duct that formed in depths of nasooptic furrow

Nasal bone

Lacrimal bone

Nasolacrimal foramen (becomes bony canal)

Part of naso-lacrimal duct within nasal cavity with slit-like opening in inferior nasal meatus

Maxilla

Uncinate process of ethmoid bone

Semilunar hiatus

Palatine bone

Hamulus

Body of sphenoid bone

Hypophyseal fossa

Vestigial remnant of Rathke's pouch

Medial pterygoid plate of sphenoid bone

Lower border of supreme nasal concha

Lower border of superior nasal concha

Superior nasal meatus

Middle nasal concha (*cut edge*) (inferior nasal concha completely removed)

Maxillary sinus with opening into semilunar hiatus (striped area represents membrane forming most of medial wall of sinus)

Growth of frontal and maxillary sinuses throughout life

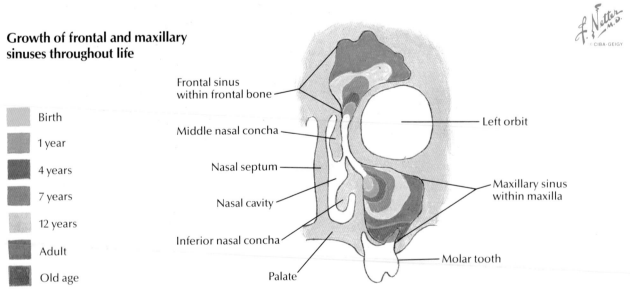

Birth

1 year

4 years

7 years

12 years

Adult

Old age

Frontal sinus within frontal bone

Middle nasal concha

Nasal septum

Nasal cavity

Inferior nasal concha

Palate

Left orbit

Maxillary sinus within maxilla

Molar tooth

PLATE 44

HEAD AND NECK

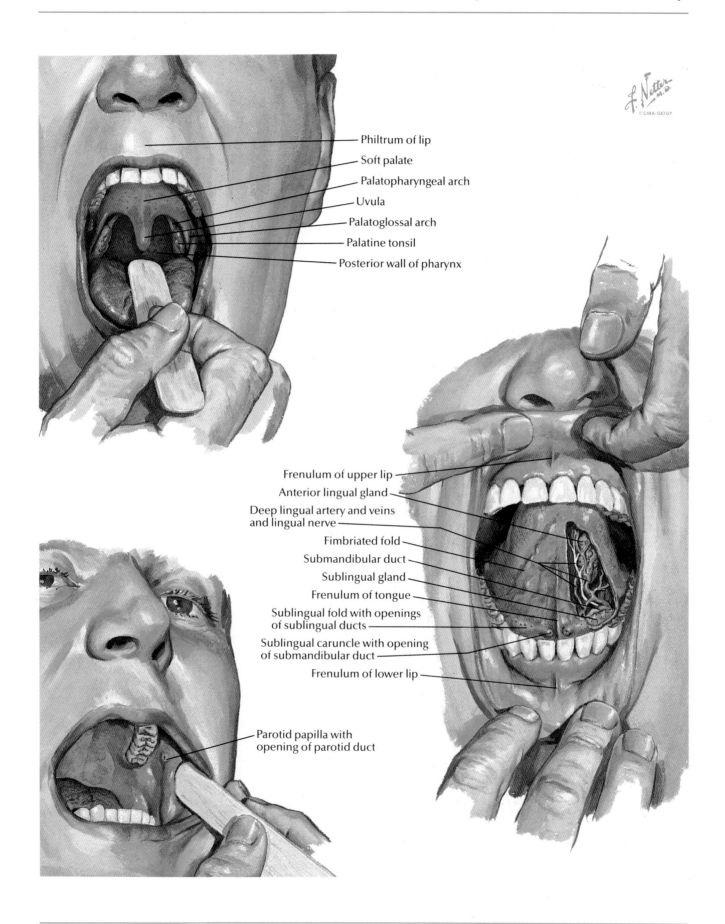

Philtrum of lip

Soft palate

Palatopharyngeal arch

Uvula

Palatoglossal arch

Palatine tonsil

Posterior wall of pharynx

Frenulum of upper lip

Anterior lingual gland

Deep lingual artery and veins and lingual nerve

Fimbriated fold

Submandibular duct

Sublingual gland

Frenulum of tongue

Sublingual fold with openings of sublingual ducts

Sublingual caruncle with opening of submandibular duct

Frenulum of lower lip

Parotid papilla with opening of parotid duct

Roof of Mouth

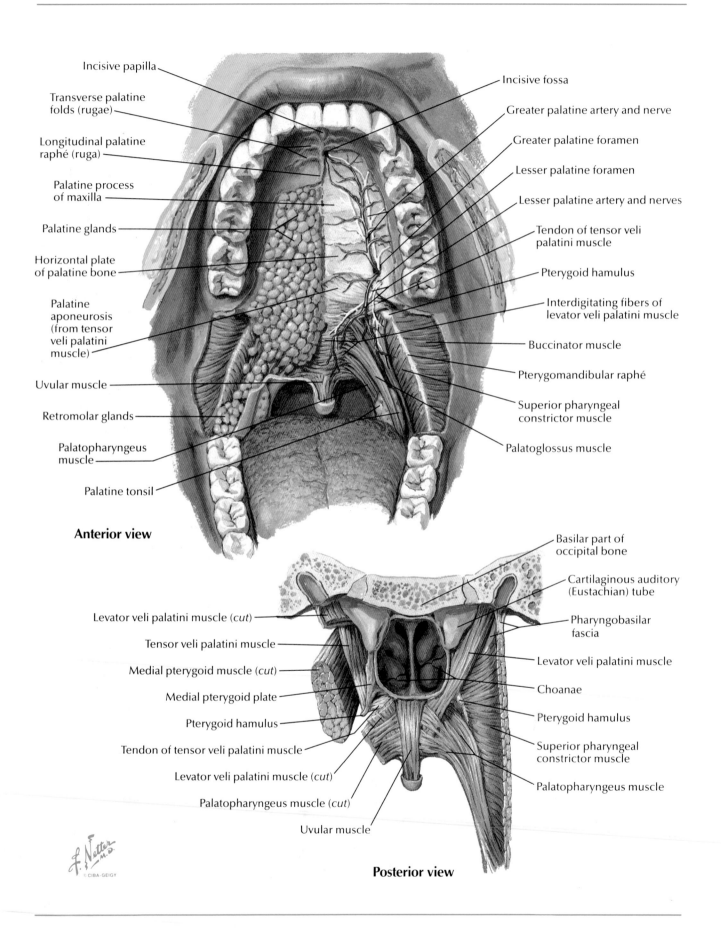

Incisive papilla

Transverse palatine folds (rugae)

Longitudinal palatine raphé (ruga)

Palatine process of maxilla

Palatine glands

Horizontal plate of palatine bone

Palatine aponeurosis (from tensor veli palatini muscle)

Uvular muscle

Retromolar glands

Palatopharyngeus muscle

Palatine tonsil

Anterior view

Incisive fossa

Greater palatine artery and nerve

Greater palatine foramen

Lesser palatine foramen

Lesser palatine artery and nerves

Tendon of tensor veli palatini muscle

Pterygoid hamulus

Interdigitating fibers of levator veli palatini muscle

Buccinator muscle

Pterygomandibular raphé

Superior pharyngeal constrictor muscle

Palatoglossus muscle

Levator veli palatini muscle (*cut*)

Tensor veli palatini muscle

Medial pterygoid muscle (*cut*)

Medial pterygoid plate

Pterygoid hamulus

Tendon of tensor veli palatini muscle

Levator veli palatini muscle (*cut*)

Palatopharyngeus muscle (*cut*)

Uvular muscle

Basilar part of occipital bone

Cartilaginous auditory (Eustachian) tube

Pharyngobasilar fascia

Levator veli palatini muscle

Choanae

Pterygoid hamulus

Superior pharyngeal constrictor muscle

Palatopharyngeus muscle

Posterior view

PLATE 46

HEAD AND NECK

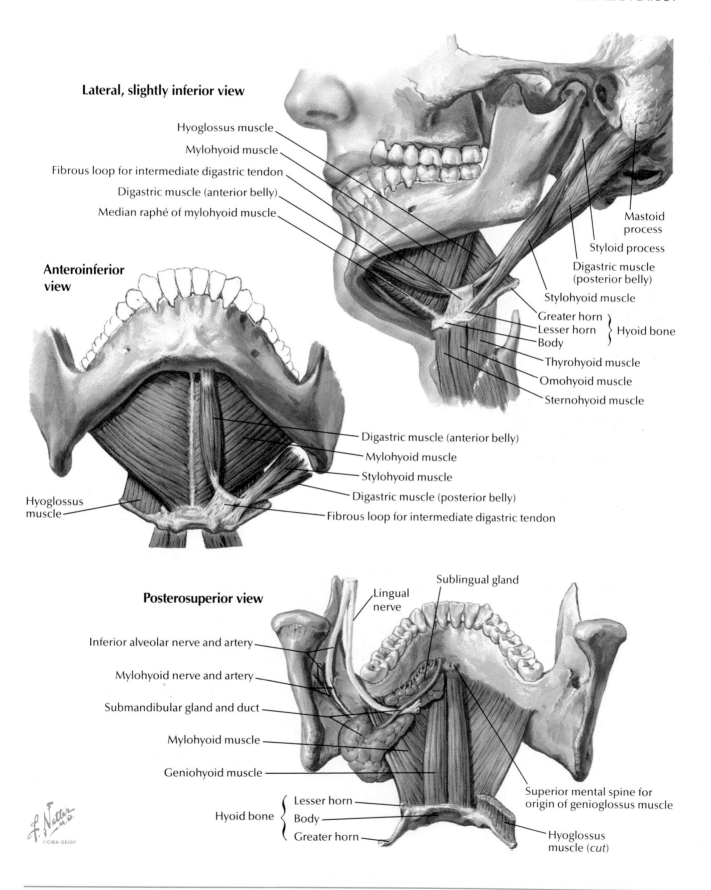

Lateral, slightly inferior view

Hyoglossus muscle
Mylohyoid muscle
Fibrous loop for intermediate digastric tendon
Digastric muscle (anterior belly)
Median raphé of mylohyoid muscle

Mastoid process
Styloid process
Digastric muscle (posterior belly)
Stylohyoid muscle
Greater horn
Lesser horn } Hyoid bone
Body
Thyrohyoid muscle
Omohyoid muscle
Sternohyoid muscle

Anteroinferior view

Digastric muscle (anterior belly)
Mylohyoid muscle
Stylohyoid muscle
Digastric muscle (posterior belly)
Fibrous loop for intermediate digastric tendon

Hyoglossus muscle

Posterosuperior view

Lingual nerve
Sublingual gland

Inferior alveolar nerve and artery
Mylohyoid nerve and artery
Submandibular gland and duct
Mylohyoid muscle
Geniohyoid muscle

Lesser horn
Hyoid bone { Body
Greater horn

Superior mental spine for origin of genioglossus muscle
Hyoglossus muscle (*cut*)

Muscles Involved in Mastication

FOR FACIAL MUSCLES SEE PLATES 20, 21

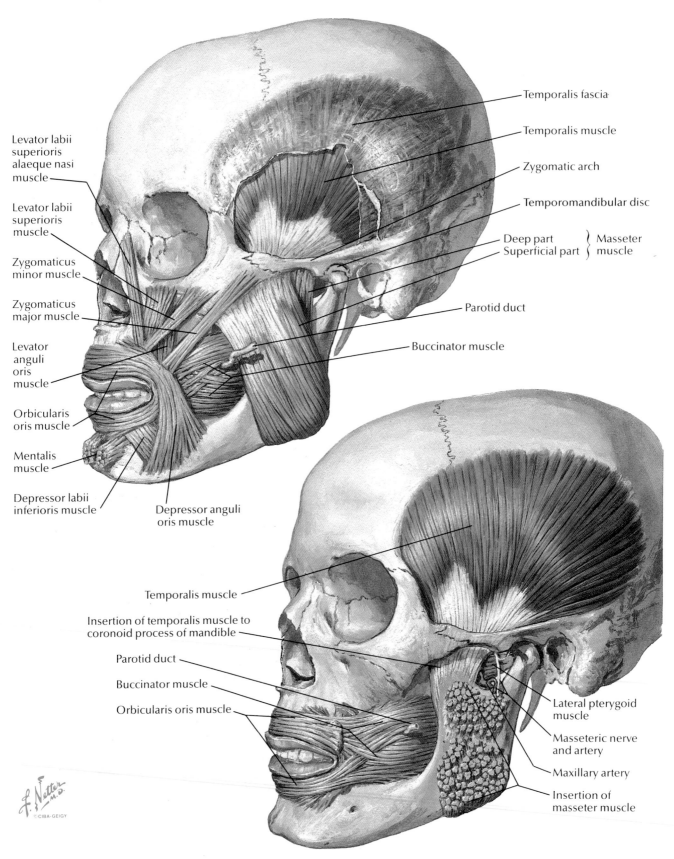

Temporalis fascia

Temporalis muscle

Zygomatic arch

Temporomandibular disc

Deep part }
Superficial part } Masseter muscle

Parotid duct

Buccinator muscle

Levator labii superioris alaeque nasi muscle

Levator labii superioris muscle

Zygomaticus minor muscle

Zygomaticus major muscle

Levator anguli oris muscle

Orbicularis oris muscle

Mentalis muscle

Depressor labii inferioris muscle

Depressor anguli oris muscle

Temporalis muscle

Insertion of temporalis muscle to coronoid process of mandible

Parotid duct

Buccinator muscle

Orbicularis oris muscle

Lateral pterygoid muscle

Masseteric nerve and artery

Maxillary artery

Insertion of masseter muscle

PLATE 48

HEAD AND NECK

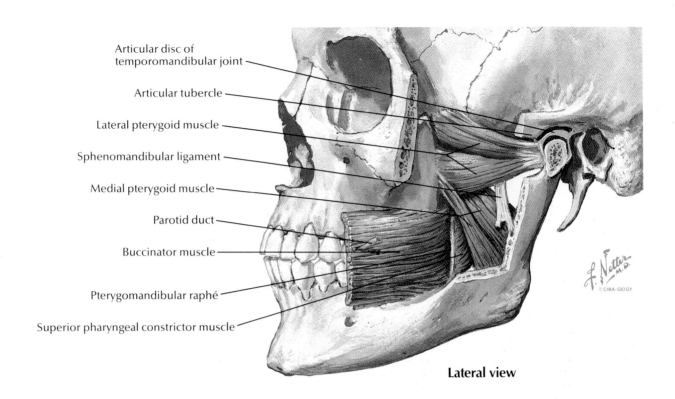

Articular disc of
temporomandibular joint

Articular tubercle

Lateral pterygoid muscle

Sphenomandibular ligament

Medial pterygoid muscle

Parotid duct

Buccinator muscle

Pterygomandibular raphé

Superior pharyngeal constrictor muscle

Lateral view

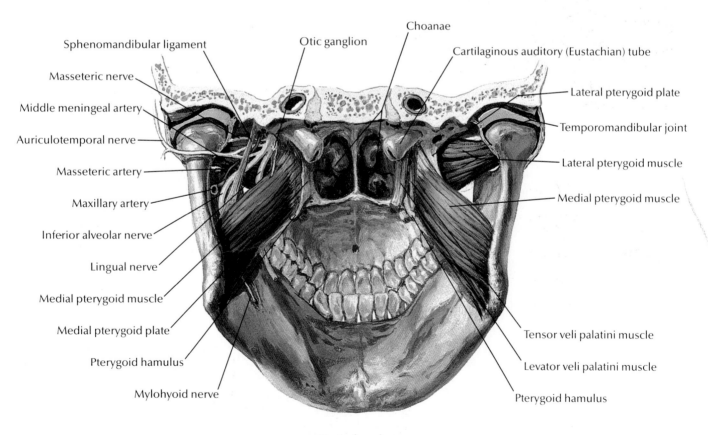

Sphenomandibular ligament

Masseteric nerve

Middle meningeal artery

Auriculotemporal nerve

Masseteric artery

Maxillary artery

Inferior alveolar nerve

Lingual nerve

Medial pterygoid muscle

Medial pterygoid plate

Pterygoid hamulus

Mylohyoid nerve

Otic ganglion

Choanae

Cartilaginous auditory (Eustachian) tube

Lateral pterygoid plate

Temporomandibular joint

Lateral pterygoid muscle

Medial pterygoid muscle

Tensor veli palatini muscle

Levator veli palatini muscle

Pterygoid hamulus

Posterior view

Teeth

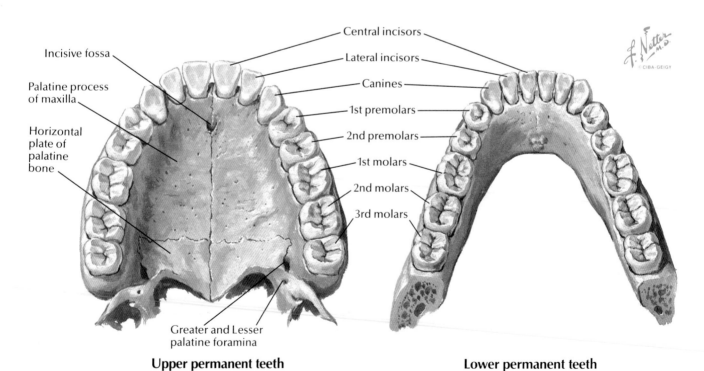

PLATE 50   **HEAD AND NECK**

Deciduous (primary) Usual age of eruption

Central incisor (8–10 months)
Lateral incisor (8–10 months)
Canine (cuspid) (16–20 months)
1st molar (15–21 months)
2nd molar (20–24 months)

2nd molar (20–24 months)
1st molar 15–21 months)
Canine (cuspid) (15–21 months)
Lateral incisor (15–21 months)
Central incisor (6–9 months)

Permanent (colored blue) Usual age of eruption

Central incisor (7th year)
Lateral incisor (8th year)
Canine (cuspid) (11th–12th year)
1st premolar (9th year)
2nd premolar (10th year)
1st molar (6th year)
2nd molar (12th–13th year)

3rd molars (17th–25th year)

2nd molar (12th–13th year)
1st molar (6th year)
2nd premolar (10th year)
1st premolar (9th year)
Canine (cuspid) (11th–12th year)
Lateral incisor (8th year)
Central incisor (7th year)

Incisive fossa
Palatine process of maxilla
Horizontal plate of palatine bone

Central incisors
Lateral incisors
Canines
1st premolars
2nd premolars
1st molars
2nd molars
3rd molars

Greater and Lesser palatine foramina

Upper permanent teeth   **Lower permanent teeth**

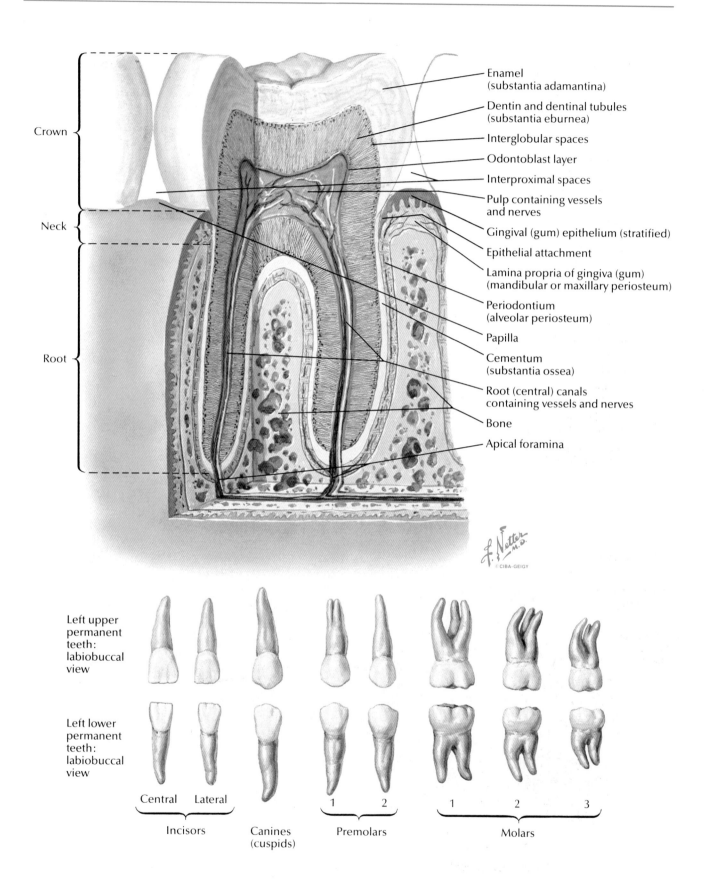

Crown

Neck

Root

Enamel
(substantia adamantina)

Dentin and dentinal tubules
(substantia eburnea)

Interglobular spaces

Odontoblast layer

Interproximal spaces

Pulp containing vessels
and nerves

Gingival (gum) epithelium (stratified)

Epithelial attachment

Lamina propria of gingiva (gum)
(mandibular or maxillary periosteum)

Periodontium
(alveolar periosteum)

Papilla

Cementum
(substantia ossea)

Root (central) canals
containing vessels and nerves

Bone

Apical foramina

Left upper
permanent
teeth:
labiobuccal
view

Left lower
permanent
teeth:
labiobuccal
view

Central   Lateral

Incisors

Canines
(cuspids)

1   2

Premolars

1   2   3

Molars

Tongue

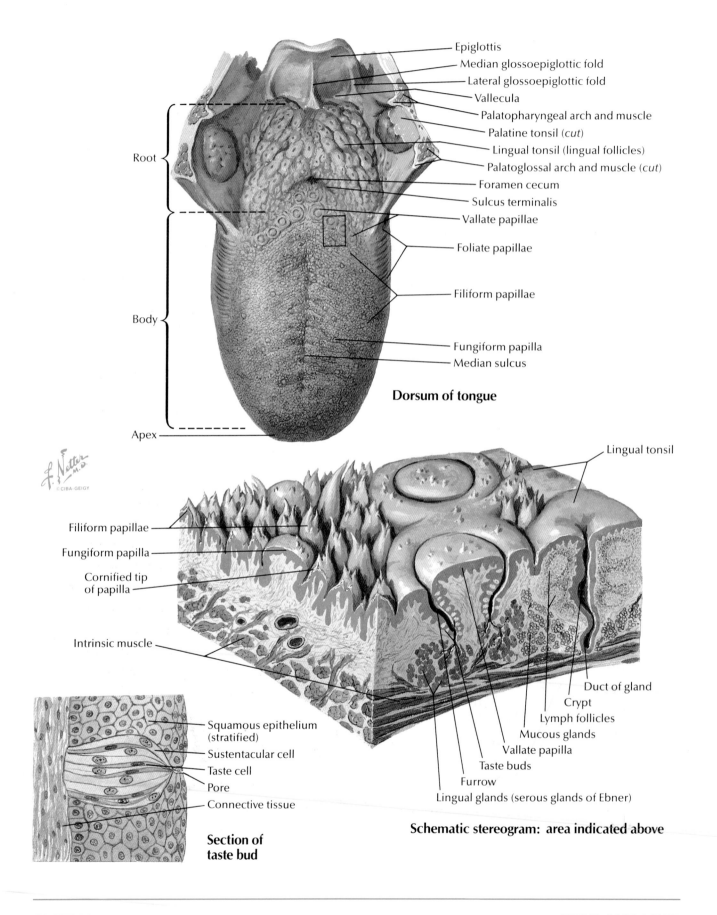

Epiglottis
Median glossoepiglottic fold
Lateral glossoepiglottic fold
Vallecula
Palatopharyngeal arch and muscle
Palatine tonsil (*cut*)
Lingual tonsil (lingual follicles)
Palatoglossal arch and muscle (*cut*)
Foramen cecum
Sulcus terminalis
Vallate papillae
Foliate papillae
Filiform papillae
Fungiform papilla
Median sulcus

Root

Body

Apex

Dorsum of tongue

Lingual tonsil

Filiform papillae
Fungiform papilla
Cornified tip of papilla

Intrinsic muscle

Squamous epithelium (stratified)
Sustentacular cell
Taste cell
Pore
Connective tissue

Section of taste bud

Duct of gland
Crypt
Lymph follicles
Mucous glands
Vallate papilla
Taste buds
Furrow
Lingual glands (serous glands of Ebner)

Schematic stereogram: area indicated above

PLATE 52

HEAD AND NECK

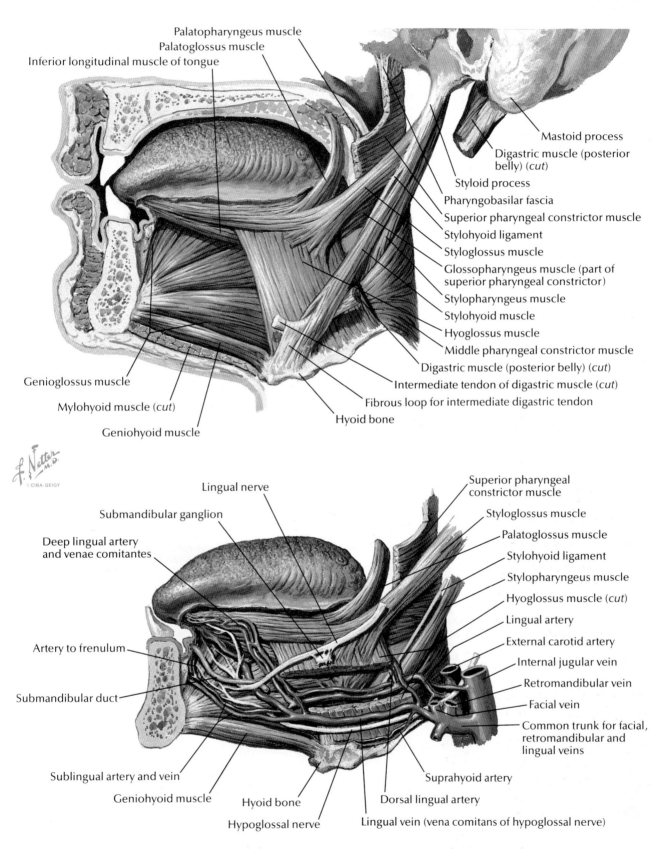

Palatopharyngeus muscle

Palatoglossus muscle

Inferior longitudinal muscle of tongue

Mastoid process

Digastric muscle (posterior belly) *(cut)*

Styloid process

Pharyngobasilar fascia

Superior pharyngeal constrictor muscle

Stylohyoid ligament

Styloglossus muscle

Glossopharyngeus muscle (part of superior pharyngeal constrictor)

Stylopharyngeus muscle

Stylohyoid muscle

Hyoglossus muscle

Middle pharyngeal constrictor muscle

Digastric muscle (posterior belly) *(cut)*

Intermediate tendon of digastric muscle *(cut)*

Fibrous loop for intermediate digastric tendon

Hyoid bone

Genioglossus muscle

Mylohyoid muscle *(cut)*

Geniohyoid muscle

Lingual nerve

Submandibular ganglion

Deep lingual artery and venae comitantes

Artery to frenulum

Submandibular duct

Superior pharyngeal constrictor muscle

Styloglossus muscle

Palatoglossus muscle

Stylohyoid ligament

Stylopharyngeus muscle

Hyoglossus muscle *(cut)*

Lingual artery

External carotid artery

Internal jugular vein

Retromandibular vein

Facial vein

Common trunk for facial, retromandibular and lingual veins

Sublingual artery and vein

Geniohyoid muscle

Hyoid bone

Hypoglossal nerve

Suprahyoid artery

Dorsal lingual artery

Lingual vein (vena comitans of hypoglossal nerve)

Tongue and Mouth: Sections

**Horizontal section
below lingula of
mandible: superior view**

Orbicularis oris muscle

Buccinator muscle

Buccopharyngeal fascia

Facial artery and vein

Pterygomandibular raphé

Lingual nerve and superior pharyngeal constrictor muscle

Masseter muscle

Palatoglossus muscle in palatoglossal arch

Palatine tonsil

Palatopharyngeus muscle in palatopharyngeal arch

Ramus of mandible

Inferior alveolar artery, vein and nerve

Medial pterygoid muscle

Styloglossus muscle

Facial nerve

Retromandibular vein

External carotid artery

Parotid gland

Stylopharyngeus muscle

Stylohyoid muscle

Sternocleidomastoid muscle

Digastric muscle (posterior belly)

Internal jugular vein, internal carotid artery,
and nerves IX, X and XII in carotid sheath

Superior cervical sympathetic ganglion

Axis (C2)

Longus capitis muscle

Prevertebral fascia

Buccopharyngeal fascia
and retropharyngeal space

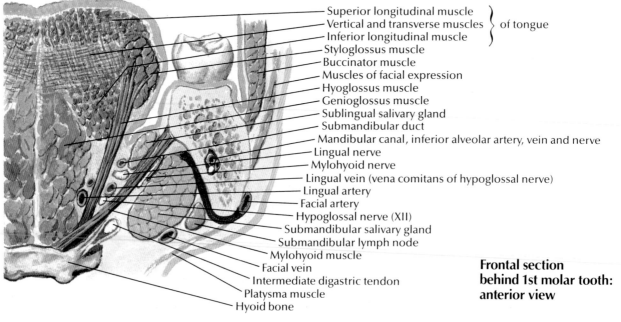

Superior longitudinal muscle
Vertical and transverse muscles } of tongue
Inferior longitudinal muscle
Styloglossus muscle
Buccinator muscle
Muscles of facial expression
Hyoglossus muscle
Genioglossus muscle
Sublingual salivary gland
Submandibular duct
Mandibular canal, inferior alveolar artery, vein and nerve
Lingual nerve
Mylohyoid nerve
Lingual vein (vena comitans of hypoglossal nerve)
Lingual artery
Facial artery
Hypoglossal nerve (XII)
Submandibular salivary gland
Submandibular lymph node
Mylohyoid muscle
Facial vein
Intermediate digastric tendon
Platysma muscle
Hyoid bone

**Frontal section
behind 1st molar tooth:
anterior view**

PLATE 54

HEAD AND NECK

Superficial temporal artery and vein and auriculotemporal nerve

Branches of facial nerve

Transverse facial artery

Accessory parotid gland

Parotid duct

Buccinator muscle (*cut*)

Masseter muscle

Lingual nerve

Submandibular ganglion

Tongue

Frenulum of tongue

Sublingual fold with openings of sublingual ducts

Sublingual caruncle with opening of submandibular duct

Sublingual gland

Submandibular duct

Sublingual artery and vein

Mylohyoid muscle (*cut*)

Digastric muscle (anterior belly)

Submandibular gland

Facial artery and vein

Hyoid bone

Parotid gland

Retromandibular vein

Digastric muscle (posterior belly)

Stylohyoid muscle

External jugular vein

Sternocleidomastoid muscle

Common trunk receiving facial, retromandibular and lingual veins

Internal jugular vein

External carotid artery

Parotid gland: totally serous

Submandibular gland: mostly serous, partially mucous

Sublingual gland: almost completely mucous

Afferent Innervation of Mouth and Pharynx

SEE ALSO PLATES 41, 46, 53, 58, 116, 117, 119, 127, 129

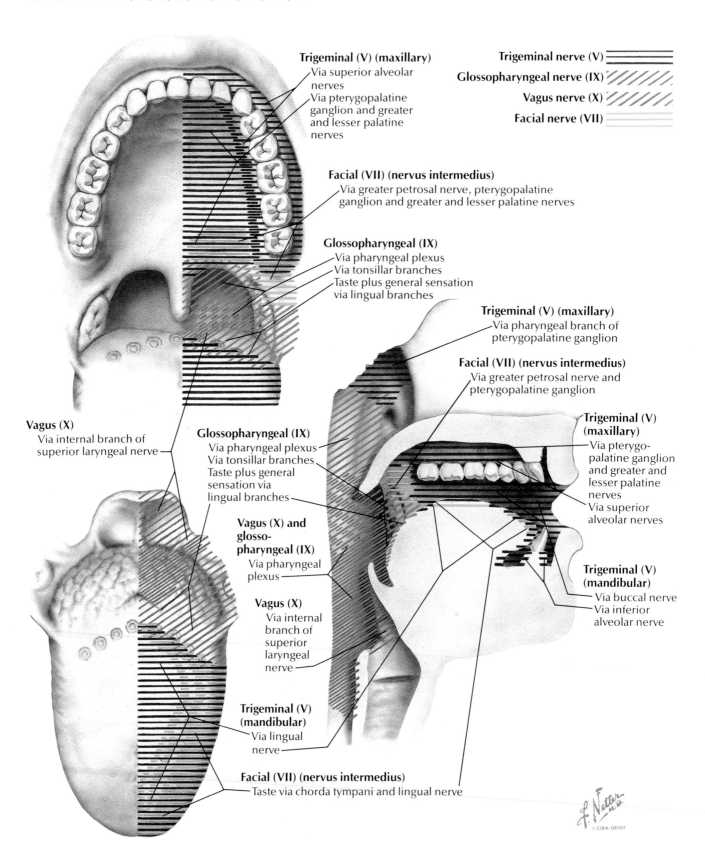

Trigeminal (V) (maxillary)
Via superior alveolar nerves
Via pterygopalatine ganglion and greater and lesser palatine nerves

Trigeminal nerve (V)
Glossopharyngeal nerve (IX)
Vagus nerve (X)
Facial nerve (VII)

Facial (VII) (nervus intermedius)
Via greater petrosal nerve, pterygopalatine ganglion and greater and lesser palatine nerves

Glossopharyngeal (IX)
Via pharyngeal plexus
Via tonsillar branches
Taste plus general sensation via lingual branches

Trigeminal (V) (maxillary)
Via pharyngeal branch of pterygopalatine ganglion

Facial (VII) (nervus intermedius)
Via greater petrosal nerve and pterygopalatine ganglion

Trigeminal (V) (maxillary)
Via pterygo-palatine ganglion and greater and lesser palatine nerves
Via superior alveolar nerves

Vagus (X)
Via internal branch of superior laryngeal nerve

Glossopharyngeal (IX)
Via pharyngeal plexus
Via tonsillar branches
Taste plus general sensation via lingual branches

Vagus (X) and glosso-pharyngeal (IX)
Via pharyngeal plexus

Vagus (X)
Via internal branch of superior laryngeal nerve

Trigeminal (V) (mandibular)
Via buccal nerve
Via inferior alveolar nerve

Trigeminal (V) (mandibular)
Via lingual nerve

Facial (VII) (nervus intermedius)
Taste via chorda tympani and lingual nerve

PLATE 56

HEAD AND NECK

Frontal sinus

Sphenoidal sinus

Nasal septum

Nasopharynx

Soft palate

Palatine glands

Hard palate

Oral cavity

Incisive canal

Palatine tonsil

Body of tongue

Oropharynx

Foramen cecum

Lingual tonsil

Genioglossus muscle

Root of tongue

Epiglottis

Mandible

Geniohyoid muscle

Hyoid bone

Hyoepiglottic ligament

Thyrohyoid membrane

Laryngopharynx (hypopharynx)

Aditus of larynx

Thyroid cartilage

Vocal fold (cord)

Transverse arytenoid muscle

Cricoid cartilage

Trachea

Esophagus

Esophageal muscles

Thyroid gland

Superficial (investing) cervical fascia

Pretracheal fascia

Suprasternal space (of Burns)

Manubrium of sternum

Sella turcica

Pharyngeal opening of auditory (Eustachian) tube

Sphenooccipital suture

Pharyngeal tonsil

Pharyngeal tubercle of occipital bone

Pharyngobasilar fascia

Anterior longitudinal ligament

Anterior atlantooccipital membrane

Apical ligament of dens

Anterior tubercle of atlas (C1)

Dens of axis (C2)

Pharyngeal constrictor muscles

Bucco-pharyngeal fascia

Retro-pharyngeal space

Prevertebral fascia and anterior longitudinal ligament

Vertebral bodies

C1

C2

C3

C4

C5

C6

C7

T1

Fauces

Medial sagittal view

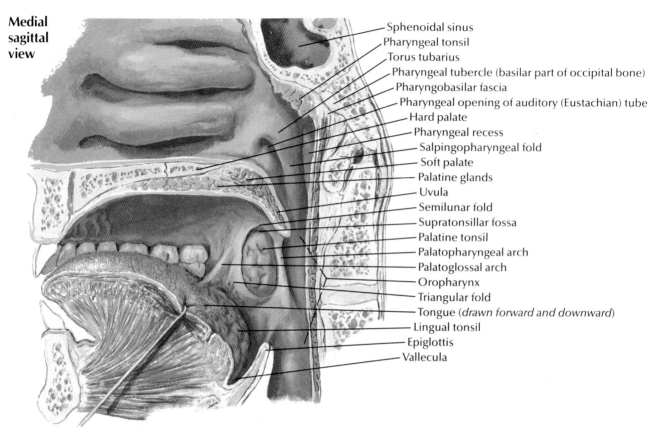

- Sphenoidal sinus
- Pharyngeal tonsil
- Torus tubarius
- Pharyngeal tubercle (basilar part of occipital bone)
- Pharyngobasilar fascia
- Pharyngeal opening of auditory (Eustachian) tube
- Hard palate
- Pharyngeal recess
- Salpingopharyngeal fold
- Soft palate
- Palatine glands
- Uvula
- Semilunar fold
- Supratonsillar fossa
- Palatine tonsil
- Palatopharyngeal arch
- Palatoglossal arch
- Oropharynx
- Triangular fold
- Tongue (*drawn forward and downward*)
- Lingual tonsil
- Epiglottis
- Vallecula

Pharyngeal mucosa removed

- Cartilaginous auditory (Eustachian) tube
- Medial pterygoid plate
- Tensor veli palatini muscle and tendon
- Levator veli palatini muscle
- Ascending palatine artery
- Ascending pharyngeal artery (pharyngeal branch)
- Lesser palatine artery
- Salpingopharyngeus muscle
- Pterygoid hamulus
- Pterygomandibular raphé
- Tonsillar branch of lesser palatine artery
- Superior pharyngeal constrictor muscle
- Tonsillar branch of ascending pharyngeal artery
- Palatoglossus muscle
- Palatopharyngeus muscle
- Tonsillar branch of ascending palatine artery
- Tonsillar branch of facial artery
- Tonsillar branch of dorsal lingual artery
- Glossopharyngeal nerve (IX) and tonsillar branch
- Stylohyoid ligament
- Hyoglossus muscle
- Middle pharyngeal constrictor muscle
- Stylopharyngeus muscle

PLATE 58

HEAD AND NECK

Medial pterygoid plate

Cartilaginous auditory (Eustachian) tube

Tensor veli palatini muscle

Pharyngobasilar fascia

Levator veli palatini muscle

Palatine aponeurosis and tendon of tensor veli palatini muscle

Pharyngeal tubercle (basilar part of occipital bone)

Pharyngobasilar fascia

Anterior longitudinal ligament

Anterior atlantooccipital membrane

Apical ligament of dens

Salpingopharyngeus muscle

Muscles of soft palate

Palatopharyngeal sphincter (Passavant's ridge)

Pterygoid hamulus

Superior pharyngeal constrictor muscle

Pterygomandibular raphé

Palatopharyngeus muscle

Buccinator muscle

Glossopharyngeus muscle (part of superior pharyngeal constrictor)

Stylopharyngeus muscle

Stylohyoid ligament

Styloglossus muscle

Middle pharyngeal constrictor muscle

Fibers to pharyngoepiglottic fold

Buccopharyngeal fascia and retropharyngeal space

Prevertebral fascia and anterior longitudinal ligament

Internal branch of superior laryngeal nerve

Longitudinal pharyngeal muscles

Inferior pharyngeal constrictor muscle

Pharyngeal aponeurosis

Cricopharyngeus muscle (part of inferior pharyngeal constrictor)

Cricoid attachment of longitudinal esophageal muscle

Circular esophageal muscle

Longitudinal esophageal muscle

C1
C2
C3
C4
C5
C6
C7

Hyoglossus muscle

Geniohyoid muscle

Mylohyoid muscle

Hyoid bone

Thyrohyoid membrane

Thyroid cartilage

Cricothyroid ligament

Corniculate and arytenoid cartilages

Cricoid cartilage

Trachea

•••••••••••• Margins of middle pharyngeal constrictor muscle

– – – – – – – Margins and attachment of inferior pharyngeal constrictor muscle

Pharynx: Opened Posterior View

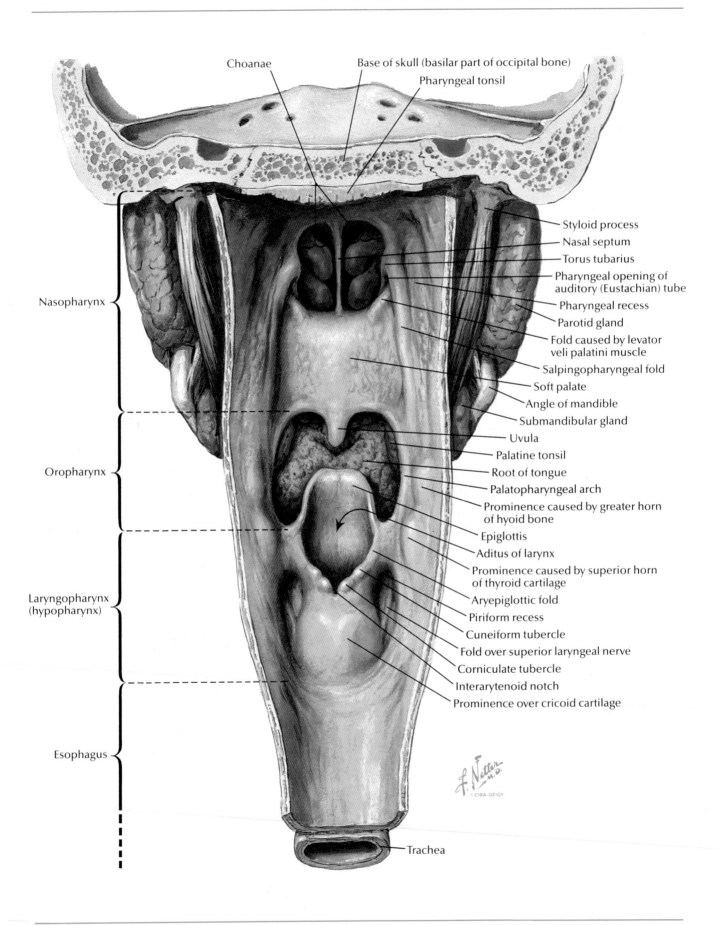

Choanae

Base of skull (basilar part of occipital bone)

Pharyngeal tonsil

Nasopharynx

Styloid process

Nasal septum

Torus tubarius

Pharyngeal opening of auditory (Eustachian) tube

Pharyngeal recess

Parotid gland

Fold caused by levator veli palatini muscle

Salpingopharyngeal fold

Soft palate

Angle of mandible

Submandibular gland

Uvula

Palatine tonsil

Oropharynx

Root of tongue

Palatopharyngeal arch

Prominence caused by greater horn of hyoid bone

Epiglottis

Aditus of larynx

Prominence caused by superior horn of thyroid cartilage

Aryepiglottic fold

Piriform recess

Cuneiform tubercle

Laryngopharynx (hypopharynx)

Fold over superior laryngeal nerve

Corniculate tubercle

Interarytenoid notch

Prominence over cricoid cartilage

Esophagus

Trachea

PLATE 60

HEAD AND NECK

Basilar part of occipital bone

Pharyngeal tubercle

Pharyngeal tonsil

Styloid process

Cartilaginous auditory (Eustachian) tube

Digastric muscle (posterior belly)

Pharyngobasilar fascia

Stylohyoid muscle

Choana

Stylopharyngeus muscle

Levator veli palatini muscle

Superior pharyngeal constrictor muscle

Accessory muscle bundle from petrous part of temporal bone

Salpingopharyngeus muscle

Uvula

Medial pterygoid muscle

Palatopharyngeus muscle

Pharyngobasilar fascia

Middle pharyngeal constrictor muscle

Pharyngeal raphé

Stylopharyngeus muscle

Superior pharyngeal constrictor muscle

Pharyngoepiglottic fold

Hyoid bone (tip of greater horn)

Aryepiglottic fold

Middle pharyngeal constrictor muscle

Inferior pharyngeal constrictor muscle (*cut edge*)

Epiglottis

Longitudinal pharyngeal muscles

Inferior pharyngeal constrictor muscle

Superior horn of thyroid cartilage

Cuneiform tubercle

Thyrohyoid membrane

Corniculate tubercle

Internal branch of superior laryngeal nerve

Transverse and oblique arytenoid muscles

Pharyngeal aponeurosis

Posterior cricoarytenoid muscle

Cricopharyngeus muscle (part of inferior pharyngeal constrictor)

Cricopharyngeus muscle (part of inferior pharyngeal constrictor)

Posterior border of thyroid cartilage lamina

Longitudinal esophageal muscle

Cricoid attachment of longitudinal esophageal muscle

Circular esophageal muscle

Muscles of Pharynx: Lateral View

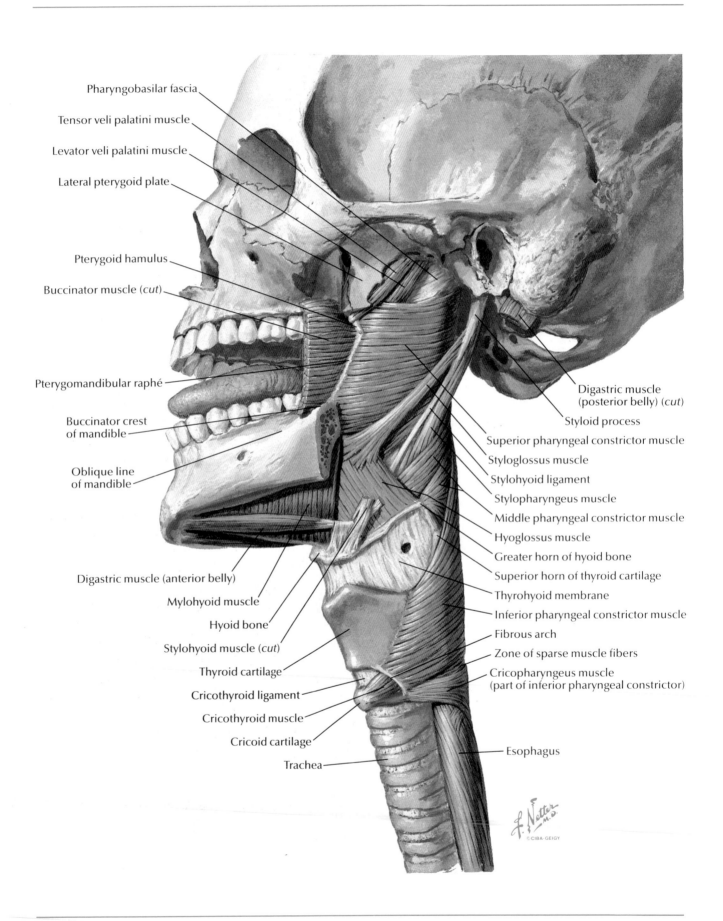

Pharyngobasilar fascia

Tensor veli palatini muscle

Levator veli palatini muscle

Lateral pterygoid plate

Pterygoid hamulus

Buccinator muscle (*cut*)

Pterygomandibular raphé

Buccinator crest of mandible

Oblique line of mandible

Digastric muscle (anterior belly)

Mylohyoid muscle

Hyoid bone

Stylohyoid muscle (*cut*)

Thyroid cartilage

Cricothyroid ligament

Cricothyroid muscle

Cricoid cartilage

Trachea

Digastric muscle (posterior belly) (*cut*)

Styloid process

Superior pharyngeal constrictor muscle

Styloglossus muscle

Stylohyoid ligament

Stylopharyngeus muscle

Middle pharyngeal constrictor muscle

Hyoglossus muscle

Greater horn of hyoid bone

Superior horn of thyroid cartilage

Thyrohyoid membrane

Inferior pharyngeal constrictor muscle

Fibrous arch

Zone of sparse muscle fibers

Cricopharyngeus muscle (part of inferior pharyngeal constrictor)

Esophagus

PLATE 62   HEAD AND NECK

From ophthalmic artery { Supraorbital artery / Supratrochlear artery

Middle meningeal artery

Deep temporal arteries

Dorsal nasal artery

Masseteric artery

Angular artery

Infraorbital artery

Sphenopalatine artery

Descending palatine artery

Posterior superior alveolar artery

Superior labial artery

Buccal artery

Buccinator muscle and parotid duct (cut)

Inferior labial artery

Superior pharyngeal constrictor muscle

Mental artery

Inferior alveolar artery and lingual branch

Facial artery

Submental artery

Mylohyoid artery

Submandibular gland

Hypoglossal nerve (XII)

Suprahyoid artery

External carotid artery

Superior laryngeal artery

Superior thyroid artery

Cricothyroid artery

Common carotid artery

Vertebral artery

Subclavian artery

Transverse facial artery (cut)

Superficial temporal artery

Maxillary artery

Posterior auricular artery

Ascending pharyngeal artery

Occipital artery and sternocleidomastoid branch

Glossopharyngeal nerve (IX)

Ascending palatine artery

Tonsillar artery

Facial artery

Lingual artery

Ascending pharyngeal artery

Internal carotid artery

Vagus nerve (X)

Superior cervical cardiac nerve

Sympathetic trunk

Anterior scalene muscle

Phrenic nerve

Middle scalene muscle

Ascending cervical artery

Inferior thyroid artery

Transverse cervical artery

Suprascapular artery

Costocervical trunk

Thyrocervical trunk

Veins of Oral and Pharyngeal Regions

SEE ALSO PLATES 17, 26, 98

Supratrochlear vein

Supraorbital vein

Nasofrontal vein

Superior ophthalmic vein

Angular vein

External nasal vein

Emissary (Vesalian) vein communicating with cavernous sinus

Infraorbital vein

Posterior superior alveolar veins

Palatine vein

Pterygoid plexus

Superior labial vein

Deep facial vein

Maxillary veins

Inferior labial vein

Mental vein

Facial vein and artery

External palatine vein

Submental vein

Submandibular gland

Vena comitans of hypoglossal nerve

Deep lingual vein coursing medial to hyoglossus muscle

Lingual vein

Communication to anterior jugular vein (*cut*)

Superior laryngeal vein

Superior thyroid vein

Thyroid gland

Middle thyroid vein

Inferior thyroid veins

Termination of anterior jugular vein (*cut*)

Left brachiocephalic vein

Occipital vein and artery

Superficial temporal vein and artery

Transverse facial vein (*cut*)

Posterior auricular vein

Retromandibular vein

External jugular vein (*cut*)

Inferior alveolar vein and artery

Occipital vein and artery

Hypoglossal nerve (XII)

Common trunk for facial, retromandibular and lingual veins

Internal jugular vein

External carotid artery

Common carotid artery

Vagus nerve (X) and sympathetic trunk

Middle scalene muscle

Anterior scalene muscle

External jugular vein (*cut*)

Transverse cervical vein (*cut*)

Suprascapular vein (*cut*)

Subclavian artery

Subclavian vein

PLATE 64

Zygomaticotemporal nerve (V$_2$)

Deep temporal nerves (V$_3$)

Masseteric nerve (V$_3$)

Mandibular nerve (V$_3$)

Nerve to medial pterygoid and tensor veli palatini muscles (V$_3$) (*cut*)

Zygomaticofacial nerve (V$_2$)

Maxillary nerve (V$_2$)

Infraorbital nerve (V$_2$)

Pterygopalatine ganglion

Greater and lesser palatine nerves (V$_2$)

Anterior, middle and posterior superior alveolar nerves (V$_2$)

Nerve to lateral pterygoid muscle (V$_3$) (*cut*)

Buccal nerve (V$_3$)

Chorda tympani nerve (VII)

Lingual nerve (V$_3$)

Medial pterygoid muscle (*cut*) (lateral pterygoid removed)

Inferior alveolar nerve (V$_3$)

Mental nerve (V$_3$)

Mylohyoid nerve (V$_3$)

Submandibular ganglion

Glossopharyngeal nerve (IX) and tonsillar branch

Hypoglossal nerve (XII)

Carotid sinus nerve (IX) and carotid body

Nerve to thyrohyoid muscle (C1, 2 via XII)

External and internal branches of superior laryngeal nerve (X)

Ansa cervicalis (C1, 2, 3) { Superior root / Inferior root

Nerves to superior and inferior bellies of omohyoid, sternohyoid and sternothyroid muscles (ansa cervicalis)

Recurrent laryngeal nerve (X)

Sympathetic trunk and middle cervical ganglion

Common carotid artery

Vertebral artery

Auriculotemporal nerve (V$_3$)

Middle meningeal artery

Superficial temporal artery (*cut*)

Facial nerve (VII) (*cut*)

Maxillary artery

Accessory nerve (XI) (*cut*)

1st cervical nerve (ventral ramus) (*cut*)

2nd cervical nerve (ventral ramus) (*cut*)

Pharyngeal plexus composed of branches from glossopharyngeal (IX), vagus (X) and sympathetic nerves

Internal carotid artery

External carotid artery

Vagus nerve (X) and superior cervical cardiac branch

4th cervical nerve (ventral ramus) (*cut*)

Phrenic nerve (C3, 4, 5)

Ascending cervical artery

Middle scalene muscle

Anterior scalene muscle

Brachial plexus (*cut*)

Thyrocervical trunk

Subclavian artery

Lymph Vessels and Nodes of Oral and Pharyngeal Regions

SEE ALSO PLATE 197

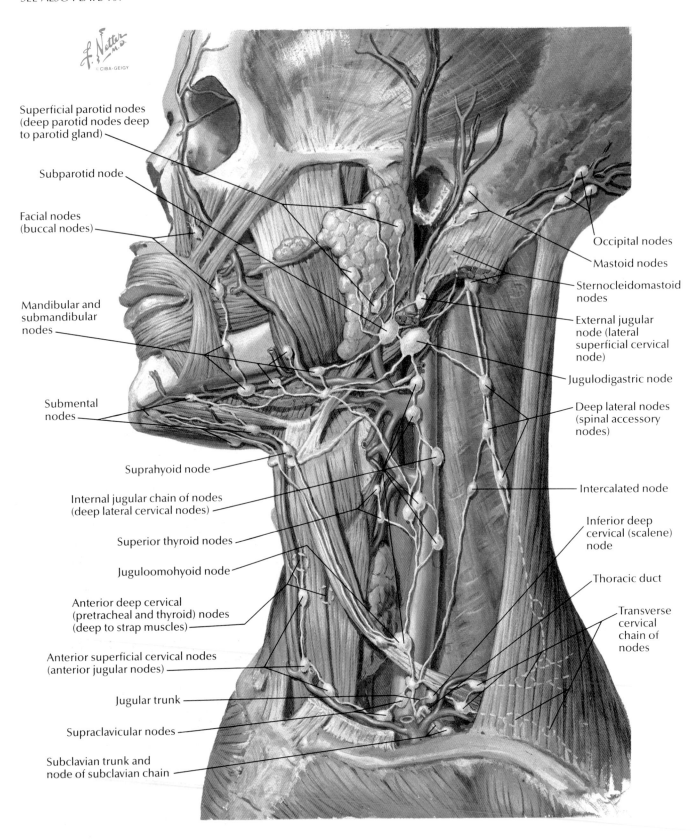

Superficial parotid nodes (deep parotid nodes deep to parotid gland)

Subparotid node

Facial nodes (buccal nodes)

Mandibular and submandibular nodes

Submental nodes

Suprahyoid node

Internal jugular chain of nodes (deep lateral cervical nodes)

Superior thyroid nodes

Juguloomohyoid node

Anterior deep cervical (pretracheal and thyroid) nodes (deep to strap muscles)

Anterior superficial cervical nodes (anterior jugular nodes)

Jugular trunk

Supraclavicular nodes

Subclavian trunk and node of subclavian chain

Occipital nodes

Mastoid nodes

Sternocleidomastoid nodes

External jugular node (lateral superficial cervical node)

Jugulodigastric node

Deep lateral nodes (spinal accessory nodes)

Intercalated node

Inferior deep cervical (scalene) node

Thoracic duct

Transverse cervical chain of nodes

PLATE 66

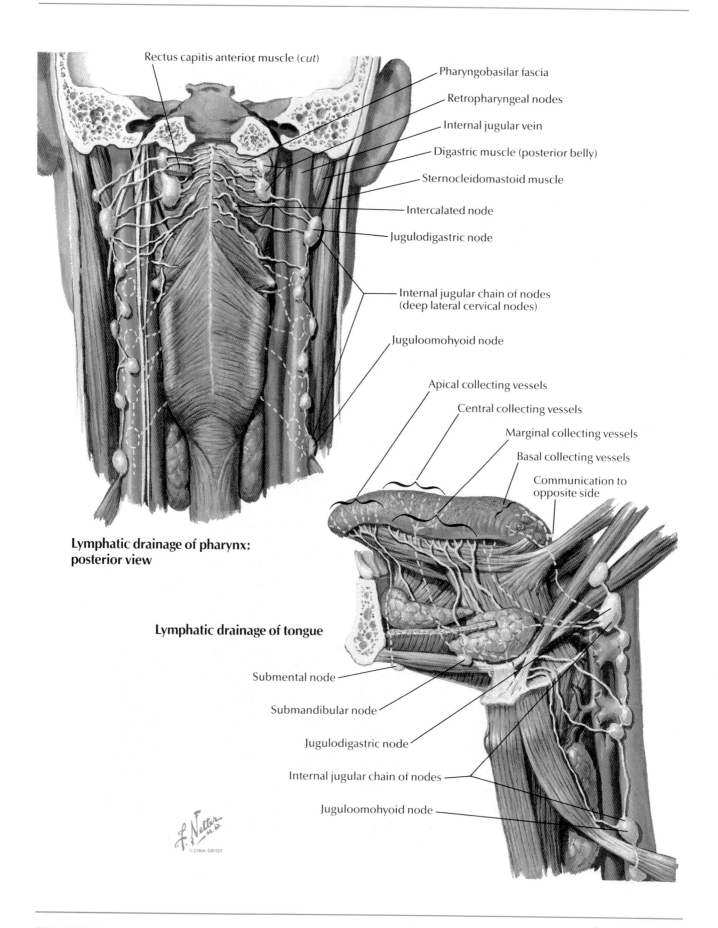

Rectus capitis anterior muscle (*cut*)

Pharyngobasilar fascia

Retropharyngeal nodes

Internal jugular vein

Digastric muscle (posterior belly)

Sternocleidomastoid muscle

Intercalated node

Jugulodigastric node

Internal jugular chain of nodes
(deep lateral cervical nodes)

Juguloomohyoid node

Apical collecting vessels

Central collecting vessels

Marginal collecting vessels

Basal collecting vessels

Communication to
opposite side

**Lymphatic drainage of pharynx:
posterior view**

Lymphatic drainage of tongue

Submental node

Submandibular node

Jugulodigastric node

Internal jugular chain of nodes

Juguloomohyoid node

Thyroid Gland: Anterior View

External carotid artery

Internal carotid artery

Superior thyroid artery and vein

Superior laryngeal artery

Thyrohyoid membrane

Ansa { Superior root
cervicalis { Inferior root

Common carotid artery

Internal jugular vein

Middle thyroid vein

Inferior thyroid veins

Ascending cervical artery

Inferior thyroid artery

Transverse cervical artery

Suprascapular artery

Thyrocervical trunk

Subclavian
artery and vein

Vagus nerve (X)

Right recurrent
laryngeal nerve

Brachiocephalic trunk

Brachiocephalic veins

Superior vena cava

Aortic arch

Hyoid bone

Superior laryngeal nerve
Internal branch
External branch

Thyroid cartilage (lamina)

Cricothyroid ligament

Cricothyroid muscles

Cricoid cartilage

Pyramidal lobe
(often absent
or small)   } Thyroid
Right lobe   gland
Left lobe
Isthmus

Pretracheal lymph nodes

Phrenic nerve

Anterior scalene muscle

Vagus nerve (X)

External jugular vein

Anterior jugular vein

1st rib (cut)

Left recurrent laryngeal nerve

Thyroid cartilage

Cricothyroid ligament

Common carotid artery

Medial margin of
sternocleidomastoid muscle

Cricothyroid muscle

Cricoid cartilage

Thyroid gland

Cupula (dome) of pleura

PLATE 68

HEAD AND NECK

Superior pharyngeal constrictor muscle

Middle pharyngeal constrictor muscle

Tip of greater horn of hyoid bone

Inferior pharyngeal constrictor muscle

Median pharyngeal raphé

Zone of sparse muscle fibers

Cricopharyngeus muscle (part of inferior pharyngeal constrictor)

Circular esophageal muscle in V-shaped area of sparse longitudinal muscle fibers (area of Laimer)

Longitudinal esophageal muscle

Inferior thyroid vein

Trachea

Inferior bulb of internal jugular vein

Vertebral artery

Left subclavian artery and vein

Internal thoracic artery and vein

Left brachiocephalic vein

Left recurrent laryngeal nerve

Arch of aorta

Left vagus nerve (X)

External carotid artery

Internal carotid artery

Facial artery

Lingual artery

Superior laryngeal nerve
Internal branch
External branch

Superior thyroid artery

Superior laryngeal artery

Common carotid artery

Vagus nerve (X)

Internal jugular vein

Thyroid gland (right lobe)

Superior parathyroid gland

Inferior parathyroid gland

Ascending cervical artery

Inferior thyroid artery

Right recurrent laryngeal nerve

Transverse cervical artery

Suprascapular artery

Thyrocervical trunk

Right subclavian artery and vein

Right brachiocephalic vein

Brachiocephalic trunk

Right vagus nerve (X)

Superior vena cava

Parathyroid Glands

SEE ALSO PLATE 74

Posterior view

Thyrohyoid membrane

Hyoid bone

Superior laryngeal nerve
Internal branch
External branch

Vagus nerve (X)

Epiglottis

Superior thyroid artery

Common carotid artery

Sheath of thyroid gland (*cut*)

Superior parathyroid gland

Left lobe of thyroid gland

Ascending cervical artery

Inferior parathyroid gland

Recurrent laryngeal nerve

Esophagus

Subclavian artery

Trachea

External carotid artery

Internal carotid artery

Superior thyroid artery

Superior laryngeal artery

Inferior pharyngeal constrictor muscle (*cut*)

Common carotid artery

Sheath of thyroid gland (*cut*)

Cricopharyngeus muscle (part of inferior pharyngeal constrictor)

Superior parathyroid gland

Right lobe of thyroid gland

Inferior parathyroid gland (may be more caudally located, even within mediastinum)

Inferior thyroid artery

Recurrent laryngeal nerve

Transverse cervical artery

Suprascapular artery

Thyrocervical trunk

Vertebral artery

Subclavian artery

Brachiocephalic trunk

Right lateral view

External carotid artery

Superior laryngeal artery

Superior thyroid artery (*cut*)

Inferior pharyngeal constrictor muscle

Common carotid artery

Internal jugular vein

Inferior thyroid artery

Recurrent laryngeal nerve

Esophagus

Internal branch of superior laryngeal nerve

External branch of superior laryngeal nerve

Superior parathyroid gland

Thyroid gland (right lobe) (*reflected*)

Inferior parathyroid gland

PLATE 70　　　　　　　　　　　　　　　　　　**HEAD AND NECK**

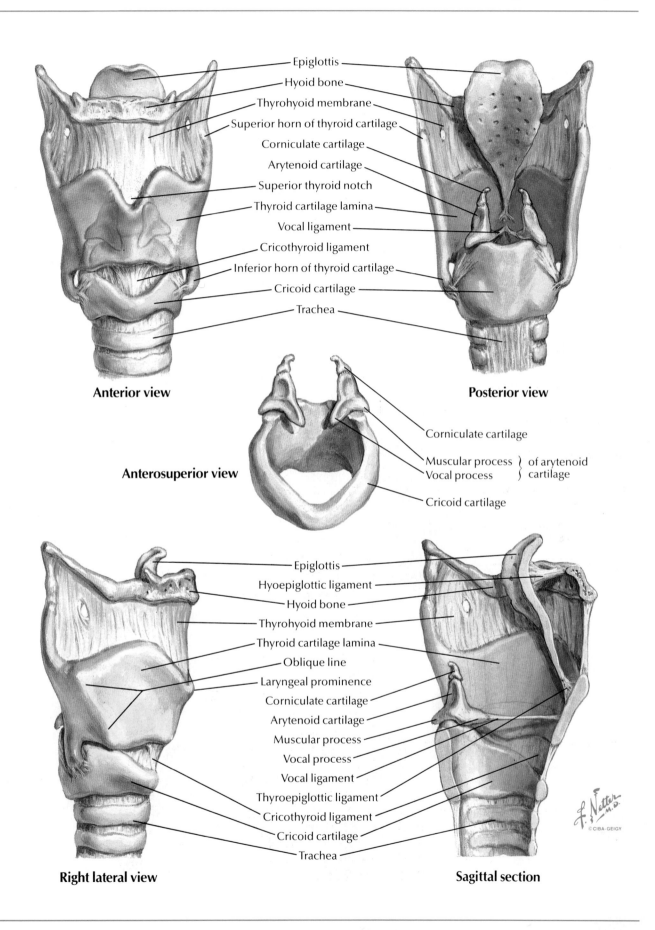

Epiglottis

Hyoid bone

Thyrohyoid membrane

Superior horn of thyroid cartilage

Corniculate cartilage

Arytenoid cartilage

Superior thyroid notch

Thyroid cartilage lamina

Vocal ligament

Cricothyroid ligament

Inferior horn of thyroid cartilage

Cricoid cartilage

Trachea

Anterior view

Posterior view

Anterosuperior view

Corniculate cartilage

Muscular process } of arytenoid
Vocal process } cartilage

Cricoid cartilage

Epiglottis

Hyoepiglottic ligament

Hyoid bone

Thyrohyoid membrane

Thyroid cartilage lamina

Oblique line

Laryngeal prominence

Corniculate cartilage

Arytenoid cartilage

Muscular process

Vocal process

Vocal ligament

Thyroepiglottic ligament

Cricothyroid ligament

Cricoid cartilage

Trachea

Right lateral view

Sagittal section

PLATE 71

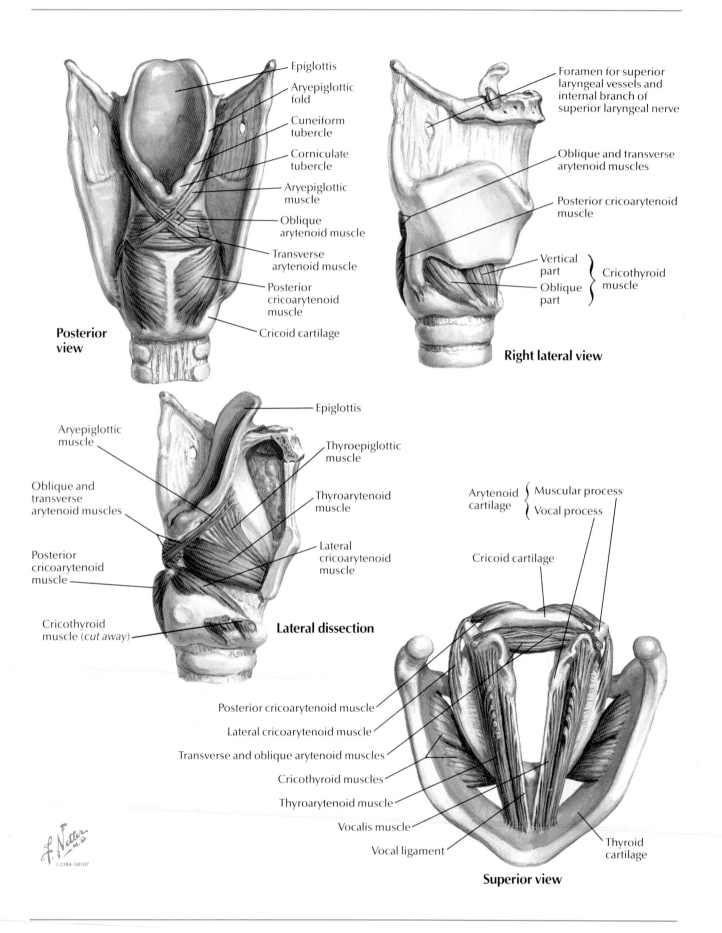

Epiglottis

Aryepiglottic fold

Cuneiform tubercle

Corniculate tubercle

Aryepiglottic muscle

Oblique arytenoid muscle

Transverse arytenoid muscle

Posterior cricoarytenoid muscle

Cricoid cartilage

Posterior view

Foramen for superior laryngeal vessels and internal branch of superior laryngeal nerve

Oblique and transverse arytenoid muscles

Posterior cricoarytenoid muscle

Vertical part

Oblique part

Cricothyroid muscle

Right lateral view

Aryepiglottic muscle

Oblique and transverse arytenoid muscles

Posterior cricoarytenoid muscle

Cricothyroid muscle (*cut away*)

Epiglottis

Thyroepiglottic muscle

Thyroarytenoid muscle

Lateral cricoarytenoid muscle

Lateral dissection

Arytenoid cartilage

Muscular process

Vocal process

Cricoid cartilage

Posterior cricoarytenoid muscle

Lateral cricoarytenoid muscle

Transverse and oblique arytenoid muscles

Cricothyroid muscles

Thyroarytenoid muscle

Vocalis muscle

Vocal ligament

Thyroid cartilage

Superior view

PLATE 72   **HEAD AND NECK**

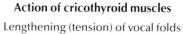

Action of cricothyroid muscles

Lengthening (tension) of vocal folds

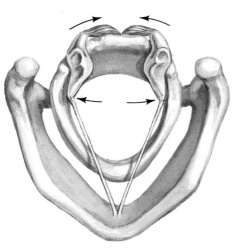

Action of posterior cricoarytenoid muscles

Abduction of vocal folds

Action of lateral cricoarytenoid muscles

Adduction of vocal folds

Action of transverse arytenoid muscle

Adduction of vocal folds

Action of vocalis and thyroarytenoid muscles

Shortening (relaxation) of vocal folds

Nerves of Larynx

SEE ALSO PLATES 68, 69, 70, 223

Superior laryngeal nerve

Internal branch

External branch

Inferior pharyngeal constrictor muscle

Cricothyroid muscle

Cricopharyngeus muscle (part of inferior pharyngeal constrictor)

Recurrent laryngeal nerve

Right lateral view

Internal branch of superior laryngeal nerve

Sensory branches to larynx

Anastomosis

Aryepiglottic muscle

Thyroepiglottic muscle

Transverse and oblique arytenoid muscles

Thyroarytenoid muscle

Vocalis muscle

Lateral cricoarytenoid muscle

Posterior cricoarytenoid muscle

Cricothyroid articular facet

Anterior and posterior branches of inferior laryngeal nerve

Recurrent laryngeal nerve

Right lateral view:
thyroid cartilage lamina removed

Right vagus nerve (X)

Anomalous right inferior laryngeal nerve (not recurrent)

Anomalous (retroesophageal) right subclavian artery

Right common carotid artery

Arch of aorta

Left vagus nerve (X)

Left common carotid artery

Left inferior laryngeal nerve

Left recurrent laryngeal nerve

Left subclavian artery

Anomalous (retroesophageal) right subclavian artery originating from left side of aortic arch

Left recurrent laryngeal nerve

Anterior view:
anomalous right inferior laryngeal nerve, not recurrent, associated with anomalous right subclavian artery

PLATE 74   **HEAD AND NECK**

Position of patient and physician

Mirror warmed over alcohol flame to prevent fogging, then tested on back of physician's hand

Technique

Mirror elevates uvula

Median glosso-epiglottic fold

Vallecula

Vocal folds (true cords)

Glottis

Trachea

Piriform recess

Interarytenoid notch

Esophagus

Root of tongue (lingual tonsil)

Epiglottis

Ventricular folds (false cords)

Vestibule

Aryepiglottic fold

Ventricle

Cuneiform tubercle

Corniculate tubercle

Normal larynx: inspiration

Normal larynx: phonation

Eyelids

Superior palpebral conjunctiva: tarsal (Meibomian) glands shining through

Pupil

Cornea

Limbus of cornea

Bulbar conjunctiva over sclera

Inferior fornix of conjunctiva

Inferior palpebral conjunctiva: tarsal glands shining through

Superior lacrimal papilla and puncta

Plica semilunaris

Lacrimal caruncle in lacrimal lake

Inferior lacrimal papilla and puncta

Levator palpebrae superioris muscle

Orbital septum

Superior tarsal (Müller's) muscle (smooth)

Superior conjunctival fornix

Orbicularis oculi muscle (palpebral part)

Superior tarsus

Tarsal (Meibomian) glands

Sebaceous glands

Cilia (lashes)

Openings of tarsal glands

Inferior tarsus

Orbicularis oculi muscle (palpebral part)

Inferior conjunctival fornix

Orbital septum

Sclera

Bulbar conjunctiva

Palpebral conjunctiva

Cornea

Lens

Anterior chamber

Iris

Posterior chamber

Frontal bone

Insertion of levator palpebrae superioris muscle

Orbital septum

Superior tarsus

Lateral palpebral ligament and overlying raphé

Inferior tarsus

Orbital septum

Zygomatic bone

Supraorbital artery and nerve

Supratrochlear artery and nerve

Dorsal nasal artery

Lacrimal sac

Medial palpebral ligament

Maxilla (frontal process)

Infraorbital artery and nerve

PLATE 76

HEAD AND NECK

Lacrimal Apparatus

SEE ALSO PLATES 40, 127

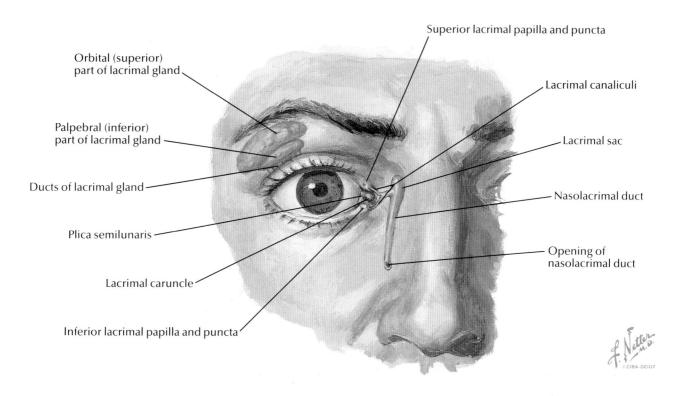

Superior lacrimal papilla and puncta

Orbital (superior) part of lacrimal gland

Lacrimal canaliculi

Palpebral (inferior) part of lacrimal gland

Lacrimal sac

Ducts of lacrimal gland

Nasolacrimal duct

Plica semilunaris

Lacrimal caruncle

Opening of nasolacrimal duct

Inferior lacrimal papilla and puncta

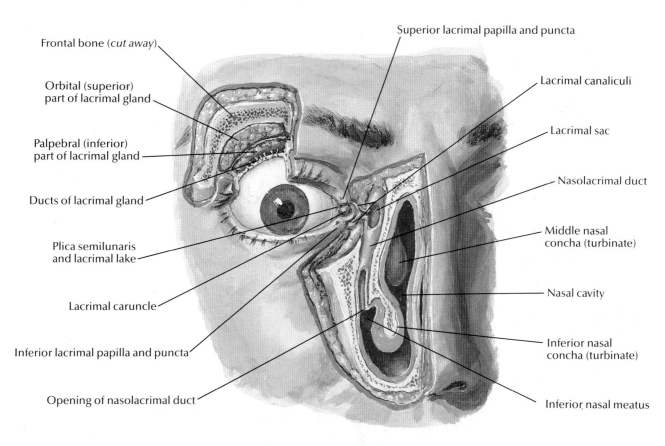

Superior lacrimal papilla and puncta

Frontal bone (*cut away*)

Orbital (superior) part of lacrimal gland

Lacrimal canaliculi

Palpebral (inferior) part of lacrimal gland

Lacrimal sac

Ducts of lacrimal gland

Nasolacrimal duct

Plica semilunaris and lacrimal lake

Middle nasal concha (turbinate)

Lacrimal caruncle

Nasal cavity

Inferior lacrimal papilla and puncta

Inferior nasal concha (turbinate)

Opening of nasolacrimal duct

Inferior nasal meatus

ORBIT AND CONTENTS

PLATE 77

Fascia of Orbit and Eyeball

Horizontal section

Medial palpebral ligament

Nasal cavity

Medial check ligament

Ethmoidal cells

Periorbita

Medial rectus muscle and sheath

Bulbar sheath (Tenon's capsule)

Sclera

Episcleral space

Optic nerve (II) and sheath

Sphenoidal sinus

Tarsus of eyelid

Palpebral conjunctiva

Bulbar conjunctiva

Cornea

Lateral palpebral ligament

Lateral check ligament

Periorbita

Sclera

Bulbar sheath (Tenon's capsule)

Episcleral space

Lateral rectus muscle and sheath

Orbital fat

Common annular tendon

Frontal section

Superior rectus muscle and sheath

Lacrimal gland

Lateral rectus muscle and sheath

Periorbita

Sclera

Bulbar sheath (Tenon's capsule)

Episcleral space

Orbital fat

Levator palpebrae superioris muscle and sheath

Superior oblique muscle and sheath

Medial rectus muscle and sheath

Periorbita

Ethmoidal cell

Sclera

Bulbar sheath (Tenon's capsule)

Inferior rectus muscle and sheath

Inferior oblique muscle and sheath

Infraorbital nerve (V₂)

Muscle attachments and nerves and vessels entering orbit

Superior orbital fissure

Lacrimal nerve (V₁)

Frontal nerve (V₁)

Trochlear nerve (IV)

Superior ophthalmic vein

Lateral rectus muscle

Superior division of oculomotor nerve (III)

Inferior orbital fissure

Abducens nerve (VI)

Levator palpebrae superioris muscle

Superior oblique muscle

Superior rectus muscle

Medial rectus muscle

Optic nerve (II)

Ophthalmic artery

} in optic canal

Inferior rectus muscle

Inferior division of oculomotor nerve (III)

Nasociliary nerve (V₁)

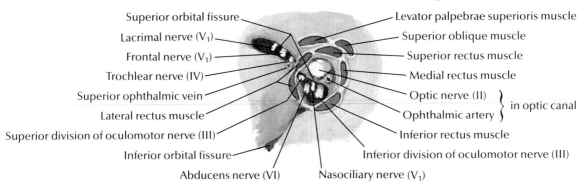

PLATE 78

HEAD AND NECK

Right lateral view

Superior oblique muscle

Levator palpebrae superioris muscle

Superior rectus muscle

Medial rectus muscle

Common annular tendon

Lateral rectus muscle (*cut*)

Inferior rectus muscle

Trochlea (pulley)

Optic nerve (II)

Lateral rectus muscle (*cut*)

Inferior oblique muscle

Superior view

Superior oblique muscle

Medial rectus muscle

Inferior rectus muscle

Common annular tendon

Superior palpebral tarsus

Levator palpebrae superioris muscle (*cut*)

Superior rectus muscle (*cut*)

Lateral rectus muscle

Optic nerve (II)

Superior rectus muscle (*cut*)

Levator palpebrae superioris muscle (*cut*)

Innervation and action of extrinsic eye muscles: anterior view

Superior oblique muscle ⎰ **Trochlear nerve (IV)**

Oculomotor nerve (III) ⎰ Levator palpebrae superioris muscle

Superior rectus muscle

Medial rectus muscle

Inferior rectus muscle

Inferior oblique muscle

Lateral rectus muscle ⎰ **Abducens nerve (VI)**

Note: arrows indicate direction of eye movement produced by each muscle

Arteries and Veins of Orbit and Eyelids

SEE ALSO PLATES 17, 98

Superior view

Supratrochlear artery

Dorsal nasal artery

Anterior meningeal artery

Anterior ethmoidal artery

Posterior ethmoidal artery

Continuation of ophthalmic artery

Muscular branch

Ophthalmic artery

Internal carotid artery

Medial palpebral artery

Lateral palpebral artery

Lacrimal gland

Supraorbital artery

Zygomatic branches

Posterior ciliary arteries

Muscular branch

Lacrimal artery

Central artery of retina

Anterior view

Frontal branch of superficial temporal artery

Superior lateral palpebral artery

Inferior lateral palpebral artery

Zygomaticofacial artery

Transverse facial artery

Infraorbital artery

Supraorbital artery

Supratrochlear artery

Dorsal nasal artery

Superior medial palpebral artery

Angular artery

Inferior medial palpebral artery

Superior and inferior palpebral arterial arches

Facial artery

(X = anastomosis of vessels from external and internal carotid arteries)

Lateral view

Supratrochlear vein

Supraorbital vein

Superior ophthalmic vein

Cavernous sinus

Inferior ophthalmic vein

Pterygoid plexus

Retromandibular vein

Nasofrontal vein

Angular vein

Vorticose veins

Facial vein

PLATE 80

Superior view

Supratrochlear nerve

Medial rectus muscle

Superior oblique muscle

Infratrochlear nerve

Nasociliary nerve

Trochlear nerve (IV)

Common annular tendon

Ophthalmic nerve (V₁)

Optic nerve (II)

Internal carotid artery and nerve plexus

Oculomotor nerve (III)

Trochlear nerve (IV)

Abducens nerve (VI)

Tentorium cerebelli

Medial branch · Lateral branch } Supraorbital nerve

Levator palpebrae superioris muscle

Superior rectus muscle

Lacrimal gland

Lacrimal nerve

Lateral rectus muscle

Frontal nerve

Maxillary nerve (V₂)

Meningeal branch of maxillary nerve

Mandibular nerve (V₃)

Lesser petrosal nerve

Meningeal branch of mandibular nerve

Greater petrosal nerve

Trigeminal (semilunar) ganglion

Tentorial (meningeal) branch of ophthalmic nerve

Superior view:
levator palpebrae superioris, superior rectus and superior oblique muscles partially cut away

Supratrochlear nerve (cut)

Supraorbital nerve branches (cut)

Infratrochlear nerve

Anterior ethmoidal nerve

Optic nerve (II)

Posterior ethmoidal nerve

Superior division of oculomotor nerve (III) (cut)

Nasociliary nerve

Internal carotid plexus

Trochlear nerve (IV) (cut)

Oculomotor nerve (III)

Abducens nerve (VI)

Long ciliary nerves

Short ciliary nerves

Lacrimal nerve

Ciliary ganglion

Parasympathetic root from oculomotor nerve

Sympathetic root from internal carotid plexus

Sensory root from nasociliary nerve

Branches to inferior and medial rectus muscles

Abducens nerve (VI)

Inferior division of oculomotor nerve (III)

Lacrimal nerve

Frontal nerve (cut)

Ophthalmic nerve (V₁)

Eyeball

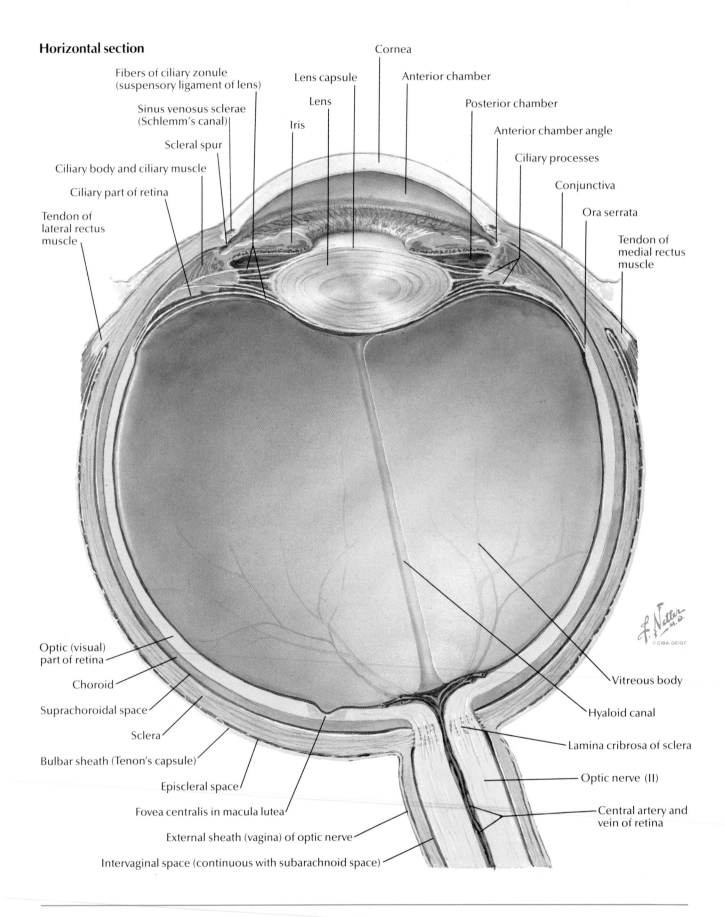

Fibers of ciliary zonule
(suspensory ligament of lens)

Sinus venosus sclerae
(Schlemm's canal)

Scleral spur

Ciliary body and ciliary muscle

Ciliary part of retina

Tendon of
lateral rectus
muscle

Iris

Lens capsule

Lens

Cornea

Anterior chamber

Posterior chamber

Anterior chamber angle

Ciliary processes

Conjunctiva

Ora serrata

Tendon of
medial rectus
muscle

Optic (visual)
part of retina

Choroid

Suprachoroidal space

Sclera

Bulbar sheath (Tenon's capsule)

Episcleral space

Fovea centralis in macula lutea

External sheath (vagina) of optic nerve

Intervaginal space (continuous with subarachnoid space)

Vitreous body

Hyaloid canal

Lamina cribrosa of sclera

Optic nerve (II)

Central artery and
vein of retina

PLATE 82

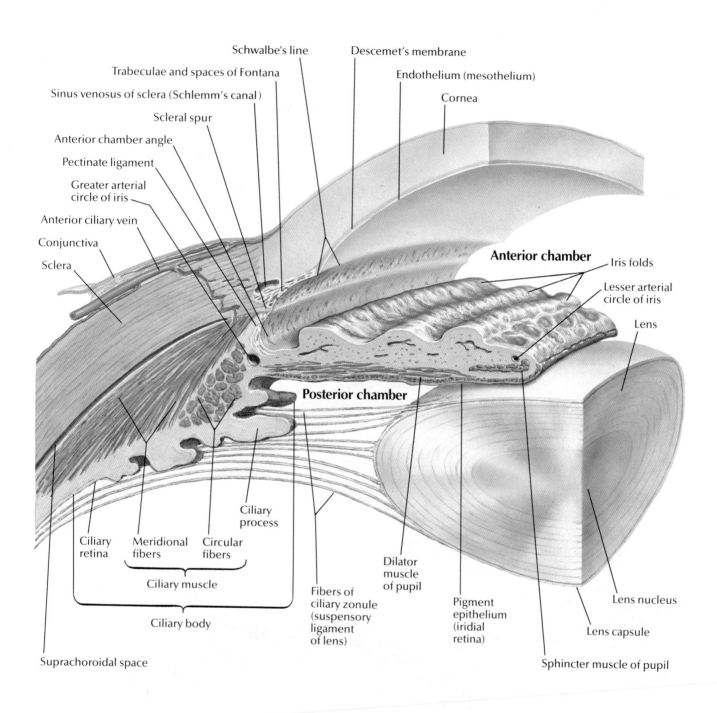

Schwalbe's line

Trabeculae and spaces of Fontana

Sinus venosus of sclera (Schlemm's canal)

Scleral spur

Anterior chamber angle

Pectinate ligament

Greater arterial circle of iris

Anterior ciliary vein

Conjunctiva

Sclera

Descemet's membrane

Endothelium (mesothelium)

Cornea

Anterior chamber

Iris folds

Lesser arterial circle of iris

Lens

Posterior chamber

Ciliary process

Ciliary retina

Meridional fibers

Circular fibers

Ciliary muscle

Ciliary body

Fibers of ciliary zonule (suspensory ligament of lens)

Dilator muscle of pupil

Pigment epithelium (iridial retina)

Lens nucleus

Lens capsule

Sphincter muscle of pupil

Suprachoroidal space

Note: for clarity only single plane of zonular fibers shown; actually fibers surround entire circumference of lens

Anterior Chamber Angle of Eye

Mirror

Contact lens

Goldmann gonioscopic mirror

Contact lens

To viewer's eye

Mirror

**Open (normal)
anterior chamber angle:
gonioscopic view**

Schwalbe's line

Schlemm's canal (*visible
if it contains blood*)

Line of scleral spur

Trabeculae

Iris

Pupil

**Closed angle:
gonioscopic view**

PLATE 84

HEAD AND NECK

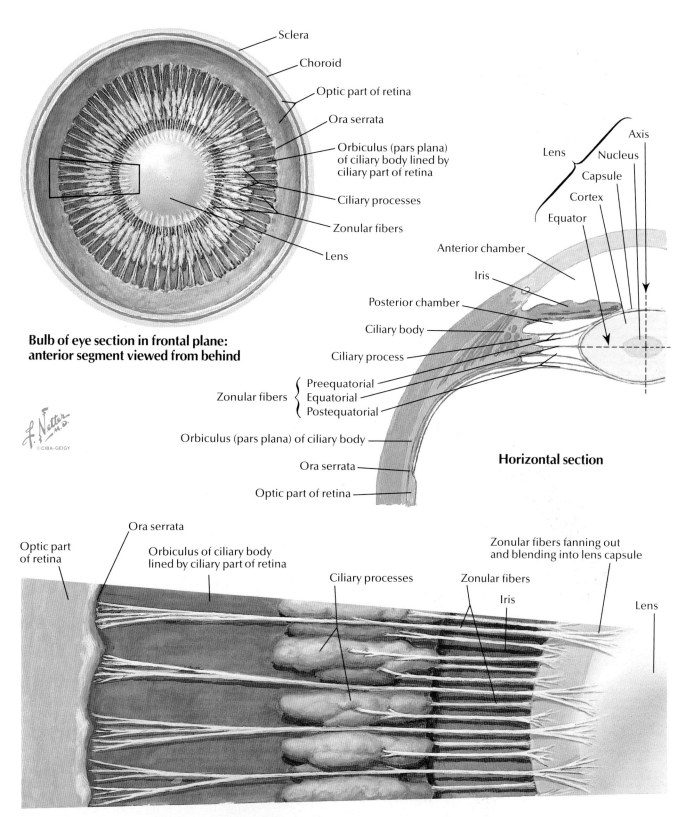

Sclera

Choroid

Optic part of retina

Ora serrata

Orbiculus (pars plana)
of ciliary body lined by
ciliary part of retina

Ciliary processes

Zonular fibers

Lens

**Bulb of eye section in frontal plane:
anterior segment viewed from behind**

Axis

Lens

Nucleus

Capsule

Cortex

Equator

Anterior chamber

Iris

Posterior chamber

Ciliary body

Ciliary process

Zonular fibers { Preequatorial
Equatorial
Postequatorial

Orbiculus (pars plana) of ciliary body

Ora serrata

Optic part of retina

Horizontal section

Ora serrata

Optic part
of retina

Orbiculus of ciliary body
lined by ciliary part of retina

Ciliary processes

Zonular fibers fanning out
and blending into lens capsule

Zonular fibers

Iris

Lens

Segment outlined in top illustration magnified to ultramicroscopic scale (semischematic)

Intrinsic Arteries and Veins of Eye

SEE ALSO PLATE 80

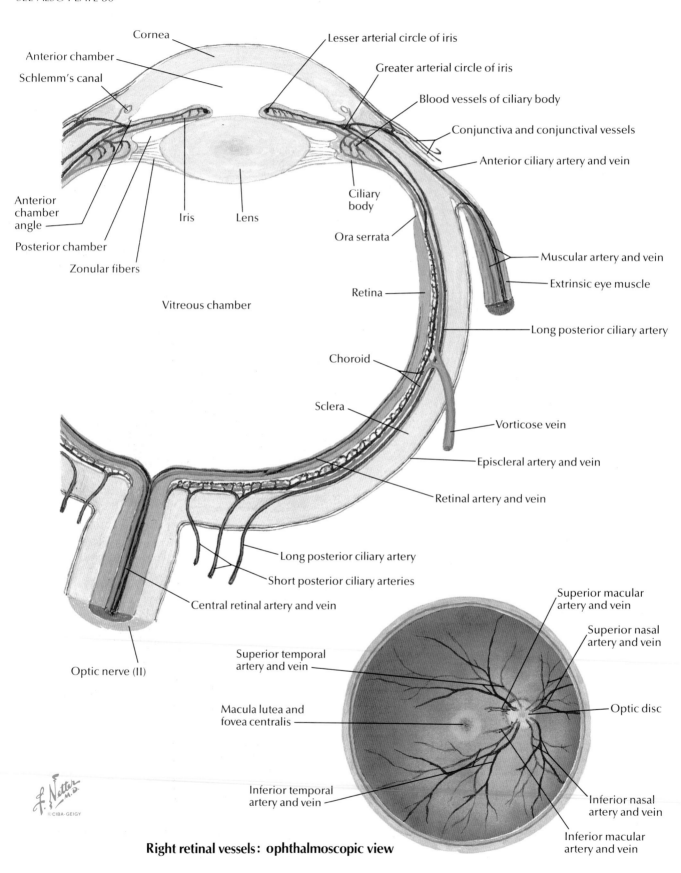

Cornea

Anterior chamber

Schlemm's canal

Anterior chamber angle

Posterior chamber

Zonular fibers

Iris

Lens

Vitreous chamber

Lesser arterial circle of iris

Greater arterial circle of iris

Blood vessels of ciliary body

Conjunctiva and conjunctival vessels

Anterior ciliary artery and vein

Ciliary body

Ora serrata

Retina

Muscular artery and vein

Extrinsic eye muscle

Long posterior ciliary artery

Choroid

Sclera

Vorticose vein

Episcleral artery and vein

Retinal artery and vein

Long posterior ciliary artery

Short posterior ciliary arteries

Central retinal artery and vein

Optic nerve (II)

Superior macular artery and vein

Superior nasal artery and vein

Superior temporal artery and vein

Macula lutea and fovea centralis

Optic disc

Inferior temporal artery and vein

Inferior nasal artery and vein

Inferior macular artery and vein

Right retinal vessels: ophthalmoscopic view

PLATE 86

Frontal section

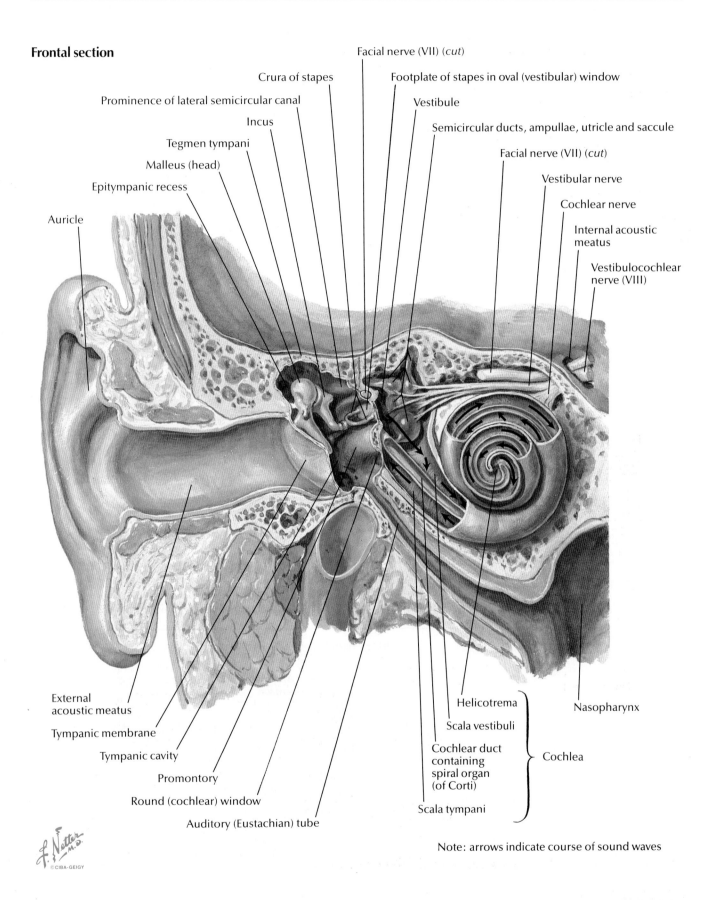

Facial nerve (VII) (*cut*)

Footplate of stapes in oval (vestibular) window

Crura of stapes

Vestibule

Prominence of lateral semicircular canal

Semicircular ducts, ampullae, utricle and saccule

Incus

Facial nerve (VII) (*cut*)

Tegmen tympani

Vestibular nerve

Malleus (head)

Cochlear nerve

Epitympanic recess

Internal acoustic meatus

Auricle

Vestibulocochlear nerve (VIII)

External acoustic meatus

Helicotrema

Nasopharynx

Tympanic membrane

Scala vestibuli

Tympanic cavity

Cochlear duct containing spiral organ (of Corti)

Cochlea

Promontory

Round (cochlear) window

Scala tympani

Auditory (Eustachian) tube

Note: arrows indicate course of sound waves

External Ear and Tympanic Cavity

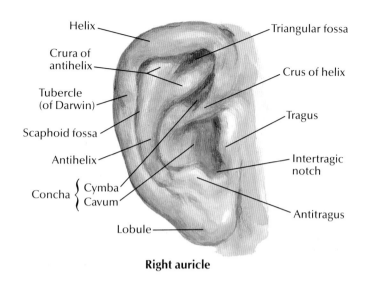

Right auricle

Labels: Helix, Crura of antihelix, Tubercle (of Darwin), Scaphoid fossa, Antihelix, Concha { Cymba, Cavum }, Lobule, Triangular fossa, Crus of helix, Tragus, Intertragic notch, Antitragus

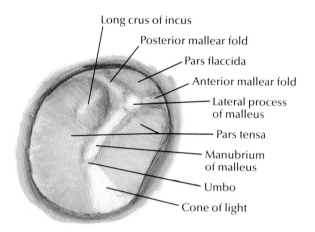

Right tympanic membrane (eardrum) viewed through speculum

Labels: Long crus of incus, Posterior mallear fold, Pars flaccida, Anterior mallear fold, Lateral process of malleus, Pars tensa, Manubrium of malleus, Umbo, Cone of light

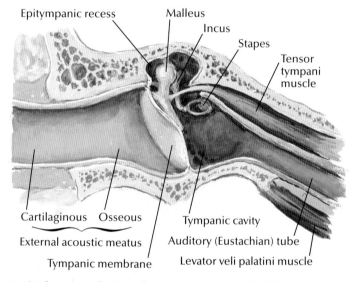

Sagittal section of external acoustic meatus and middle ear

Labels: Epitympanic recess, Malleus, Incus, Stapes, Tensor tympani muscle, Cartilaginous, Osseous, External acoustic meatus, Tympanic membrane, Tympanic cavity, Auditory (Eustachian) tube, Levator veli palatini muscle

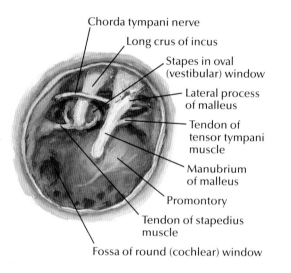

View into tympanic cavity after removal of tympanic membrane

Labels: Chorda tympani nerve, Long crus of incus, Stapes in oval (vestibular) window, Lateral process of malleus, Tendon of tensor tympani muscle, Manubrium of malleus, Promontory, Tendon of stapedius muscle, Fossa of round (cochlear) window

Auditory ossicles

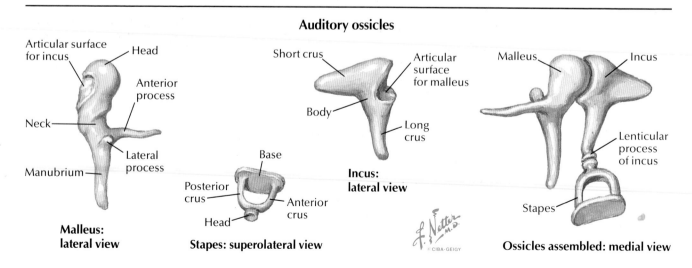

Malleus: lateral view

Labels: Articular surface for incus, Head, Anterior process, Neck, Lateral process, Manubrium

Stapes: superolateral view

Labels: Base, Posterior crus, Anterior crus, Head

Incus: lateral view

Labels: Short crus, Articular surface for malleus, Body, Long crus

Ossicles assembled: medial view

Labels: Malleus, Incus, Lenticular process of incus, Stapes

f. Netter M.D.
©CIBA-GEIGY

PLATE 88

HEAD AND NECK

Lateral wall of tympanic cavity: medial (internal) view

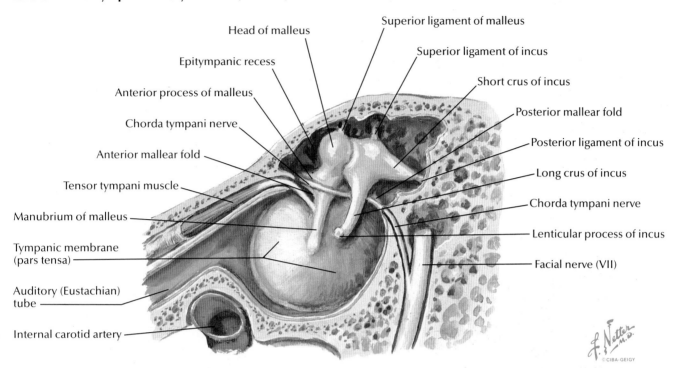

Head of malleus

Superior ligament of malleus

Superior ligament of incus

Epitympanic recess

Short crus of incus

Anterior process of malleus

Posterior mallear fold

Chorda tympani nerve

Posterior ligament of incus

Anterior mallear fold

Long crus of incus

Tensor tympani muscle

Chorda tympani nerve

Manubrium of malleus

Lenticular process of incus

Tympanic membrane (pars tensa)

Facial nerve (VII)

Auditory (Eustachian) tube

Internal carotid artery

Medial wall of tympanic cavity: lateral view

Prominence of lateral semicircular canal

Prominence of facial canal

Tympanic (mastoid) antrum

Geniculum of facial nerve

Greater petrosal nerve

Footplate of stapes in fossa of oval (vestibular) window

Tensor tympani muscle (*tendon cut*)

Crura of stapes

Auditory (Eustachian) tube

Pyramidal eminence

Levator veli palatini muscle

Chorda tympani nerve (*cut*)

Mastoid cells

Tendon of stapedius muscle

Promontory with tympanic nerve (of Jacobson) and plexus under mucosa

Fossa of round (cochlear) window

Jugular fossa

Internal carotid artery

Facial nerve (VII) in stylomastoid foramen

Tympanic cells

Osseous and Membranous Labyrinths

SEE ALSO PLATE 118

Right osseous labyrinth, anterolateral view: surrounding cancellous bone removed

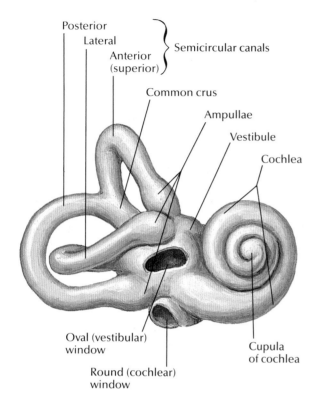

Posterior
Lateral
Anterior (superior) } Semicircular canals

Common crus

Ampullae

Vestibule

Cochlea

Oval (vestibular) window

Round (cochlear) window

Cupula of cochlea

Dissected right osseous labyrinth: membranous labyrinth removed

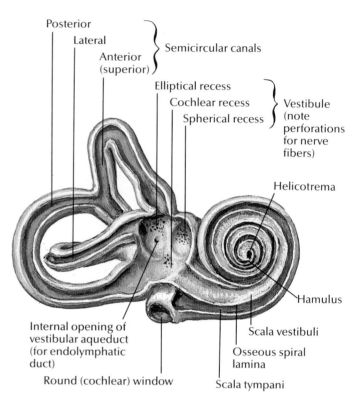

Posterior
Lateral
Anterior (superior) } Semicircular canals

Elliptical recess
Cochlear recess
Spherical recess } Vestibule (note perforations for nerve fibers)

Helicotrema

Hamulus

Internal opening of vestibular aqueduct (for endolymphatic duct)

Round (cochlear) window

Scala vestibuli

Osseous spiral lamina

Scala tympani

Right membranous labyrinth with nerves: posteromedial view

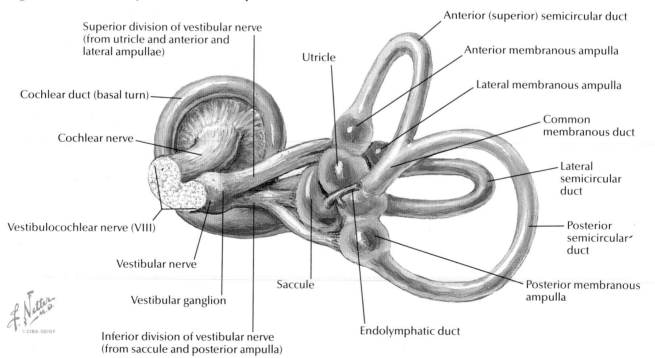

Superior division of vestibular nerve (from utricle and anterior and lateral ampullae)

Cochlear duct (basal turn)

Cochlear nerve

Vestibulocochlear nerve (VIII)

Vestibular nerve

Vestibular ganglion

Inferior division of vestibular nerve (from saccule and posterior ampulla)

Saccule

Endolymphatic duct

Utricle

Anterior (superior) semicircular duct

Anterior membranous ampulla

Lateral membranous ampulla

Common membranous duct

Lateral semicircular duct

Posterior semicircular duct

Posterior membranous ampulla

PLATE 90

HEAD AND NECK

Osseous and membranous labyrinths: schema

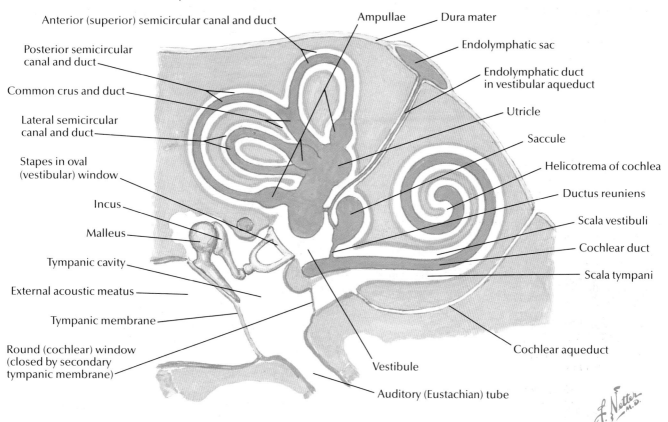

Anterior (superior) semicircular canal and duct

Ampullae

Dura mater

Posterior semicircular canal and duct

Endolymphatic sac

Endolymphatic duct in vestibular aqueduct

Common crus and duct

Utricle

Lateral semicircular canal and duct

Saccule

Helicotrema of cochlea

Stapes in oval (vestibular) window

Ductus reuniens

Incus

Scala vestibuli

Malleus

Cochlear duct

Tympanic cavity

Scala tympani

External acoustic meatus

Tympanic membrane

Round (cochlear) window (closed by secondary tympanic membrane)

Cochlear aqueduct

Vestibule

Auditory (Eustachian) tube

Section through turn of cochlea

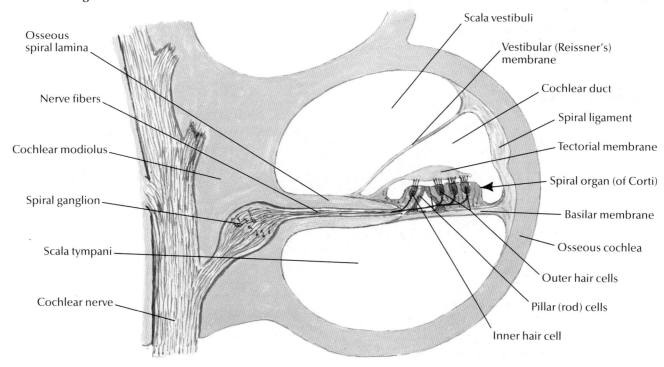

Osseous spiral lamina

Scala vestibuli

Vestibular (Reissner's) membrane

Nerve fibers

Cochlear duct

Cochlear modiolus

Spiral ligament

Tectorial membrane

Spiral ganglion

Spiral organ (of Corti)

Basilar membrane

Scala tympani

Osseous cochlea

Outer hair cells

Cochlear nerve

Pillar (rod) cells

Inner hair cell

Orientation of Labyrinth in Skull

Superior projection of right osseous labyrinth on floor of skull

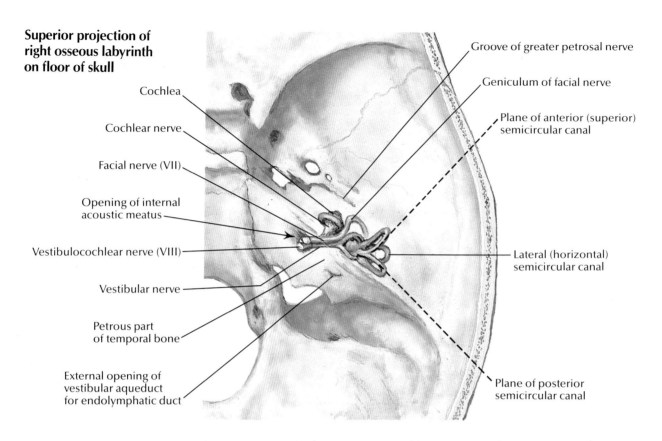

Cochlea

Cochlear nerve

Facial nerve (VII)

Opening of internal acoustic meatus

Vestibulocochlear nerve (VIII)

Vestibular nerve

Petrous part of temporal bone

External opening of vestibular aqueduct for endolymphatic duct

Groove of greater petrosal nerve

Geniculum of facial nerve

Plane of anterior (superior) semicircular canal

Lateral (horizontal) semicircular canal

Plane of posterior semicircular canal

Lateral projection of right membranous labyrinth

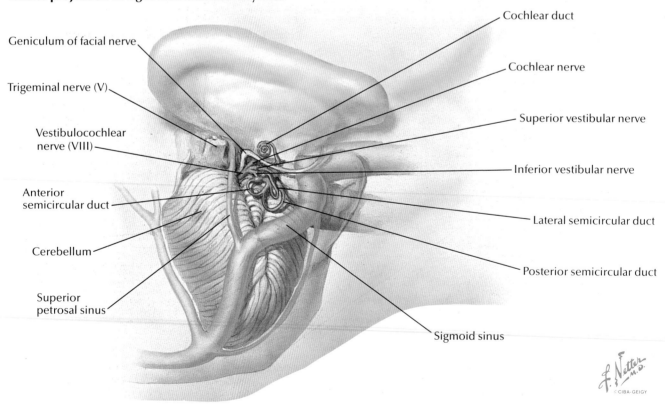

Geniculum of facial nerve

Trigeminal nerve (V)

Vestibulocochlear nerve (VIII)

Anterior semicircular duct

Cerebellum

Superior petrosal sinus

Cochlear duct

Cochlear nerve

Superior vestibular nerve

Inferior vestibular nerve

Lateral semicircular duct

Posterior semicircular duct

Sigmoid sinus

PLATE 92

HEAD AND NECK

Cartilage of auditory tube at base of skull: inferior view

Hamulus of medial pterygoid plate

Lateral pterygoid plate

Scaphoid fossa

Foramen ovale

Foramen spinosum

Spine of sphenoid bone

Internal carotid artery entering carotid canal

Mastoid process

Palatine process of maxilla

Horizontal plate of palatine bone

Choana

Lateral lamina } of cartilage
Medial lamina } of auditory tube

Foramen lacerum

Petrous part of temporal bone

Occipital condyle

Foramen magnum

Section through cartilage of auditory tube with tube closed

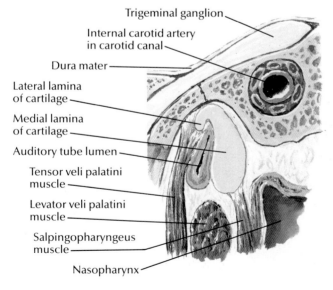

Trigeminal ganglion

Internal carotid artery in carotid canal

Dura mater

Lateral lamina of cartilage

Medial lamina of cartilage

Auditory tube lumen

Tensor veli palatini muscle

Levator veli palatini muscle

Salpingopharyngeus muscle

Nasopharynx

Auditory tube closed by elastic recoil of cartilage, tissue turgidity and tension of salpingopharyngeus muscles

Section through cartilage of auditory tube with tube open

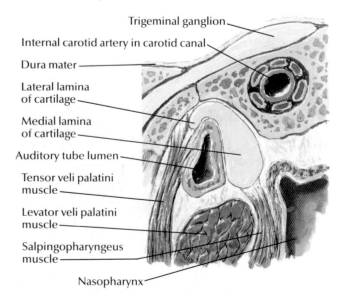

Trigeminal ganglion

Internal carotid artery in carotid canal

Dura mater

Lateral lamina of cartilage

Medial lamina of cartilage

Auditory tube lumen

Tensor veli palatini muscle

Levator veli palatini muscle

Salpingopharyngeus muscle

Nasopharynx

Lumen opened chiefly when attachment of tensor veli palatini muscle pulls wall of tube laterally during swallowing

Meninges and Diploic Veins

SEE ALSO PLATE 17

Coronal dissection

Diploic veins

Superior sagittal sinus

Emissary vein

Frontal and parietal tributaries of superficial temporal vein

Frontal and parietal branches of superficial temporal artery

Granular foveola (indentation of skull by arachnoid granulation)

Venous lacuna

Inferior sagittal sinus

Arachnoid granulation

Cerebral vein penetrates subdural space to enter sinus

Dura mater (two layers)

Epidural space (potential)

Arachnoid

Subarachnoid space

Pia mater

Middle meningeal artery and vein

Deep, middle and superficial temporal arteries and veins

Thalamostriate, superior choroidal and internal cerebral veins and choroid plexus of lateral ventricle

Deep and superficial middle cerebral veins

Diploic and emissary veins of skull

Frontal diploic vein

Anterior temporal diploic vein

Parietal emissary vein

Posterior temporal diploic vein

Occipital emissary vein

Occipital diploic vein

Mastoid emissary vein

PLATE 94

Frontal (anterior) and parietal (posterior) branches of middle meningeal artery

Middle meningeal artery

Anterior meningeal branch of anterior ethmoidal artery

Arachnoid granulations

Opening of superior cerebral vein

Venous lacuna

Superior sagittal sinus

Dura mater

Mastoid branch of occipital artery

Meningeal branches of ascending pharyngeal artery

Mastoid branch of occipital artery

Middle meningeal artery

Recurrent meningeal branch of lacrimal (ophthalmic) artery

Accessory meningeal artery

Anterior meningeal branch of anterior ethmoidal artery

Posterior ethmoidal artery

Internal carotid artery and its meningohypophyseal trunk (*phantom*)

Middle meningeal artery

Accessory meningeal artery

Superficial temporal artery

Maxillary artery

Posterior auricular artery

Occipital artery

External carotid artery

Anterior and posterior meningeal branches of vertebral artery

Tentorial, cavernous sinus and meningeal branches of meningohypophyseal trunk

Meninges and Superficial Cerebral Veins

FOR DEEP VEINS OF BRAIN SEE PLATE 138

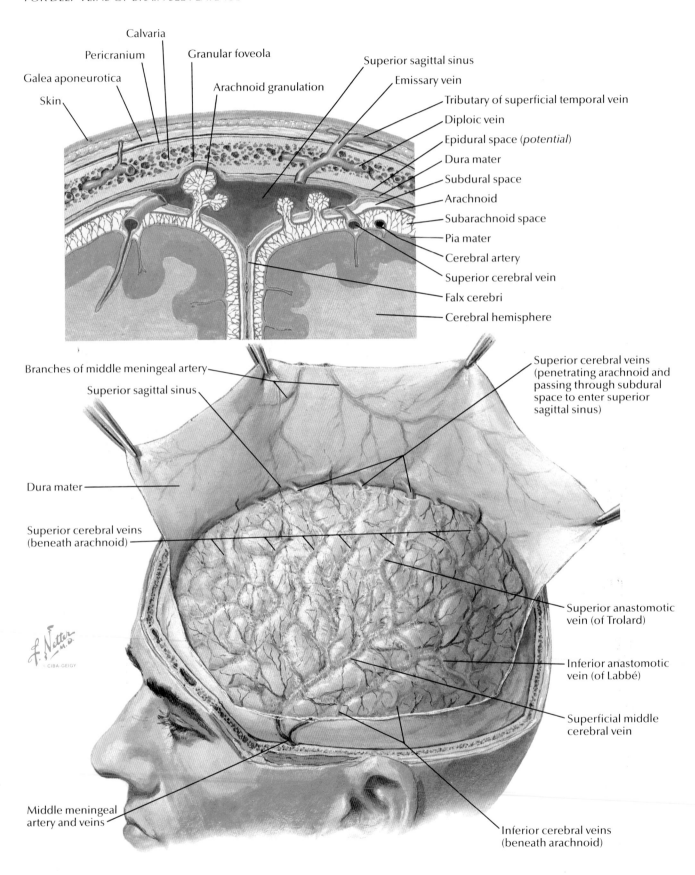

Skin

Galea aponeurotica

Pericranium

Calvaria

Granular foveola

Arachnoid granulation

Superior sagittal sinus

Emissary vein

Tributary of superficial temporal vein

Diploic vein

Epidural space (*potential*)

Dura mater

Subdural space

Arachnoid

Subarachnoid space

Pia mater

Cerebral artery

Superior cerebral vein

Falx cerebri

Cerebral hemisphere

Branches of middle meningeal artery

Superior sagittal sinus

Superior cerebral veins (penetrating arachnoid and passing through subdural space to enter superior sagittal sinus)

Dura mater

Superior cerebral veins (beneath arachnoid)

Superior anastomotic vein (of Trolard)

Inferior anastomotic vein (of Labbé)

Superficial middle cerebral vein

Middle meningeal artery and veins

Inferior cerebral veins (beneath arachnoid)

PLATE 96   **HEAD AND NECK**

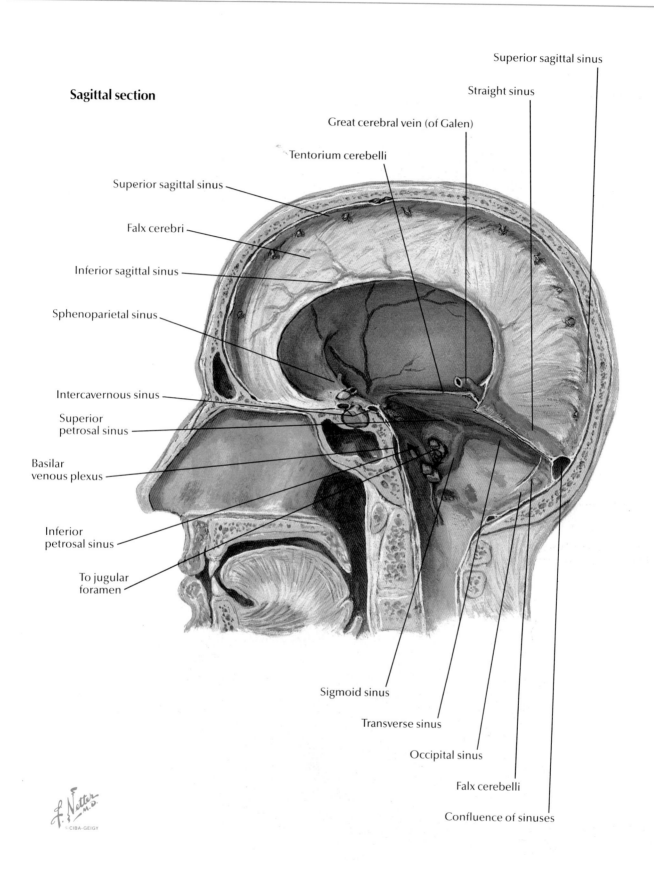

Sagittal section

Superior sagittal sinus

Straight sinus

Great cerebral vein (of Galen)

Tentorium cerebelli

Superior sagittal sinus

Falx cerebri

Inferior sagittal sinus

Sphenoparietal sinus

Intercavernous sinus

Superior petrosal sinus

Basilar venous plexus

Inferior petrosal sinus

To jugular foramen

Sigmoid sinus

Transverse sinus

Occipital sinus

Falx cerebelli

Confluence of sinuses

Venous Sinuses of Dura Mater (continued)

SEE ALSO PLATE 80

Horizontal section: superior view

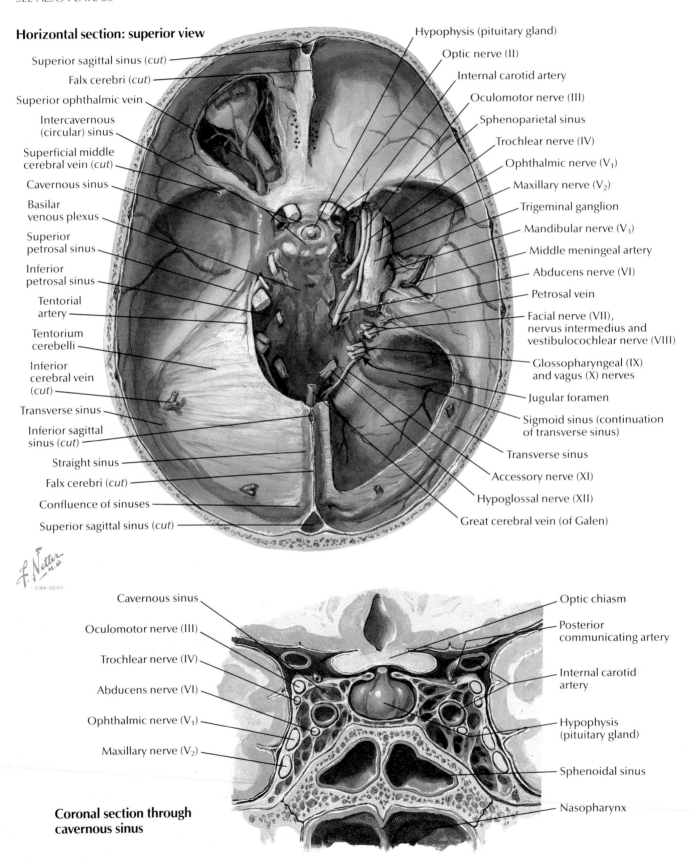

Superior sagittal sinus (*cut*)

Falx cerebri (*cut*)

Superior ophthalmic vein

Intercavernous (circular) sinus

Superficial middle cerebral vein (*cut*)

Cavernous sinus

Basilar venous plexus

Superior petrosal sinus

Inferior petrosal sinus

Tentorial artery

Tentorium cerebelli

Inferior cerebral vein (*cut*)

Transverse sinus

Inferior sagittal sinus (*cut*)

Straight sinus

Falx cerebri (*cut*)

Confluence of sinuses

Superior sagittal sinus (*cut*)

Hypophysis (pituitary gland)

Optic nerve (II)

Internal carotid artery

Oculomotor nerve (III)

Sphenoparietal sinus

Trochlear nerve (IV)

Ophthalmic nerve (V₁)

Maxillary nerve (V₂)

Trigeminal ganglion

Mandibular nerve (V₃)

Middle meningeal artery

Abducens nerve (VI)

Petrosal vein

Facial nerve (VII), nervus intermedius and vestibulocochlear nerve (VIII)

Glossopharyngeal (IX) and vagus (X) nerves

Jugular foramen

Sigmoid sinus (continuation of transverse sinus)

Transverse sinus

Accessory nerve (XI)

Hypoglossal nerve (XII)

Great cerebral vein (of Galen)

Cavernous sinus

Oculomotor nerve (III)

Trochlear nerve (IV)

Abducens nerve (VI)

Ophthalmic nerve (V₁)

Maxillary nerve (V₂)

Coronal section through cavernous sinus

Optic chiasm

Posterior communicating artery

Internal carotid artery

Hypophysis (pituitary gland)

Sphenoidal sinus

Nasopharynx

PLATE 98   **HEAD AND NECK**

Central sulcus (of Rolando)
Precentral gyrus
Precentral sulcus
Superior frontal gyrus
Superior frontal sulcus
Middle frontal gyrus
Inferior frontal sulcus
Inferior frontal gyrus
Opercular part
Triangular part
Orbital part
Frontal pole

Lateral sulcus (of Sylvius) { Anterior ramus
Ascending ramus
Posterior ramus

Temporal pole

Postcentral gyrus
Postcentral sulcus
Superior parietal lobule
Intraparietal sulcus
Inferior parietal lobule
Supramarginal gyrus
Angular gyrus
Parieto-occipital sulcus
Occipital pole
Calcarine sulcus
Lunate sulcus (inconstant)
Transverse occipital sulcus
Preoccipital notch
Inferior temporal gyrus

Superior temporal gyrus
Superior temporal sulcus
Middle temporal gyrus
Inferior temporal sulcus

Frontal lobe
Parietal lobe
Temporal lobe
Occipital lobe

Frontoparietal operculum
Frontal operculum
Orbital operculum

Insula (island of Reil) { Short gyri
Central sulcus
Limen
Long gyrus
Circular sulcus

Temporal operculum

Cerebrum: Medial Views

FOR HYPOPHYSIS SEE PLATE 140

Sagittal section of brain in situ

Cingulate gyrus
Cingulate sulcus
Medial frontal gyrus
Sulcus of corpus callosum
Fornix
Septum pellucidum
Interventricular foramen (of Monro)
Interthalamic adhesion
Thalamus (3rd ventricle)
Subcallosal (parolfactory) area
Anterior commissure
Paraterminal gyrus
Hypothalamic sulcus
Lamina terminalis
Optic recess
Optic chiasm
Tuber cinereum
Hypophysis (pituitary gland)
Mamillary body
Cerebral peduncle
Pons
Cerebral aqueduct (of Sylvius)

Precentral sulcus
Central sulcus (of Rolando)
Paracentral lobule
Corpus callosum
Precuneus
Superior sagittal sinus
Choroid plexus of 3rd ventricle
Stria medullaris of thalamus
Parietooccipital sulcus
Cuneus
Habenular commissure
Pineal body
Posterior commissure
Calcarine sulcus
Straight sinus in tentorium cerebelli
Great cerebral vein (of Galen)
Superior colliculus
Inferior colliculus
Quadrigeminal (tectal) lamina
Cerebellum
Superior medullary velum
4th ventricle and choroid plexus
Inferior medullary velum
Medulla oblongata

Medial surface of cerebral hemisphere: brainstem excised

Cingulate gyrus
Mamillothalamic fasciculus
Mamillary body
Uncus
Optic nerve (II)
Olfactory tract
Collateral sulcus
Rhinal sulcus
Medial occipitotemporal gyrus
Occipitotemporal sulcus
Lateral occipitotemporal gyrus

Genu
Rostrum } of
Trunk   corpus callosum
Splenium }
Isthmus of cingulate gyrus
Parietooccipital sulcus
Cuneus
Calcarine sulcus
Lingual gyrus
Crus   }
Body   } of fornix
Column }
Fimbria of hippocampus
Dentate gyrus
Parahippocampal gyrus

PLATE 100

HEAD AND NECK

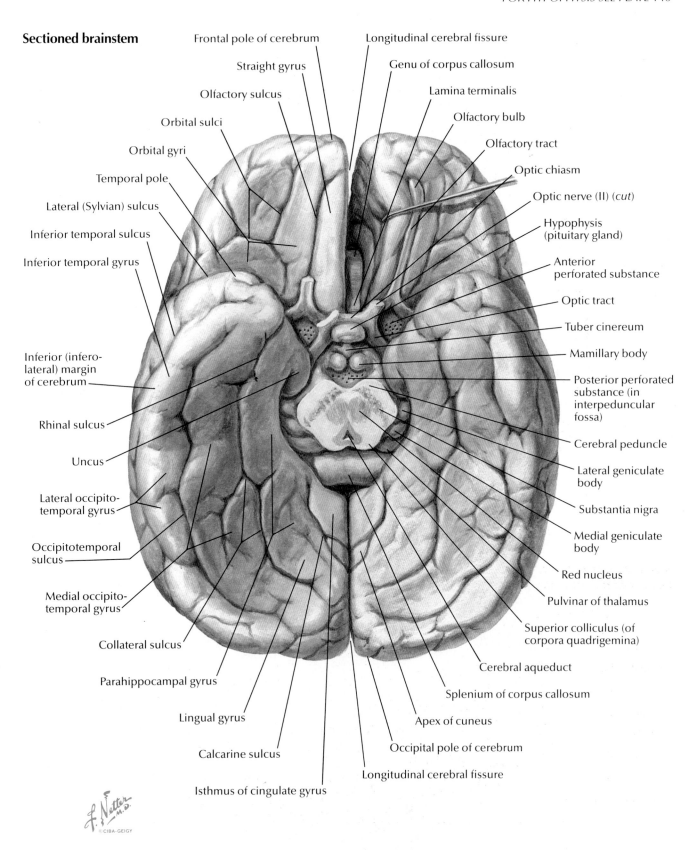

Sectioned brainstem

Frontal pole of cerebrum

Straight gyrus

Olfactory sulcus

Orbital sulci

Orbital gyri

Temporal pole

Lateral (Sylvian) sulcus

Inferior temporal sulcus

Inferior temporal gyrus

Inferior (infero-lateral) margin of cerebrum

Rhinal sulcus

Uncus

Lateral occipito-temporal gyrus

Occipitotemporal sulcus

Medial occipito-temporal gyrus

Collateral sulcus

Parahippocampal gyrus

Lingual gyrus

Calcarine sulcus

Isthmus of cingulate gyrus

Longitudinal cerebral fissure

Genu of corpus callosum

Lamina terminalis

Olfactory bulb

Olfactory tract

Optic chiasm

Optic nerve (II) (cut)

Hypophysis (pituitary gland)

Anterior perforated substance

Optic tract

Tuber cinereum

Mamillary body

Posterior perforated substance (in interpeduncular fossa)

Cerebral peduncle

Lateral geniculate body

Substantia nigra

Medial geniculate body

Red nucleus

Pulvinar of thalamus

Superior colliculus (of corpora quadrigemina)

Cerebral aqueduct

Splenium of corpus callosum

Apex of cuneus

Occipital pole of cerebrum

Longitudinal cerebral fissure

Ventricles of Brain

Left lateral phantom view

Right lateral ventricle

Frontal (anterior) horn

Central part

Temporal (inferior) horn

Occipital (posterior) horn

Left lateral ventricle

Cerebral aqueduct (of Sylvius)

4th ventricle

Left lateral aperture (foramen of Luschka)

Left lateral recess

Median aperture (foramen of Magendie)

Central canal of spinal cord

Left interventricular foramen (of Monro)

3rd ventricle

Optic recess

Interthalamic adhesion

Infundibular recess

Pineal recess

Suprapineal recess

Corpus callosum

Septum pellucidum

Lateral ventricle

Body of caudate nucleus

Choroid plexus of lateral ventricle

Stria terminalis

Superior thalamostriate vein

Body of fornix

Internal cerebral vein

Tela choroidea of 3rd ventricle

Choroid plexus of 3rd ventricle

Thalamus

Putamen

Globus pallidus

Lentiform nucleus

Internal capsule

3rd ventricle and interthalamic adhesion

Hypothalamus

Tail of caudate nucleus

Optic tract

Choroid plexus of lateral ventricle

Temporal (inferior) horn of lateral ventricle

Fimbria of hippocampus

Hippocampus

Dentate gyrus

Parahippocampal gyrus

White arrow in left interventricular foramen (of Monro)

—— Ependyma

—— Pia mater

Coronal section of brain: posterior view

PLATE 102

HEAD AND NECK

Choroid plexus of lateral ventricle (*phantom*)

Cistern of corpus callosum

Dura mater

Arachnoid

Superior sagittal sinus

Subarachnoid space

Arachnoid granulations

Interventricular foramen (of Monro)

Chiasmatic cistern

Choroid plexus of 3rd ventricle

Interpeduncular cistern

Cerebral aqueduct (of Sylvius)

Pontine cistern

Lateral aperture (foramen of Luschka)

Choroid plexus of 4th ventricle

Dura mater

Arachnoid

Subarachnoid space

Central canal of spinal cord

Cistern of great cerebral vein

Cerebellomedullary cistern

Median aperture (foramen of Magendie)

Basal Ganglia

Horizontal sections through cerebrum

Genu of corpus callosum

Lateral ventricle

Septum pellucidum

Column of fornix

Insula (island of Reil)

Interthalamic adhesion

Thalamus

Crus of fornix

Choroid plexus of lateral ventricle

Splenium of corpus callosum

Head of caudate nucleus

Anterior limb
Genu
Posterior limb
} of internal capsule

Putamen
Globus pallidus
} Lentiform nucleus

3rd ventricle

External capsule

Claustrum

Retrolenticular part of internal capsule

Tail of caudate nucleus

Hippocampus and fimbria

Occipital (posterior) horn of lateral ventricle

Habenula

Pineal body

Organization of basal ganglia

Caudate nucleus · Putamen · Globus pallidus

Striatum · Lentiform nucleus

Corpus striatum · Claustrum

Basal ganglia

Cleft for internal capsule

Caudate nucleus { Body / Head

Levels of sections above { A / B

Lentiform nucleus (globus pallidus medial to putamen)

Amygdaloid body

Thalamus

Pulvinar

Medial geniculate body

Lateral geniculate body

Tail of caudate nucleus

Interrelationship of thalamus, lentiform nucleus, caudate nucleus and amygdaloid body (schema): left lateral view

PLATE 104

HEAD AND NECK

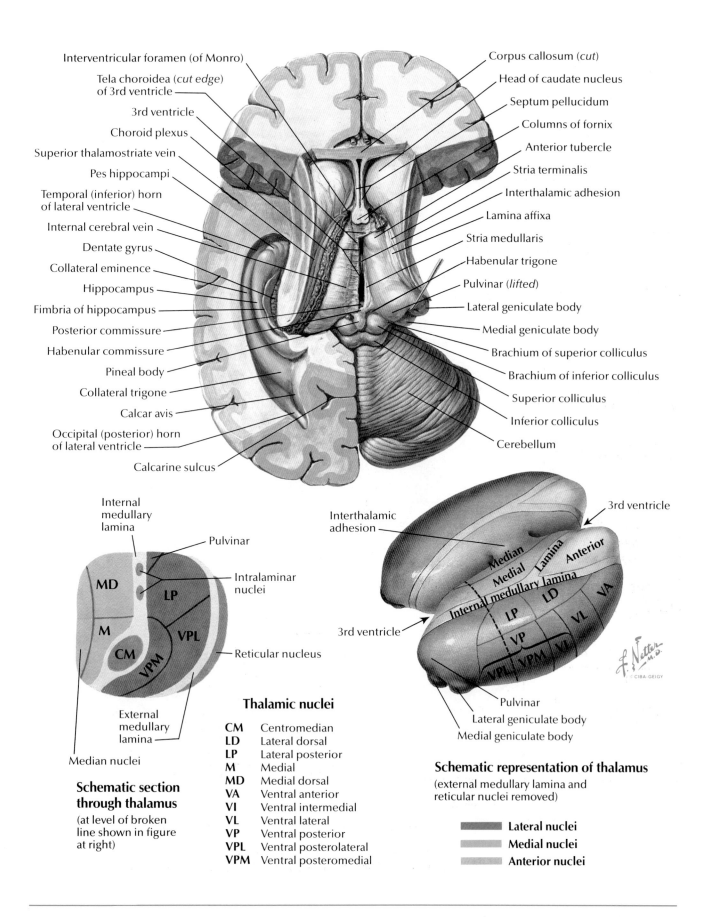

Interventricular foramen (of Monro)

Tela choroidea (*cut edge*) of 3rd ventricle

3rd ventricle

Choroid plexus

Superior thalamostriate vein

Pes hippocampi

Temporal (inferior) horn of lateral ventricle

Internal cerebral vein

Dentate gyrus

Collateral eminence

Hippocampus

Fimbria of hippocampus

Posterior commissure

Habenular commissure

Pineal body

Collateral trigone

Calcar avis

Occipital (posterior) horn of lateral ventricle

Calcarine sulcus

Corpus callosum (*cut*)

Head of caudate nucleus

Septum pellucidum

Columns of fornix

Anterior tubercle

Stria terminalis

Interthalamic adhesion

Lamina affixa

Stria medullaris

Habenular trigone

Pulvinar (*lifted*)

Lateral geniculate body

Medial geniculate body

Brachium of superior colliculus

Brachium of inferior colliculus

Superior colliculus

Inferior colliculus

Cerebellum

Internal medullary lamina

Pulvinar

Intralaminar nuclei

MD

LP

M

VPL

CM

VPM

Reticular nucleus

External medullary lamina

Median nuclei

Interthalamic adhesion

3rd ventricle

Median

Medial

Lamina

Anterior

Internal medullary lamina

LD

VA

LP

VL

VP

VI

VPL VPM

3rd ventricle

Pulvinar

Lateral geniculate body

Medial geniculate body

Thalamic nuclei

CM	Centromedian
LD	Lateral dorsal
LP	Lateral posterior
M	Medial
MD	Medial dorsal
VA	Ventral anterior
VI	Ventral intermedial
VL	Ventral lateral
VP	Ventral posterior
VPL	Ventral posterolateral
VPM	Ventral posteromedial

Schematic section through thalamus

(at level of broken line shown in figure at right)

Schematic representation of thalamus

(external medullary lamina and reticular nuclei removed)

■ **Lateral nuclei**
■ **Medial nuclei**
■ **Anterior nuclei**

Hippocampus and Fornix

Superior dissection

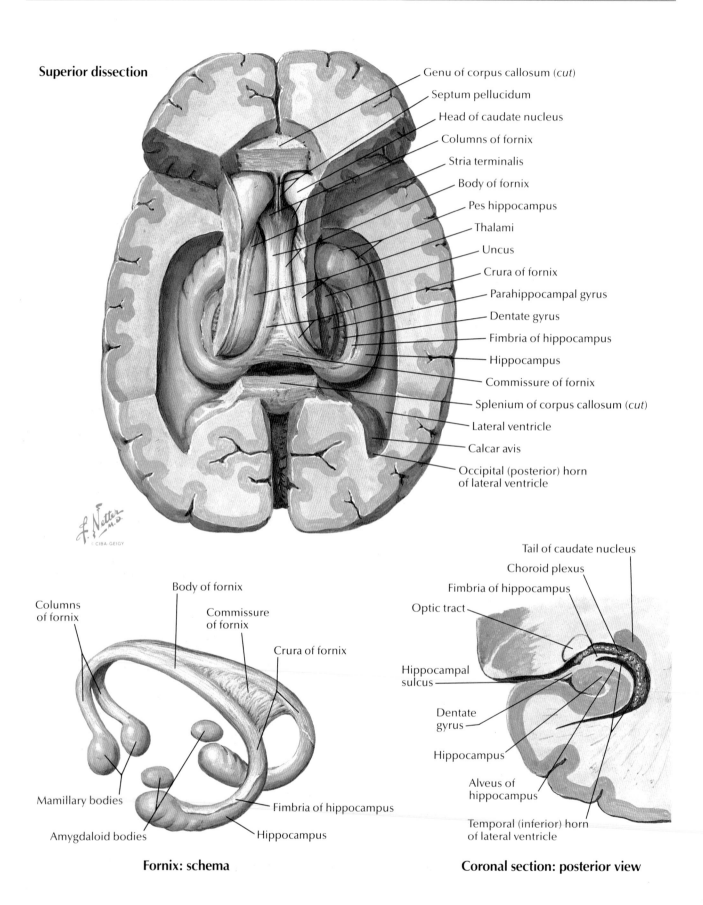

Genu of corpus callosum (*cut*)

Septum pellucidum

Head of caudate nucleus

Columns of fornix

Stria terminalis

Body of fornix

Pes hippocampus

Thalami

Uncus

Crura of fornix

Parahippocampal gyrus

Dentate gyrus

Fimbria of hippocampus

Hippocampus

Commissure of fornix

Splenium of corpus callosum (*cut*)

Lateral ventricle

Calcar avis

Occipital (posterior) horn of lateral ventricle

Body of fornix

Columns of fornix

Commissure of fornix

Crura of fornix

Mamillary bodies

Amygdaloid bodies

Fimbria of hippocampus

Hippocampus

Fornix: schema

Tail of caudate nucleus

Choroid plexus

Fimbria of hippocampus

Optic tract

Hippocampal sulcus

Dentate gyrus

Hippocampus

Alveus of hippocampus

Temporal (inferior) horn of lateral ventricle

Coronal section: posterior view

PLATE 106

HEAD AND NECK

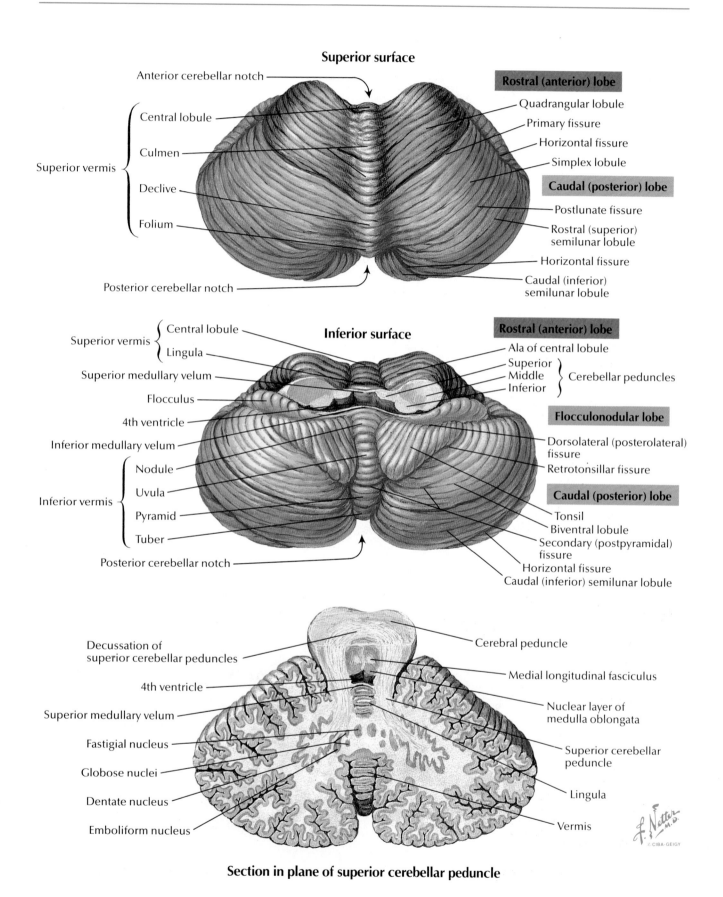

Superior surface

Anterior cerebellar notch

Superior vermis
- Central lobule
- Culmen
- Declive
- Folium

Posterior cerebellar notch

Rostral (anterior) lobe
- Quadrangular lobule
- Primary fissure
- Horizontal fissure
- Simplex lobule

Caudal (posterior) lobe
- Postlunate fissure
- Rostral (superior) semilunar lobule
- Horizontal fissure
- Caudal (inferior) semilunar lobule

Inferior surface

Superior vermis
- Central lobule
- Lingula

Superior medullary velum

Flocculus

4th ventricle

Inferior medullary velum

Inferior vermis
- Nodule
- Uvula
- Pyramid
- Tuber

Posterior cerebellar notch

Rostral (anterior) lobe
- Ala of central lobule
- Superior
- Middle — Cerebellar peduncles
- Inferior

Flocculonodular lobe
- Dorsolateral (posterolateral) fissure
- Retrotonsillar fissure

Caudal (posterior) lobe
- Tonsil
- Biventral lobule
- Secondary (postpyramidal) fissure
- Horizontal fissure
- Caudal (inferior) semilunar lobule

Decussation of superior cerebellar peduncles

4th ventricle

Superior medullary velum

Fastigial nucleus

Globose nuclei

Dentate nucleus

Emboliform nucleus

Cerebral peduncle

Medial longitudinal fasciculus

Nuclear layer of medulla oblongata

Superior cerebellar peduncle

Lingula

Vermis

Section in plane of superior cerebellar peduncle

Brainstem

Posterolateral view

Pulvinars of thalamus

Pineal body

Superior colliculi

Inferior colliculi

Trochlear nerve (IV)

Superior medullary velum

Superior cerebellar peduncle

Rhomboid fossa of 4th ventricle

Glossopharyngeal (IX) and vagus (X) nerves

Cuneate tubercle

Gracile tubercle

Dorsal roots of 1st spinal nerve (C1)

Fasciculus cuneatus

Fasciculus gracilis

Thalamus (*cut surface*)

Lateral geniculate body

Optic tract

Medial geniculate body

Brachia of superior and inferior colliculi

Cerebral peduncle

Pons

Trigeminal nerve (V)

Middle cerebellar peduncle

Vestibulocochlear nerve (VIII)

Facial nerve (VII)

Inferior cerebellar peduncle

Hypoglossal nerve (XII)

Accessory nerve (XI)

Anterior view

Optic chiasm

Optic tract

Tuber cinereum

Cerebral peduncle

Lateral geniculate body

Posterior perforated substance

Pons

Middle cerebellar peduncle

Olive

Pyramid

Ventral roots of 1st spinal nerve (C1)

Pyramidal decussation

Olfactory tract

Anterior perforated substance

Infundibulum (pituitary stalk)

Mamillary bodies

Temporal lobe (*cut surface*)

Oculomotor nerve (III)

Trochlear nerve (IV)

Trigeminal nerve (V)

Abducens nerve (VI)

Facial nerve (VII) and nervus intermedius

Vestibulocochlear nerve (VIII)

Flocculus of cerebellum

Choroid plexus of 4th ventricle

Glossopharyngeal nerve (IX)

Vagus nerve (X)

Hypoglossal nerve (XII)

Accessory nerve (XI)

PLATE 108   **HEAD AND NECK**

Fourth Ventricle and Cerebellum

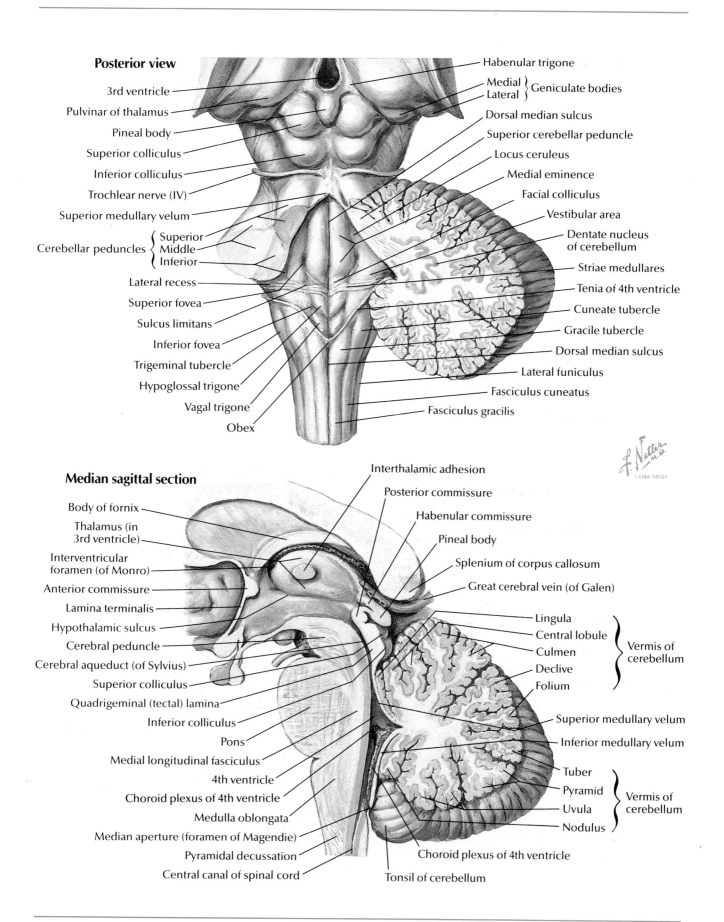

Posterior view

3rd ventricle
Pulvinar of thalamus
Pineal body
Superior colliculus
Inferior colliculus
Trochlear nerve (IV)
Superior medullary velum
Cerebellar peduncles { Superior / Middle / Inferior
Lateral recess
Superior fovea
Sulcus limitans
Inferior fovea
Trigeminal tubercle
Hypoglossal trigone
Vagal trigone
Obex

Habenular trigone
Medial } Geniculate bodies
Lateral }
Dorsal median sulcus
Superior cerebellar peduncle
Locus ceruleus
Medial eminence
Facial colliculus
Vestibular area
Dentate nucleus of cerebellum
Striae medullares
Tenia of 4th ventricle
Cuneate tubercle
Gracile tubercle
Dorsal median sulcus
Lateral funiculus
Fasciculus cuneatus
Fasciculus gracilis

Median sagittal section

Body of fornix
Thalamus (in 3rd ventricle)
Interventricular foramen (of Monro)
Anterior commissure
Lamina terminalis
Hypothalamic sulcus
Cerebral peduncle
Cerebral aqueduct (of Sylvius)
Superior colliculus
Quadrigeminal (tectal) lamina
Inferior colliculus
Pons
Medial longitudinal fasciculus
4th ventricle
Choroid plexus of 4th ventricle
Medulla oblongata
Median aperture (foramen of Magendie)
Pyramidal decussation
Central canal of spinal cord

Interthalamic adhesion
Posterior commissure
Habenular commissure
Pineal body
Splenium of corpus callosum
Great cerebral vein (of Galen)
Lingula
Central lobule } Vermis of cerebellum
Culmen
Declive
Folium
Superior medullary velum
Inferior medullary velum
Tuber
Pyramid } Vermis of cerebellum
Uvula
Nodulus
Choroid plexus of 4th ventricle
Tonsil of cerebellum

Cranial Nerve Nuclei in Brainstem: Schema

Posterior phantom view

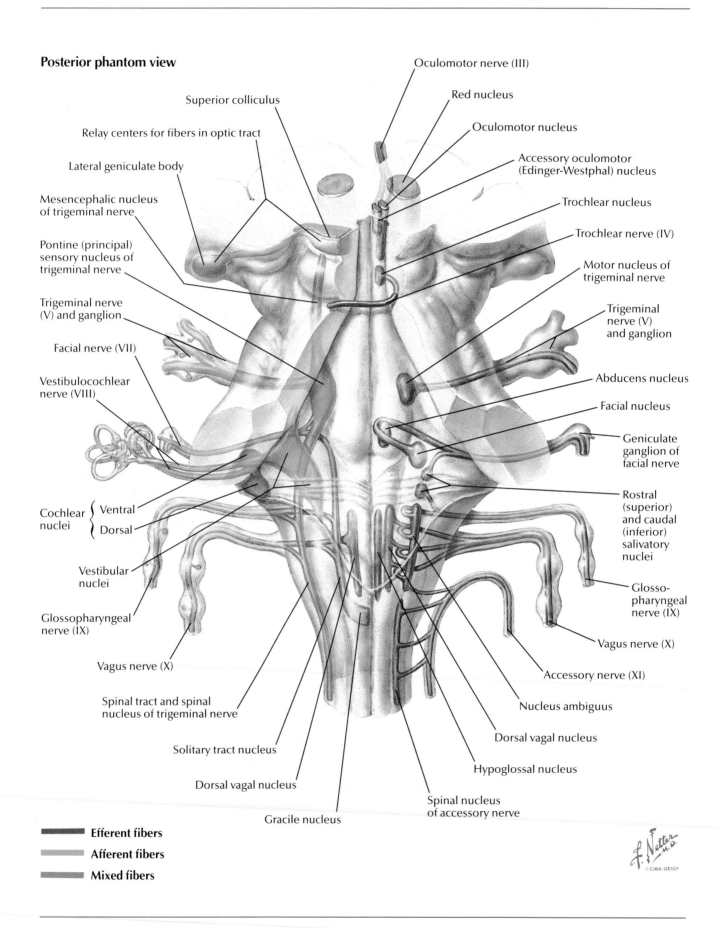

Oculomotor nerve (III)

Red nucleus

Oculomotor nucleus

Accessory oculomotor (Edinger-Westphal) nucleus

Trochlear nucleus

Trochlear nerve (IV)

Motor nucleus of trigeminal nerve

Trigeminal nerve (V) and ganglion

Abducens nucleus

Facial nucleus

Geniculate ganglion of facial nerve

Rostral (superior) and caudal (inferior) salivatory nuclei

Glosso-pharyngeal nerve (IX)

Vagus nerve (X)

Accessory nerve (XI)

Nucleus ambiguus

Dorsal vagal nucleus

Hypoglossal nucleus

Spinal nucleus of accessory nerve

Superior colliculus

Relay centers for fibers in optic tract

Lateral geniculate body

Mesencephalic nucleus of trigeminal nerve

Pontine (principal) sensory nucleus of trigeminal nerve

Trigeminal nerve (V) and ganglion

Facial nerve (VII)

Vestibulocochlear nerve (VIII)

Cochlear { Ventral / Dorsal } nuclei

Vestibular nuclei

Glossopharyngeal nerve (IX)

Vagus nerve (X)

Spinal tract and spinal nucleus of trigeminal nerve

Solitary tract nucleus

Dorsal vagal nucleus

Gracile nucleus

▬▬ **Efferent fibers**

▬▬ **Afferent fibers**

▬▬ **Mixed fibers**

PLATE 110

HEAD AND NECK

Medial dissection

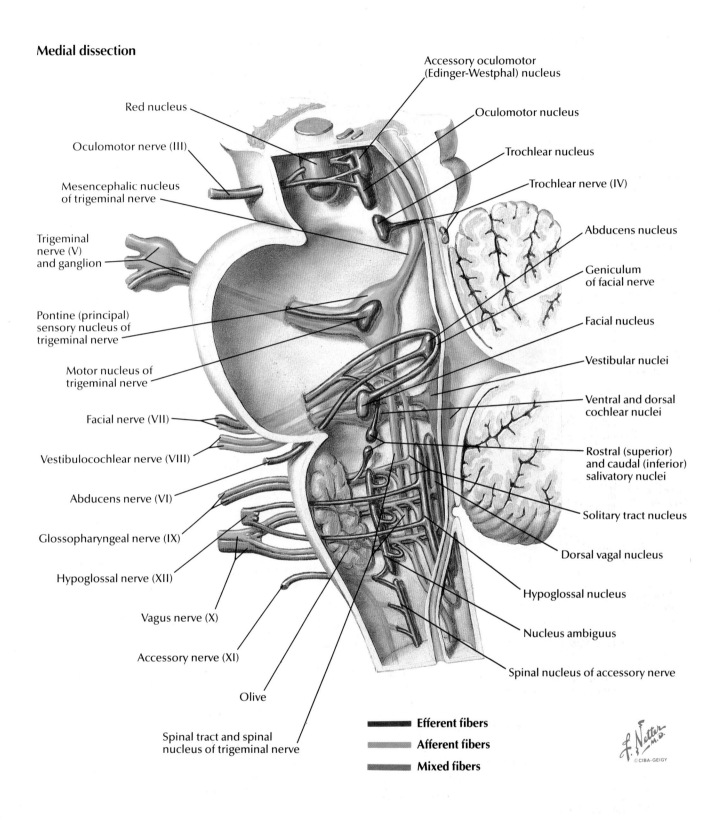

Red nucleus

Oculomotor nerve (III)

Mesencephalic nucleus of trigeminal nerve

Trigeminal nerve (V) and ganglion

Pontine (principal) sensory nucleus of trigeminal nerve

Motor nucleus of trigeminal nerve

Facial nerve (VII)

Vestibulocochlear nerve (VIII)

Abducens nerve (VI)

Glossopharyngeal nerve (IX)

Hypoglossal nerve (XII)

Vagus nerve (X)

Accessory nerve (XI)

Olive

Spinal tract and spinal nucleus of trigeminal nerve

Accessory oculomotor (Edinger-Westphal) nucleus

Oculomotor nucleus

Trochlear nucleus

Trochlear nerve (IV)

Abducens nucleus

Geniculum of facial nerve

Facial nucleus

Vestibular nuclei

Ventral and dorsal cochlear nuclei

Rostral (superior) and caudal (inferior) salivatory nuclei

Solitary tract nucleus

Dorsal vagal nucleus

Hypoglossal nucleus

Nucleus ambiguus

Spinal nucleus of accessory nerve

Efferent fibers

Afferent fibers

Mixed fibers

Cranial Nerves (Motor and Sensory Distribution): Schema

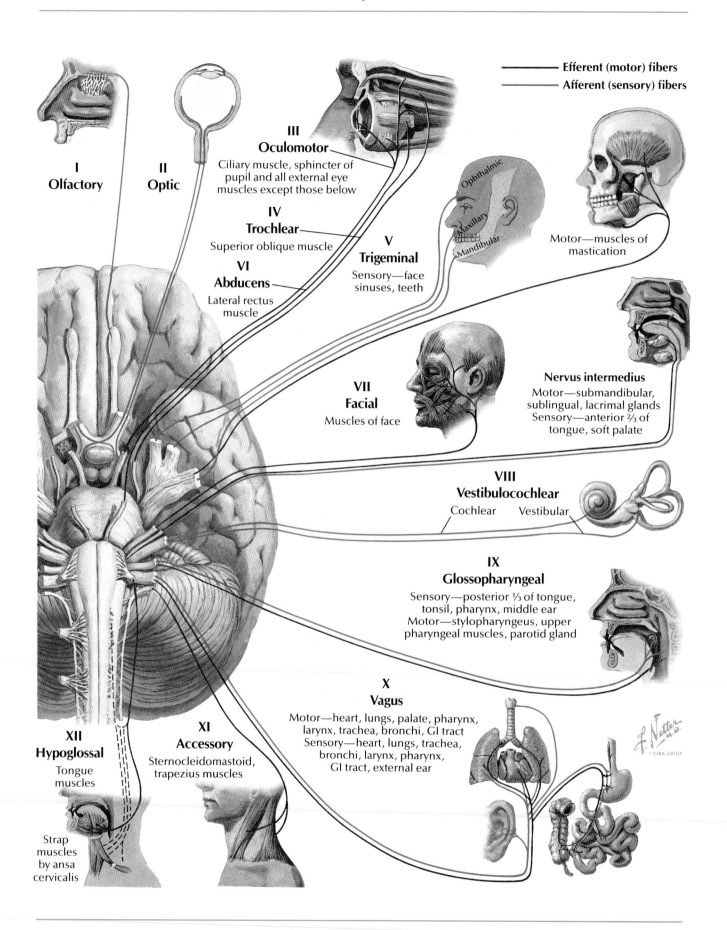

Efferent (motor) fibers
Afferent (sensory) fibers

I
Olfactory

II
Optic

III
Oculomotor
Ciliary muscle, sphincter of pupil and all external eye muscles except those below

IV
Trochlear
Superior oblique muscle

V
Trigeminal
Sensory—face sinuses, teeth

Ophthalmic
Maxillary
Mandibular

VI
Abducens
Lateral rectus muscle

Motor—muscles of mastication

VII
Facial
Muscles of face

Nervus intermedius
Motor—submandibular, sublingual, lacrimal glands
Sensory—anterior ⅔ of tongue, soft palate

VIII
Vestibulocochlear
Cochlear   Vestibular

IX
Glossopharyngeal
Sensory—posterior ⅓ of tongue, tonsil, pharynx, middle ear
Motor—stylopharyngeus, upper pharyngeal muscles, parotid gland

X
Vagus
Motor—heart, lungs, palate, pharynx, larynx, trachea, bronchi, GI tract
Sensory—heart, lungs, trachea, bronchi, larynx, pharynx, GI tract, external ear

XII
Hypoglossal
Tongue muscles

Strap muscles by ansa cervicalis

XI
Accessory
Sternocleidomastoid, trapezius muscles

PLATE 112

HEAD AND NECK

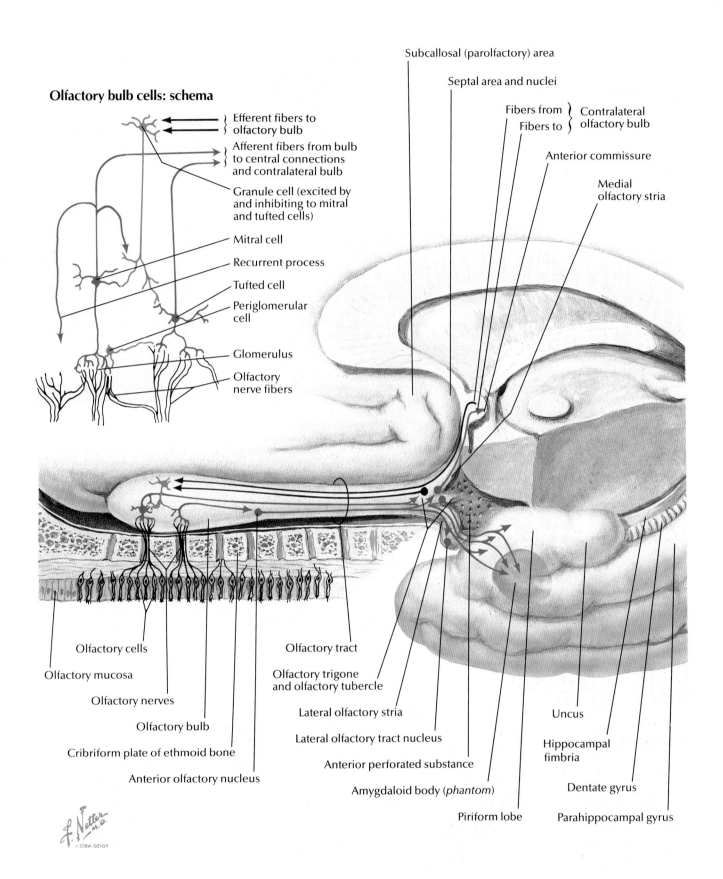

Olfactory bulb cells: schema

Efferent fibers to olfactory bulb

Afferent fibers from bulb to central connections and contralateral bulb

Granule cell (excited by and inhibiting to mitral and tufted cells)

Mitral cell

Recurrent process

Tufted cell

Periglomerular cell

Glomerulus

Olfactory nerve fibers

Subcallosal (parolfactory) area

Septal area and nuclei

Fibers from } Contralateral
Fibers to } olfactory bulb

Anterior commissure

Medial olfactory stria

Olfactory cells

Olfactory mucosa

Olfactory nerves

Olfactory bulb

Cribriform plate of ethmoid bone

Anterior olfactory nucleus

Olfactory tract

Olfactory trigone and olfactory tubercle

Lateral olfactory stria

Lateral olfactory tract nucleus

Anterior perforated substance

Amygdaloid body (*phantom*)

Piriform lobe

Uncus

Hippocampal fimbria

Dentate gyrus

Parahippocampal gyrus

Optic Nerve (Visual Pathway): Schema

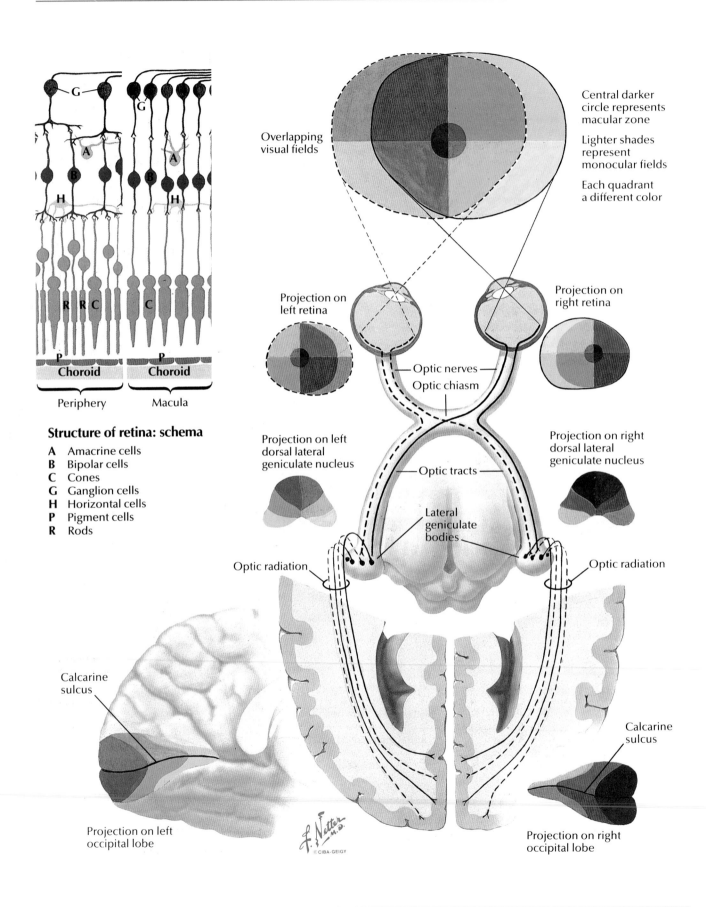

G

A

B

H

R R C

P
Choroid

Periphery

C

P
Choroid

Macula

Structure of retina: schema

A Amacrine cells
B Bipolar cells
C Cones
G Ganglion cells
H Horizontal cells
P Pigment cells
R Rods

Overlapping
visual fields

Central darker
circle represents
macular zone

Lighter shades
represent
monocular fields

Each quadrant
a different color

Projection on
left retina

Projection on
right retina

Optic nerves
Optic chiasm

Projection on left
dorsal lateral
geniculate nucleus

Projection on right
dorsal lateral
geniculate nucleus

Optic tracts

Lateral
geniculate
bodies

Optic radiation

Optic radiation

Calcarine
sulcus

Calcarine
sulcus

Projection on left
occipital lobe

Projection on right
occipital lobe

PLATE 114

HEAD AND NECK

SEE ALSO PLATES 81, 126, 153

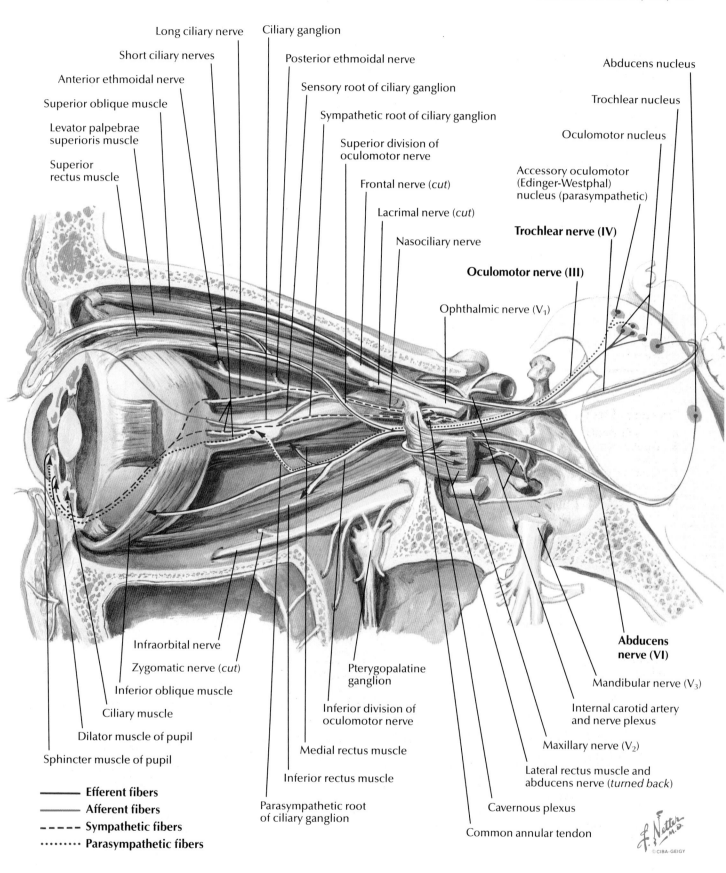

Long ciliary nerve

Short ciliary nerves

Anterior ethmoidal nerve

Superior oblique muscle

Levator palpebrae superioris muscle

Superior rectus muscle

Ciliary ganglion

Posterior ethmoidal nerve

Sensory root of ciliary ganglion

Sympathetic root of ciliary ganglion

Superior division of oculomotor nerve

Frontal nerve (*cut*)

Lacrimal nerve (*cut*)

Nasociliary nerve

Abducens nucleus

Trochlear nucleus

Oculomotor nucleus

Accessory oculomotor (Edinger-Westphal) nucleus (parasympathetic)

Trochlear nerve (IV)

Oculomotor nerve (III)

Ophthalmic nerve (V_1)

Infraorbital nerve

Zygomatic nerve (*cut*)

Inferior oblique muscle

Ciliary muscle

Dilator muscle of pupil

Sphincter muscle of pupil

Pterygopalatine ganglion

Inferior division of oculomotor nerve

Medial rectus muscle

Inferior rectus muscle

Parasympathetic root of ciliary ganglion

Abducens nerve (VI)

Mandibular nerve (V_3)

Internal carotid artery and nerve plexus

Maxillary nerve (V_2)

Lateral rectus muscle and abducens nerve (*turned back*)

Cavernous plexus

Common annular tendon

——— **Efferent fibers**

——— **Afferent fibers**

- - - - **Sympathetic fibers**

·········· **Parasympathetic fibers**

Trigeminal Nerve: Schema

SEE ALSO PLATES 18, 37, 38, 40, 41, 153

—— Efferent fibers
—— Afferent fibers
······ Proprioceptive fibers
······ Parasympathetic fibers
–––– Sympathetic fibers

Ophthalmic nerve (V₁)
Tentorial (meningeal) branch
Nasociliary nerve
Lacrimal nerve
Sensory root of ciliary ganglion
Frontal nerve
Ciliary ganglion
Posterior ethmoidal nerve
Long ciliary nerve
Short ciliary nerves
Anterior ethmoidal nerve
Supraorbital nerve
Supratrochlear nerve
Infratrochlear nerve
Internal nasal branches and
External nasal branches of anterior ethmoidal nerve

Trigeminal nerve (V) and ganglion
Motor nucleus
Mesencephalic nucleus
Pontine (principal) nucleus
Spinal tract and nucleus

Maxillary nerve (V₂)
Meningeal branch
Zygomaticotemporal nerve
Zygomaticofacial nerve
Zygomatic nerve
Infraorbital nerve
Pterygopalatine ganglion
Superior alveolar branches of infraorbital nerve
Nasal branches (posterior superior lateral, nasopalatine and posterior superior medial)
Nerve (Vidian) of pterygoid canal (from facial nerve [VII] and carotid plexus)
Pharyngeal branch
Greater and lesser palatine nerves
Deep temporal nerves (to temporalis muscle)
Lateral pterygoid and masseteric nerves
Tensor veli palatini and medial pterygoid nerves
Buccal nerve
Mental nerve
Inferior dental plexus
Lingual nerve

Facial nerve (VII)
Chorda tympani nerve

Superficial temporal branches
Articular and auricular branches
Auriculotemporal nerve
Parotid branches
Meningeal branch
Lesser petrosal nerve (from glossopharyngeal nerve [IX])

Submandibular ganglion
Mylohyoid nerve
Mandibular nerve (V₃)
Inferior alveolar nerve
Otic ganglion
Tensor tympani nerve

PLATE 116

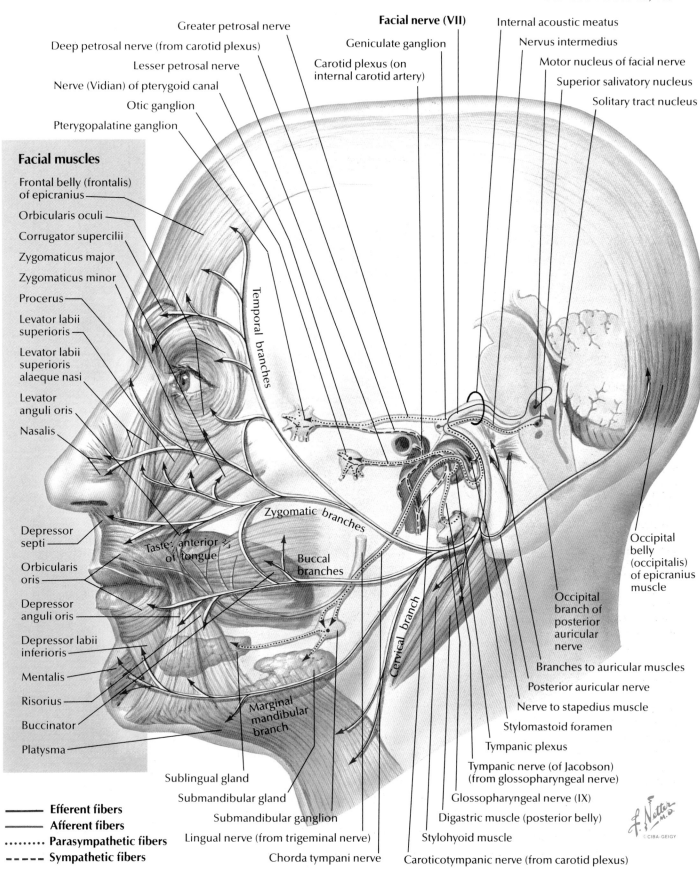

Greater petrosal nerve

Deep petrosal nerve (from carotid plexus)

Lesser petrosal nerve

Nerve (Vidian) of pterygoid canal

Otic ganglion

Pterygopalatine ganglion

Facial nerve (VII)

Geniculate ganglion

Carotid plexus (on internal carotid artery)

Internal acoustic meatus

Nervus intermedius

Motor nucleus of facial nerve

Superior salivatory nucleus

Solitary tract nucleus

Facial muscles

Frontal belly (frontalis) of epicranius

Orbicularis oculi

Corrugator supercilii

Zygomaticus major

Zygomaticus minor

Procerus

Levator labii superioris

Levator labii superioris alaeque nasi

Levator anguli oris

Nasalis

Depressor septi

Orbicularis oris

Depressor anguli oris

Depressor labii inferioris

Mentalis

Risorius

Buccinator

Platysma

Temporal branches

Zygomatic branches

Taste: anterior ⅔ of tongue

Buccal branches

Cervical branch

Marginal mandibular branch

Sublingual gland

Submandibular gland

Submandibular ganglion

Lingual nerve (from trigeminal nerve)

Chorda tympani nerve

Occipital belly (occipitalis) of epicranius muscle

Occipital branch of posterior auricular nerve

Branches to auricular muscles

Posterior auricular nerve

Nerve to stapedius muscle

Stylomastoid foramen

Tympanic plexus

Tympanic nerve (of Jacobson) (from glossopharyngeal nerve)

Glossopharyngeal nerve (IX)

Digastric muscle (posterior belly)

Stylohyoid muscle

Caroticotympanic nerve (from carotid plexus)

———— **Efferent fibers**

———— **Afferent fibers**

········· **Parasympathetic fibers**

- - - - - **Sympathetic fibers**

Vestibulocochlear Nerve: Schema

Afferent fibers

Facial canal

Geniculate ganglion of facial nerve

Greater petrosal nerve

Spiral ganglion of cochlea

Vestibular nerve

Cochlear nerve

Motor root of facial nerve and nervus intermedius

Vestibulocochlear nerve (VIII)

Medulla oblongata (cross section)

Tympanic cavity

Chorda tympani nerve

Head of malleus

Incus

Internal acoustic meatus

Vestibular nuclei

Medial

Rostral (superior)

Caudal (inferior)

Lateral

Ventral

Dorsal
} Cochlear nuclei

Inferior cerebellar peduncle (to cerebellum)

Vestibular ganglion

Superior division
Inferior division
} of vestibular nerve

Saccule

Ampulla of posterior semicircular duct

Utricle

Ampulla of superior semicircular duct

Ampulla of lateral semicircular duct

PLATE 118

HEAD AND NECK

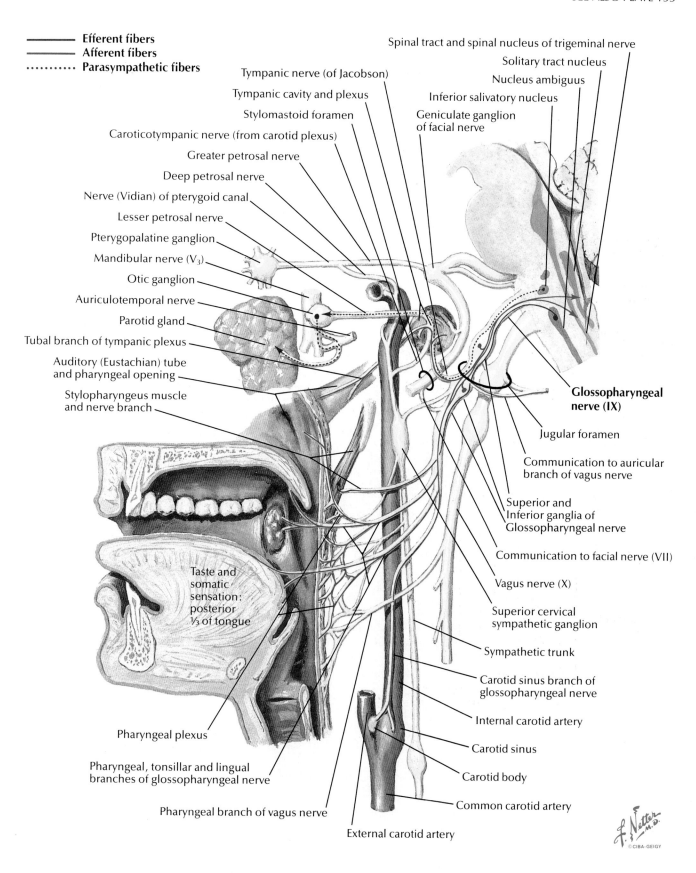

Efferent fibers
Afferent fibers
Parasympathetic fibers

Tympanic nerve (of Jacobson)

Tympanic cavity and plexus

Stylomastoid foramen

Caroticotympanic nerve (from carotid plexus)

Greater petrosal nerve

Deep petrosal nerve

Nerve (Vidian) of pterygoid canal

Lesser petrosal nerve

Pterygopalatine ganglion

Mandibular nerve (V₃)

Otic ganglion

Auriculotemporal nerve

Parotid gland

Tubal branch of tympanic plexus

Auditory (Eustachian) tube and pharyngeal opening

Stylopharyngeus muscle and nerve branch

Taste and somatic sensation: posterior ⅓ of tongue

Pharyngeal plexus

Pharyngeal, tonsillar and lingual branches of glossopharyngeal nerve

Pharyngeal branch of vagus nerve

External carotid artery

Spinal tract and spinal nucleus of trigeminal nerve

Solitary tract nucleus

Nucleus ambiguus

Inferior salivatory nucleus

Geniculate ganglion of facial nerve

Glossopharyngeal nerve (IX)

Jugular foramen

Communication to auricular branch of vagus nerve

Superior and Inferior ganglia of Glossopharyngeal nerve

Communication to facial nerve (VII)

Vagus nerve (X)

Superior cervical sympathetic ganglion

Sympathetic trunk

Carotid sinus branch of glossopharyngeal nerve

Internal carotid artery

Carotid sinus

Carotid body

Common carotid artery

Vagus Nerve: Schema

SEE ALSO PLATE 153

Glossopharyngeal nerve (IX)

Meningeal branch of vagus nerve

Auricular branch of vagus nerve

Auditory (Eustachian) tube

Levator veli palatini muscle

Salpingopharyngeus muscle

Palatoglossus muscle

Palatopharyngeus muscle

Superior pharyngeal constrictor muscle

Stylopharyngeus muscle

Middle pharyngeal constrictor muscle

Inferior pharyngeal constrictor muscle

Cricothyroid muscle

Trachea

Esophagus

Right subclavian artery

Right recurrent laryngeal nerve

Heart

Hepatic branch of anterior vagal trunk (in lesser omentum)

Celiac branches from anterior and posterior vagal trunks to celiac plexus

Celiac and superior mesenteric ganglia and celiac plexus

Hepatic plexus

Gallbladder and bile ducts

Liver

Pyloric branch from hepatic plexus

Pancreas

Duodenum

Ascending colon

Cecum

Appendix

Dorsal vagal nucleus (parasympathetic and visceral afferent)

Solitary tract nucleus (visceral afferents including taste)

Spinal tract and spinal nucleus of trigeminal nerve (somatic afferent)

Nucleus ambiguus (motor to pharyngeal and laryngeal muscles)

Cranial root of accessory nerve

Vagus nerve (X)

Jugular foramen

Superior ganglion of vagus nerve

Inferior ganglion of vagus nerve

Pharyngeal branch of vagus nerve (motor to muscles of palate and lower pharynx; sensory to lower pharynx)

Communicating branch of vagus nerve to carotid sinus branch of glossopharyngeal nerve

Pharyngeal plexus

Superior laryngeal nerve:
Internal branch (sensory and parasympathetic)
External branch (motor to cricothyroid muscle)

Superior cervical cardiac branch of vagus nerve

Inferior cervical cardiac branch of vagus nerve

Thoracic cardiac branch of vagus nerve

Left recurrent laryngeal nerve (motor to muscles of larynx except cricothyroid; sensory and parasympathetic to larynx below vocal folds; parasympathetic, efferent and afferent to upper esophagus and trachea)

Pulmonary plexus

Cardiac plexus

Esophageal plexus

Anterior vagal trunk

Gastric branches of anterior vagal trunk (branches from posterior trunk behind stomach)

Vagal branches (parasympathetic motor, secretomotor and afferent fibers) accompany superior mesenteric artery and its branches usually as far as left colic (splenic) flexure

Small intestine

—— **Efferent fibers**
—— **Afferent fibers**
······· **Parasympathetic fibers**

PLATE 120

Nucleus ambiguus

Vagus nerve (X)

Cranial root of accessory nerve (joins vagus nerve and via recurrent laryngeal nerve supplies muscles of larynx, except cricothyroid)

Spinal root of accessory nerve

Foramen magnum

Jugular foramen

Superior ganglion of vagus nerve

Accessory nerve (XI)

Internal branch of accessory nerve

Inferior ganglion of vagus nerve

1st spinal nerve (C1)

2nd spinal nerve (C2)

External branch of accessory nerve (to sternocleidomastoid and trapezius muscles)

Sternocleidomastoid muscle (*cut*)

3rd spinal nerve (C3)

4th spinal nerve (C4)

Trapezius muscle

—— **Efferent fibers**
—— **Proprioceptive fibers**

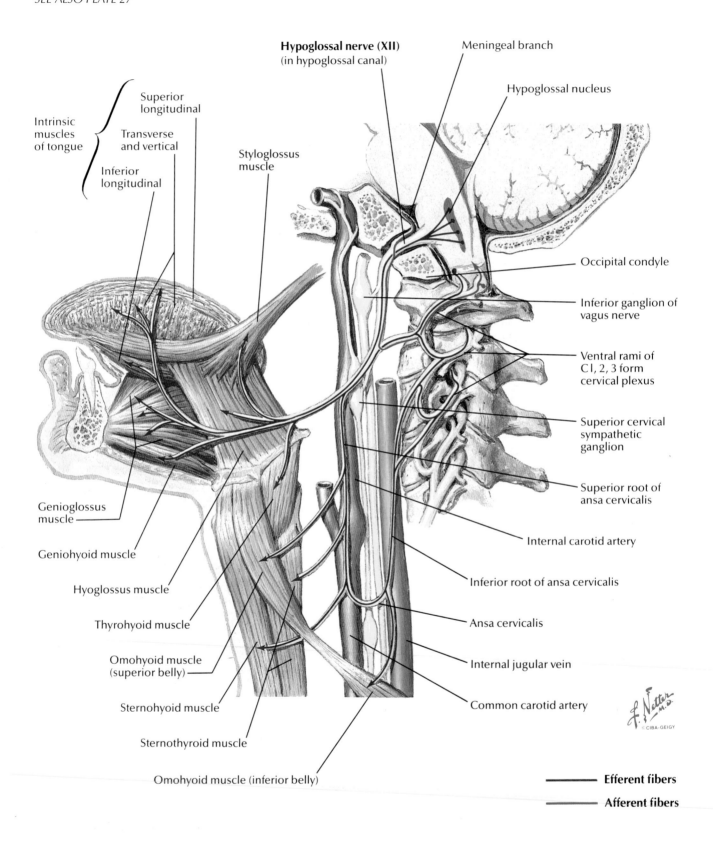

Hypoglossal nerve (XII)
(in hypoglossal canal)

Meningeal branch

Hypoglossal nucleus

Intrinsic muscles of tongue
- Superior longitudinal
- Transverse and vertical
- Inferior longitudinal

Styloglossus muscle

Occipital condyle

Inferior ganglion of vagus nerve

Ventral rami of CI, 2, 3 form cervical plexus

Superior cervical sympathetic ganglion

Superior root of ansa cervicalis

Internal carotid artery

Genioglossus muscle

Geniohyoid muscle

Hyoglossus muscle

Thyrohyoid muscle

Omohyoid muscle (superior belly)

Sternohyoid muscle

Sternothyroid muscle

Omohyoid muscle (inferior belly)

Inferior root of ansa cervicalis

Ansa cervicalis

Internal jugular vein

Common carotid artery

Efferent fibers

Afferent fibers

PLATE 122

HEAD AND NECK

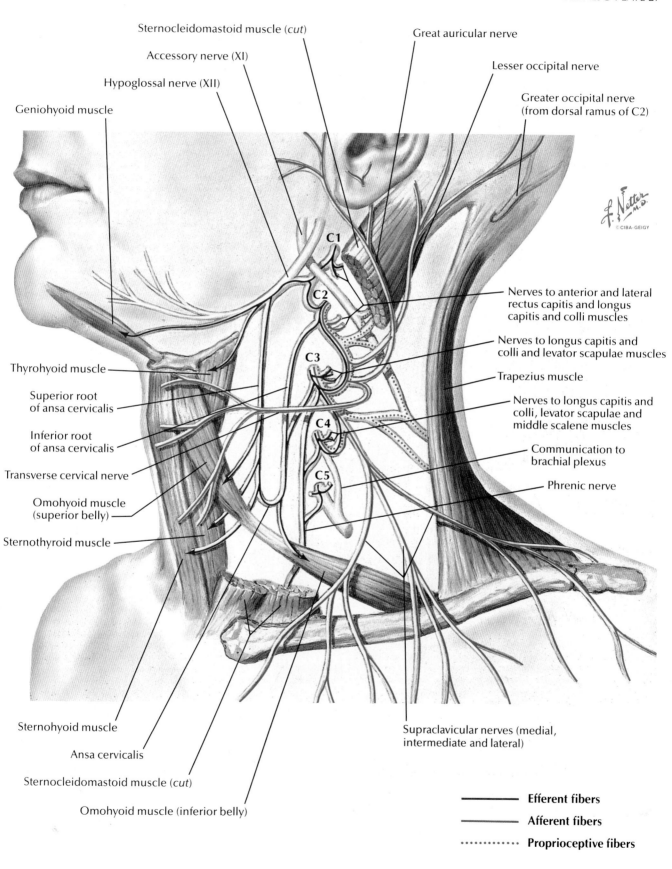

Sternocleidomastoid muscle (*cut*)

Accessory nerve (XI)

Hypoglossal nerve (XII)

Geniohyoid muscle

Great auricular nerve

Lesser occipital nerve

Greater occipital nerve (from dorsal ramus of C2)

C1

C2

C3

C4

C5

Nerves to anterior and lateral rectus capitis and longus capitis and colli muscles

Nerves to longus capitis and colli and levator scapulae muscles

Trapezius muscle

Nerves to longus capitis and colli, levator scapulae and middle scalene muscles

Communication to brachial plexus

Phrenic nerve

Thyrohyoid muscle

Superior root of ansa cervicalis

Inferior root of ansa cervicalis

Transverse cervical nerve

Omohyoid muscle (superior belly)

Sternothyroid muscle

Sternohyoid muscle

Ansa cervicalis

Sternocleidomastoid muscle (*cut*)

Omohyoid muscle (inferior belly)

Supraclavicular nerves (medial, intermediate and lateral)

——— Efferent fibers

——— Afferent fibers

·············· Proprioceptive fibers

Autonomic Nerves in Neck

SEE ALSO PLATES 65, 119, 120, 152, 198, 214, 228, 304

Internal carotid nerve

Glossopharyngeal nerve (IX)

Laryngopharyngeal sympathetic branch

Vagus nerve (X) (*cut*)

Superior cervical sympathetic ganglion

C1

C2

C3

C4

Gray rami communicantes

C5

C6

C7

C8

Subclavian artery

Pharyngeal plexus

Superior pharyngeal branch of vagus nerve

External carotid artery and plexus

Superior laryngeal nerve

Internal carotid artery and carotid sinus branch of glossopharyngeal nerve

Carotid body

Carotid sinus

Superior cervical cardiac branch of vagus nerve

Superior cervical sympathetic cardiac nerve

Phrenic nerve (*cut*)

Middle cervical sympathetic ganglion

Common carotid artery and plexus

Middle cervical sympathetic cardiac nerve

Vertebral ganglion

Vertebral artery and plexus

Recurrent laryngeal nerve

Cervicothoracic (stellate) ganglion

Ansa subclavia

Vagus nerve (X) (*cut*)

Inferior cervical sympathetic cardiac nerve

Thoracic sympathetic and vagal cardiac nerves

PLATE 124

HEAD AND NECK

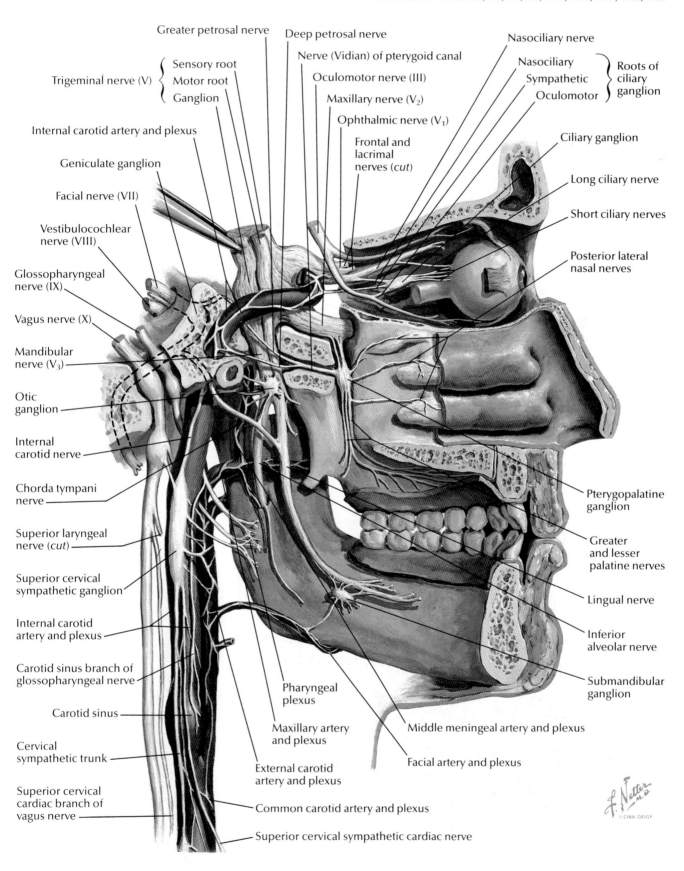

Greater petrosal nerve

Deep petrosal nerve

Nasociliary nerve

Nerve (Vidian) of pterygoid canal

Nasociliary

Roots of ciliary ganglion

Trigeminal nerve (V) { Sensory root Motor root Ganglion }

Oculomotor nerve (III)

Sympathetic

Oculomotor

Maxillary nerve (V₂)

Internal carotid artery and plexus

Ophthalmic nerve (V₁)

Ciliary ganglion

Geniculate ganglion

Frontal and lacrimal nerves (*cut*)

Long ciliary nerve

Facial nerve (VII)

Short ciliary nerves

Vestibulocochlear nerve (VIII)

Posterior lateral nasal nerves

Glossopharyngeal nerve (IX)

Vagus nerve (X)

Mandibular nerve (V₃)

Otic ganglion

Internal carotid nerve

Pterygopalatine ganglion

Chorda tympani nerve

Superior laryngeal nerve (*cut*)

Greater and lesser palatine nerves

Superior cervical sympathetic ganglion

Lingual nerve

Internal carotid artery and plexus

Inferior alveolar nerve

Carotid sinus branch of glossopharyngeal nerve

Pharyngeal plexus

Submandibular ganglion

Carotid sinus

Cervical sympathetic trunk

Maxillary artery and plexus

Middle meningeal artery and plexus

Superior cervical cardiac branch of vagus nerve

External carotid artery and plexus

Facial artery and plexus

Common carotid artery and plexus

Superior cervical sympathetic cardiac nerve

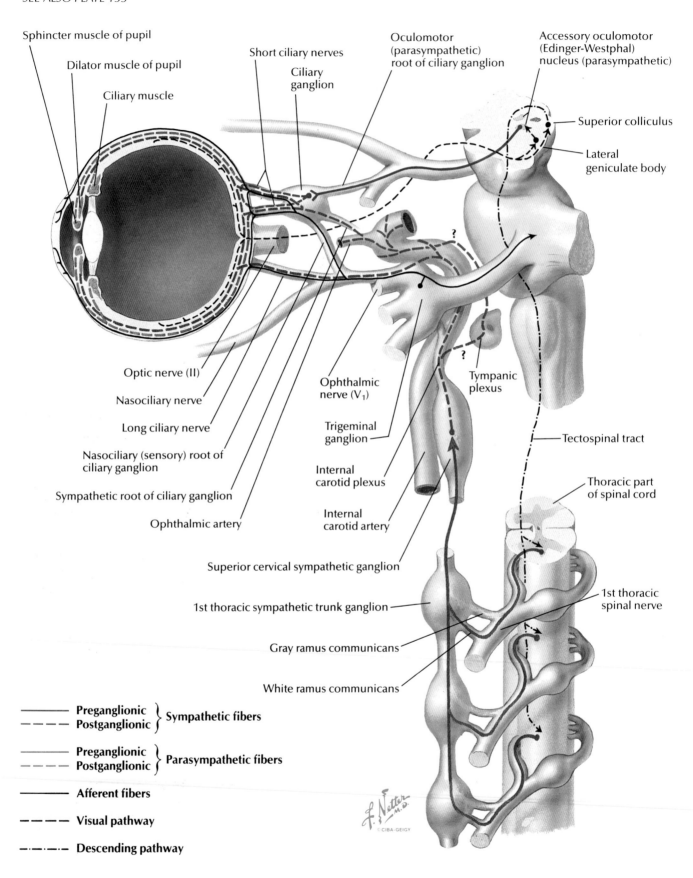

Sphincter muscle of pupil

Dilator muscle of pupil

Ciliary muscle

Short ciliary nerves

Ciliary ganglion

Oculomotor (parasympathetic) root of ciliary ganglion

Accessory oculomotor (Edinger-Westphal) nucleus (parasympathetic)

Superior colliculus

Lateral geniculate body

Optic nerve (II)

Nasociliary nerve

Long ciliary nerve

Nasociliary (sensory) root of ciliary ganglion

Sympathetic root of ciliary ganglion

Ophthalmic artery

Ophthalmic nerve (V_1)

Trigeminal ganglion

Internal carotid plexus

Internal carotid artery

Superior cervical sympathetic ganglion

1st thoracic sympathetic trunk ganglion

Gray ramus communicans

White ramus communicans

Tympanic plexus

Tectospinal tract

Thoracic part of spinal cord

1st thoracic spinal nerve

———— **Preganglionic** } **Sympathetic fibers**
– – – – **Postganglionic** }

———— **Preganglionic** } **Parasympathetic fibers**
– – – – **Postganglionic** }

———— **Afferent fibers**

– – – – **Visual pathway**

–·–·– **Descending pathway**

PLATE 126

HEAD AND NECK

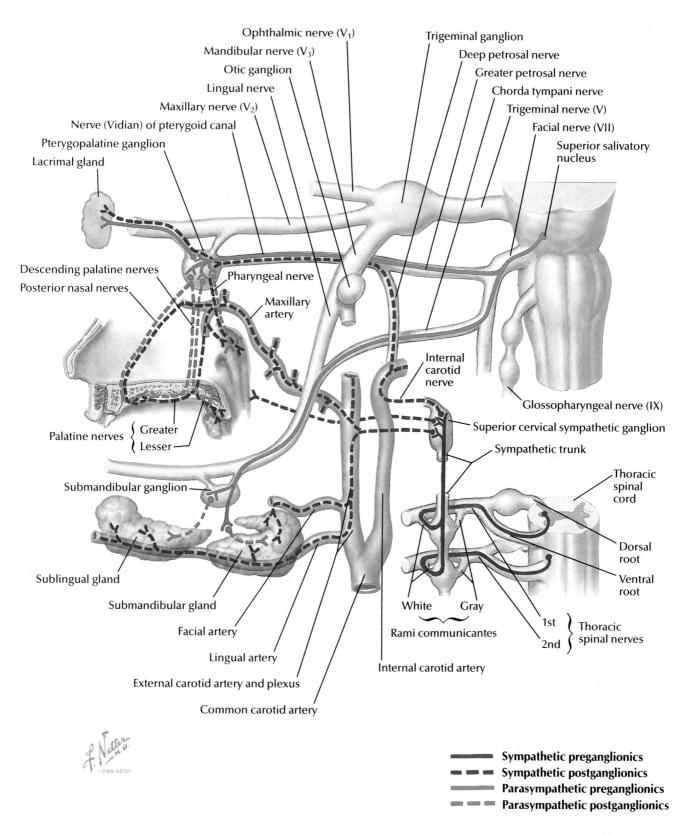

Ophthalmic nerve (V₁)

Mandibular nerve (V₃)

Otic ganglion

Lingual nerve

Maxillary nerve (V₂)

Nerve (Vidian) of pterygoid canal

Pterygopalatine ganglion

Lacrimal gland

Trigeminal ganglion

Deep petrosal nerve

Greater petrosal nerve

Chorda tympani nerve

Trigeminal nerve (V)

Facial nerve (VII)

Superior salivatory nucleus

Descending palatine nerves

Posterior nasal nerves

Pharyngeal nerve

Maxillary artery

Internal carotid nerve

Glossopharyngeal nerve (IX)

Superior cervical sympathetic ganglion

Sympathetic trunk

Palatine nerves { Greater / Lesser }

Submandibular ganglion

Thoracic spinal cord

Sublingual gland

Dorsal root

Ventral root

Submandibular gland

Facial artery

Lingual artery

White   Gray

Rami communicantes

1st } Thoracic spinal nerves
2nd

External carotid artery and plexus

Internal carotid artery

Common carotid artery

Sympathetic preganglionics
Sympathetic postganglionics
Parasympathetic preganglionics
Parasympathetic postganglionics

Otic Ganglion: Schema

SEE ALSO PLATE 153

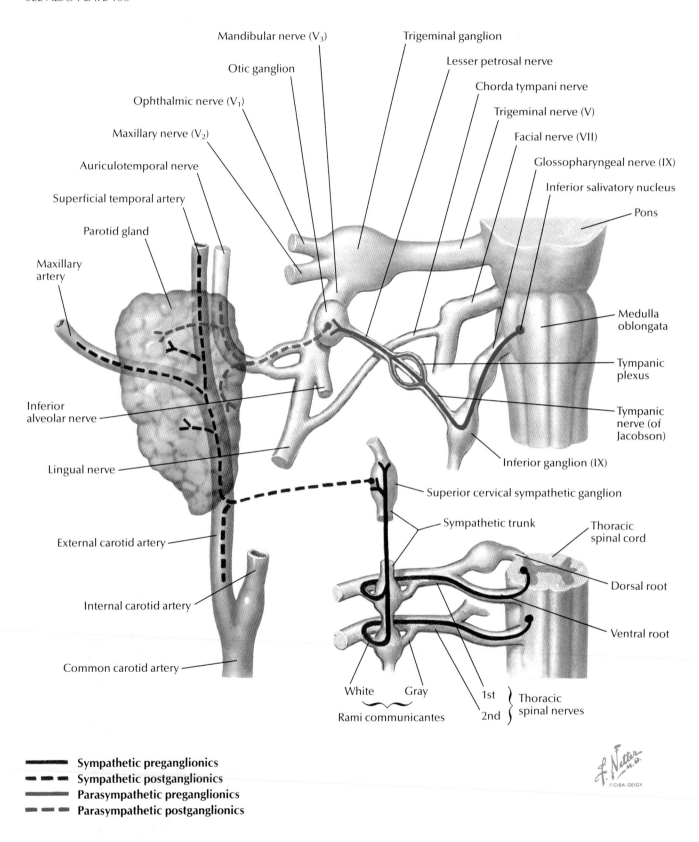

Mandibular nerve (V₃)

Otic ganglion

Ophthalmic nerve (V₁)

Maxillary nerve (V₂)

Auriculotemporal nerve

Superficial temporal artery

Parotid gland

Maxillary artery

Inferior alveolar nerve

Lingual nerve

External carotid artery

Internal carotid artery

Common carotid artery

Trigeminal ganglion

Lesser petrosal nerve

Chorda tympani nerve

Trigeminal nerve (V)

Facial nerve (VII)

Glossopharyngeal nerve (IX)

Inferior salivatory nucleus

Pons

Medulla oblongata

Tympanic plexus

Tympanic nerve (of Jacobson)

Inferior ganglion (IX)

Superior cervical sympathetic ganglion

Sympathetic trunk

Thoracic spinal cord

Dorsal root

Ventral root

White   Gray

Rami communicantes

1st
2nd } Thoracic spinal nerves

▬▬▬▬ Sympathetic preganglionics
▬ ▬ ▬ Sympathetic postganglionics
▬▬▬▬ Parasympathetic preganglionics
▭ ▬ ▬ Parasympathetic postganglionics

PLATE 128

Taste Pathways: Schema

SEE ALSO PLATES 41, 89, 117, 119, 120

——————— Usual pathway

- - - - - - - Accessory pathway

Ventral posteromedial (VPM) nucleus of thalamus

Sensory cortex (just below face area)

Lateral hypothalamic area

Amygdaloid body

Pontine taste area

Trigeminal nerve (V)

Trigeminal (semilunar) ganglion

Ophthalmic nerve (V₁)

Maxillary nerve (V₂)

Mandibular nerve (V₃)

Pterygopalatine ganglion

Nerve (Vidian) of pterygoid canal

Lingual nerve

Fungiform papillae

Foliate papillae

Vallate papillae

Epiglottis

Larynx

Mesencephalic nucleus and Motor nucleus of trigeminal nerve

Pons

Greater petrosal nerve

Geniculate ganglion

Facial nerve (VII) and Nervus intermedius

Nucleus of solitary tract (rostral part)

Glossopharyngeal nerve (IX)

Medulla oblongata (lower part)

Petrosal (inferior) ganglion of glossopharyngeal nerve

Nodose (inferior) ganglion of vagus nerve

Vagus nerve (X)

Otic ganglion

Chorda tympani nerve

Superior laryngeal nerve

Arteries to Brain and Meninges

SEE ALSO PLATES 28, 29

Left middle meningeal artery

Posterior cerebral artery

Superior cerebellar artery

Basilar artery

Left internal acoustic (labyrinthine) artery

Mastoid branch of left occipital artery

Anterior inferior cerebellar artery

Meningeal branch of left ascending pharyngeal artery

Posterior inferior cerebellar artery

Left and right vertebral arteries

Posterior meningeal branch of vertebral artery

Anterior meningeal branch of vertebral artery

Posterior auricular artery

Occipital artery

Internal carotid artery

Carotid sinus

Carotid body

Vertebral artery

Transverse process of C6

Deep cervical artery

Highest intercostal artery

Costocervical trunk

Subclavian artery

Middle cerebral artery

Anterior cerebral artery

Anterior communicating artery

Ophthalmic artery

Posterior communicating artery

Cavernous sinus

Middle meningeal artery

Maxillary artery

Superficial temporal artery

External carotid artery

Facial artery

Lingual artery

Ascending pharyngeal artery

Superior laryngeal artery

Superior thyroid artery

Common carotid artery

Ascending cervical artery *(cut)*

Inferior thyroid artery

Thyrocervical trunk

Brachiocephalic trunk

Internal thoracic artery

PLATE 130   **HEAD AND NECK**

Anterior cerebral artery

Middle cerebral artery

Posterior communicating artery

Caroticotympanic branch of internal carotid artery

Posterior cerebral artery

Superior cerebellar artery

Anterior tympanic artery

Middle meningeal artery

Maxillary artery

Basilar artery

Anterior inferior cerebellar artery

Posterior inferior cerebellar artery

External carotid artery

Internal carotid artery

Superior thyroid artery

Common carotid artery

Vertebral artery

Ascending cervical artery

Inferior thyroid artery

Thyrocervical trunk

Subclavian artery

Brachiocephalic trunk

Anterior communicating artery

Ophthalmic artery

Supraorbital artery

Supratrochlear artery

Lacrimal artery

Dorsal nasal artery

Middle meningeal artery

Angular artery

Superficial temporal artery

Posterior auricular artery

Facial artery

Occipital artery

Lingual artery

Ascending pharyngeal artery

Anterior spinal artery

Spinal (radicular) branches

Vertebral artery

Common carotid artery

Deep cervical artery

Transverse cervical artery

Suprascapular artery

Highest intercostal artery

Costocervical trunk

Subclavian artery

Internal thoracic artery

Aorta {
Arch
Descending
Ascending
}

Anastomoses

1 Right–Left
2 Carotid–Vertebral
3 Internal carotid–External carotid
4 Subclavian–Carotid
5 Subclavian–Vertebral

CEREBRAL VASCULATURE

PLATE 131

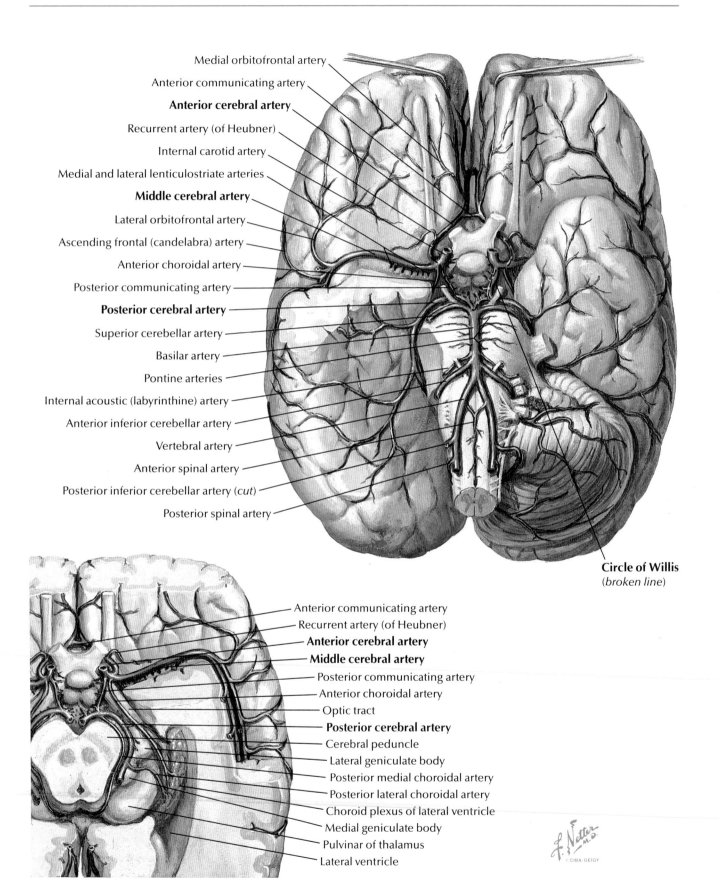

Medial orbitofrontal artery

Anterior communicating artery

Anterior cerebral artery

Recurrent artery (of Heubner)

Internal carotid artery

Medial and lateral lenticulostriate arteries

Middle cerebral artery

Lateral orbitofrontal artery

Ascending frontal (candelabra) artery

Anterior choroidal artery

Posterior communicating artery

Posterior cerebral artery

Superior cerebellar artery

Basilar artery

Pontine arteries

Internal acoustic (labyrinthine) artery

Anterior inferior cerebellar artery

Vertebral artery

Anterior spinal artery

Posterior inferior cerebellar artery (*cut*)

Posterior spinal artery

Circle of Willis
(*broken line*)

Anterior communicating artery

Recurrent artery (of Heubner)

Anterior cerebral artery

Middle cerebral artery

Posterior communicating artery

Anterior choroidal artery

Optic tract

Posterior cerebral artery

Cerebral peduncle

Lateral geniculate body

Posterior medial choroidal artery

Posterior lateral choroidal artery

Choroid plexus of lateral ventricle

Medial geniculate body

Pulvinar of thalamus

Lateral ventricle

PLATE 132

HEAD AND NECK

Vessels dissected out: inferior view

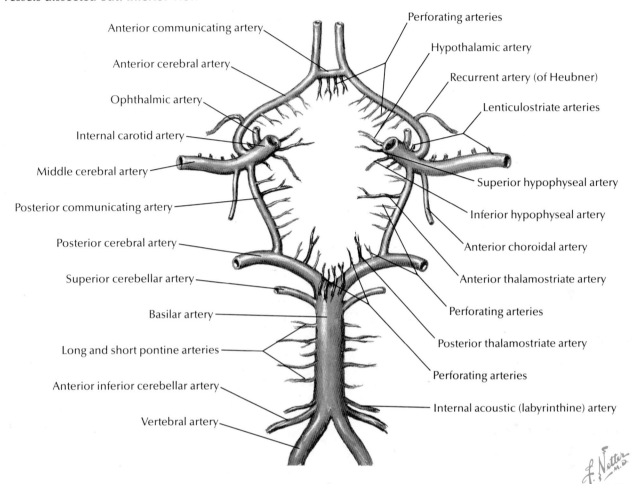

Anterior communicating artery
Anterior cerebral artery
Ophthalmic artery
Internal carotid artery
Middle cerebral artery
Posterior communicating artery
Posterior cerebral artery
Superior cerebellar artery
Basilar artery
Long and short pontine arteries
Anterior inferior cerebellar artery
Vertebral artery

Perforating arteries
Hypothalamic artery
Recurrent artery (of Heubner)
Lenticulostriate arteries
Superior hypophyseal artery
Inferior hypophyseal artery
Anterior choroidal artery
Anterior thalamostriate artery
Perforating arteries
Posterior thalamostriate artery
Perforating arteries
Internal acoustic (labyrinthine) artery

Vessels in situ: inferior view

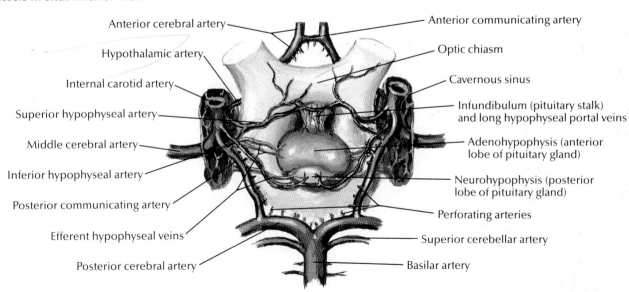

Anterior cerebral artery
Hypothalamic artery
Internal carotid artery
Superior hypophyseal artery
Middle cerebral artery
Inferior hypophyseal artery
Posterior communicating artery
Efferent hypophyseal veins
Posterior cerebral artery

Anterior communicating artery
Optic chiasm
Cavernous sinus
Infundibulum (pituitary stalk) and long hypophyseal portal veins
Adenohypophysis (anterior lobe of pituitary gland)
Neurohypophysis (posterior lobe of pituitary gland)
Perforating arteries
Superior cerebellar artery
Basilar artery

Corpus callosum

Medial and lateral lenticulostriate arteries

Lateral orbitofrontal artery

Ascending frontal (candelabra) artery

Precentral (pre-Rolandic) and central (Rolandic) arteries

Anterior and posterior parietal arteries

Angular artery

Temporal arteries (anterior, middle and posterior)

Middle cerebral artery and branches (deep in lateral cerebral [Sylvian] sulcus)

Anterior communicating artery

Posterior communicating artery

Anterior inferior cerebellar artery

Posterior spinal artery

Paracentral artery

Medial frontal branches

Pericallosal artery

Callosomarginal artery

Frontopolar artery

Anterior cerebral arteries

Medial orbitofrontal artery

Recurrent artery (of Heubner)

Internal carotid artery

Anterior choroidal artery

Posterior cerebral artery

Superior cerebellar artery

Basilar and pontine arteries

Internal acoustic (labyrinthine) artery

Vertebral artery

Posterior inferior cerebellar artery

Anterior spinal artery

Falx cerebri

Corpus striatum (caudate and lentiform nuclei)

Medial and lateral lenticulostriate arteries

Insula (island of Reil)

Limen of insula

Precentral (pre-Rolandic), central (Rolandic) and parietal arteries

Lateral cerebral (Sylvian) sulcus

Temporal arteries

Temporal lobe

Middle cerebral artery

Internal carotid artery

Callosomarginal arteries and Pericallosal arteries (branches of anterior cerebral arteries)

Trunk of corpus callosum

Internal capsule

Septum pellucidum

Rostrum of corpus callosum

Anterior cerebral arteries

Recurrent artery (of Heubner)

Anterior communicating artery

Optic chiasm

PLATE 134

HEAD AND NECK

Anterior parietal (postcentral) artery

Central (Rolandic) artery

Precentral (pre-Rolandic) artery

Ascending frontal (candelabra) artery

Terminal branches of anterior cerebral artery

Lateral orbitofrontal artery

Left middle cerebral artery

Left anterior cerebral artery

Anterior communicating artery

Right anterior cerebral artery

Left internal carotid artery

Posterior parietal artery

Angular artery

Terminal branches of posterior cerebral artery

Posterior temporal artery

Middle temporal artery

Anterior temporal artery

Medial frontal branches { Posterior / Middle / Anterior

Pericallosal artery

Paracentral artery

Cingular branches

Right posterior cerebral artery

Callosomarginal artery

Frontopolar artery

Right anterior cerebral artery

Medial orbito-frontal artery

Anterior communicating artery (*cut*)

Recurrent artery (of Heubner)

Right internal carotid artery

Precuneal artery

Posterior pericallosal artery

Parietooccipital artery

Calcarine artery

Posterior temporal artery

Anterior temporal artery

Posterior communicating artery

Arteries of Posterior Cranial Fossa

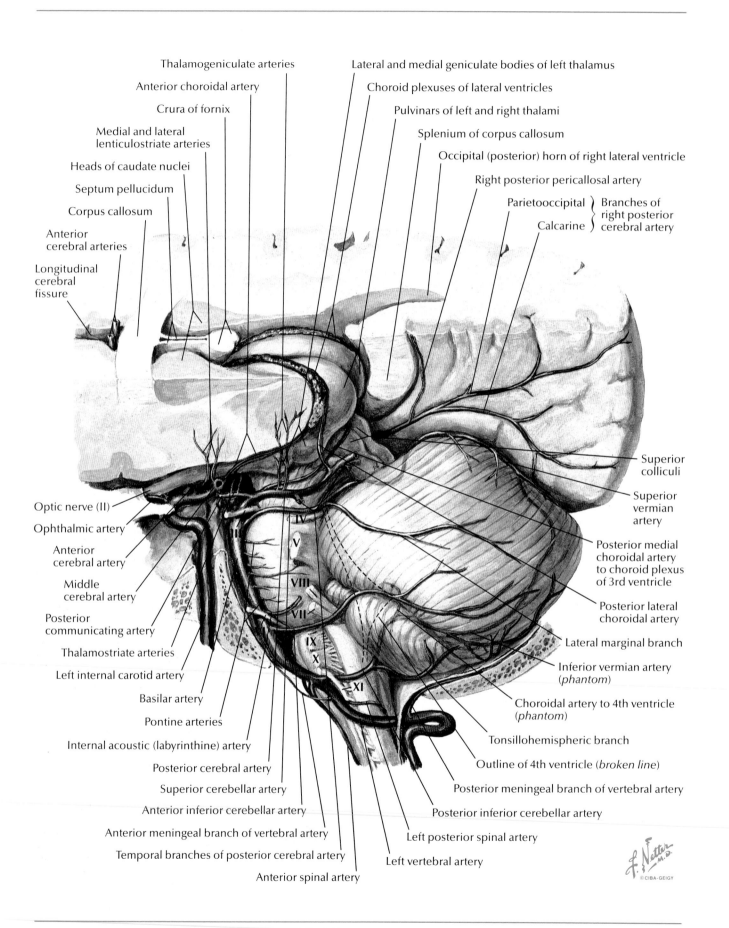

Thalamogeniculate arteries

Anterior choroidal artery

Crura of fornix

Medial and lateral lenticulostriate arteries

Heads of caudate nuclei

Septum pellucidum

Corpus callosum

Anterior cerebral arteries

Longitudinal cerebral fissure

Lateral and medial geniculate bodies of left thalamus

Choroid plexuses of lateral ventricles

Pulvinars of left and right thalami

Splenium of corpus callosum

Occipital (posterior) horn of right lateral ventricle

Right posterior pericallosal artery

Parietooccipital ⎱ Branches of
Calcarine ⎰ right posterior cerebral artery

Optic nerve (II)

Ophthalmic artery

Anterior cerebral artery

Middle cerebral artery

Posterior communicating artery

Thalamostriate arteries

Left internal carotid artery

Basilar artery

Pontine arteries

Internal acoustic (labyrinthine) artery

Posterior cerebral artery

Superior cerebellar artery

Anterior inferior cerebellar artery

Anterior meningeal branch of vertebral artery

Temporal branches of posterior cerebral artery

Anterior spinal artery

II

IV

V

VIII

VII

IX

X

XI

Superior colliculi

Superior vermian artery

Posterior medial choroidal artery to choroid plexus of 3rd ventricle

Posterior lateral choroidal artery

Lateral marginal branch

Inferior vermian artery (phantom)

Choroidal artery to 4th ventricle (phantom)

Tonsillohemispheric branch

Outline of 4th ventricle (broken line)

Posterior meningeal branch of vertebral artery

Posterior inferior cerebellar artery

Left posterior spinal artery

Left vertebral artery

PLATE 136

HEAD AND NECK

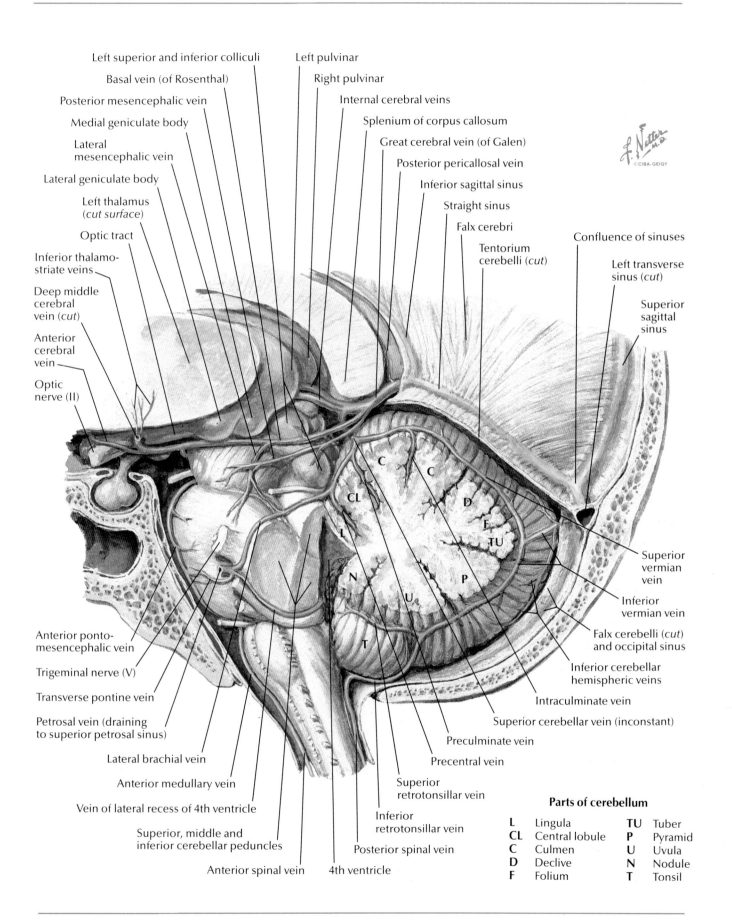

Left superior and inferior colliculi
Basal vein (of Rosenthal)
Posterior mesencephalic vein
Medial geniculate body
Lateral mesencephalic vein
Lateral geniculate body
Left thalamus (*cut surface*)
Optic tract
Inferior thalamo-striate veins
Deep middle cerebral vein (*cut*)
Anterior cerebral vein
Optic nerve (II)

Left pulvinar
Right pulvinar
Internal cerebral veins
Splenium of corpus callosum
Great cerebral vein (of Galen)
Posterior pericallosal vein
Inferior sagittal sinus
Straight sinus
Falx cerebri
Tentorium cerebelli (*cut*)

Confluence of sinuses
Left transverse sinus (*cut*)
Superior sagittal sinus

Anterior ponto-mesencephalic vein
Trigeminal nerve (V)
Transverse pontine vein
Petrosal vein (draining to superior petrosal sinus)
Lateral brachial vein
Anterior medullary vein
Vein of lateral recess of 4th ventricle
Superior, middle and inferior cerebellar peduncles
Anterior spinal vein

4th ventricle

Inferior retrotonsillar vein
Posterior spinal vein
Superior retrotonsillar vein
Precentral vein
Preculminate vein
Superior cerebellar vein (inconstant)
Intraculminate vein
Inferior cerebellar hemispheric veins
Falx cerebelli (*cut*) and occipital sinus
Inferior vermian vein
Superior vermian vein

Parts of cerebellum

L	Lingula	**TU**	Tuber
CL	Central lobule	**P**	Pyramid
C	Culmen	**U**	Uvula
D	Declive	**N**	Nodule
F	Folium	**T**	Tonsil

Deep Veins of Brain

FOR SUPERFICIAL VEINS OF BRAIN SEE PLATE 96

Longitudinal cerebral fissure
Anterior cerebral veins
Rostrum of corpus callosum
Septum pellucidum
Anterior septal vein
Head of caudate nucleus
Anterior terminal caudate vein
Caudate veins
Interventricular foramen (of Monro)
Columns of fornix
Superior thalamostriate vein
Superior choroidal vein and choroid plexus of lateral ventricle
Thalamus
Tela choroidea of 3rd ventricle
Direct lateral vein
Posterior terminal caudate vein
Internal cerebral veins
Basal vein (of Rosenthal)
Great cerebral vein (of Galen)
Inferior sagittal sinus
Straight sinus
Tentorium cerebelli
Transverse sinus
Confluence of sinuses
Superior sagittal sinus

Dissection: superior view

Anterior cerebral vein
Superficial middle cerebral vein (draining to sphenoparietal sinus)
Deep middle cerebral vein
Cerebral peduncle
Basal vein (of Rosenthal)
Lateral geniculate body
Medial geniculate body
Pulvinar of thalamus
Splenium of corpus callosum
Great cerebral vein (of Galen)

Uncal vein
Optic chiasm
Inferior cerebral veins
Inferior anastomotic vein (of Labbé)

Dissection: inferior view

PLATE 138

HEAD AND NECK

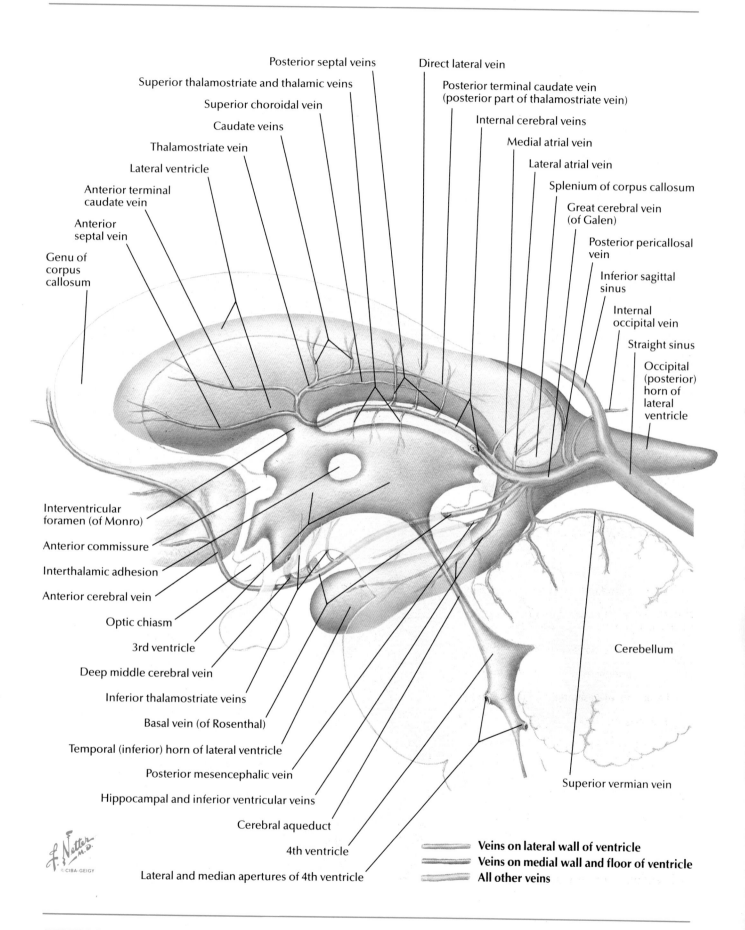

Posterior septal veins

Superior thalamostriate and thalamic veins

Superior choroidal vein

Caudate veins

Thalamostriate vein

Lateral ventricle

Anterior terminal caudate vein

Anterior septal vein

Genu of corpus callosum

Direct lateral vein

Posterior terminal caudate vein (posterior part of thalamostriate vein)

Internal cerebral veins

Medial atrial vein

Lateral atrial vein

Splenium of corpus callosum

Great cerebral vein (of Galen)

Posterior pericallosal vein

Inferior sagittal sinus

Internal occipital vein

Straight sinus

Occipital (posterior) horn of lateral ventricle

Interventricular foramen (of Monro)

Anterior commissure

Interthalamic adhesion

Anterior cerebral vein

Optic chiasm

3rd ventricle

Deep middle cerebral vein

Inferior thalamostriate veins

Basal vein (of Rosenthal)

Temporal (inferior) horn of lateral ventricle

Posterior mesencephalic vein

Hippocampal and inferior ventricular veins

Cerebral aqueduct

4th ventricle

Lateral and median apertures of 4th ventricle

Cerebellum

Superior vermian vein

Veins on lateral wall of ventricle
Veins on medial wall and floor of ventricle
All other veins

Hypothalamus and Hypophysis

SEE ALSO PLATES 100, 101

Septum pellucidum

Thalamus

Fornix

Hypothalamic sulcus

Anterior commissure

Principal nuclei of hypothalamus

Paraventricular

Posterior

Dorsomedial

Supraoptic

Ventromedial

Tuberal

Mamillary

Optic chiasm

Infundibulum (pituitary stalk)

Hypophysis (pituitary gland)

Mamillothalamic tract

Dorsal longitudinal fasciculus and other descending pathways

Lamina terminalis

Paraventricular hypothalamic nucleus

Supraoptic hypothalamic nucleus

Supraopticohypophyseal tract

Tuberohypophyseal tract

Hypothalamohypophyseal tract

Infundibulum (pituitary stalk)

Hypothalamic sulcus

Mamillary body

Tuberal hypothalamic nucleus

Adenohypophysis (anterior lobe of pituitary gland)

Pars infundibularis (pars tuberalis)

Fibrous trabecula

Pars intermedia

Pars distalis

Cleft

Median eminence of tuber cinereum

Infundibular stem

Infundibular process

Neurohypophysis (posterior lobe of pituitary gland)

PLATE 140　　　　　　　　　　　　　　　　　　　　　**HEAD AND NECK**

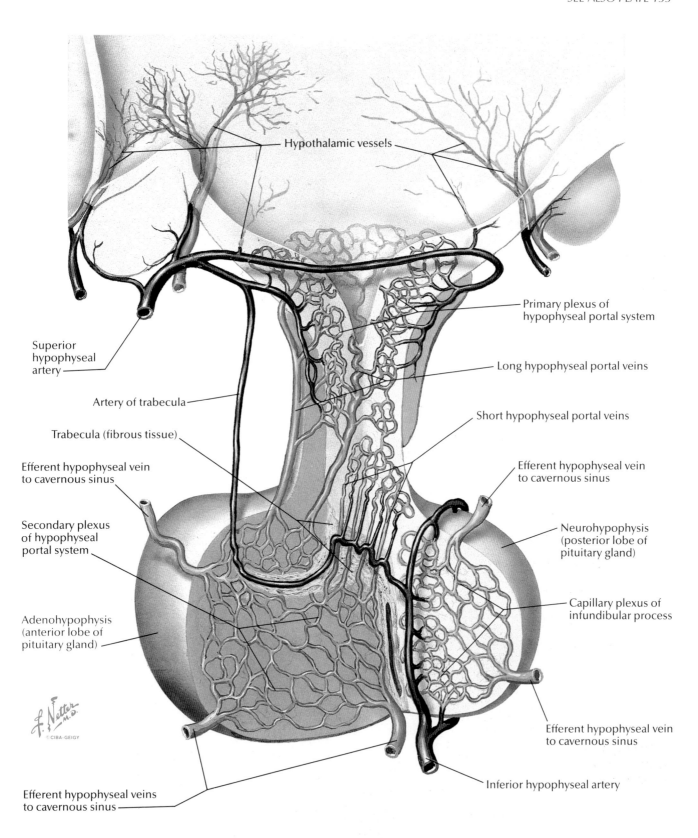

Hypothalamic vessels

Primary plexus of hypophyseal portal system

Superior hypophyseal artery

Long hypophyseal portal veins

Artery of trabecula

Short hypophyseal portal veins

Trabecula (fibrous tissue)

Efferent hypophyseal vein to cavernous sinus

Efferent hypophyseal vein to cavernous sinus

Secondary plexus of hypophyseal portal system

Neurohypophysis (posterior lobe of pituitary gland)

Adenohypophysis (anterior lobe of pituitary gland)

Capillary plexus of infundibular process

Efferent hypophyseal vein to cavernous sinus

Efferent hypophyseal veins to cavernous sinus

Inferior hypophyseal artery

Section II

BACK AND SPINAL CORD

Anterior view

Atlas (C1)

Axis (C2)

C7

T1

T12

L1

L5

Sacrum (S1–5)

Coccyx

Left lateral view

Atlas (C1)

Axis (C2)

C7

T1

T12

L1

L5

Sacrum (S1–5)

Coccyx

Posterior view

Atlas (C1)

Axis (C2)

Cervical vertebrae

C7

T1

Thoracic vertebrae

T12

L1

Lumbar vertebrae

L5

Sacrum (S1–5)

Coccyx

Thoracic Vertebrae

SEE ALSO PLATE 172

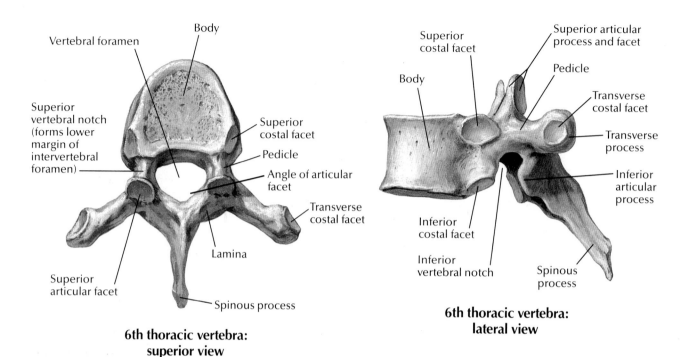

Vertebral foramen

Body

Superior vertebral notch (forms lower margin of intervertebral foramen)

Superior costal facet

Pedicle

Angle of articular facet

Transverse costal facet

Superior articular facet

Lamina

Spinous process

6th thoracic vertebra: superior view

Superior costal facet

Body

Superior articular process and facet

Pedicle

Transverse costal facet

Transverse process

Inferior articular process

Inferior costal facet

Inferior vertebral notch

Spinous process

6th thoracic vertebra: lateral view

Vertebral canal

Superior articular process and facet

7th rib

Spinous process (T 7)

Transverse process (T 9)

Inferior articular process (T 9)

Lamina

Spinous process (T 9)

7th, 8th and 9th thoracic vertebrae: posterior view

Body

Superior articular process and facet

Transverse process

Costal facet

Spinous process

Inferior articular process and facet

12th thoracic vertebra: lateral view

F. Netter M.D.
© CIBA-GEIGY

PLATE 143

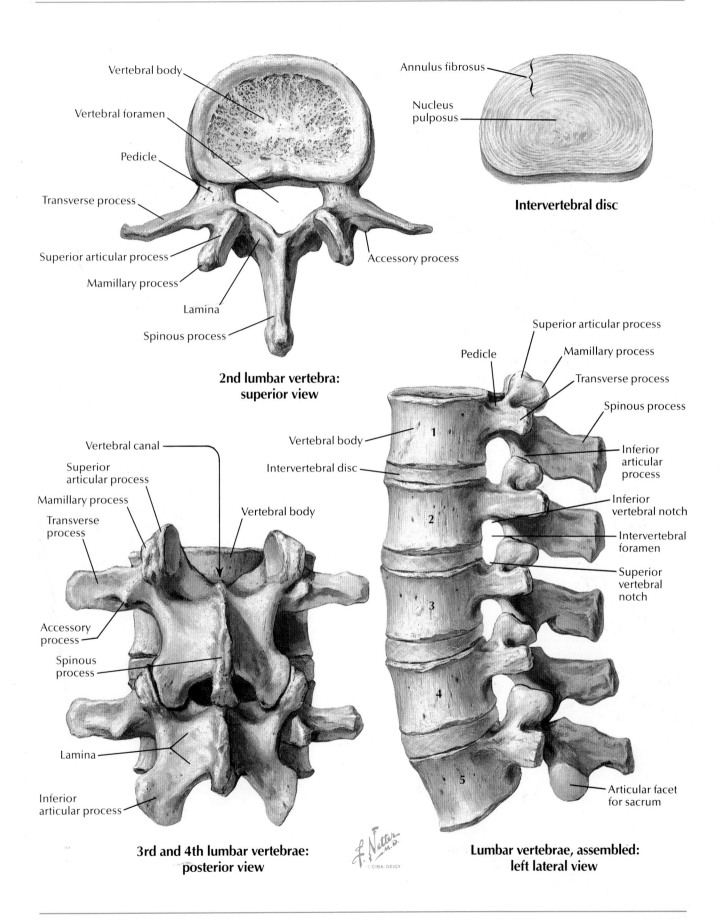

Vertebral body

Vertebral foramen

Pedicle

Transverse process

Superior articular process

Mamillary process

Lamina

Spinous process

**2nd lumbar vertebra:
superior view**

Annulus fibrosus

Nucleus
pulposus

Intervertebral disc

Vertebral canal

Superior
articular process

Mamillary process

Transverse
process

Accessory
process

Spinous
process

Vertebral body

Lamina

Inferior
articular process

**3rd and 4th lumbar vertebrae:
posterior view**

Accessory process

Pedicle

Superior articular process

Mamillary process

Transverse process

Spinous process

Vertebral body

Intervertebral disc

Inferior
articular
process

Inferior
vertebral notch

Intervertebral
foramen

Superior
vertebral
notch

Articular facet
for sacrum

**Lumbar vertebrae, assembled:
left lateral view**

Sacrum and Coccyx

SEE ALSO PLATES 142, 147, 231, 334, 335, 336

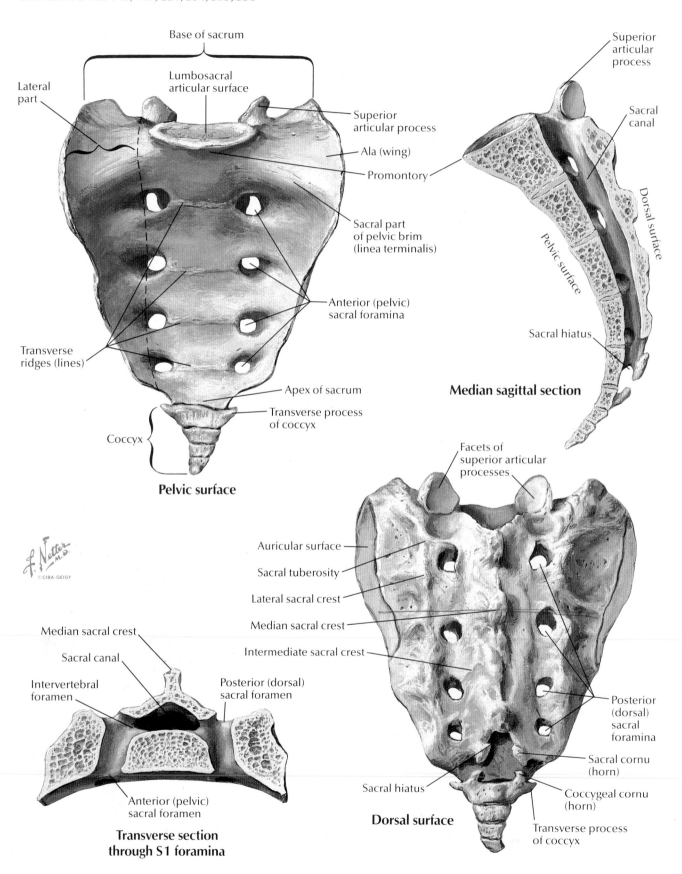

Base of sacrum

Lateral part

Lumbosacral articular surface

Superior articular process

Ala (wing)

Promontory

Sacral part of pelvic brim (linea terminalis)

Anterior (pelvic) sacral foramina

Transverse ridges (lines)

Apex of sacrum

Transverse process of coccyx

Coccyx

Pelvic surface

Superior articular process

Sacral canal

Dorsal surface

Pelvic surface

Sacral hiatus

Median sagittal section

Facets of superior articular processes

Auricular surface

Sacral tuberosity

Lateral sacral crest

Median sacral crest

Intermediate sacral crest

Posterior (dorsal) sacral foramina

Sacral cornu (horn)

Sacral hiatus

Coccygeal cornu (horn)

Transverse process of coccyx

Dorsal surface

Median sacral crest

Sacral canal

Intervertebral foramen

Posterior (dorsal) sacral foramen

Anterior (pelvic) sacral foramen

Transverse section through S1 foramina

PLATE 145

BACK AND SPINAL CORD

Left lateral view (*partially sectioned*)

Anterior longitudinal ligament

Lumbar vertebral body

Intervertebral disc

Anterior longitudinal ligament

Posterior longitudinal ligament

Inferior articular process

Capsule of zygapophyseal joint (*partially opened*)

Superior articular process

Transverse process

Spinous process

Ligamentum flavum

Interspinous ligament

Supraspinous ligament

Intervertebral foramen

Anterior vertebral segments: posterior view (*pedicles sectioned*)

Pedicle (*cut surface*)

Posterior surface of vertebral bodies

Posterior longitudinal ligament

Intervertebral disc

Posterior vertebral segments: anterior view

Pedicle (*cut surface*)

Ligamentum flavum

Lamina

Superior articular process

Transverse process

Inferior articular facet

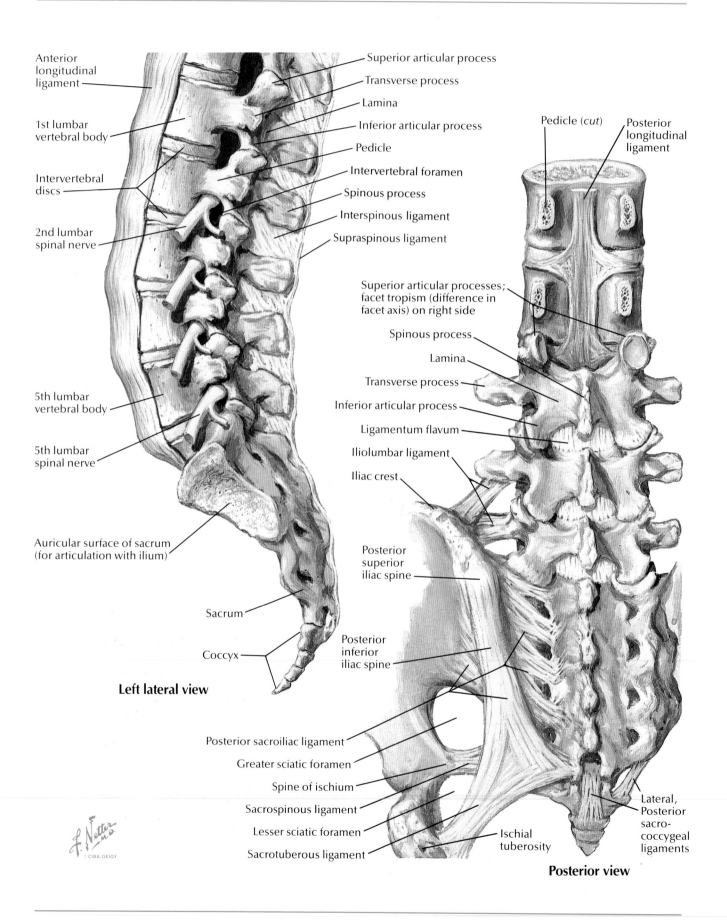

Anterior longitudinal ligament

1st lumbar vertebral body

Intervertebral discs

2nd lumbar spinal nerve

5th lumbar vertebral body

5th lumbar spinal nerve

Auricular surface of sacrum (for articulation with ilium)

Sacrum

Coccyx

Left lateral view

Superior articular process

Transverse process

Lamina

Inferior articular process

Pedicle

Intervertebral foramen

Spinous process

Interspinous ligament

Supraspinous ligament

Pedicle (cut)

Posterior longitudinal ligament

Superior articular processes; facet tropism (difference in facet axis) on right side

Spinous process

Lamina

Transverse process

Inferior articular process

Ligamentum flavum

Iliolumbar ligament

Iliac crest

Posterior superior iliac spine

Posterior inferior iliac spine

Posterior sacroiliac ligament

Greater sciatic foramen

Spine of ischium

Sacrospinous ligament

Lesser sciatic foramen

Sacrotuberous ligament

Ischial tuberosity

Lateral, Posterior sacro-coccygeal ligaments

Posterior view

PLATE 147

BACK AND SPINAL CORD

Base of skull

1st cervical nerve

2nd cervical vertebra (axis)

8th cervical nerve

1st thoracic nerve

1st rib

Intercostal nerves

12th thoracic nerve

12th rib

Subcostal nerve

Conus medullaris

1st lumbar nerve

Cauda equina

5th lumbar nerve

1st sacral nerve

Sacrum (*cut away*)

Internal filum terminale (pial)

Termination of dural sac

External filum terminale (dural)

5th sacral nerve

Coccygeal nerve

1st cervical vertebra (atlas)

Cervical plexus

7th cervical vertebra

1st thoracic vertebra

Brachial plexus

Spinal dura mater

Filaments of spinal nerve roots (T7 and T8)

12th thoracic vertebra

1st lumbar vertebra

Iliohypogastric nerve

Ilioinguinal nerve

Lumbar plexus

5th lumbar vertebra

Femoral nerve

Sacral plexus

Superior and inferior gluteal nerves

Sciatic nerve

Posterior femoral cutaneous nerve

Pudendal nerve

Coccyx

©CIBA-GEIGY

Relation of Spinal Nerve Roots to Vertebrae

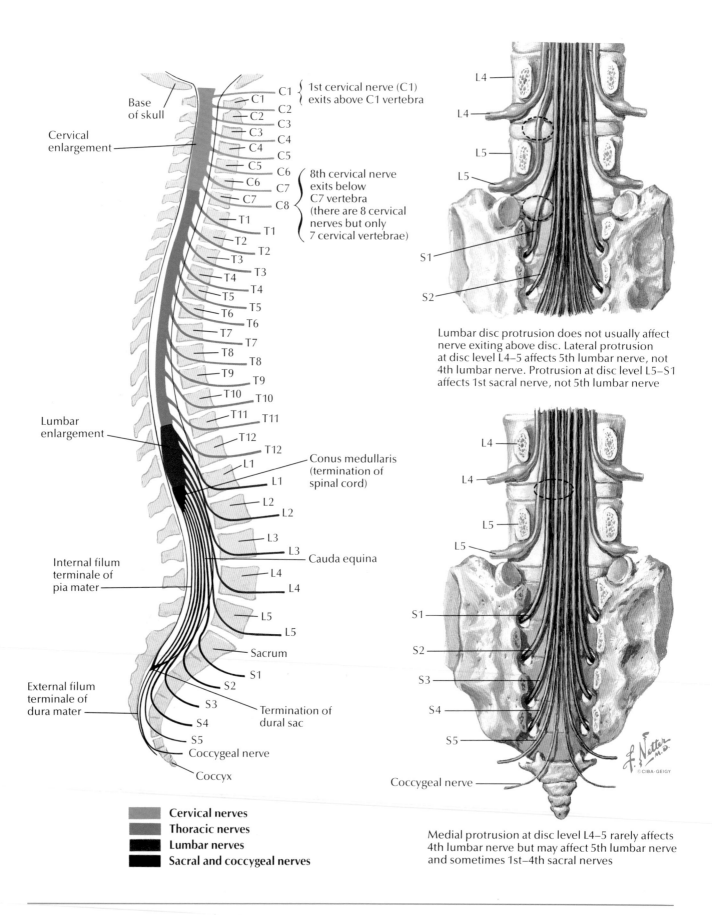

Base of skull

Cervical enlargement

C1 — 1st cervical nerve (C1) exits above C1 vertebra

8th cervical nerve exits below C7 vertebra (there are 8 cervical nerves but only 7 cervical vertebrae)

Lumbar enlargement

Conus medullaris (termination of spinal cord)

Cauda equina

Internal filum terminale of pia mater

Sacrum

Termination of dural sac

External filum terminale of dura mater

Coccygeal nerve

Coccyx

Cervical nerves
Thoracic nerves
Lumbar nerves
Sacral and coccygeal nerves

Lumbar disc protrusion does not usually affect nerve exiting above disc. Lateral protrusion at disc level L4–5 affects 5th lumbar nerve, not 4th lumbar nerve. Protrusion at disc level L5–S1 affects 1st sacral nerve, not 5th lumbar nerve

Medial protrusion at disc level L4–5 rarely affects 4th lumbar nerve but may affect 5th lumbar nerve and sometimes 1st–4th sacral nerves

PLATE 149

BACK AND SPINAL CORD

Schematic demarcation of dermatomes shown as distinct segments. There is actually considerable overlap between any two adjacent dermatomes

Levels of principal dermatomes

C5	Clavicles
C5, 6, 7	Lateral parts of upper limbs
C8, T1	Medial sides of upper limbs
C6	Thumb
C6, 7, 8	Hand
C8	Ring and little fingers
T4	Level of nipples
T10	Level of umbilicus
T12	Inguinal or groin regions
L1, 2, 3, 4	Anterior and inner surfaces of lower limbs
L4, 5, S1	Foot
L4	Medial side of great toe
S1, 2, L5	Posterior and outer surfaces of lower limbs
S1	Lateral margin of foot and little toe
S2, 3, 4	Perineum

Spinal Cord Cross Sections: Fiber Tracts

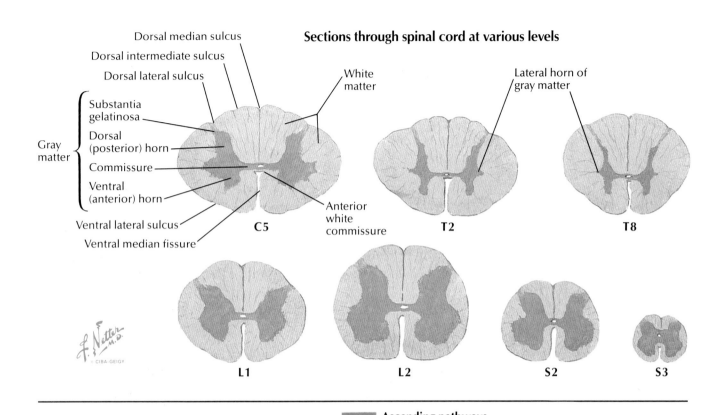

Sections through spinal cord at various levels

Dorsal median sulcus

Dorsal intermediate sulcus

Dorsal lateral sulcus

White matter

Lateral horn of gray matter

Gray matter
- Substantia gelatinosa
- Dorsal (posterior) horn
- Commissure
- Ventral (anterior) horn

Ventral lateral sulcus

Ventral median fissure

Anterior white commissure

C5   **T2**   **T8**

L1   **L2**   **S2**   **S3**

Principal fiber tracts of spinal cord

Ascending pathways
Descending pathways
Fibers passing in both directions

Fasciculus gracilis

Fasciculus cuneatus

Dorsolateral tract (fasciculus) (of Lissauer)

Dorsal (posterior) spinocerebellar tract

Lateral spinothalamic tract and spinoreticular tract

Ventral (anterior) spinocerebellar tract

Spinoolivary tract

Spinotectal tract

Ventral (anterior) spinothalamic tract

Fasciculus proprius

Septomarginal fasciculus (oval bundle)

Interfascicular fasciculus (comma tract)

Lateral corticospinal (pyramidal) tract (crossed)

Rubrospinal tract

Lateral (medullary) reticulospinal tract

Ventral (anterior) or medial (pontine) reticulospinal tract

Vestibulospinal tract

Ventral (anterior) corticospinal tract (direct)

Tectospinal tract

Medial longitudinal (sulcomarginal) fasciculi

PLATE 151

BACK AND SPINAL CORD

Autonomic Nervous System: General Topography

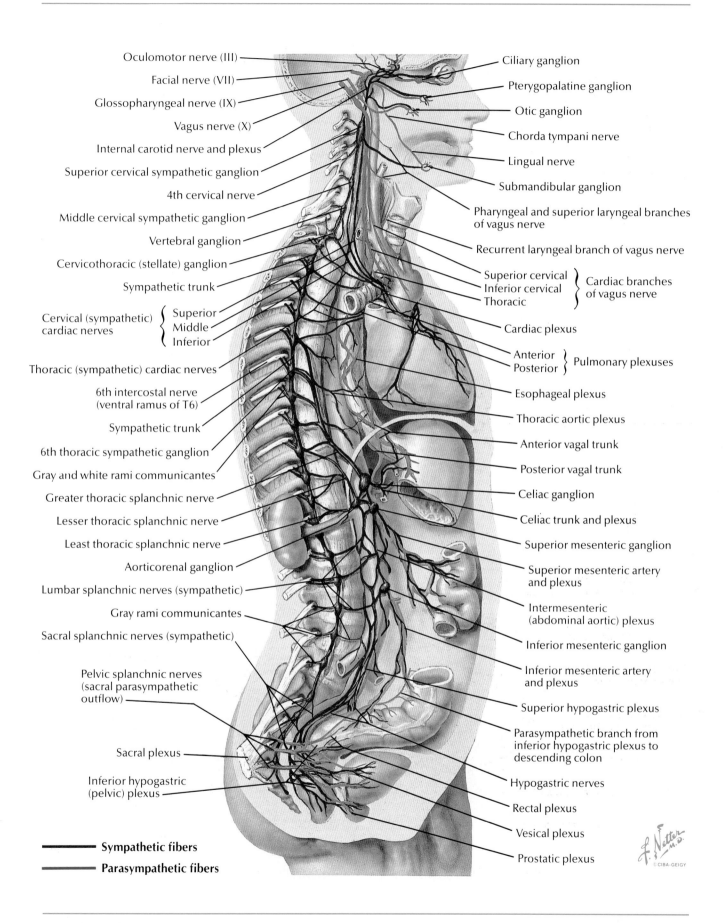

Oculomotor nerve (III)
Facial nerve (VII)
Glossopharyngeal nerve (IX)
Vagus nerve (X)
Internal carotid nerve and plexus
Superior cervical sympathetic ganglion
4th cervical nerve
Middle cervical sympathetic ganglion
Vertebral ganglion
Cervicothoracic (stellate) ganglion
Sympathetic trunk
Cervical (sympathetic) cardiac nerves { Superior Middle Inferior
Thoracic (sympathetic) cardiac nerves
6th intercostal nerve (ventral ramus of T6)
Sympathetic trunk
6th thoracic sympathetic ganglion
Gray and white rami communicantes
Greater thoracic splanchnic nerve
Lesser thoracic splanchnic nerve
Least thoracic splanchnic nerve
Aorticorenal ganglion
Lumbar splanchnic nerves (sympathetic)
Gray rami communicantes
Sacral splanchnic nerves (sympathetic)
Pelvic splanchnic nerves (sacral parasympathetic outflow)
Sacral plexus
Inferior hypogastric (pelvic) plexus

Ciliary ganglion
Pterygopalatine ganglion
Otic ganglion
Chorda tympani nerve
Lingual nerve
Submandibular ganglion
Pharyngeal and superior laryngeal branches of vagus nerve
Recurrent laryngeal branch of vagus nerve
Superior cervical Inferior cervical Thoracic } Cardiac branches of vagus nerve
Cardiac plexus
Anterior Posterior } Pulmonary plexuses
Esophageal plexus
Thoracic aortic plexus
Anterior vagal trunk
Posterior vagal trunk
Celiac ganglion
Celiac trunk and plexus
Superior mesenteric ganglion
Superior mesenteric artery and plexus
Intermesenteric (abdominal aortic) plexus
Inferior mesenteric ganglion
Inferior mesenteric artery and plexus
Superior hypogastric plexus
Parasympathetic branch from inferior hypogastric plexus to descending colon
Hypogastric nerves
Rectal plexus
Vesical plexus
Prostatic plexus

——— Sympathetic fibers
——— Parasympathetic fibers

Autonomic Nervous System: Schema

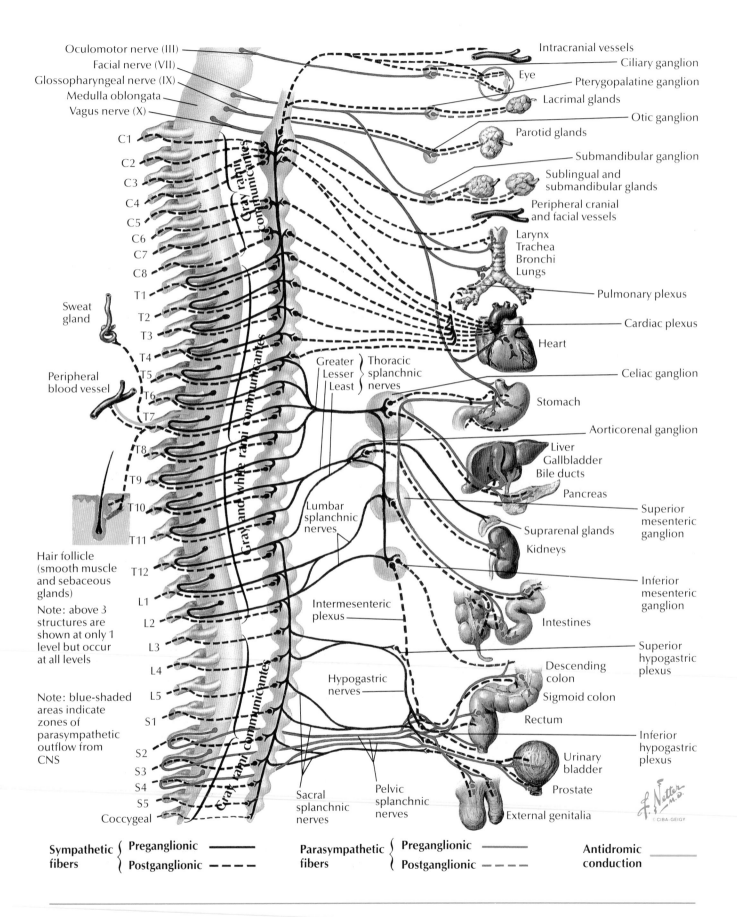

Oculomotor nerve (III)
Facial nerve (VII)
Glossopharyngeal nerve (IX)
Medulla oblongata
Vagus nerve (X)

Intracranial vessels
Ciliary ganglion
Eye
Pterygopalatine ganglion
Lacrimal glands
Otic ganglion
Parotid glands
Submandibular ganglion
Sublingual and submandibular glands
Peripheral cranial and facial vessels
Larynx Trachea Bronchi Lungs
Pulmonary plexus
Cardiac plexus
Heart
Celiac ganglion
Stomach
Aorticorenal ganglion
Liver Gallbladder Bile ducts
Pancreas
Superior mesenteric ganglion
Suprarenal glands
Kidneys
Inferior mesenteric ganglion
Intestines
Superior hypogastric plexus
Descending colon
Sigmoid colon
Rectum
Inferior hypogastric plexus
Urinary bladder
Prostate
External genitalia

C1
C2
C3
C4
C5
C6
C7
C8
T1
T2
T3
T4
T5
T6
T7
T8
T9
T10
T11
T12
L1
L2
L3
L4
L5
S1
S2
S3
S4
S5
Coccygeal

Gray rami communicantes
Gray and white rami communicantes
Gray rami communicantes

Sweat gland

Peripheral blood vessel

Greater Lesser Least } Thoracic splanchnic nerves

Lumbar splanchnic nerves

Intermesenteric plexus

Hypogastric nerves

Sacral splanchnic nerves
Pelvic splanchnic nerves

Hair follicle (smooth muscle and sebaceous glands)

Note: above 3 structures are shown at only 1 level but occur at all levels

Note: blue-shaded areas indicate zones of parasympathetic outflow from CNS

Sympathetic fibers { Preganglionic ——— Postganglionic – – –

Parasympathetic fibers { Preganglionic ——— Postganglionic – – –

Antidromic conduction

PLATE 153

BACK AND SPINAL CORD

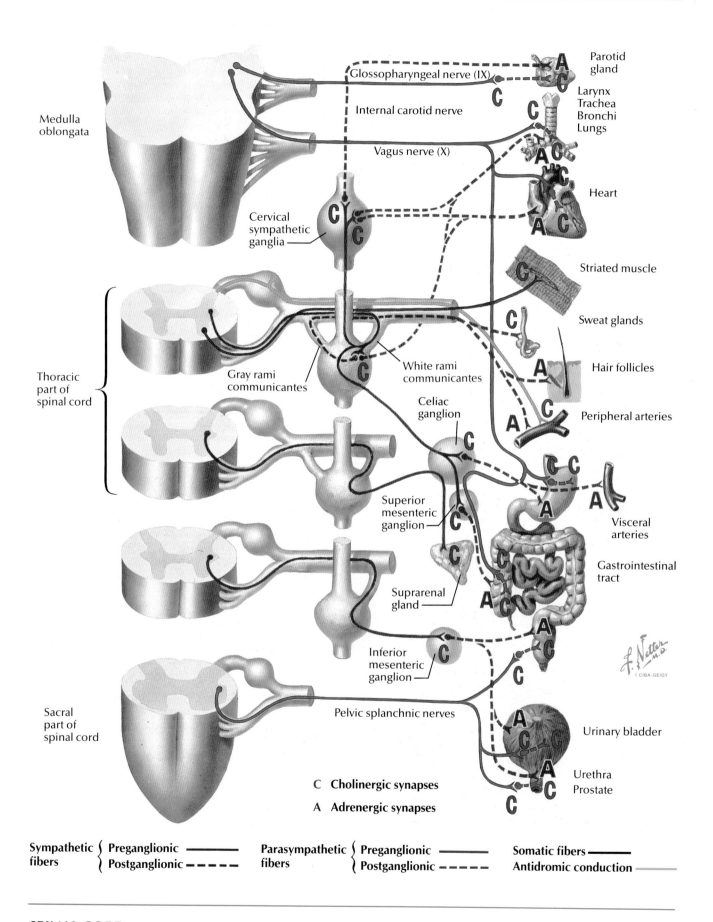

Medulla oblongata

Glossopharyngeal nerve (IX)

Internal carotid nerve

Vagus nerve (X)

Cervical sympathetic ganglia

Thoracic part of spinal cord

Gray rami communicantes

White rami communicantes

Celiac ganglion

Superior mesenteric ganglion

Suprarenal gland

Inferior mesenteric ganglion

Sacral part of spinal cord

Pelvic splanchnic nerves

Parotid gland

Larynx Trachea Bronchi Lungs

Heart

Striated muscle

Sweat glands

Hair follicles

Peripheral arteries

Visceral arteries

Gastrointestinal tract

Urinary bladder

Urethra Prostate

C **Cholinergic synapses**

A **Adrenergic synapses**

Sympathetic fibers { **Preganglionic** —— **Postganglionic** - - - -   **Parasympathetic fibers** { **Preganglionic** —— **Postganglionic** - - - -   **Somatic fibers** —— **Antidromic conduction** ——

Spinal Membranes and Nerve Roots

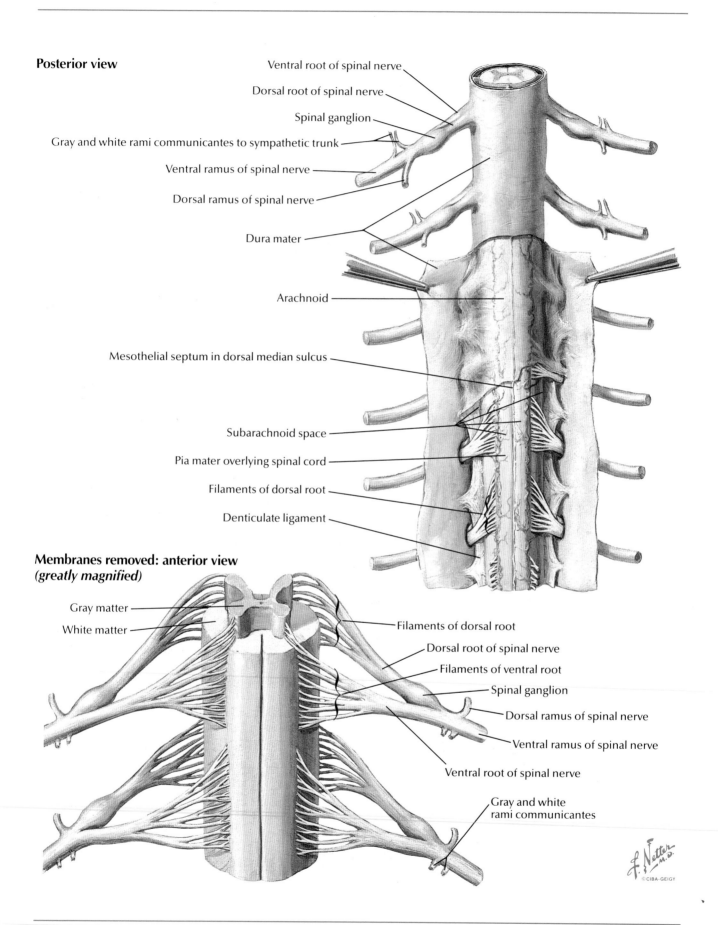

Posterior view

Ventral root of spinal nerve

Dorsal root of spinal nerve

Spinal ganglion

Gray and white rami communicantes to sympathetic trunk

Ventral ramus of spinal nerve

Dorsal ramus of spinal nerve

Dura mater

Arachnoid

Mesothelial septum in dorsal median sulcus

Subarachnoid space

Pia mater overlying spinal cord

Filaments of dorsal root

Denticulate ligament

Membranes removed: anterior view
(greatly magnified)

Gray matter

White matter

Filaments of dorsal root

Dorsal root of spinal nerve

Filaments of ventral root

Spinal ganglion

Dorsal ramus of spinal nerve

Ventral ramus of spinal nerve

Ventral root of spinal nerve

Gray and white
rami communicantes

PLATE 155

BACK AND SPINAL CORD

Section through thoracic vertebra

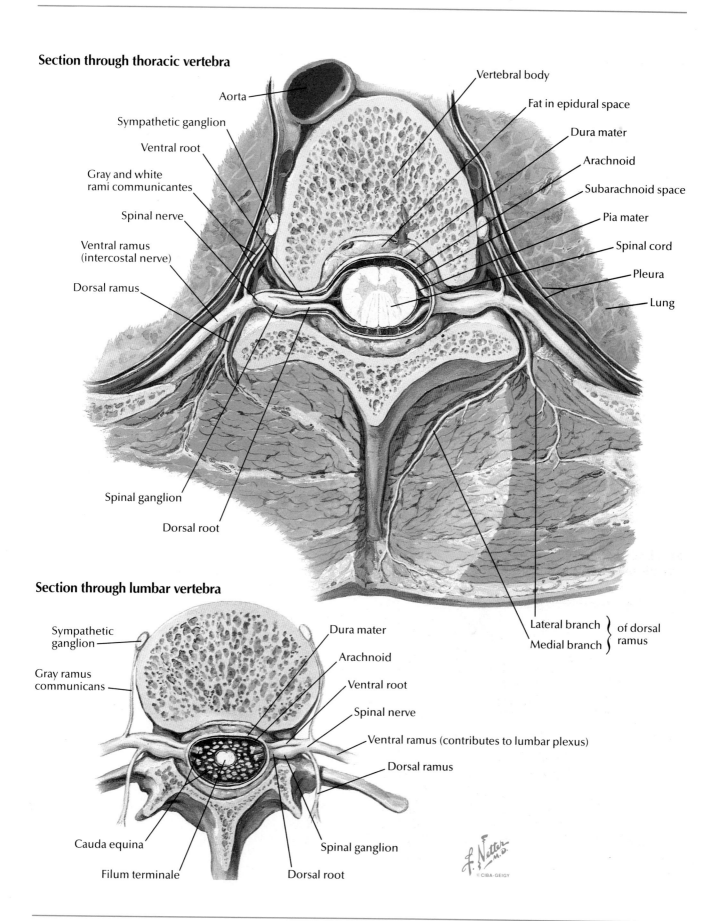

Aorta

Sympathetic ganglion

Ventral root

Gray and white rami communicantes

Spinal nerve

Ventral ramus (intercostal nerve)

Dorsal ramus

Spinal ganglion

Dorsal root

Vertebral body

Fat in epidural space

Dura mater

Arachnoid

Subarachnoid space

Pia mater

Spinal cord

Pleura

Lung

Lateral branch } of dorsal
Medial branch } ramus

Section through lumbar vertebra

Sympathetic ganglion

Gray ramus communicans

Cauda equina

Filum terminale

Dura mater

Arachnoid

Ventral root

Spinal nerve

Ventral ramus (contributes to lumbar plexus)

Dorsal ramus

Spinal ganglion

Dorsal root

Arteries of Spinal Cord: Schema

SEE ALSO PLATE 131

Anterior view

Posterior view

Posterior cerebral artery

Superior cerebellar artery

Basilar artery

Anterior inferior cerebellar artery

Posterior inferior cerebellar artery

Anterior spinal artery

Vertebral artery

Anterior radicular arteries

Ascending cervical artery

Deep cervical artery

Subclavian artery

Anterior radicular artery

Posterior intercostal artery

Pial plexus

Artery of Adamkiewicz (major anterior radicular artery)

Posterior intercostal artery

Anterior radicular artery

Lumbar artery

Anastomotic loops to posterior spinal arteries

Cauda equina arteries

Lateral (or middle) sacral artery

Cervical vertebrae

Thoracic vertebrae

Lumbar vertebrae

Sacrum

Posterior inferior cerebellar artery

Posterior spinal arteries

Vertebral artery

Posterior radicular arteries

Deep cervical artery

Ascending cervical artery

Subclavian artery

Posterior radicular arteries

Posterior intercostal arteries

Posterior radicular arteries

Lumbar arteries

Anastomotic loops to anterior spinal artery

Lateral (or middle) sacral artery

PLATE 157

Posterior spinal arteries

Anterior spinal artery

Anterior radicular artery

Posterior radicular artery

Branch to vertebral body
and dura mater

Spinal branch

Dorsal branch of
posterior intercostal artery

Posterior intercostal artery

Paravertebral anastomoses

Prevertebral anastomoses

Aorta

**Section through thoracic level:
anterosuperior view**

Sulcal (central) branches
to right side of spinal cord

Anterior radicular artery

Pial arterial plexus

Posterior radicular artery

Anterior spinal artery

Arterial distribution: schema

Right posterior spinal artery

Peripheral branches from pial plexus

Sulcal (central) branches
to left side of spinal cord

Left posterior spinal artery

Zone supplied by penetrating
branches from pial plexus

Zone supplied by central branches

Zone supplied by both
central branches and branches
from pial plexus

Posterior radicular artery

Anterior radicular artery

Pial arterial plexus

Veins of Spinal Cord

Anterior external venous plexus

Anterior internal venous plexus

Basivertebral vein

Posterior internal venous plexus

Intervertebral vein

Posterior external venous plexus

Anterior external venous plexus

Basivertebral vein

Anterior internal venous plexus

Anterior and posterior radicular veins

Intervertebral vein

Posterior internal venous plexus

Posterior external venous plexus

Anterior spinal vein

Anterior sulcal (central) vein

Basivertebral vein

Anterior internal venous plexus

Intervertebral vein

Anterior radicular vein

Posterior radicular vein

Pial venous plexus

Posterior sulcal (central) vein

Posterior spinal vein

Posterior internal venous plexus

PLATE 159

BACK AND SPINAL CORD

Muscles of Back: Superficial Layers

Superior nuchal line of skull

Spinous process (C2)

Sternocleidomastoid muscle

Posterior (lateral) triangle of neck

Trapezius muscle

Spine of scapula

Deltoid muscle

Infraspinatus fascia

Teres minor muscle

Teres major muscle

Latissimus dorsi muscle

Spinous process (T12)

Thoracolumbar fascia

External abdominal oblique muscle

Internal abdominal oblique muscle in lumbar (Petit's) triangle

Iliac crest

Fascia (gluteal aponeurosis) over gluteus medius muscle

Gluteus maximus muscle

Semispinalis capitis muscle

Splenius capitis muscle

Spinous process (C7)

Splenius cervicis muscle

Levator scapulae muscle

Rhomboideus minor muscle (cut)

Supraspinatus muscle

Serratus posterior superior muscle

Rhomboideus major muscle (cut)

Infraspinatus fascia (over infraspinatus muscle)

Teres minor and major muscles

Latissimus dorsi muscle (cut)

Serratus anterior muscle

Serratus posterior inferior muscle

12th rib

Erector spinae muscle

External abdominal oblique muscle

Internal abdominal oblique muscle

MUSCLES AND NERVES

PLATE 160

Muscles of Back: Intermediate Layers

Superior nuchal line of skull

Posterior tubercle of atlas (C1)

Longissimus capitis muscle

Semispinalis capitis muscle

Splenius capitis and splenius cervicis muscles

Serratus posterior superior muscle

Erector spinae muscle
- Iliocostalis muscle
- Longissimus muscle
- Spinalis muscle

Serratus posterior inferior muscle

Aponeurosis of transversus abdominis muscle

Internal abdominal oblique muscle

External abdominal oblique muscle (cut)

Iliac crest

Rectus capitis posterior minor muscle

Superior obliquus capitis muscle

Rectus capitis posterior major muscle

Inferior obliquus capitis muscle

Longissimus capitis muscle

Semispinalis capitis muscle (cut)

Spinalis cervicis muscle

Spinous process (C7)

Longissimus cervicis muscle

Iliocostalis cervicis muscle

Iliocostalis thoracis muscle

Hook

Spinalis thoracis muscle

Longissimus thoracis muscle

Iliocostalis lumborum muscle

Spinous process (T12)

Transversus abdominis muscle and aponeurosis

Thoracolumbar fascia (cut edge)

PLATE 161

BACK AND SPINAL CORD

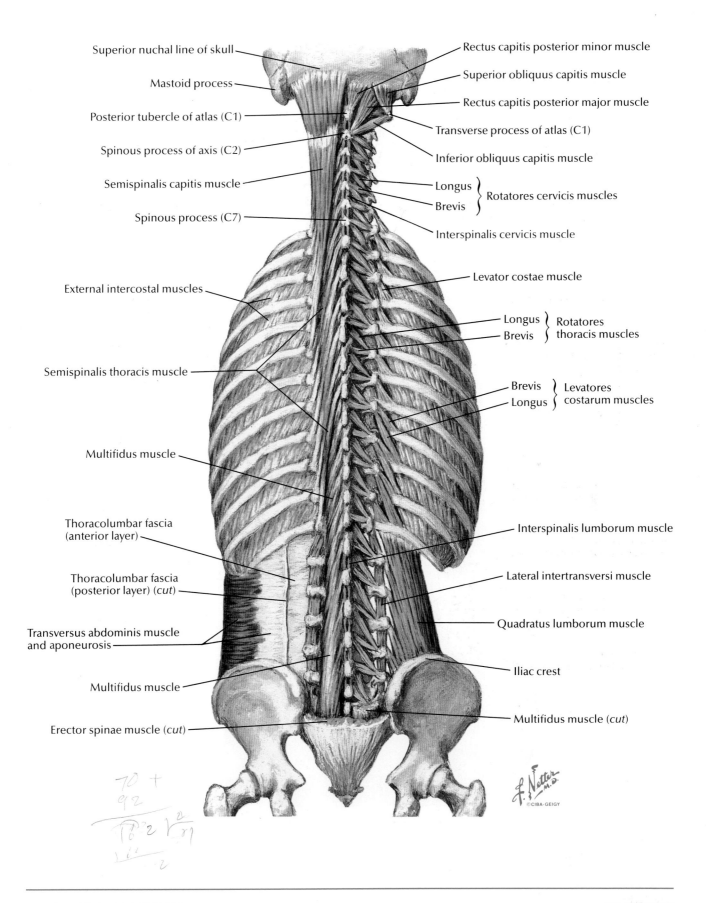

Superior nuchal line of skull

Mastoid process

Posterior tubercle of atlas (C1)

Spinous process of axis (C2)

Semispinalis capitis muscle

Spinous process (C7)

External intercostal muscles

Semispinalis thoracis muscle

Multifidus muscle

Thoracolumbar fascia (anterior layer)

Thoracolumbar fascia (posterior layer) (cut)

Transversus abdominis muscle and aponeurosis

Multifidus muscle

Erector spinae muscle (cut)

Rectus capitis posterior minor muscle

Superior obliquus capitis muscle

Rectus capitis posterior major muscle

Transverse process of atlas (C1)

Inferior obliquus capitis muscle

Longus } Rotatores cervicis muscles
Brevis }

Interspinalis cervicis muscle

Levator costae muscle

Longus } Rotatores
Brevis } thoracis muscles

Brevis } Levatores
Longus } costarum muscles

Interspinalis lumborum muscle

Lateral intertransversi muscle

Quadratus lumborum muscle

Iliac crest

Multifidus muscle (cut)

Nerves of Back

SEE ALSO PLATES 166, 179, 237, 241

Accessory nerve (XI)

Trapezius muscle (*reflected*)

Levator scapulae muscle

Transverse cervical artery (descending branch) and vein

Subtrapezial plexus

Supraspinatus muscle

Spine of scapula

Infraspinatus fascia

Rhomboideus minor muscle

Rhomboideus major muscle

Latissimus dorsi muscle

Spinous process of 12th thoracic vertebra

Thoracolumbar fascia

Gluteus maximus muscle

Greater occipital nerve (dorsal ramus of C2)

3rd occipital nerve (dorsal ramus of C3)

Lesser occipital nerve } Cervical plexus (ventral rami of C2, 3)

Great auricular nerve }

Trapezius muscle

Spinal nerves (medial cutaneous branches of dorsal rami of C4–T6; C7, 8 are minimal)

Deltoid muscle

Infraspinatus fascia

Teres minor and major muscles

Superior lateral brachial cutaneous nerve from axillary nerve (C5, 6)

Spinal nerves (lateral cutaneous branches of dorsal rami of T7–12)

Spinal nerves (lateral cutaneous branches of ventral intercostal rami)

External abdominal oblique muscle

Iliac crest

Iliohypogastric nerve (ventral ramus of L1)

Superior cluneal nerves (dorsal rami of L1, 2, 3)

Middle cluneal nerves (dorsal rami of S1, 2, 3)

Inferior cluneal nerves from posterior femoral cutaneous nerve (S1, 2, 3)

f. Netter m.d.

©CIBA-GEIGY

PLATE 163

BACK AND SPINAL CORD

Rectus capitis posterior minor muscle

Rectus capitis posterior major muscle

Semispinalis capitis muscle
(*cut and reflected*)

Vertebral artery

Superior obliquus
capitis muscle

Suboccipital nerve
(dorsal ramus of C1)

Posterior arch
of atlas (C1)

Occipital artery

Inferior obliquus
capitis muscle

Dorsal ramus of C2

Splenius capitis muscle
(*cut and reflected*)

Dorsal ramus of C3

Longissimus capitis muscle

Splenius cervicis muscle

Semispinalis cervicis muscle

Semispinalis capitis muscle (*cut*)

Splenius capitis muscle (*cut*)

Galea aponeurotica

Occipital belly (occipitalis) of
epicranius muscle

Greater occipital nerve
(dorsal ramus of C2)

Occipital artery

3rd occipital nerve
(dorsal ramus of C3)

Semispinalis capitis
and splenius capitis
muscles in posterior
(lateral) triangle of neck

Posterior auricular artery

Great auricular nerve
(cervical plexus C2, 3)

Lesser occipital nerve
(cervical plexus C2, 3)

Sternocleidomastoid muscle

Trapezius muscle

Medial cutaneous branches
of dorsal rami of C4, 5, 6

MUSCLES AND NERVES

PLATE 164

Lumbar Region of Back: Cross Section

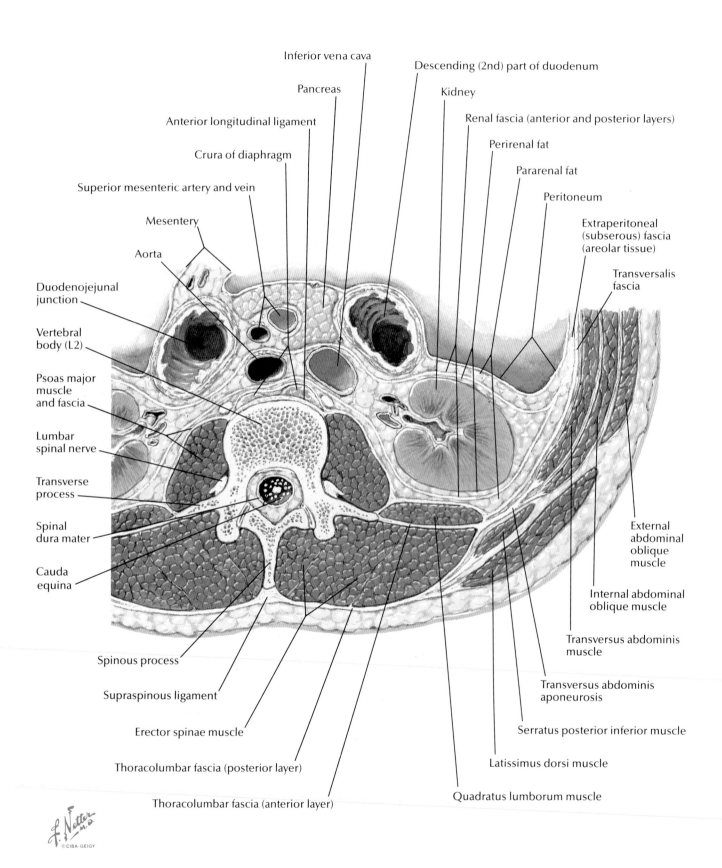

Inferior vena cava

Pancreas

Descending (2nd) part of duodenum

Kidney

Anterior longitudinal ligament

Renal fascia (anterior and posterior layers)

Crura of diaphragm

Perirenal fat

Superior mesenteric artery and vein

Pararenal fat

Mesentery

Peritoneum

Aorta

Extraperitoneal (subserous) fascia (areolar tissue)

Duodenojejunal junction

Transversalis fascia

Vertebral body (L2)

Psoas major muscle and fascia

Lumbar spinal nerve

Transverse process

Spinal dura mater

Cauda equina

External abdominal oblique muscle

Internal abdominal oblique muscle

Spinous process

Transversus abdominis muscle

Supraspinous ligament

Transversus abdominis aponeurosis

Erector spinae muscle

Serratus posterior inferior muscle

Thoracolumbar fascia (posterior layer)

Latissimus dorsi muscle

Thoracolumbar fascia (anterior layer)

Quadratus lumborum muscle

PLATE 165

BACK AND SPINAL CORD

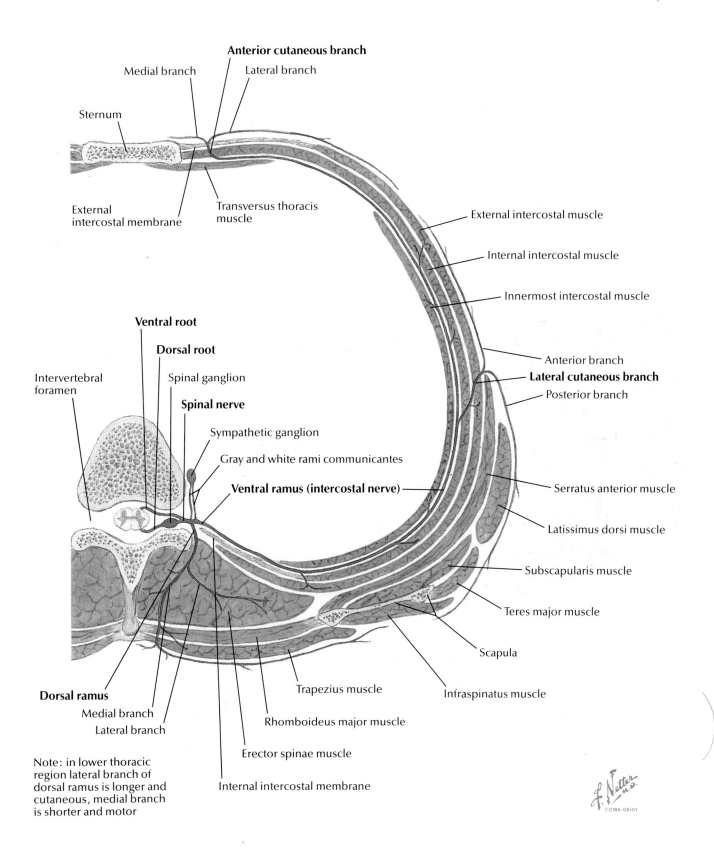

Anterior cutaneous branch

Medial branch

Lateral branch

Sternum

External intercostal membrane

Transversus thoracis muscle

External intercostal muscle

Internal intercostal muscle

Innermost intercostal muscle

Ventral root

Dorsal root

Spinal ganglion

Spinal nerve

Sympathetic ganglion

Gray and white rami communicantes

Ventral ramus (intercostal nerve)

Intervertebral foramen

Anterior branch

Lateral cutaneous branch

Posterior branch

Serratus anterior muscle

Latissimus dorsi muscle

Subscapularis muscle

Teres major muscle

Scapula

Infraspinatus muscle

Dorsal ramus

Medial branch

Lateral branch

Trapezius muscle

Rhomboideus major muscle

Erector spinae muscle

Internal intercostal membrane

Note: in lower thoracic region lateral branch of dorsal ramus is longer and cutaneous, medial branch is shorter and motor

Section III

THORAX

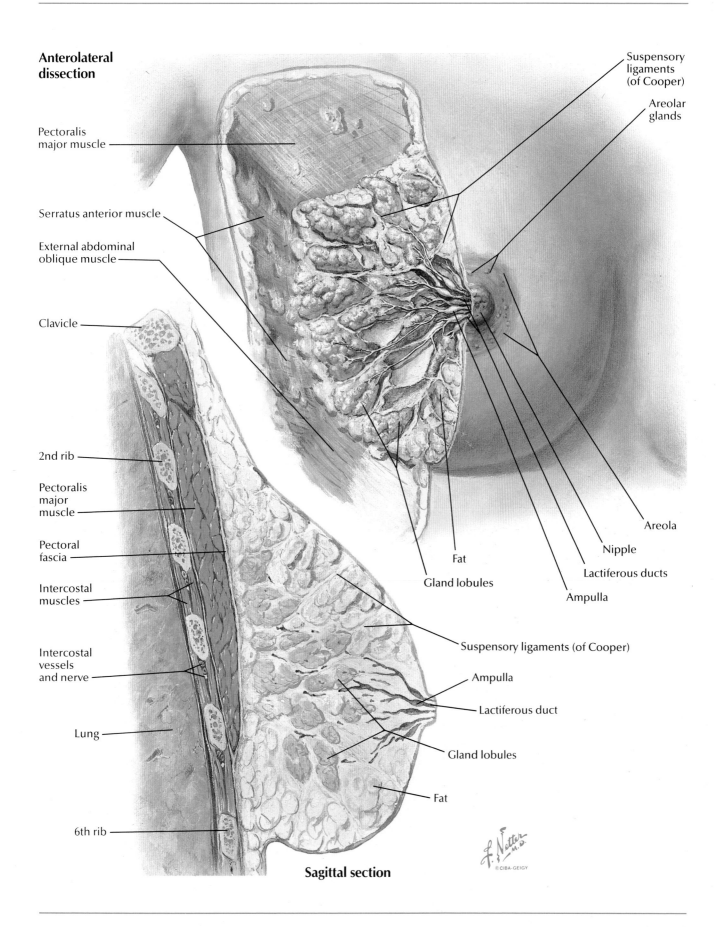

Anterolateral dissection

Pectoralis major muscle

Serratus anterior muscle

External abdominal oblique muscle

Clavicle

2nd rib

Pectoralis major muscle

Pectoral fascia

Intercostal muscles

Intercostal vessels and nerve

Lung

6th rib

Suspensory ligaments (of Cooper)

Areolar glands

Areola

Nipple

Lactiferous ducts

Ampulla

Fat

Gland lobules

Suspensory ligaments (of Cooper)

Ampulla

Lactiferous duct

Gland lobules

Fat

Sagittal section

Arteries of Mammary Gland

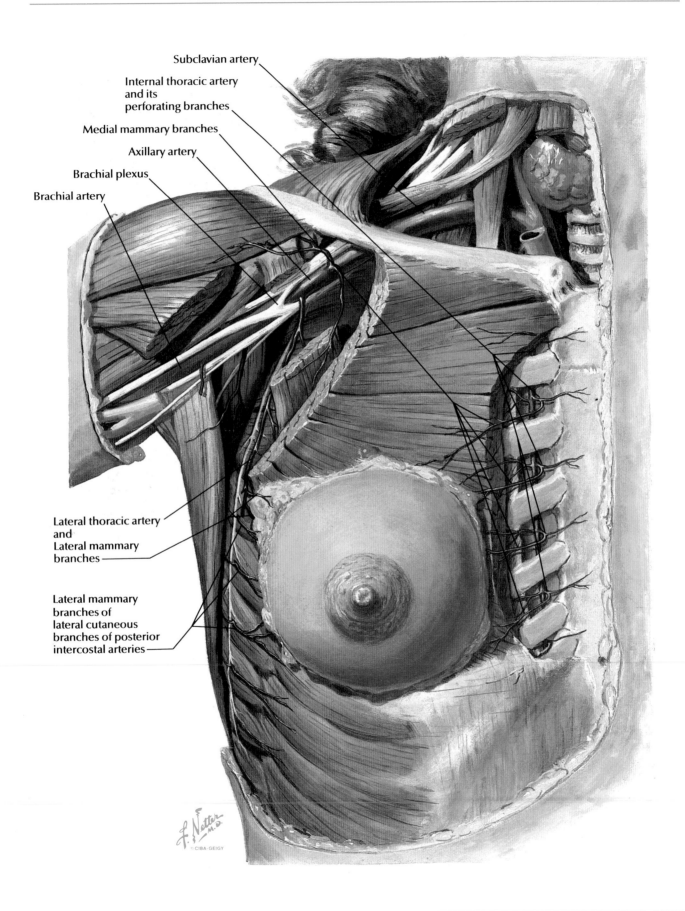

Subclavian artery

Internal thoracic artery and its perforating branches

Medial mammary branches

Axillary artery

Brachial plexus

Brachial artery

Lateral thoracic artery and Lateral mammary branches

Lateral mammary branches of lateral cutaneous branches of posterior intercostal arteries

PLATE 168

THORAX

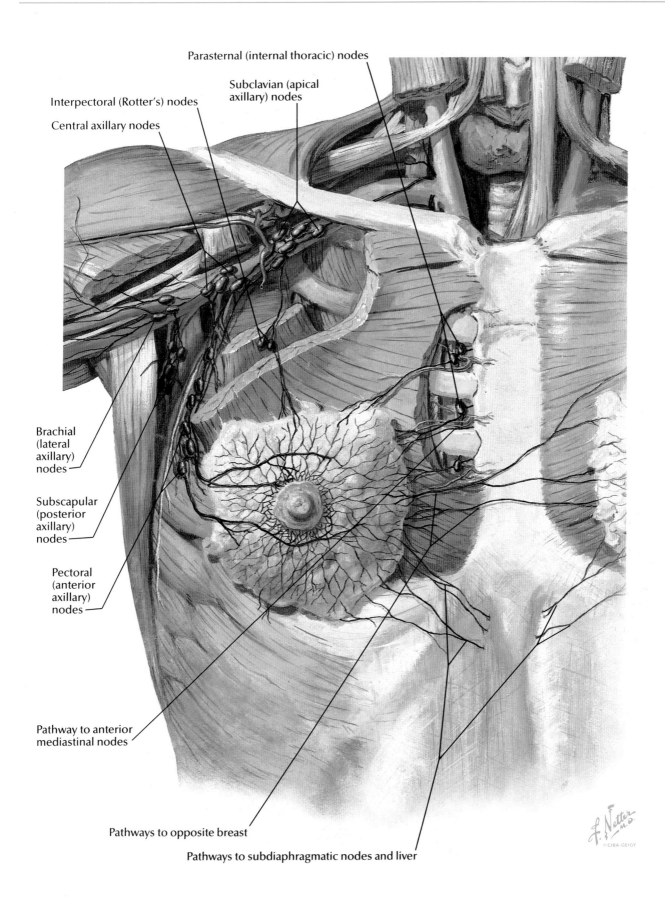

Parasternal (internal thoracic) nodes

Subclavian (apical axillary) nodes

Interpectoral (Rotter's) nodes

Central axillary nodes

Brachial (lateral axillary) nodes

Subscapular (posterior axillary) nodes

Pectoral (anterior axillary) nodes

Pathway to anterior mediastinal nodes

Pathways to opposite breast

Pathways to subdiaphragmatic nodes and liver

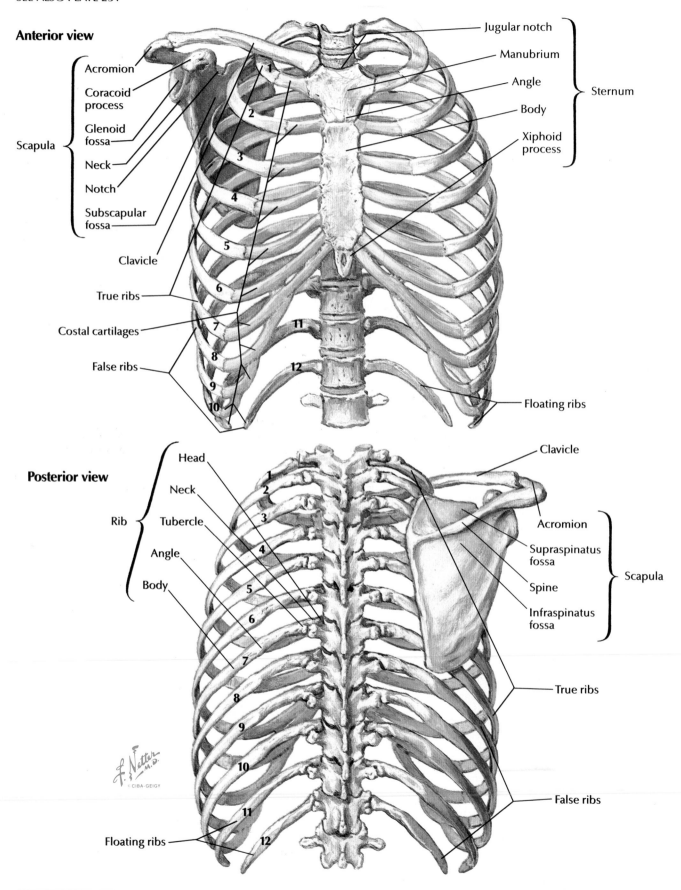

Anterior view

Scapula
- Acromion
- Coracoid process
- Glenoid fossa
- Neck
- Notch
- Subscapular fossa

Clavicle

True ribs

Costal cartilages

False ribs

Jugular notch

Manubrium

Angle

Body

Xiphoid process

Sternum

1
2
3
4
5
6
7
8
9
10
11
12

Floating ribs

Posterior view

Rib
- Head
- Neck
- Tubercle
- Angle
- Body

Clavicle

Acromion

Supraspinatus fossa

Spine

Infraspinatus fossa

Scapula

True ribs

False ribs

Floating ribs

1
2
3
4
5
6
7
8
9
10
11
12

PLATE 170

THORAX

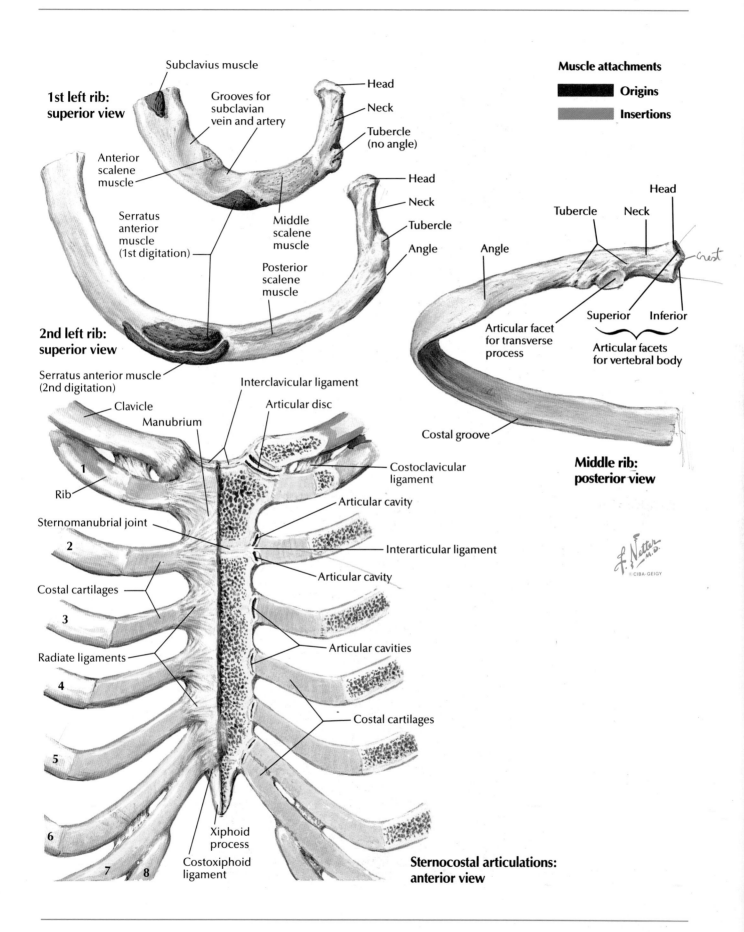

Muscle attachments

▮ **Origins**
▮ **Insertions**

1st left rib: superior view

Subclavius muscle

Grooves for subclavian vein and artery

Anterior scalene muscle

Head

Neck

Tubercle (no angle)

Serratus anterior muscle (1st digitation)

Middle scalene muscle

Head

Neck

Tubercle

Angle

Posterior scalene muscle

2nd left rib: superior view

Serratus anterior muscle (2nd digitation)

Tubercle

Neck

Head

Angle

Articular facet for transverse process

Superior Inferior

Articular facets for vertebral body

crest

Costal groove

Middle rib: posterior view

Clavicle

Manubrium

Interclavicular ligament

Articular disc

1

Rib

Sternomanubrial joint

2

Costal cartilages

3

Radiate ligaments

4

5

6

7 8

Xiphoid process

Costoxiphoid ligament

Costoclavicular ligament

Articular cavity

Interarticular ligament

Articular cavity

Articular cavities

Costal cartilages

Sternocostal articulations: anterior view

F. Netter M.D.
© CIBA-GEIGY

Costovertebral Joints

SEE ALSO PLATE 143

Anterior longitudinal ligament

Inferior costal articular facet for head of rib

Interarticular ligament

Superior costal articular facet for head of rib

Radiate ligament

Costal facet of transverse process for tubercle of rib

Lateral costotransverse ligament

Intertransverse ligament

Superior costotransverse ligament

Left lateral view

Superior costovertebral articular facet of rib head

Interarticular ligament

Radiate ligament

Synovial cavities

Superior costotransverse ligament (*cut*)

Costotransverse ligament

Lateral costotransverse ligament

Transverse section: superior view

Superior costal articular facet for head of rib

Transverse process (*cut off*)

Radiate ligament

Costotransverse ligament

Lateral costotransverse ligament

Superior costotransverse ligament

Intertransverse ligament

Right posterolateral view

PLATE 172

THORAX

Scalene muscles
Anterior
Middle

Cervical rib compresses subclavian artery: poststenotic dilatation

Cervical rib adheres to 1st thoracic rib by dense fibrous band

Lowest cord of brachial plexus elevated by cervical rib

C1
C2
C3
C4
C5
C6
C7
T1

C5
C6
C7
C8
T1

Normal morphology

Rudimentary 1st thoracic rib with postfixed brachial plexus

C4
C5
C6
C7
T1

C6
C7
C8
T1
T2

C5
C6
C7
C8
T1

Note: cervical rib also often asymptomatic

Anterior Thoracic Wall

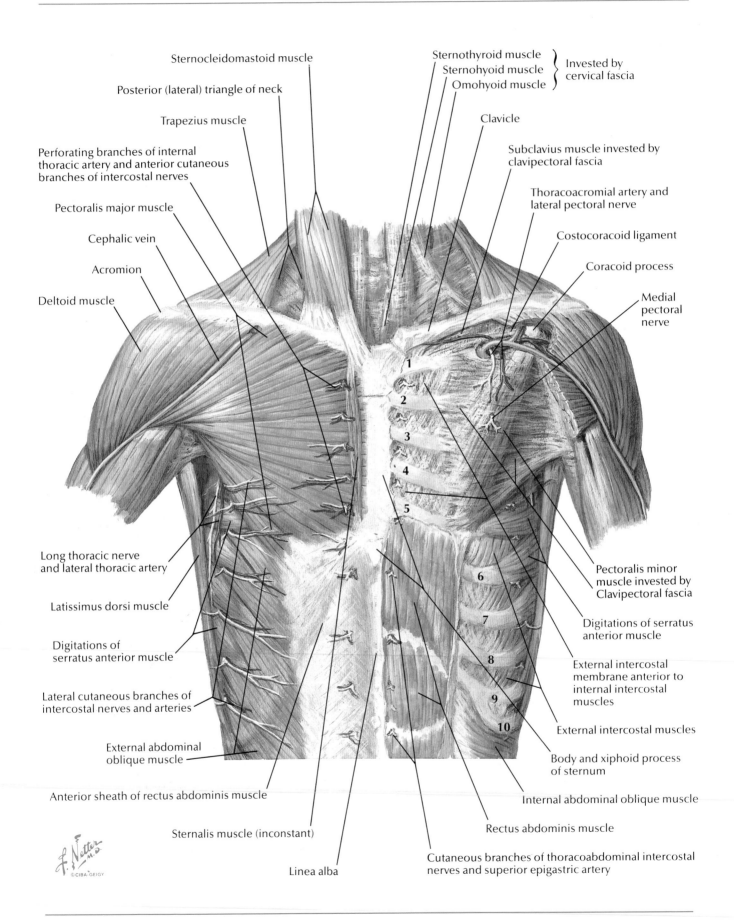

Sternocleidomastoid muscle

Posterior (lateral) triangle of neck

Trapezius muscle

Perforating branches of internal thoracic artery and anterior cutaneous branches of intercostal nerves

Pectoralis major muscle

Cephalic vein

Acromion

Deltoid muscle

Sternothyroid muscle
Sternohyoid muscle } Invested by
Omohyoid muscle } cervical fascia

Clavicle

Subclavius muscle invested by clavipectoral fascia

Thoracoacromial artery and lateral pectoral nerve

Costocoracoid ligament

Coracoid process

Medial pectoral nerve

Long thoracic nerve and lateral thoracic artery

Latissimus dorsi muscle

Digitations of serratus anterior muscle

Lateral cutaneous branches of intercostal nerves and arteries

External abdominal oblique muscle

Anterior sheath of rectus abdominis muscle

Sternalis muscle (inconstant)

Linea alba

Pectoralis minor muscle invested by Clavipectoral fascia

Digitations of serratus anterior muscle

External intercostal membrane anterior to internal intercostal muscles

External intercostal muscles

Body and xiphoid process of sternum

Internal abdominal oblique muscle

Rectus abdominis muscle

Cutaneous branches of thoracoabdominal intercostal nerves and superior epigastric artery

PLATE 174

THORAX

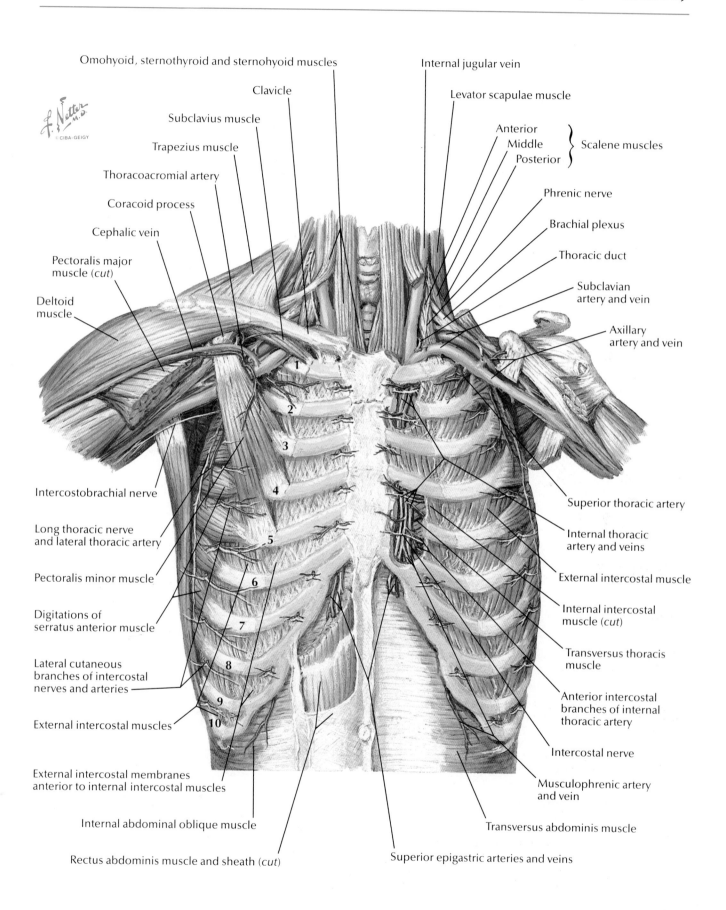

Omohyoid, sternothyroid and sternohyoid muscles

Clavicle

Subclavius muscle

Trapezius muscle

Thoracoacromial artery

Coracoid process

Cephalic vein

Pectoralis major muscle (cut)

Deltoid muscle

Intercostobrachial nerve

Long thoracic nerve and lateral thoracic artery

Pectoralis minor muscle

Digitations of serratus anterior muscle

Lateral cutaneous branches of intercostal nerves and arteries

External intercostal muscles

External intercostal membranes anterior to internal intercostal muscles

Internal abdominal oblique muscle

Rectus abdominis muscle and sheath (cut)

Internal jugular vein

Levator scapulae muscle

Anterior
Middle
Posterior } Scalene muscles

Phrenic nerve

Brachial plexus

Thoracic duct

Subclavian artery and vein

Axillary artery and vein

Superior thoracic artery

Internal thoracic artery and veins

External intercostal muscle

Internal intercostal muscle (cut)

Transversus thoracis muscle

Anterior intercostal branches of internal thoracic artery

Intercostal nerve

Musculophrenic artery and vein

Transversus abdominis muscle

Superior epigastric arteries and veins

Sternothyroid muscle

Sternohyoid muscle

Internal jugular vein

Anterior scalene muscle

Subclavian artery and vein

Clavicle (cut)

Brachiocephalic vein

Phrenic nerve and pericardiacophrenic artery and vein

Internal thoracic artery and vein

Anterior intercostal arteries and veins and intercostal nerve

Perforating branches of internal thoracic artery and vein and anterior cutaneous branch of intercostal nerve

Body of sternum

Diaphragm

Slips of costal origin of diaphragm

Transversus abdominis muscle

Sternal origin of diaphragm

Xiphoid process

Manubrium of sternum

Common carotid artery

Inferior thyroid artery

Vertebral artery

Brachiocephalic trunk

Subclavian artery and vein

Brachiocephalic vein

Internal thoracic artery and vein

Anterior intercostal arteries and veins and intercostal nerve

Internal intercostal muscles

Innermost intercostal muscles

Transversus thoracis muscle

Musculophrenic artery and vein

Transversus abdominis muscle

Internal thoracic artery and veins

Superior epigastric artery and veins

PLATE 176

THORAX

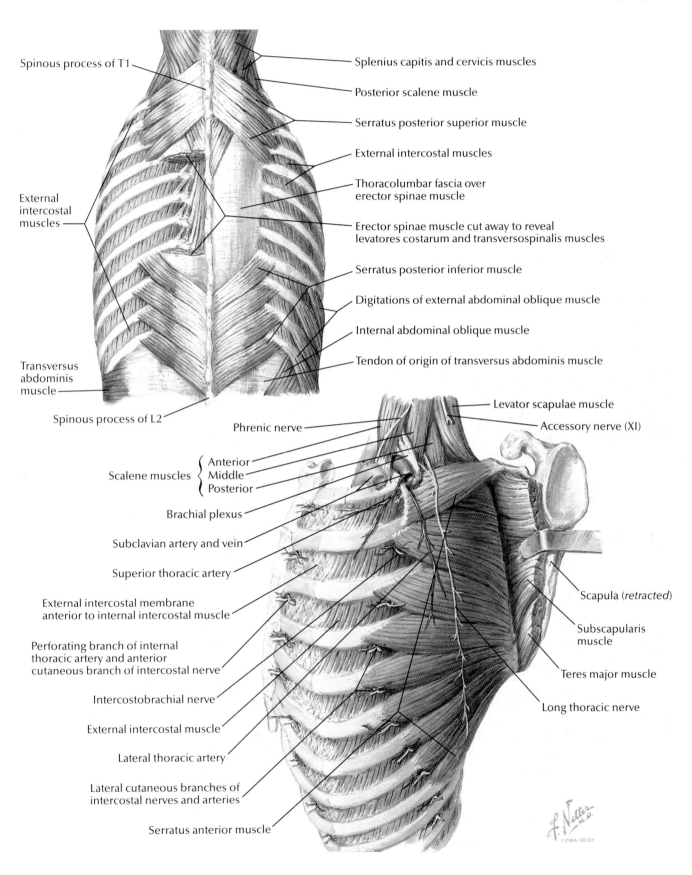

Spinous process of T1

Splenius capitis and cervicis muscles

Posterior scalene muscle

Serratus posterior superior muscle

External intercostal muscles

Thoracolumbar fascia over erector spinae muscle

Erector spinae muscle cut away to reveal levatores costarum and transversospinalis muscles

External intercostal muscles

Serratus posterior inferior muscle

Digitations of external abdominal oblique muscle

Internal abdominal oblique muscle

Tendon of origin of transversus abdominis muscle

Transversus abdominis muscle

Spinous process of L2

Levator scapulae muscle

Phrenic nerve

Accessory nerve (XI)

Scalene muscles { Anterior / Middle / Posterior

Brachial plexus

Subclavian artery and vein

Superior thoracic artery

Scapula (*retracted*)

Subscapularis muscle

External intercostal membrane anterior to internal intercostal muscle

Perforating branch of internal thoracic artery and anterior cutaneous branch of intercostal nerve

Teres major muscle

Intercostobrachial nerve

Long thoracic nerve

External intercostal muscle

Lateral thoracic artery

Lateral cutaneous branches of intercostal nerves and arteries

Serratus anterior muscle

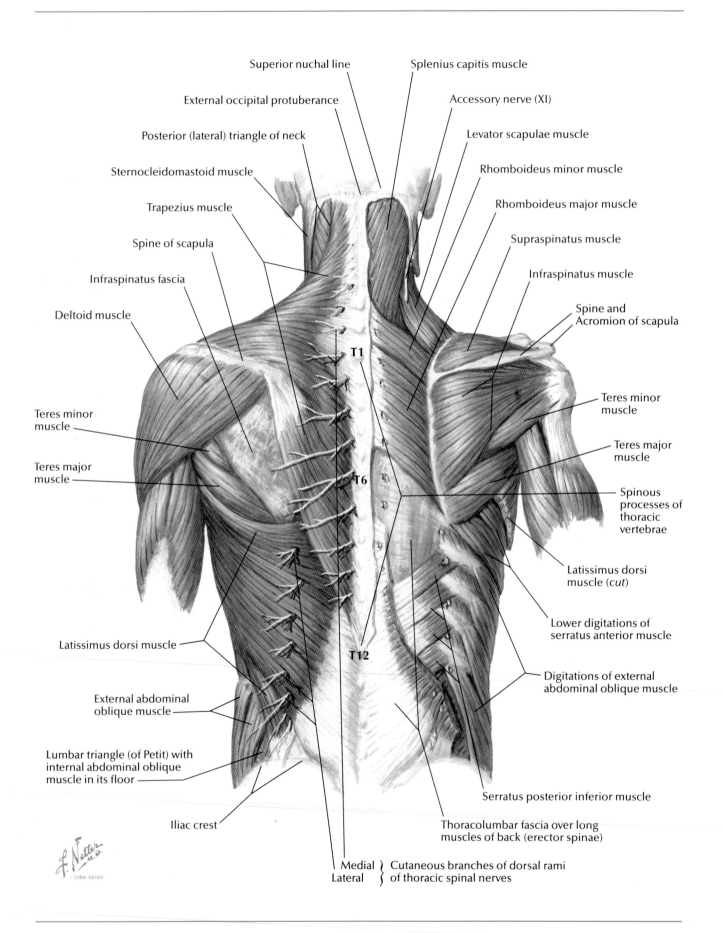

Superior nuchal line

External occipital protuberance

Posterior (lateral) triangle of neck

Sternocleidomastoid muscle

Trapezius muscle

Spine of scapula

Infraspinatus fascia

Deltoid muscle

Teres minor muscle

Teres major muscle

Latissimus dorsi muscle

External abdominal oblique muscle

Lumbar triangle (of Petit) with internal abdominal oblique muscle in its floor

Iliac crest

Splenius capitis muscle

Accessory nerve (XI)

Levator scapulae muscle

Rhomboideus minor muscle

Rhomboideus major muscle

Supraspinatus muscle

Infraspinatus muscle

Spine and Acromion of scapula

Teres minor muscle

Teres major muscle

Spinous processes of thoracic vertebrae

Latissimus dorsi muscle (cut)

Lower digitations of serratus anterior muscle

Digitations of external abdominal oblique muscle

Serratus posterior inferior muscle

Thoracolumbar fascia over long muscles of back (erector spinae)

T1

T6

T12

Medial } Cutaneous branches of dorsal rami
Lateral } of thoracic spinal nerves

PLATE 178

THORAX

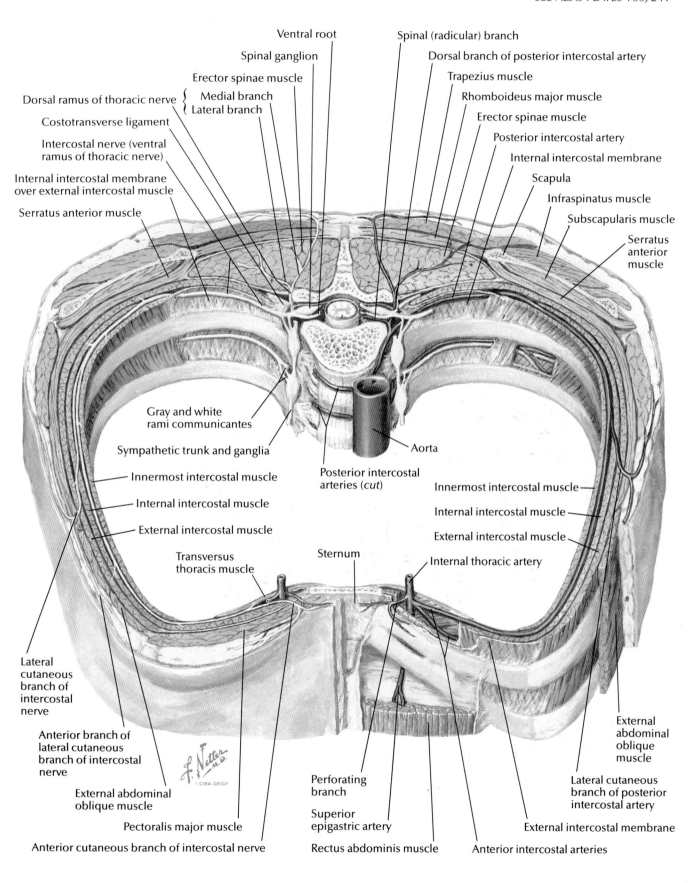

Ventral root

Spinal ganglion

Erector spinae muscle

Dorsal ramus of thoracic nerve { Medial branch
Lateral branch

Costotransverse ligament

Intercostal nerve (ventral ramus of thoracic nerve)

Internal intercostal membrane over external intercostal muscle

Serratus anterior muscle

Spinal (radicular) branch

Dorsal branch of posterior intercostal artery

Trapezius muscle

Rhomboideus major muscle

Erector spinae muscle

Posterior intercostal artery

Internal intercostal membrane

Scapula

Infraspinatus muscle

Subscapularis muscle

Serratus anterior muscle

Gray and white rami communicantes

Sympathetic trunk and ganglia

Innermost intercostal muscle

Internal intercostal muscle

External intercostal muscle

Transversus thoracis muscle

Sternum

Posterior intercostal arteries (*cut*)

Aorta

Innermost intercostal muscle

Internal intercostal muscle

External intercostal muscle

Internal thoracic artery

Lateral cutaneous branch of intercostal nerve

Anterior branch of lateral cutaneous branch of intercostal nerve

External abdominal oblique muscle

Pectoralis major muscle

Anterior cutaneous branch of intercostal nerve

Perforating branch

Superior epigastric artery

Rectus abdominis muscle

External abdominal oblique muscle

Lateral cutaneous branch of posterior intercostal artery

External intercostal membrane

Anterior intercostal arteries

SEE ALSO PLATES 218, 219

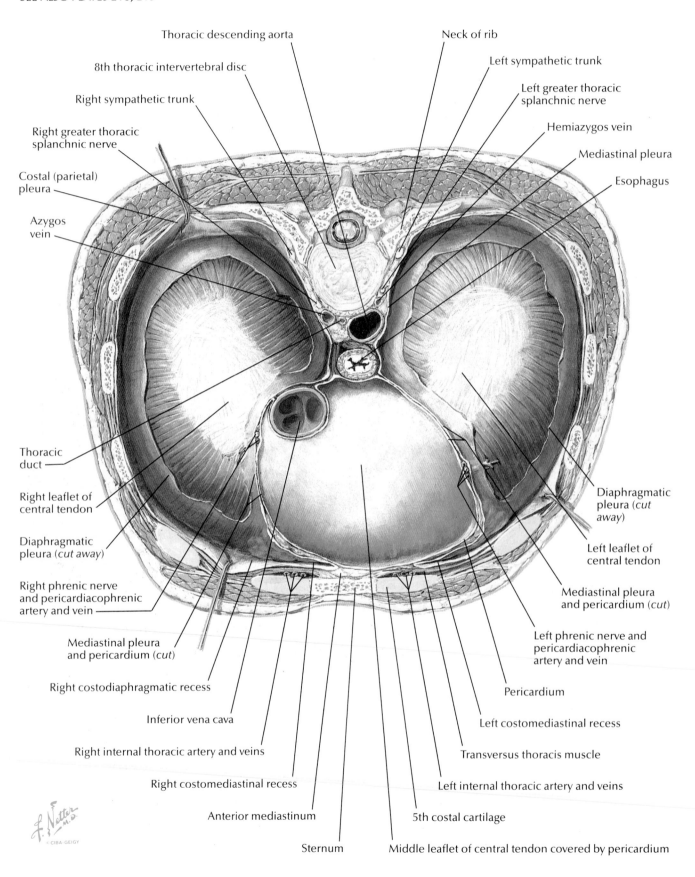

Thoracic descending aorta

Neck of rib

8th thoracic intervertebral disc

Left sympathetic trunk

Right sympathetic trunk

Left greater thoracic splanchnic nerve

Right greater thoracic splanchnic nerve

Hemiazygos vein

Costal (parietal) pleura

Mediastinal pleura

Azygos vein

Esophagus

Thoracic duct

Right leaflet of central tendon

Diaphragmatic pleura (*cut away*)

Right phrenic nerve and pericardiacophrenic artery and vein

Diaphragmatic pleura (*cut away*)

Left leaflet of central tendon

Mediastinal pleura and pericardium (*cut*)

Mediastinal pleura and pericardium (*cut*)

Left phrenic nerve and pericardiacophrenic artery and vein

Right costodiaphragmatic recess

Pericardium

Inferior vena cava

Left costomediastinal recess

Right internal thoracic artery and veins

Transversus thoracis muscle

Right costomediastinal recess

Left internal thoracic artery and veins

Anterior mediastinum

5th costal cartilage

Sternum

Middle leaflet of central tendon covered by pericardium

PLATE 180

THORAX

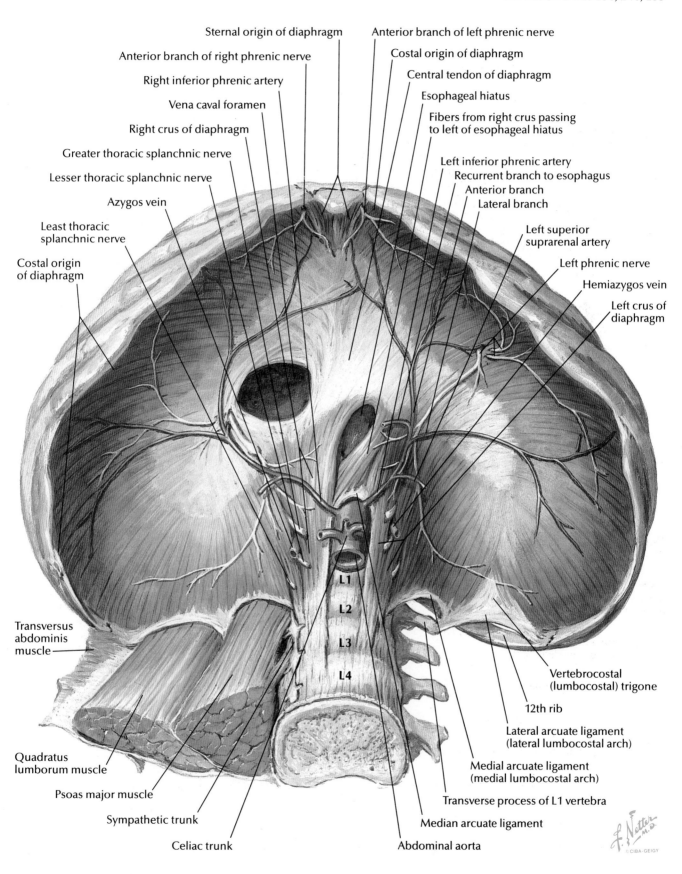

Sternal origin of diaphragm

Anterior branch of right phrenic nerve

Right inferior phrenic artery

Vena caval foramen

Right crus of diaphragm

Greater thoracic splanchnic nerve

Lesser thoracic splanchnic nerve

Azygos vein

Least thoracic splanchnic nerve

Costal origin of diaphragm

Anterior branch of left phrenic nerve

Costal origin of diaphragm

Central tendon of diaphragm

Esophageal hiatus

Fibers from right crus passing to left of esophageal hiatus

Left inferior phrenic artery

Recurrent branch to esophagus

Anterior branch

Lateral branch

Left superior suprarenal artery

Left phrenic nerve

Hemiazygos vein

Left crus of diaphragm

Transversus abdominis muscle

Quadratus lumborum muscle

Psoas major muscle

Sympathetic trunk

Celiac trunk

L1

L2

L3

L4

Vertebrocostal (lumbocostal) trigone

12th rib

Lateral arcuate ligament (lateral lumbocostal arch)

Medial arcuate ligament (medial lumbocostal arch)

Transverse process of L1 vertebra

Median arcuate ligament

Abdominal aorta

Ventral rami { C3 / C4 / C5

C3 / C4 / C5 } Ventral rami

Anterior scalene muscle

Right common carotid artery

Brachial plexus

Right phrenic nerve

Right subclavian artery

Right vagus nerve (X)

Right internal thoracic artery (*cut*)

Brachiocephalic trunk

Right pericardiaco-phrenic artery (*cut*)

Superior vena cava

Root of right lung

Pericardial branch of phrenic nerve

Mediastinal pleura

Diaphragmatic pleura (*cut*)

Anterior scalene muscle

Brachial plexus

Left phrenic nerve

Left subclavian artery

Left vagus nerve (X)

Left common carotid artery

Left internal thoracic artery (*cut*)

Thoracic cardiac nerves

Left pericardiaco-phrenic artery (*cut*)

Left recurrent laryngeal nerve

Root of left lung

Mediastinal pleura

Phrenicoabdominal branches of phrenic nerves to inferior surface of diaphragm

Phrenic nerves (efferent and afferent)

Lower intercostal nerves (afferent only from peripheral part of diaphragm)

PLATE 182

THORAX

Muscles of inspiration

Accessory

Sternocleidomastoid
(elevates sternum)

Scalenes
  Anterior
  Middle
  Posterior
(elevate and fix
upper ribs)

Principal

External intercostals
(elevate ribs, thus
increasing width of
thoracic cavity)

Interchondral part
of internal intercostals
(also elevates ribs)

Diaphragm
(domes descend, thus
increasing longitudinal
dimension of thoracic
cavity; also elevates
lower ribs)

Muscles of expiration

Quiet breathing

Expiration results from
passive recoil of lungs

Active breathing

Internal intercostals,
except interchondral
part

Abdominal muscles
(depress lower ribs,
compress abdominal
contents, thus pushing
up diaphragm)
Rectus abdominis
External oblique
Internal oblique
Transversus abdominis

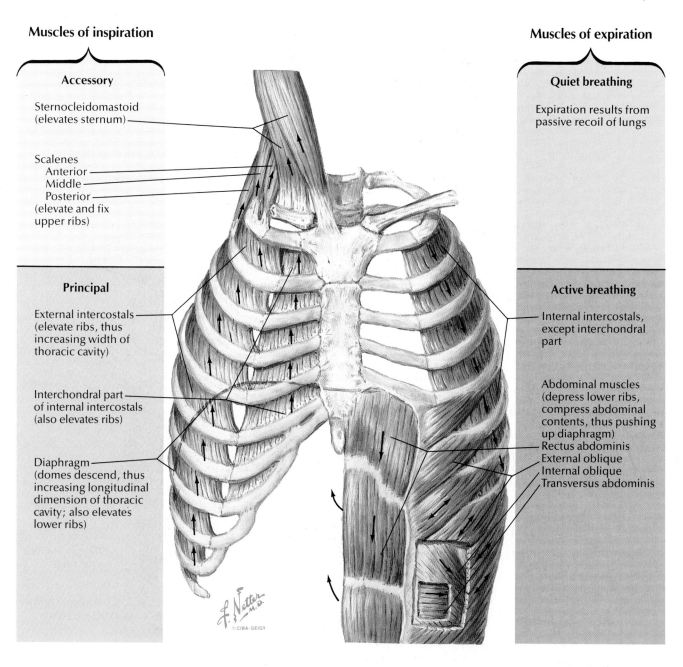

Topography of Lungs: Anterior View

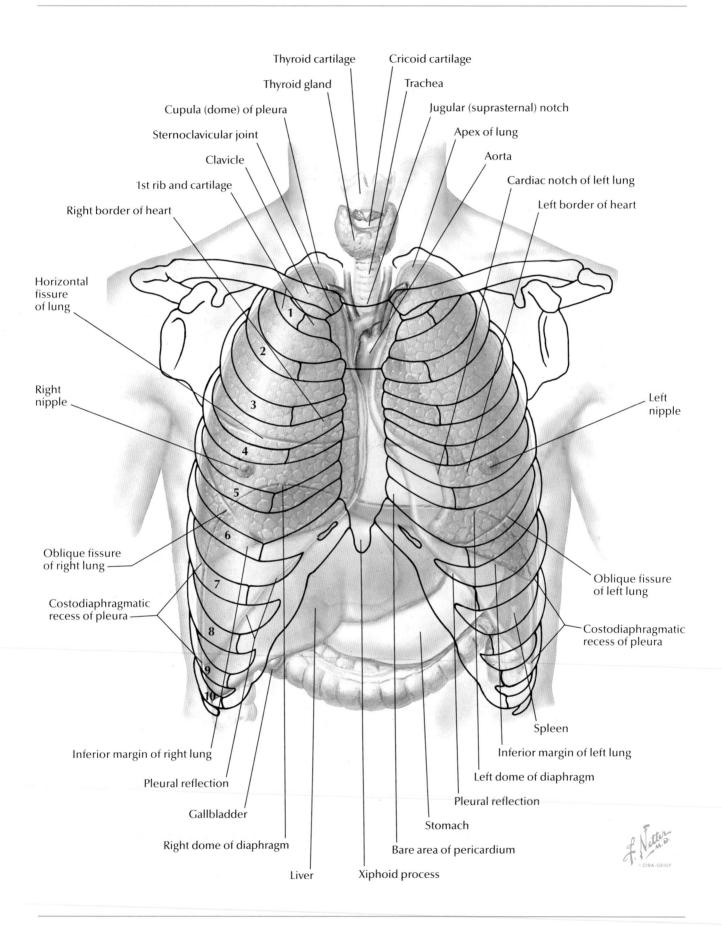

Thyroid cartilage

Cricoid cartilage

Thyroid gland

Trachea

Cupula (dome) of pleura

Jugular (suprasternal) notch

Sternoclavicular joint

Apex of lung

Clavicle

Aorta

1st rib and cartilage

Cardiac notch of left lung

Right border of heart

Left border of heart

Horizontal fissure of lung

Right nipple

Left nipple

Oblique fissure of right lung

Oblique fissure of left lung

Costodiaphragmatic recess of pleura

Costodiaphragmatic recess of pleura

1

2

3

4

5

6

7

8

9

10

Spleen

Inferior margin of right lung

Inferior margin of left lung

Pleural reflection

Left dome of diaphragm

Gallbladder

Pleural reflection

Right dome of diaphragm

Stomach

Liver

Xiphoid process

Bare area of pericardium

PLATE 184

THORAX

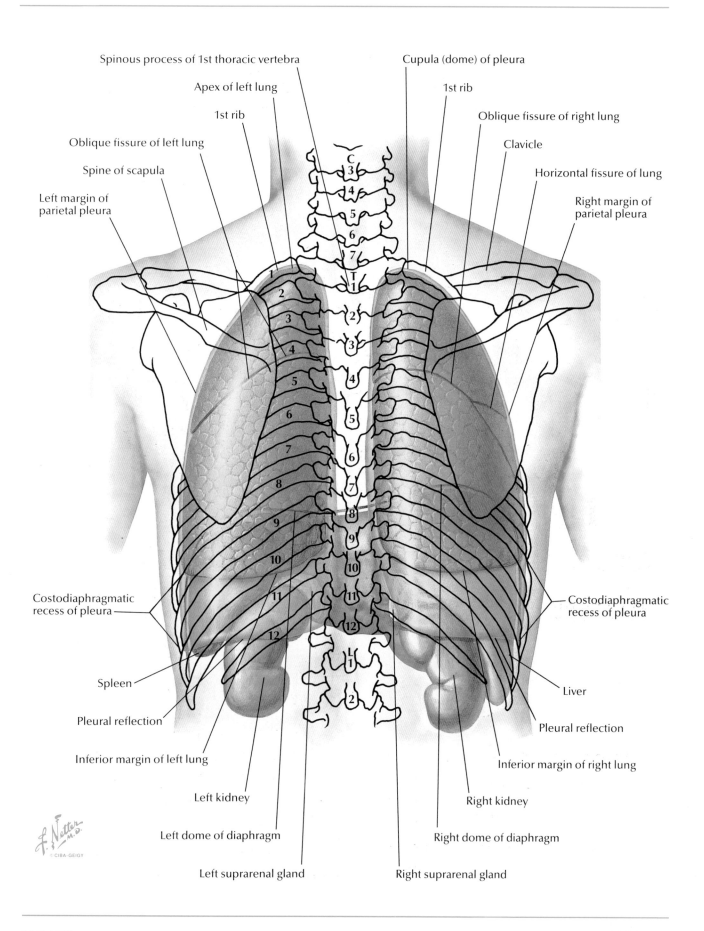

Spinous process of 1st thoracic vertebra

Apex of left lung

1st rib

Oblique fissure of left lung

Spine of scapula

Left margin of parietal pleura

Cupula (dome) of pleura

1st rib

Oblique fissure of right lung

Clavicle

Horizontal fissure of lung

Right margin of parietal pleura

Costodiaphragmatic recess of pleura

Costodiaphragmatic recess of pleura

Spleen

Pleural reflection

Inferior margin of left lung

Left kidney

Left dome of diaphragm

Left suprarenal gland

Liver

Pleural reflection

Inferior margin of right lung

Right kidney

Right dome of diaphragm

Right suprarenal gland

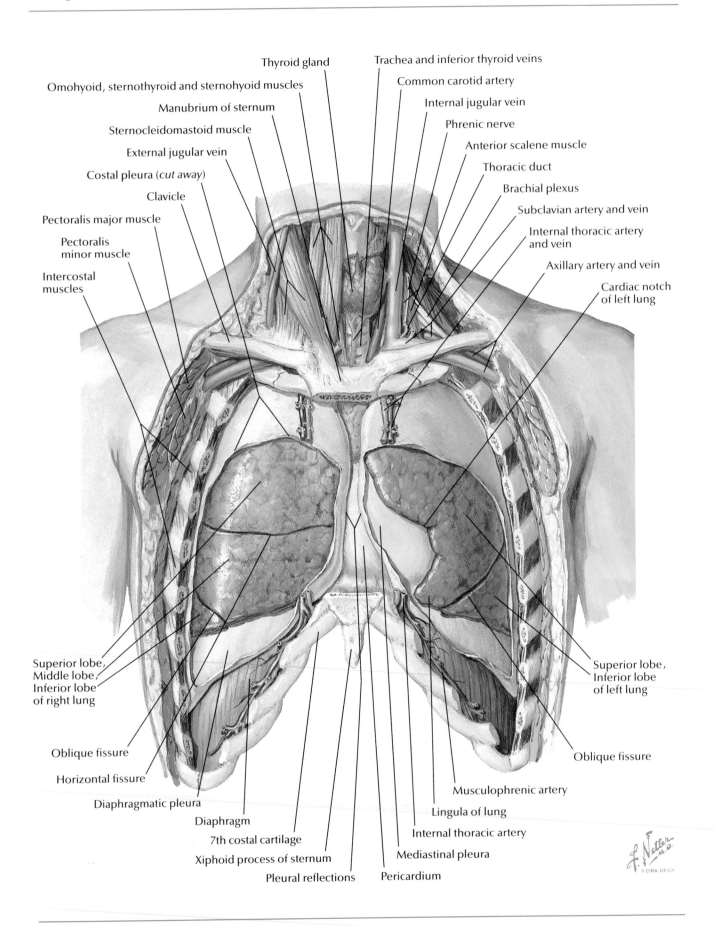

Thyroid gland

Omohyoid, sternothyroid and sternohyoid muscles

Manubrium of sternum

Sternocleidomastoid muscle

External jugular vein

Costal pleura (cut away)

Clavicle

Pectoralis major muscle

Pectoralis minor muscle

Intercostal muscles

Trachea and inferior thyroid veins

Common carotid artery

Internal jugular vein

Phrenic nerve

Anterior scalene muscle

Thoracic duct

Brachial plexus

Subclavian artery and vein

Internal thoracic artery and vein

Axillary artery and vein

Cardiac notch of left lung

Superior lobe,
Middle lobe,
Inferior lobe
of right lung

Superior lobe,
Inferior lobe
of left lung

Oblique fissure

Horizontal fissure

Diaphragmatic pleura

Diaphragm

7th costal cartilage

Xiphoid process of sternum

Pleural reflections

Pericardium

Mediastinal pleura

Internal thoracic artery

Lingula of lung

Musculophrenic artery

Oblique fissure

PLATE 186

THORAX

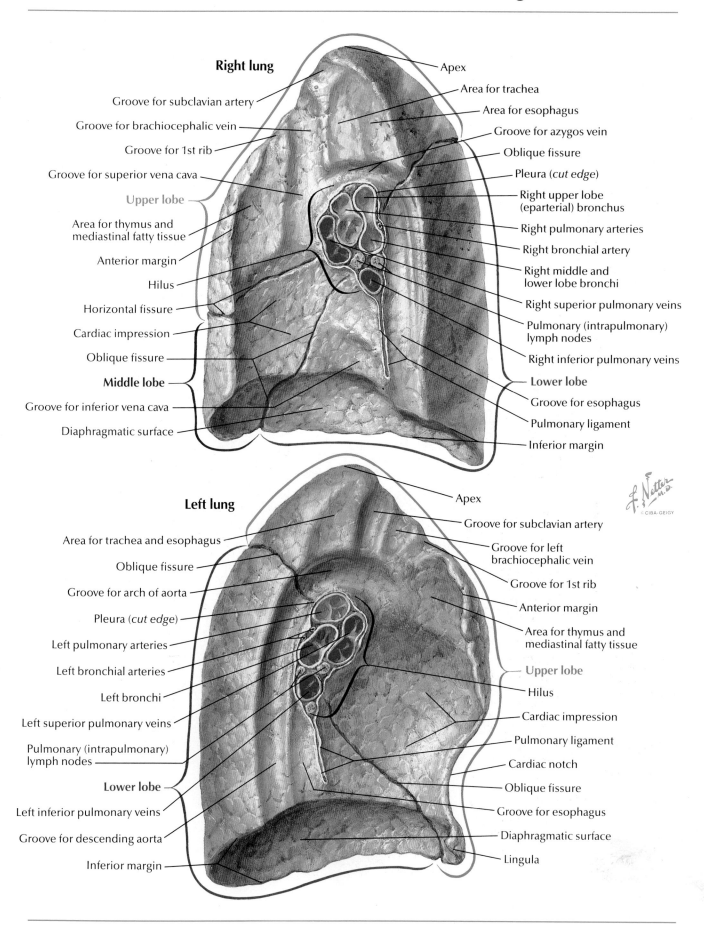

Right lung

- Groove for subclavian artery
- Groove for brachiocephalic vein
- Groove for 1st rib
- Groove for superior vena cava
- Upper lobe
- Area for thymus and mediastinal fatty tissue
- Anterior margin
- Hilus
- Horizontal fissure
- Cardiac impression
- Oblique fissure
- **Middle lobe**
- Groove for inferior vena cava
- Diaphragmatic surface

- Apex
- Area for trachea
- Area for esophagus
- Groove for azygos vein
- Oblique fissure
- Pleura (*cut edge*)
- Right upper lobe (eparterial) bronchus
- Right pulmonary arteries
- Right bronchial artery
- Right middle and lower lobe bronchi
- Right superior pulmonary veins
- Pulmonary (intrapulmonary) lymph nodes
- Right inferior pulmonary veins
- **Lower lobe**
- Groove for esophagus
- Pulmonary ligament
- Inferior margin

Left lung

- Area for trachea and esophagus
- Oblique fissure
- Groove for arch of aorta
- Pleura (*cut edge*)
- Left pulmonary arteries
- Left bronchial arteries
- Left bronchi
- Left superior pulmonary veins
- Pulmonary (intrapulmonary) lymph nodes
- **Lower lobe**
- Left inferior pulmonary veins
- Groove for descending aorta
- Inferior margin

- Apex
- Groove for subclavian artery
- Groove for left brachiocephalic vein
- Groove for 1st rib
- Anterior margin
- Area for thymus and mediastinal fatty tissue
- Upper lobe
- Hilus
- Cardiac impression
- Pulmonary ligament
- Cardiac notch
- Oblique fissure
- Groove for esophagus
- Diaphragmatic surface
- Lingula

F. Netter M.D.
©CIBA-GEIGY

Bronchopulmonary Segments

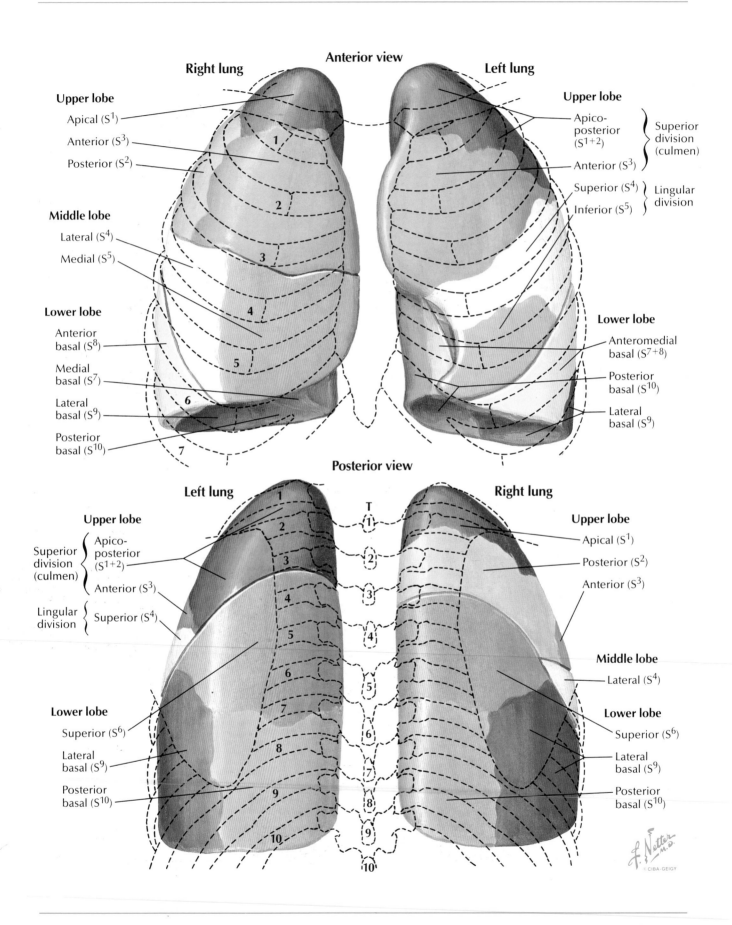

Anterior view

Right lung

Left lung

Upper lobe
- Apical (S^1)
- Anterior (S^3)
- Posterior (S^2)

Middle lobe
- Lateral (S^4)
- Medial (S^5)

Lower lobe
- Anterior basal (S^8)
- Medial basal (S^7)
- Lateral basal (S^9)
- Posterior basal (S^{10})

Upper lobe
- Apico-posterior (S^{1+2}) } Superior division (culmen)
- Anterior (S^3) }
- Superior (S^4) } Lingular division
- Inferior (S^5) }

Lower lobe
- Anteromedial basal (S^{7+8})
- Posterior basal (S^{10})
- Lateral basal (S^9)

Posterior view

Left lung

Right lung

Upper lobe
- Superior division (culmen) { Apico-posterior (S^{1+2})
- Anterior (S^3)
- Lingular division { Superior (S^4)

Lower lobe
- Superior (S^6)
- Lateral basal (S^9)
- Posterior basal (S^{10})

Upper lobe
- Apical (S^1)
- Posterior (S^2)
- Anterior (S^3)

Middle lobe
- Lateral (S^4)

Lower lobe
- Superior (S^6)
- Lateral basal (S^9)
- Posterior basal (S^{10})

F. Netter M.D.
© CIBA-GEIGY

PLATE 188

THORAX

Lateral views

Right lung

Left lung

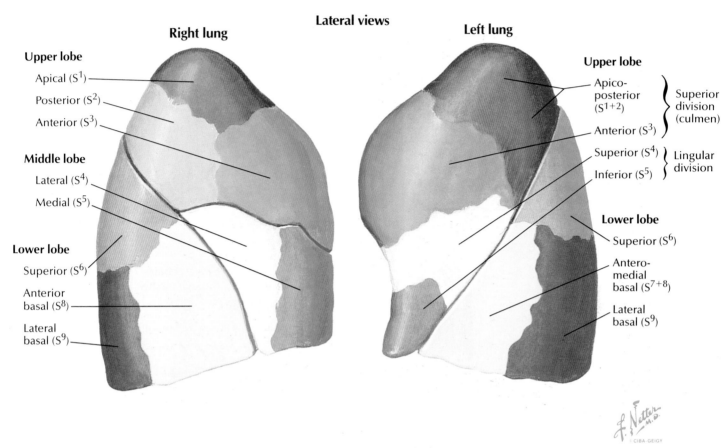

Upper lobe

Apical (S^1)

Posterior (S^2)

Anterior (S^3)

Middle lobe

Lateral (S^4)

Medial (S^5)

Lower lobe

Superior (S^6)

Anterior basal (S^8)

Lateral basal (S^9)

Upper lobe

Apico-posterior (S^{1+2}) } Superior division (culmen)

Anterior (S^3)

Superior (S^4) } Lingular division

Inferior (S^5)

Lower lobe

Superior (S^6)

Antero-medial basal (S^{7+8})

Lateral basal (S^9)

Medial views

Right lung

Left lung

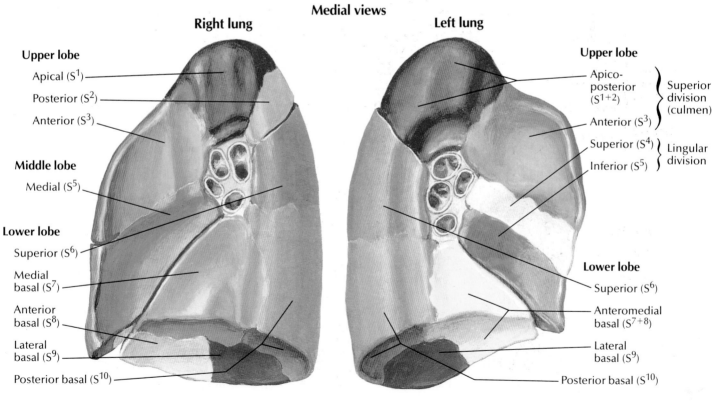

Upper lobe

Apical (S^1)

Posterior (S^2)

Anterior (S^3)

Middle lobe

Medial (S^5)

Lower lobe

Superior (S^6)

Medial basal (S^7)

Anterior basal (S^8)

Lateral basal (S^9)

Posterior basal (S^{10})

Upper lobe

Apico-posterior (S^{1+2}) } Superior division (culmen)

Anterior (S^3)

Superior (S^4) } Lingular division

Inferior (S^5)

Lower lobe

Superior (S^6)

Anteromedial basal (S^{7+8})

Lateral basal (S^9)

Posterior basal (S^{10})

Trachea and Major Bronchi

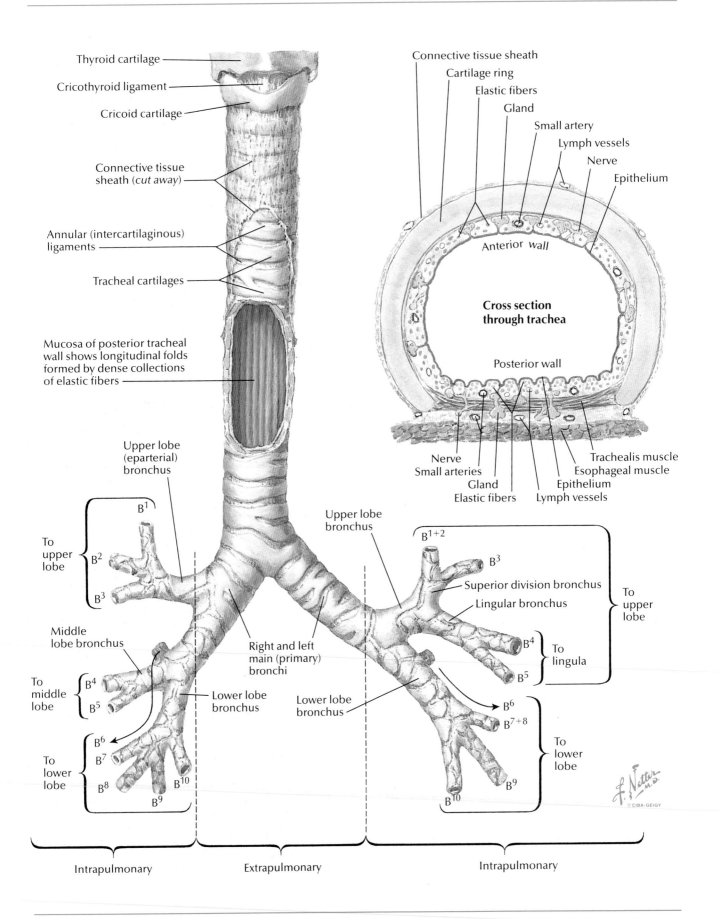

Thyroid cartilage

Cricothyroid ligament

Cricoid cartilage

Connective tissue sheath (*cut away*)

Annular (intercartilaginous) ligaments

Tracheal cartilages

Mucosa of posterior tracheal wall shows longitudinal folds formed by dense collections of elastic fibers

Connective tissue sheath

Cartilage ring

Elastic fibers

Gland

Small artery

Lymph vessels

Nerve

Epithelium

Anterior *wall*

Cross section through trachea

Posterior wall

Nerve

Small arteries

Gland

Elastic fibers

Trachealis muscle

Esophageal muscle

Epithelium

Lymph vessels

Upper lobe (eparterial) bronchus

B^1

To upper lobe

B^2

B^3

Upper lobe bronchus

B^{1+2}

B^3

Superior division bronchus

Lingular bronchus

To upper lobe

Middle lobe bronchus

To middle lobe

B^4

B^5

Right and left main (primary) bronchi

Lower lobe bronchus

Lower lobe bronchus

B^4

To lingula

B^5

B^6

B^{7+8}

To lower lobe

B^6

B^7

To lower lobe

B^8

B^{10}

B^9

B^9

B^{10}

Intrapulmonary

Extrapulmonary

Intrapulmonary

PLATE 190

THORAX

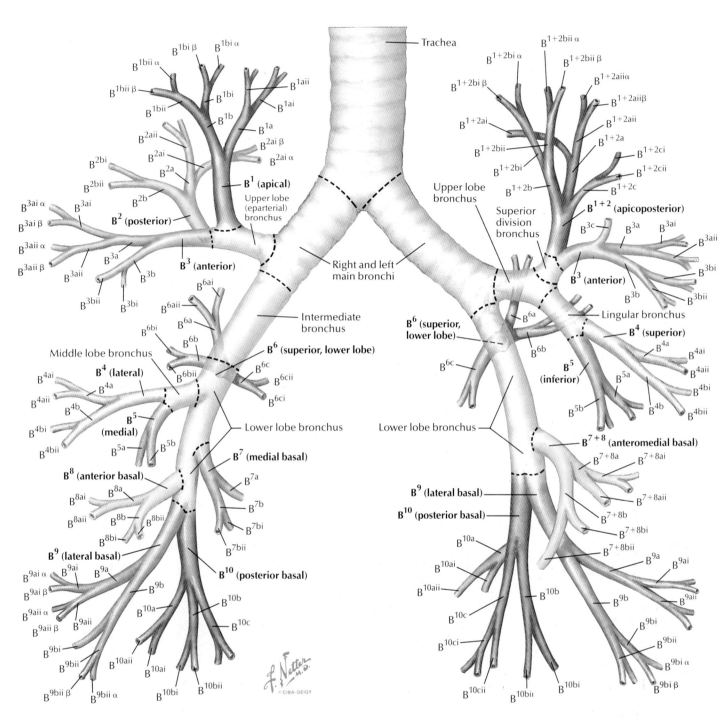

Nomenclature in common usage for bronchopulmonary segments (Plates 188 and 189) is that of Jackson and Huber, and segmental bronchi are named accordingly. Ikeda proposed nomenclature (as demonstrated here) for bronchial subdivisions as far as 6th generation. For simplification in this illustration, only some bronchial subdivisions are labeled as far as 5th or 6th generation. Segmental bronchi (B) are numbered from 1 to 10 in each lung, corresponding to pulmonary segments. In left lung, B^1

and B^2 are combined as are B^7 and B^8. Subsegmental, or 4th order, bronchi are indicated by addition of lower case letters a, b or c when an additional branch is present. Fifth order bronchi are designated by Roman numerals i (anterior) or ii (posterior), and 6th order bronchi by Greek letters α or β. Several texts use alternate numbers (as proposed by Boyden) for segmental bronchi.

Variations of standard bronchial pattern shown here are common, especially in peripheral airways

Intrapulmonary Airways: Schema

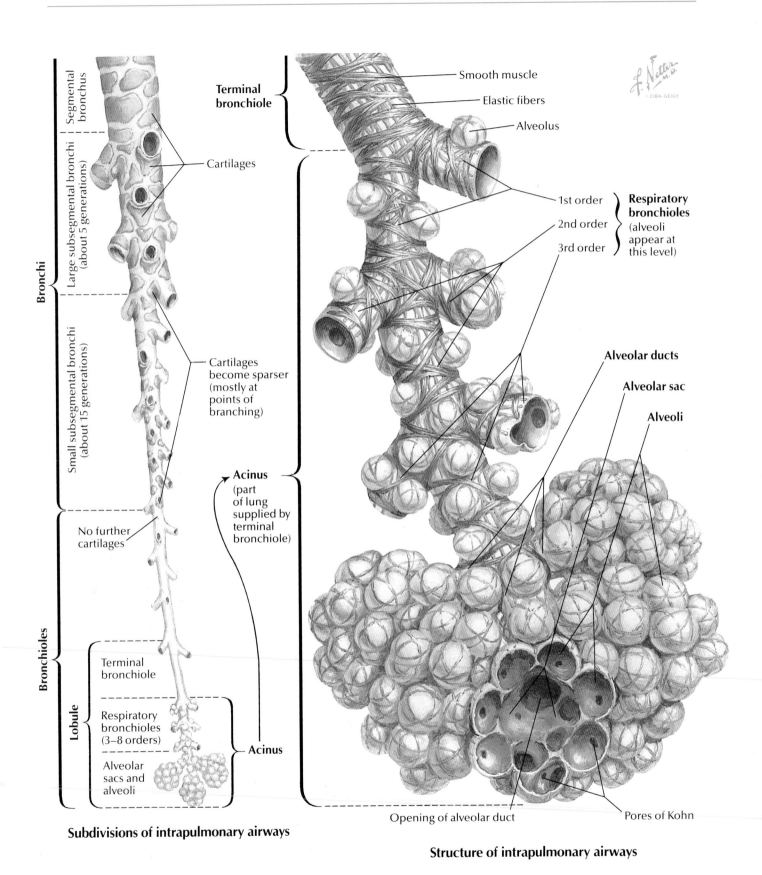

Subdivisions of intrapulmonary airways

Bronchi
- Segmental bronchus
- Large subsegmental bronchi (about 5 generations)
- Small subsegmental bronchi (about 15 generations)

Cartilages

Cartilages become sparser (mostly at points of branching)

No further cartilages

Bronchioles

Lobule
- Terminal bronchiole
- Respiratory bronchioles (3–8 orders)
- Alveolar sacs and alveoli

Acinus (part of lung supplied by terminal bronchiole)

Acinus

Structure of intrapulmonary airways

Terminal bronchiole

Smooth muscle

Elastic fibers

Alveolus

1st order
2nd order
3rd order

Respiratory bronchioles (alveoli appear at this level)

Alveolar ducts

Alveolar sac

Alveoli

Opening of alveolar duct

Pores of Kohn

PLATE 192

THORAX

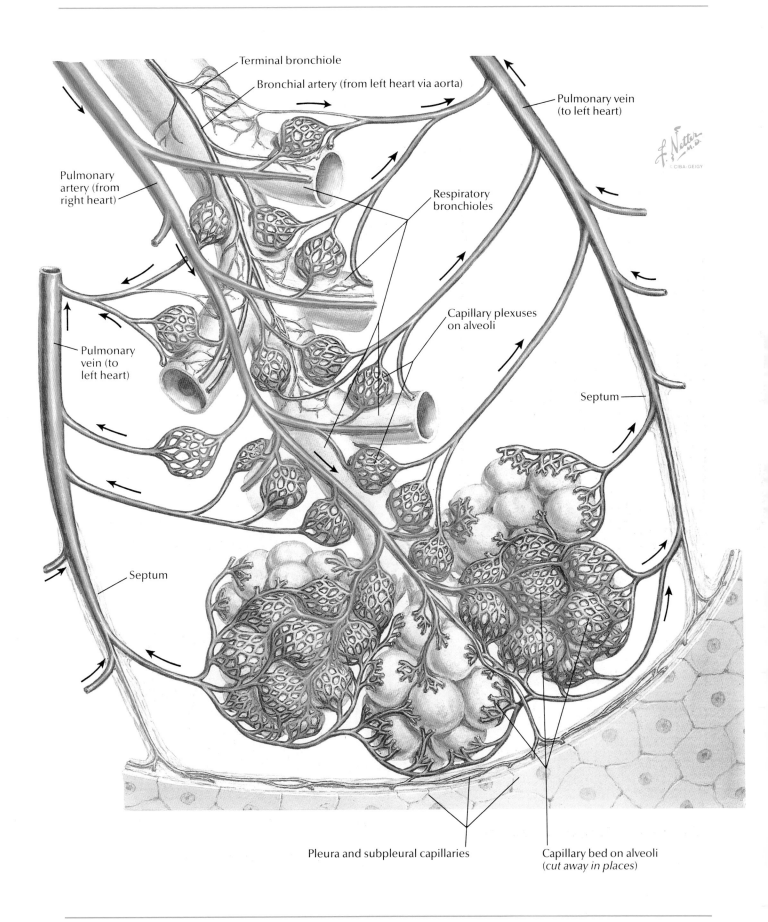

Terminal bronchiole

Bronchial artery (from left heart via aorta)

Pulmonary vein (to left heart)

Pulmonary artery (from right heart)

Respiratory bronchioles

Pulmonary vein (to left heart)

Capillary plexuses on alveoli

Septum

Septum

Pleura and subpleural capillaries

Capillary bed on alveoli (*cut away in places*)

Pulmonary Arteries and Veins

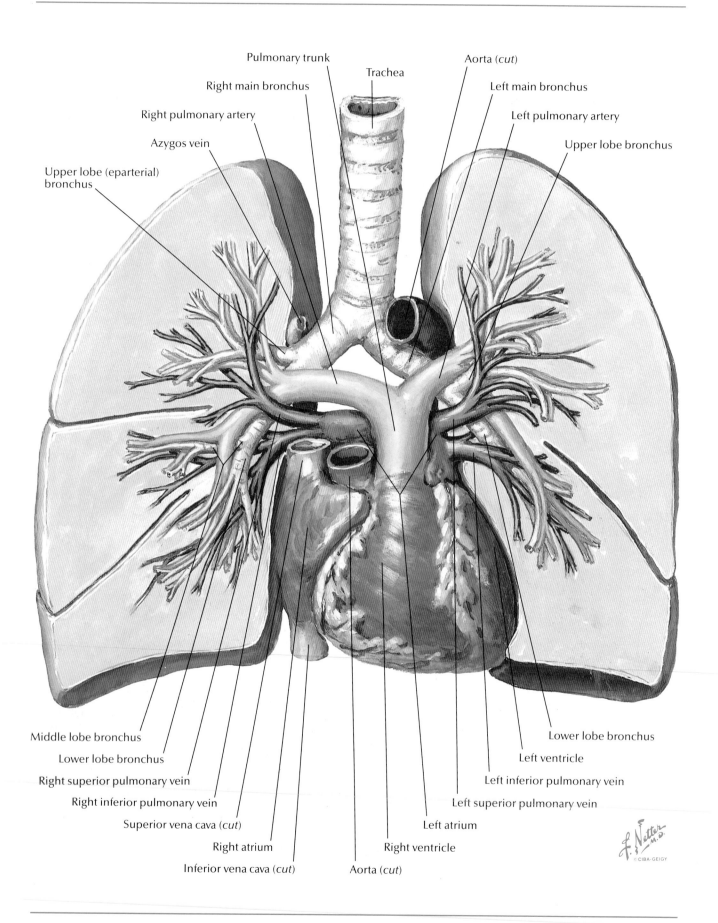

Pulmonary trunk

Trachea

Aorta (*cut*)

Right main bronchus

Left main bronchus

Right pulmonary artery

Left pulmonary artery

Azygos vein

Upper lobe bronchus

Upper lobe (eparterial) bronchus

Middle lobe bronchus

Lower lobe bronchus

Lower lobe bronchus

Left ventricle

Right superior pulmonary vein

Left inferior pulmonary vein

Right inferior pulmonary vein

Left superior pulmonary vein

Superior vena cava (*cut*)

Right atrium

Left atrium

Inferior vena cava (*cut*)

Right ventricle

Aorta (*cut*)

PLATE 194

THORAX

Main Bronchi With Pulmonary Arteries and Veins In Situ

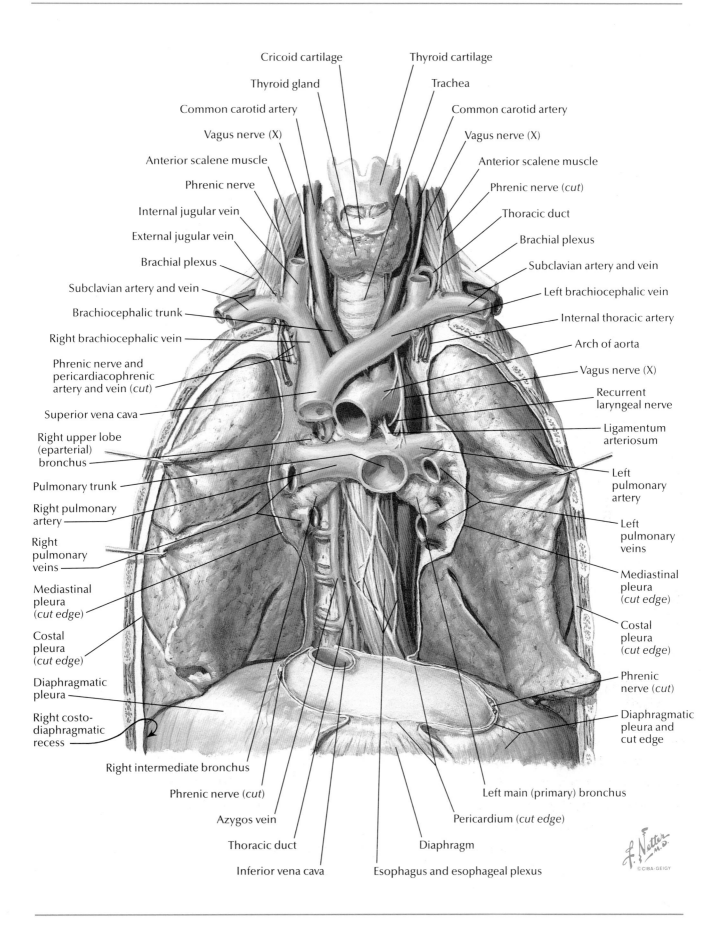

Cricoid cartilage

Thyroid gland

Common carotid artery

Vagus nerve (X)

Anterior scalene muscle

Phrenic nerve

Internal jugular vein

External jugular vein

Brachial plexus

Subclavian artery and vein

Brachiocephalic trunk

Right brachiocephalic vein

Phrenic nerve and pericardiacophrenic artery and vein (*cut*)

Superior vena cava

Right upper lobe (eparterial) bronchus

Pulmonary trunk

Right pulmonary artery

Right pulmonary veins

Mediastinal pleura (*cut edge*)

Costal pleura (*cut edge*)

Diaphragmatic pleura

Right costo-diaphragmatic recess

Right intermediate bronchus

Phrenic nerve (*cut*)

Azygos vein

Thoracic duct

Inferior vena cava

Thyroid cartilage

Trachea

Common carotid artery

Vagus nerve (X)

Anterior scalene muscle

Phrenic nerve (*cut*)

Thoracic duct

Brachial plexus

Subclavian artery and vein

Left brachiocephalic vein

Internal thoracic artery

Arch of aorta

Vagus nerve (X)

Recurrent laryngeal nerve

Ligamentum arteriosum

Left pulmonary artery

Left pulmonary veins

Mediastinal pleura (*cut edge*)

Costal pleura (*cut edge*)

Phrenic nerve (*cut*)

Diaphragmatic pleura and cut edge

Left main (primary) bronchus

Pericardium (*cut edge*)

Diaphragm

Esophagus and esophageal plexus

Bronchial Arteries and Veins

- Esophagus
- Trachea (*pulled to left by hook*)
- 3rd right posterior intercostal (1st aortic intercostal) artery
- Right bronchial artery
- Right main (primary) bronchus
- Left main (primary) bronchus (*pulled to right by hook*)
- Superior left bronchial artery
- Aorta (*pulled aside by hook*)
- Inferior left bronchial artery
- Esophageal artery

Variations in bronchial arteries

Right and left bronchial arteries originating from aorta by single stem

Only single bronchial artery to each bronchus (normally, two to left bronchus)

Bronchial veins

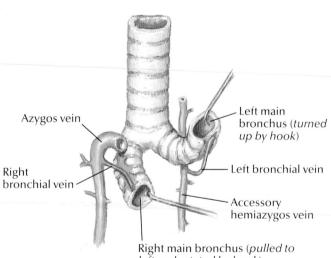

- Azygos vein
- Right bronchial vein
- Left main bronchus (*turned up by hook*)
- Left bronchial vein
- Accessory hemiazygos vein
- Right main bronchus (*pulled to left and rotated by hook*)

PLATE 196

THORAX

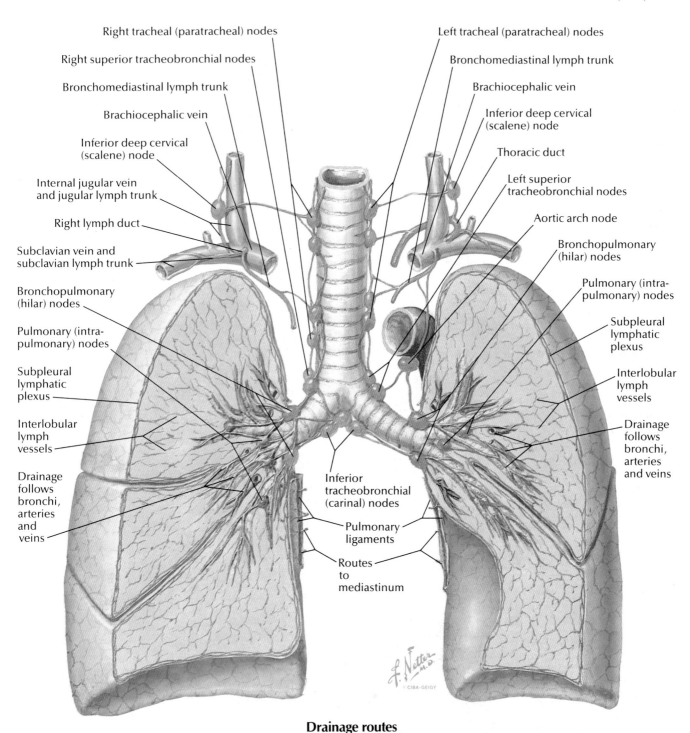

Right tracheal (paratracheal) nodes

Right superior tracheobronchial nodes

Bronchomediastinal lymph trunk

Brachiocephalic vein

Inferior deep cervical (scalene) node

Internal jugular vein and jugular lymph trunk

Right lymph duct

Subclavian vein and subclavian lymph trunk

Bronchopulmonary (hilar) nodes

Pulmonary (intra-pulmonary) nodes

Subpleural lymphatic plexus

Interlobular lymph vessels

Drainage follows bronchi, arteries and veins

Left tracheal (paratracheal) nodes

Bronchomediastinal lymph trunk

Brachiocephalic vein

Inferior deep cervical (scalene) node

Thoracic duct

Left superior tracheobronchial nodes

Aortic arch node

Bronchopulmonary (hilar) nodes

Pulmonary (intra-pulmonary) nodes

Subpleural lymphatic plexus

Interlobular lymph vessels

Drainage follows bronchi, arteries and veins

Inferior tracheobronchial (carinal) nodes

Pulmonary ligaments

Routes to mediastinum

Drainage routes

Right lung: All lobes drain to intrapulmonary and broncho-pulmonary (hilar) nodes, then to inferior tracheobronchial (carinal) nodes, right superior tracheobronchial nodes and to right tracheal nodes on way to brachiocephalic vein via bronchomediastinal lymph trunk and/or scalene node. **Left lung:** Upper lobe drains to pulmonary and hilar nodes, carinal nodes, left superior tracheobronchial nodes, left tracheal nodes and/or aortic arch node, then to brachio-cephalic vein via left bronchomediastinal trunk and thoracic duct. Left lower lobe drains also to pulmonary and hilar nodes and to carinal nodes, but then mostly to right superior tracheobronchial nodes, where it follows same route as lymph from right lung

SEE ALSO PLATES 124, 125, 152, 304

Cervicothoracic (stellate) ganglion

Ansa subclavia

Cervical cardiac nerves (sympathetic and vagal)

Thoracic sympathetic cardiac nerves

Sympathetic trunk

Vagus nerve (X) (cut) and branches to cardiac and pulmonary plexuses

Thoracic sympathetic cardiac nerves

Anterior pulmonary plexus

Posterior pulmonary plexus (protruding from behind right bronchus)

6th intercostal nerve

Gray and white rami communicantes

6th thoracic sympathetic ganglion

Greater thoracic splanchnic nerve

Sympathetic branch to esophageal plexus

Thoracic duct

Lesser thoracic splanchnic nerve

Least thoracic splanchnic nerve

Azygos vein (cut)

Inferior vena cava (cut)

Recurrent laryngeal nerve

Cervical cardiac nerves (sympathetic and vagal)

Vagus nerve (X) (cut)

Thoracic sympathetic cardiac nerves

Recurrent laryngeal nerve

Thoracic cardiac branch of vagus nerve

Cardiac plexus

Anterior pulmonary plexus

Posterior pulmonary plexus (protruding from behind left bronchus)

Sympathetic trunk

Thoracic aortic plexus

Esophageal plexus

8th intercostal nerve

Gray and white rami communicantes

Greater thoracic splanchnic nerve

Lesser thoracic splanchnic nerve

Anterior vagal trunk

Diaphragm (pulled down)

PLATE 198

THORAX

SEE ALSO PLATE 153

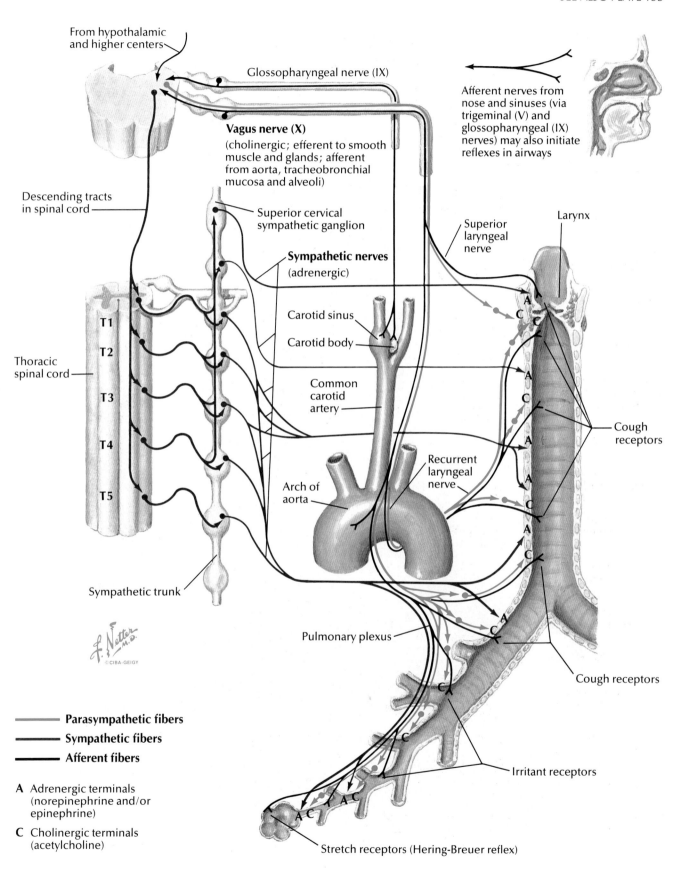

From hypothalamic and higher centers

Glossopharyngeal nerve (IX)

Afferent nerves from nose and sinuses (via trigeminal (V) and glossopharyngeal (IX) nerves) may also initiate reflexes in airways

Vagus nerve (X) (cholinergic; efferent to smooth muscle and glands; afferent from aorta, tracheobronchial mucosa and alveoli)

Descending tracts in spinal cord

Superior cervical sympathetic ganglion

Superior laryngeal nerve

Larynx

Sympathetic nerves (adrenergic)

Thoracic spinal cord

T1

T2

T3

T4

T5

Carotid sinus

Carotid body

Common carotid artery

Cough receptors

Recurrent laryngeal nerve

Arch of aorta

Sympathetic trunk

Cough receptors

Pulmonary plexus

Irritant receptors

Stretch receptors (Hering-Breuer reflex)

— Parasympathetic fibers
— **Sympathetic fibers**
— **Afferent fibers**

A Adrenergic terminals (norepinephrine and/or epinephrine)

C Cholinergic terminals (acetylcholine)

Heart In Situ

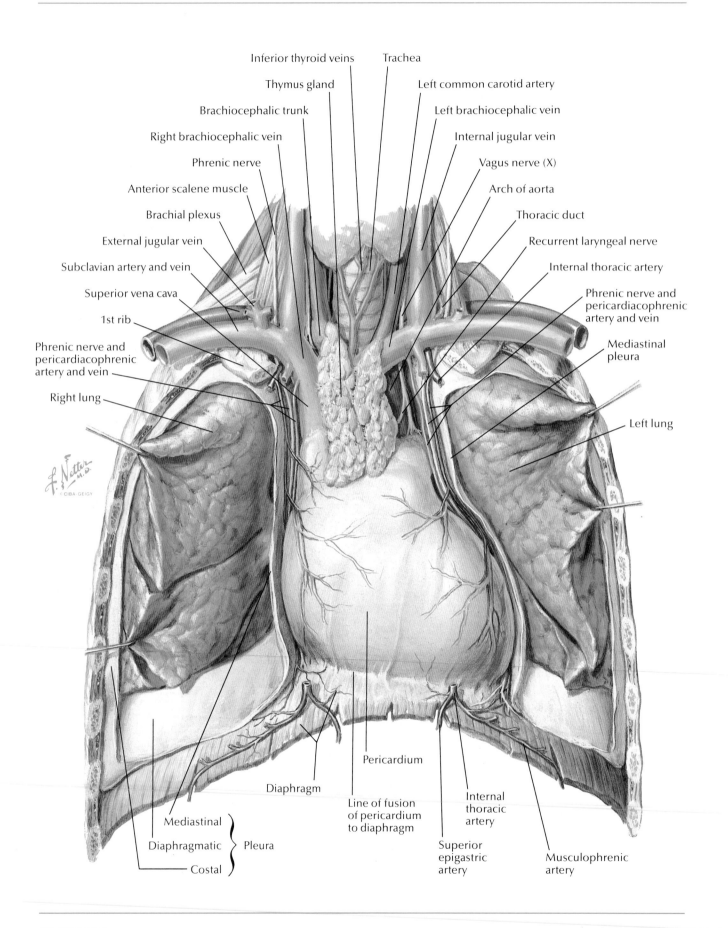

Inferior thyroid veins

Trachea

Thymus gland

Left common carotid artery

Brachiocephalic trunk

Left brachiocephalic vein

Right brachiocephalic vein

Internal jugular vein

Phrenic nerve

Vagus nerve (X)

Anterior scalene muscle

Arch of aorta

Brachial plexus

Thoracic duct

External jugular vein

Recurrent laryngeal nerve

Subclavian artery and vein

Internal thoracic artery

Superior vena cava

Phrenic nerve and pericardiacophrenic artery and vein

1st rib

Mediastinal pleura

Phrenic nerve and pericardiacophrenic artery and vein

Right lung

Left lung

Pericardium

Diaphragm

Internal thoracic artery

Line of fusion of pericardium to diaphragm

Mediastinal

Superior epigastric artery

Musculophrenic artery

Diaphragmatic } Pleura

Costal

PLATE 200

THORAX

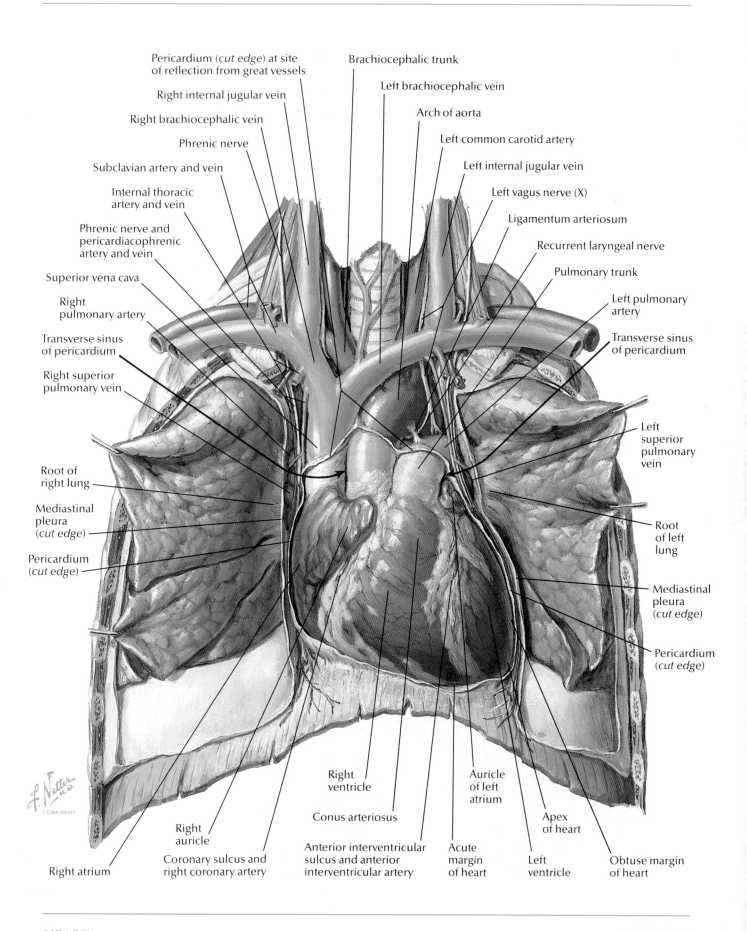

Pericardium (*cut edge*) at site of reflection from great vessels

Right internal jugular vein

Right brachiocephalic vein

Phrenic nerve

Subclavian artery and vein

Internal thoracic artery and vein

Phrenic nerve and pericardiacophrenic artery and vein

Superior vena cava

Right pulmonary artery

Transverse sinus of pericardium

Right superior pulmonary vein

Root of right lung

Mediastinal pleura (*cut edge*)

Pericardium (*cut edge*)

Brachiocephalic trunk

Left brachiocephalic vein

Arch of aorta

Left common carotid artery

Left internal jugular vein

Left vagus nerve (X)

Ligamentum arteriosum

Recurrent laryngeal nerve

Pulmonary trunk

Left pulmonary artery

Transverse sinus of pericardium

Left superior pulmonary vein

Root of left lung

Mediastinal pleura (*cut edge*)

Pericardium (*cut edge*)

Right ventricle

Conus arteriosus

Right auricle

Coronary sulcus and right coronary artery

Right atrium

Anterior interventricular sulcus and anterior interventricular artery

Auricle of left atrium

Acute margin of heart

Apex of heart

Left ventricle

Obtuse margin of heart

Heart: Basal and Diaphragmatic Surfaces

Right pulmonary artery

Left pulmonary artery

Left auricle

Left superior pulmonary vein

Left atrium

Left inferior pulmonary vein

Pericardial reflection

Oblique vein of left atrium

Coronary sinus

Left ventricle

Apex

Arch of aorta

Right auricle

Superior vena cava

Right superior pulmonary vein

Right atrium

Sulcus terminalis

Right inferior pulmonary vein

Coronary sulcus

Inferior vena cava

Right ventricle

Base of heart: posterior view

Left subclavian artery

Left common carotid artery

Left pulmonary artery

Left superior pulmonary vein

Left auricle

Left inferior pulmonary vein

Oblique vein of left atrium

Left atrium

Pericardial reflection

Coronary sinus

Left ventricle

Brachiocephalic trunk

Superior vena cava

Arch of aorta

Right pulmonary artery

Right superior pulmonary vein

Right inferior pulmonary vein

Sulcus terminalis

Right atrium

Inferior vena cava

Coronary sulcus and right coronary artery

Posterior interventricular sulcus and posterior interventricular branch of right coronary artery (posterior descending artery)

Right ventricle

Diaphragmatic surface: posteroinferior view

PLATE 202

THORAX

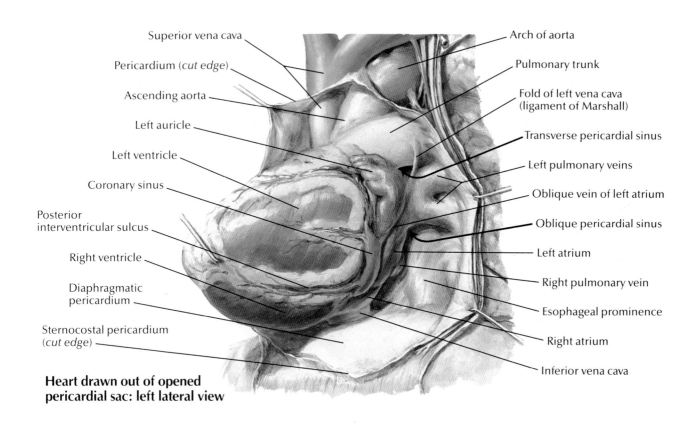

Superior vena cava

Pericardium (*cut edge*)

Ascending aorta

Left auricle

Left ventricle

Coronary sinus

Posterior interventricular sulcus

Right ventricle

Diaphragmatic pericardium

Sternocostal pericardium (*cut edge*)

Arch of aorta

Pulmonary trunk

Fold of left vena cava (ligament of Marshall)

Transverse pericardial sinus

Left pulmonary veins

Oblique vein of left atrium

Oblique pericardial sinus

Left atrium

Right pulmonary vein

Esophageal prominence

Right atrium

Inferior vena cava

Heart drawn out of opened pericardial sac: left lateral view

Right phrenic nerve and pericardiacophrenic vessels

Superior vena cava

Transverse pericardial sinus

Superior vena cava

Right pulmonary veins

Mediastinal pleura (*cut edge*)

Pericardium (*cut edge*)

Inferior vena cava

Line of fusion of pericardium to diaphragm

Arch of aorta

Ascending aorta

Mediastinal pleura (*cut edge*)

Left phrenic nerve and pericardiacophrenic vessels

Pulmonary trunk (bifurcation)

Left lung

Left pulmonary veins

Pericardium (*cut edge*)

Oblique pericardial sinus

Esophageal prominence

Diaphragmatic pericardium

Pericardial sac with heart removed: anterior view

Coronary Arteries and Cardiac Veins

Branch to sinoatrial (SA) node (superior vena cava branch)

Anterior right atrial branch of right coronary artery

Right coronary artery

Anterior cardiac veins

Small cardiac vein

Right marginal branch of right coronary artery

Left coronary artery

Circumflex branch of left coronary artery

Great cardiac vein

Anterior interventricular branch (left anterior descending) of left coronary artery

Sternocostal surface

Oblique vein of left atrium

Great cardiac vein

Circumflex branch of left coronary artery

Coronary sinus

Posterior left ventricular branch

Posterior vein of left ventricle

Middle cardiac vein

Branch to sinoatrial (SA) node (superior vena cava branch)

Sinoatrial (SA) node

Small cardiac vein

Right coronary artery

Posterior interventricular branch of right coronary artery (posterior descending artery)

Right marginal branch

Diaphragmatic surface

PLATE 204

THORAX

Anterior interventricular (left anterior descending) branch of left coronary artery very short. Apical part of sternocostal surface supplied by branches from posterior interventricular (posterior descending) branch of right coronary artery curving around apex

Posterior interventricular (posterior descending) branch derived from circumflex branch of left coronary artery instead of from right coronary artery

Posterior interventricular (posterior descending) branch absent. Area supplied chiefly by small branches from circumflex branch of left coronary artery and from right coronary artery

Posterior interventricular (posterior descending) branch absent. Area supplied chiefly by elongated anterior interventricular (left anterior descending) branch curving around apex

Coronary Arteries: Arteriographic Views

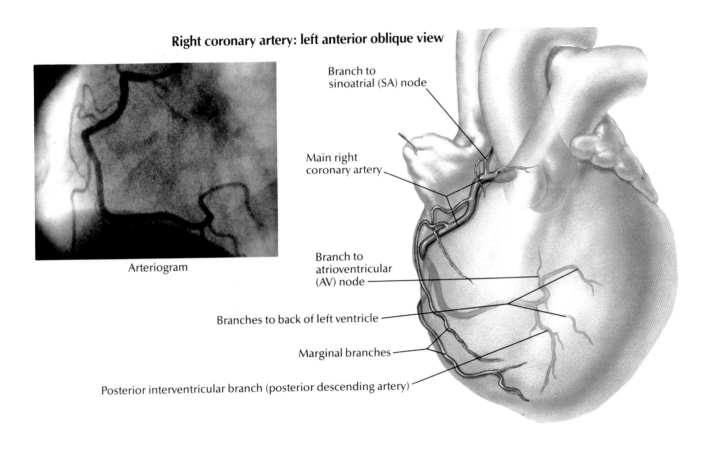

Right coronary artery: left anterior oblique view

Branch to sinoatrial (SA) node

Main right coronary artery

Branch to atrioventricular (AV) node

Branches to back of left ventricle

Marginal branches

Posterior interventricular branch (posterior descending artery)

Arteriogram

Right coronary artery: right anterior oblique view

Branch to sinoatrial (SA) node

Conus arteriosus branch

Main right coronary artery

Marginal branches

Arteriogram

Branch to atrioventricular (AV) node

Branches to back of left ventricle

Posterior interventricular branch (posterior descending artery)

PLATE 206

THORAX

Left coronary artery: left anterior oblique view

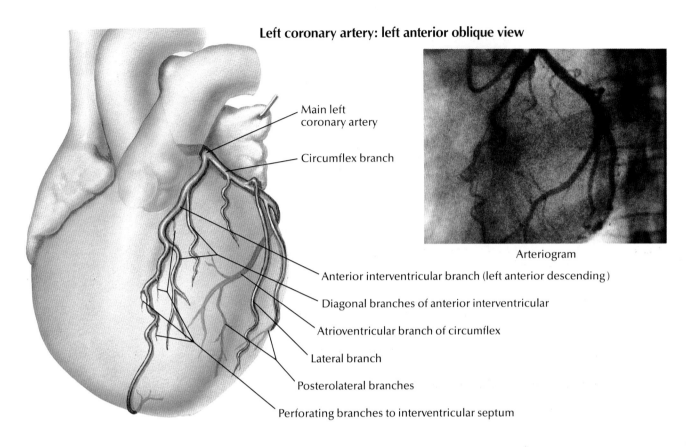

Main left coronary artery

Circumflex branch

Arteriogram

Anterior interventricular branch (left anterior descending)

Diagonal branches of anterior interventricular

Atrioventricular branch of circumflex

Lateral branch

Posterolateral branches

Perforating branches to interventricular septum

Left coronary artery: right anterior oblique view

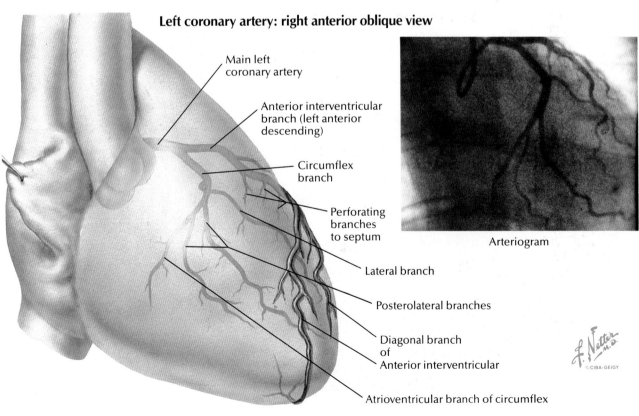

Main left coronary artery

Anterior interventricular branch (left anterior descending)

Circumflex branch

Perforating branches to septum

Arteriogram

Lateral branch

Posterolateral branches

Diagonal branch of Anterior interventricular

Atrioventricular branch of circumflex

Right Atrium and Ventricle

Ascending aorta

Superior vena cava

Right pulmonary artery

Pericardial reflection

Right superior pulmonary vein

Left atrium

Right inferior pulmonary vein

Interatrial septum

Limbus of fossa ovalis

Fossa ovalis

Valve (Eustachian) of inferior vena cava

Inferior vena cava

Pulmonary trunk

Right auricle

Conus arteriosus

Crista terminalis

Membranous septum

Septal (medial) cusp of tricuspid valve

Pectinate muscles

Opening of coronary sinus

Valve (Thebesian) of coronary sinus

Opened right atrium: right lateral view

Pericardial reflection

Aorta

Transverse pericardial sinus

Superior vena cava

Right auricle

Right atrium

Parietal band

Membranous septum

Tricuspid valve
- Anterior cusp
- Septal (medial) cusp
- Posterior cusp

Chordae tendineae

Posterior papillary muscle

Anterior papillary muscle

Trabeculae carneae

Pulmonary trunk

Transverse pericardial sinus

Anterior semilunar cusp

Right semilunar cusp — Pulmonary valve

Left semilunar cusp

Conus arteriosus

Supraventricular crest

Septal (medial) papillary muscle

Interventricular septum

Septal band — Septomarginal trabecula

Moderator band

Opened right ventricle: anterior view

PLATE 208

THORAX

Transverse sinus of pericardium

Fold of left vena cava
(ligament of Marshall)

Left auricle

Oblique vein of left atrium

Mitral
valve { Posterior cusp

Anterior
(aortic) cusp

Anterior papillary muscle

Chordae tendineae

Posterior papillary muscle

Pericardial
reflection

Arch of aorta

Ligamentum
arteriosum

Left pulmonary
artery

Right pulmonary
artery

Left pulmonary veins

Left atrium

Right pulmonary
veins

Coronary
sinus

Inferior
vena cava

**Flap opened in posterolateral
wall of left ventricle**

Left auricle

Conus arteriosus

Aortic
valve {
Left semilunar cusp

Right semilunar cusp

Posterior semilunar cusp

Membranous
septum {
Interventricular
part

Atrioventricular
part

Muscular part of
interventricular
septum

Mitral valve
(*cut away*)

Note: broken line
indicates level
of origin of
tricuspid valve

Arch of aorta

Left pulmonary
artery

Right pulmonary
artery

Left superior
pulmonary vein

Valve of
foramen ovale

Right pulmonary
veins

Left atrium

Coronary sinus

Inferior vena cava

**Section through left atrium and ventricle
with mitral valve cut away**

Valves of Heart

Pulmonary valve
- Anterior semilunar cusp
- Right semilunar cusp
- Left semilunar cusp

Aortic valve
- Right (coronary) semilunar cusp
- Left (coronary) semilunar cusp
- Posterior (noncoronary) semilunar cusp

Mitral valve
- Anterior (aortic) cusp
- Commissural cusps
- Posterior cusp

Annulus fibrosus

Conus arteriosus

Left fibrous trigone

Membranous septum
- Interventricular part (*broken line*)
- Atrio-ventricular part

Tricuspid valve
- Anterior cusp
- Septal (medial) cusp
- Posterior cusp

Annulus fibrosus

Right fibrous trigone

Artery to atrioventricular (AV) node

**Heart in diastole:
viewed from base with atria removed**

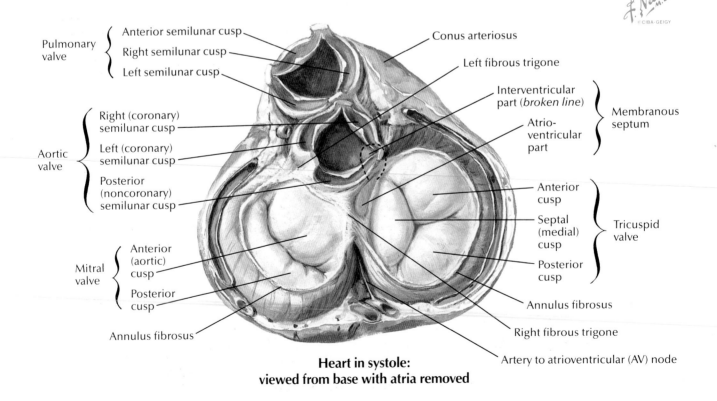

Pulmonary valve
- Anterior semilunar cusp
- Right semilunar cusp
- Left semilunar cusp

Aortic valve
- Right (coronary) semilunar cusp
- Left (coronary) semilunar cusp
- Posterior (noncoronary) semilunar cusp

Mitral valve
- Anterior (aortic) cusp
- Posterior cusp

Annulus fibrosus

Conus arteriosus

Left fibrous trigone

Membranous septum
- Interventricular part (*broken line*)
- Atrio-ventricular part

Tricuspid valve
- Anterior cusp
- Septal (medial) cusp
- Posterior cusp

Annulus fibrosus

Right fibrous trigone

Artery to atrioventricular (AV) node

**Heart in systole:
viewed from base with atria removed**

PLATE 210

THORAX

Ascending aorta

Aortic sinuses (of Valsalva)

Opening of
right coronary artery

Membranous septum { Interventricular part / Atrioventricular part

Note: broken line indicates level of origin of tricuspid valve on opposite side of septum

Muscular interventricular septum

Opening of left coronary artery

Nodule (Arantii) of semilunar valve

Lunula

Left semilunar cusp

Posterior semilunar cusp } Aortic valve

Right semilunar cusp

Anterior papillary muscle

Anterior (aortic) cusp of mitral valve

Aortic valve

Inferior vena cava

Right atrium

Coronary sinus

Chordae tendineae

Septal (medial) papillary muscle

Posterior papillary muscle (*sectioned*)

Septal band of septomarginal trabecula

Atrioventricular part

Interventricular part (*behind valve*) } Membranous septum

Posterior cusp

Anterior cusp } Tricuspid valve

Septal cusp

Posterior papillary muscle (*sectioned*)

Anterior papillary muscle

Tricuspid (right atrioventricular) valve

Left atrium

Chordae tendineae

Anterior papillary muscle (*sectioned*)

Posterior papillary muscle

Anterior cusp

Posterior cusp } Mitral valve

Commissural cusps

Anterior papillary muscle (*sectioned*)

Fibrous (Albini's) nodules

Mitral (left atrioventricular) valve

f. Netter
©CIBA-GEIGY

Atria, Ventricles and Interventricular Septum

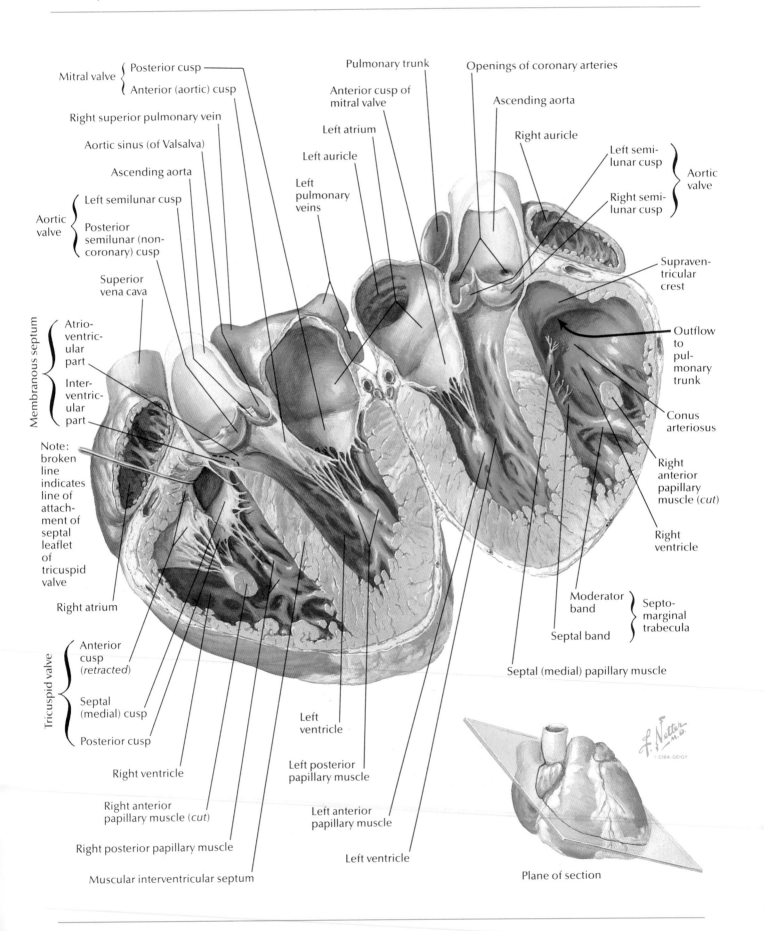

Mitral valve {
- Posterior cusp
- Anterior (aortic) cusp
}

Right superior pulmonary vein

Aortic sinus (of Valsalva)

Ascending aorta

Aortic valve {
- Left semilunar cusp
- Posterior semilunar (non-coronary) cusp
}

Superior vena cava

Membranous septum {
Atrio-ventricular part

Inter-ventricular part
}

Note: broken line indicates line of attachment of septal leaflet of tricuspid valve

Right atrium

Tricuspid valve {
Anterior cusp (retracted)

Septal (medial) cusp

Posterior cusp
}

Right ventricle

Right anterior papillary muscle (cut)

Right posterior papillary muscle

Muscular interventricular septum

Pulmonary trunk

Anterior cusp of mitral valve

Left atrium

Left auricle

Left pulmonary veins

Openings of coronary arteries

Ascending aorta

Right auricle

Left semilunar cusp
Right semilunar cusp
} Aortic valve

Supraventricular crest

Outflow to pulmonary trunk

Conus arteriosus

Right anterior papillary muscle (cut)

Right ventricle

Moderator band
Septal band
} Septomarginal trabecula

Septal (medial) papillary muscle

Left ventricle

Left posterior papillary muscle

Left anterior papillary muscle

Left ventricle

Plane of section

PLATE 212

THORAX

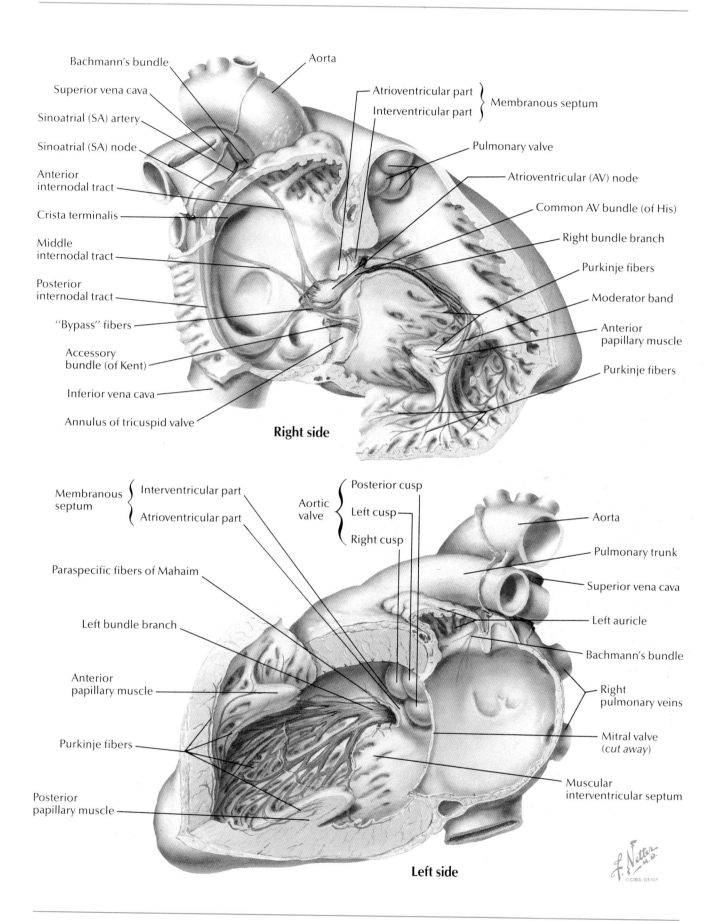

Bachmann's bundle

Aorta

Superior vena cava

Atrioventricular part

Interventricular part

Membranous septum

Sinoatrial (SA) artery

Sinoatrial (SA) node

Pulmonary valve

Anterior internodal tract

Atrioventricular (AV) node

Crista terminalis

Common AV bundle (of His)

Middle internodal tract

Right bundle branch

Purkinje fibers

Posterior internodal tract

Moderator band

"Bypass" fibers

Anterior papillary muscle

Accessory bundle (of Kent)

Purkinje fibers

Inferior vena cava

Annulus of tricuspid valve

Right side

Membranous septum

Interventricular part

Atrioventricular part

Aortic valve

Posterior cusp

Left cusp

Right cusp

Aorta

Pulmonary trunk

Paraspecific fibers of Mahaim

Superior vena cava

Left bundle branch

Left auricle

Bachmann's bundle

Anterior papillary muscle

Right pulmonary veins

Purkinje fibers

Mitral valve (*cut away*)

Posterior papillary muscle

Muscular interventricular septum

Left side

Nerves of Heart

SEE ALSO PLATES 124, 152, 198

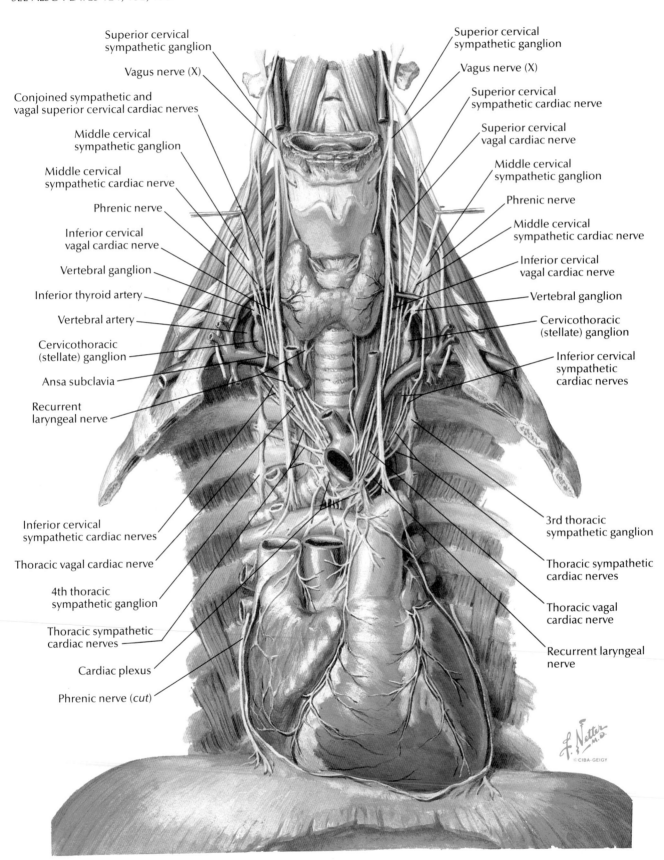

Superior cervical sympathetic ganglion

Vagus nerve (X)

Conjoined sympathetic and vagal superior cervical cardiac nerves

Middle cervical sympathetic ganglion

Middle cervical sympathetic cardiac nerve

Phrenic nerve

Inferior cervical vagal cardiac nerve

Vertebral ganglion

Inferior thyroid artery

Vertebral artery

Cervicothoracic (stellate) ganglion

Ansa subclavia

Recurrent laryngeal nerve

Inferior cervical sympathetic cardiac nerves

Thoracic vagal cardiac nerve

4th thoracic sympathetic ganglion

Thoracic sympathetic cardiac nerves

Cardiac plexus

Phrenic nerve (cut)

Superior cervical sympathetic ganglion

Vagus nerve (X)

Superior cervical sympathetic cardiac nerve

Superior cervical vagal cardiac nerve

Middle cervical sympathetic ganglion

Phrenic nerve

Middle cervical sympathetic cardiac nerve

Inferior cervical vagal cardiac nerve

Vertebral ganglion

Cervicothoracic (stellate) ganglion

Inferior cervical sympathetic cardiac nerves

3rd thoracic sympathetic ganglion

Thoracic sympathetic cardiac nerves

Thoracic vagal cardiac nerve

Recurrent laryngeal nerve

PLATE 214

Superior cervical sympathetic ganglion

Superior cervical sympathetic cardiac nerve

Middle cervical sympathetic ganglion

Middle cervical sympathetic cardiac nerve

Vertebral ganglion

Ansa subclavia

Cervicothoracic (stellate) ganglion

1st thoracic (intercostal) nerve

Inferior cervical sympathetic cardiac nerve

Thoracic vagal cardiac nerve

2nd thoracic sympathetic ganglion

White ramus communicans

Gray ramus communicans

Thoracic sympathetic cardiac nerves

4th thoracic sympathetic ganglion

Dorsal vagal nucleus

Nucleus of solitary tract

Medulla oblongata

Vagus nerves

Superior cervical vagal cardiac nerves

Inferior cervical vagal cardiac nerves

Ascending connections

T1

T2

T3

T4

Cardiac plexus

——————— Sympathetic preganglionic
– – – – – – Sympathetic postganglionic
——————— Vagal preganglionic
– – – – – – Vagal postganglionic
——————— Sympathetic afferent
——————— Vagal afferent

Innervation of Blood Vessels: Schema

SEE ALSO PLATE 153

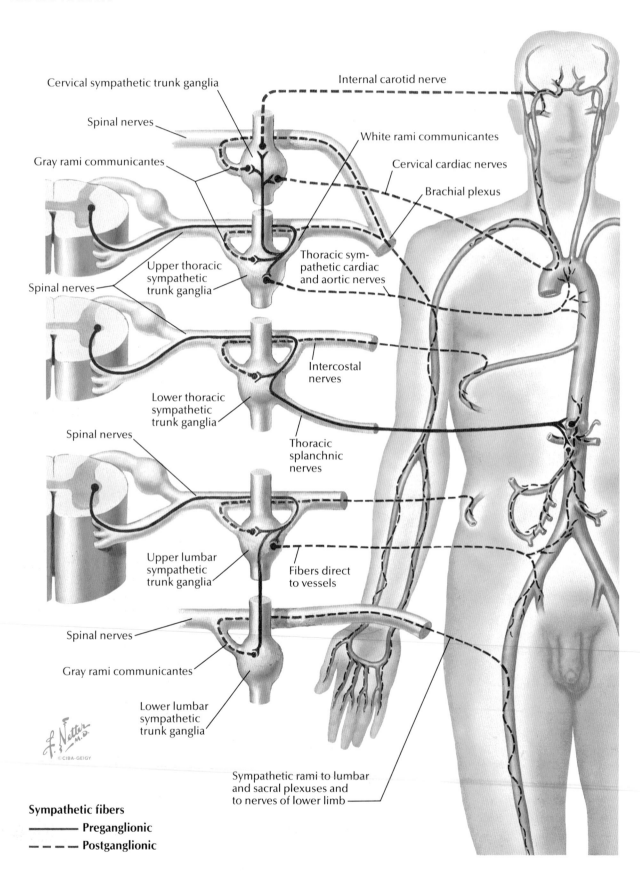

Cervical sympathetic trunk ganglia

Internal carotid nerve

Spinal nerves

White rami communicantes

Gray rami communicantes

Cervical cardiac nerves

Brachial plexus

Upper thoracic sympathetic trunk ganglia

Thoracic sympathetic cardiac and aortic nerves

Spinal nerves

Intercostal nerves

Lower thoracic sympathetic trunk ganglia

Spinal nerves

Thoracic splanchnic nerves

Upper lumbar sympathetic trunk ganglia

Fibers direct to vessels

Spinal nerves

Gray rami communicantes

Lower lumbar sympathetic trunk ganglia

Sympathetic rami to lumbar and sacral plexuses and to nerves of lower limb

Sympathetic fibers

———— **Preganglionic**

– – – – **Postganglionic**

PLATE 216

THORAX

FOR OBLITERATED UMBILICAL VESSELS SEE PLATE 236

Prenatal circulation

Pulmonary trunk

Superior vena cava

Right pulmonary artery

Right pulmonary vein

Foramen ovale

Hepatic vein

Ductus venosus

Liver

Portal vein

Umbilical vein

Umbilical arteries

Aorta

Ductus arteriosus

Left pulmonary artery

Left pulmonary vein

Inferior vena cava

Aorta

Celiac trunk

Superior mesenteric artery

Kidney

Gut

Ligamentum arteriosum (obliterated ductus arteriosus)

Fossa ovalis (obliterated foramen ovale)

Ligamentum venosum (obliterated ductus venosus)

Ligamentum teres (round ligament) of liver (obliterated umbilical vein)

Medial umbilical ligaments (obliterated umbilical arteries)

Postnatal circulation

Mediastinum: Right Lateral View

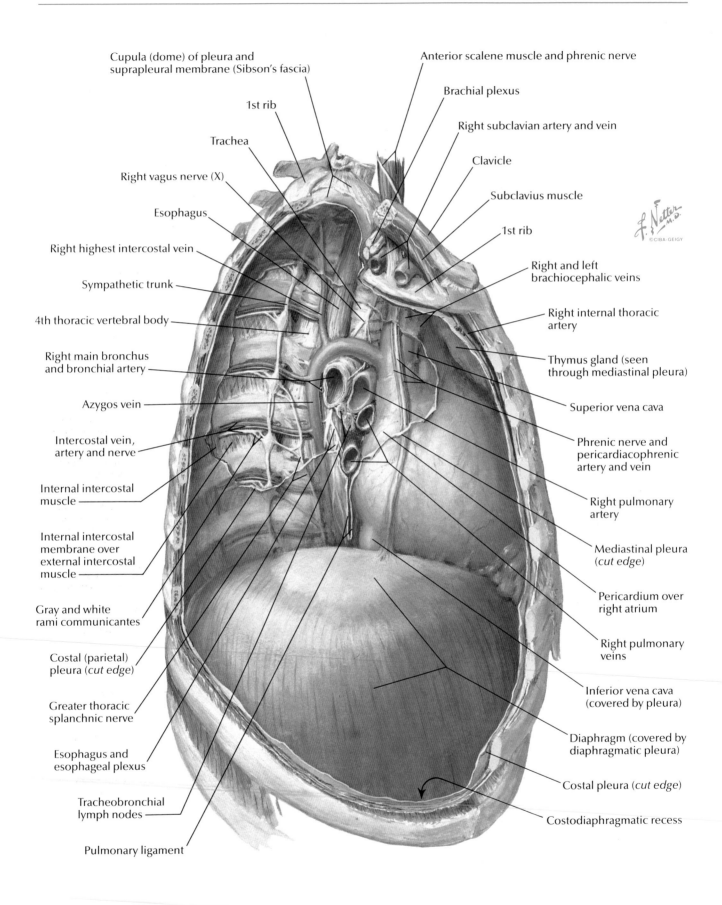

Cupula (dome) of pleura and suprapleural membrane (Sibson's fascia)

1st rib

Trachea

Right vagus nerve (X)

Esophagus

Right highest intercostal vein

Sympathetic trunk

4th thoracic vertebral body

Right main bronchus and bronchial artery

Azygos vein

Intercostal vein, artery and nerve

Internal intercostal muscle

Internal intercostal membrane over external intercostal muscle

Gray and white rami communicantes

Costal (parietal) pleura (cut edge)

Greater thoracic splanchnic nerve

Esophagus and esophageal plexus

Tracheobronchial lymph nodes

Pulmonary ligament

Anterior scalene muscle and phrenic nerve

Brachial plexus

Right subclavian artery and vein

Clavicle

Subclavius muscle

1st rib

Right and left brachiocephalic veins

Right internal thoracic artery

Thymus gland (seen through mediastinal pleura)

Superior vena cava

Phrenic nerve and pericardiacophrenic artery and vein

Right pulmonary artery

Mediastinal pleura (cut edge)

Pericardium over right atrium

Right pulmonary veins

Inferior vena cava (covered by pleura)

Diaphragm (covered by diaphragmatic pleura)

Costal pleura (cut edge)

Costodiaphragmatic recess

PLATE 218

THORAX

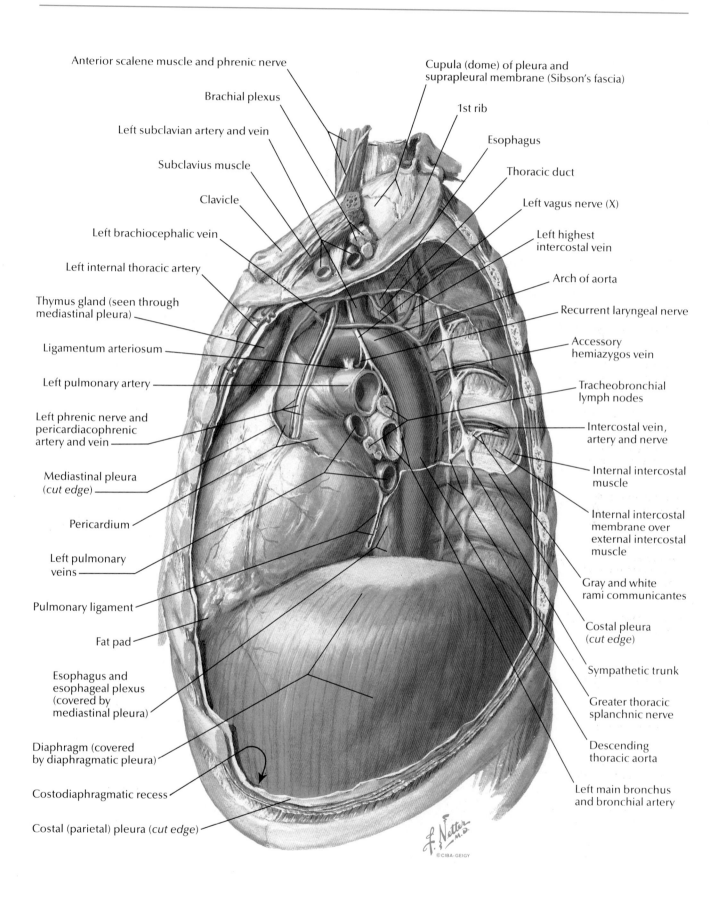

Anterior scalene muscle and phrenic nerve

Brachial plexus

Left subclavian artery and vein

Subclavius muscle

Clavicle

Left brachiocephalic vein

Left internal thoracic artery

Thymus gland (seen through mediastinal pleura)

Ligamentum arteriosum

Left pulmonary artery

Left phrenic nerve and pericardiacophrenic artery and vein

Mediastinal pleura (*cut edge*)

Pericardium

Left pulmonary veins

Pulmonary ligament

Fat pad

Esophagus and esophageal plexus (covered by mediastinal pleura)

Diaphragm (covered by diaphragmatic pleura)

Costodiaphragmatic recess

Costal (parietal) pleura (*cut edge*)

Cupula (dome) of pleura and suprapleural membrane (Sibson's fascia)

1st rib

Esophagus

Thoracic duct

Left vagus nerve (X)

Left highest intercostal vein

Arch of aorta

Recurrent laryngeal nerve

Accessory hemiazygos vein

Tracheobronchial lymph nodes

Intercostal vein, artery and nerve

Internal intercostal muscle

Internal intercostal membrane over external intercostal muscle

Gray and white rami communicantes

Costal pleura (*cut edge*)

Sympathetic trunk

Greater thoracic splanchnic nerve

Descending thoracic aorta

Left main bronchus and bronchial artery

Esophagus In Situ

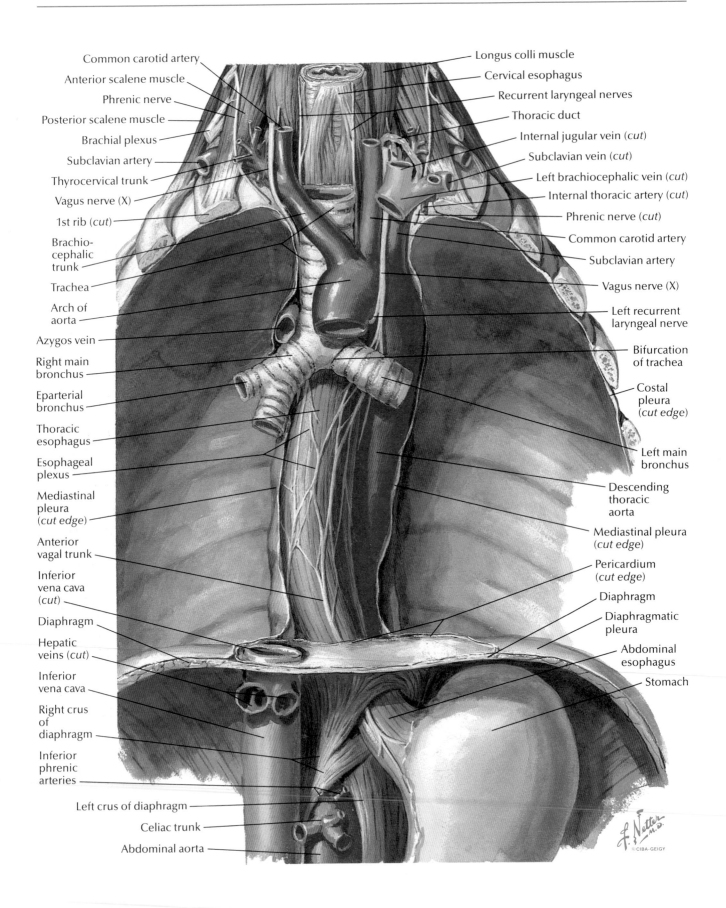

Common carotid artery

Anterior scalene muscle

Phrenic nerve

Posterior scalene muscle

Brachial plexus

Subclavian artery

Thyrocervical trunk

Vagus nerve (X)

1st rib (cut)

Brachio-
cephalic
trunk

Trachea

Arch of
aorta

Azygos vein

Right main
bronchus

Eparterial
bronchus

Thoracic
esophagus

Esophageal
plexus

Mediastinal
pleura
(cut edge)

Anterior
vagal trunk

Inferior
vena cava
(cut)

Diaphragm

Hepatic
veins (cut)

Inferior
vena cava

Right crus
of
diaphragm

Inferior
phrenic
arteries

Left crus of diaphragm

Celiac trunk

Abdominal aorta

Longus colli muscle

Cervical esophagus

Recurrent laryngeal nerves

Thoracic duct

Internal jugular vein (cut)

Subclavian vein (cut)

Left brachiocephalic vein (cut)

Internal thoracic artery (cut)

Phrenic nerve (cut)

Common carotid artery

Subclavian artery

Vagus nerve (X)

Left recurrent
laryngeal nerve

Bifurcation
of trachea

Costal
pleura
(cut edge)

Left main
bronchus

Descending
thoracic
aorta

Mediastinal pleura
(cut edge)

Pericardium
(cut edge)

Diaphragm

Diaphragmatic
pleura

Abdominal
esophagus

Stomach

PLATE 220

THORAX

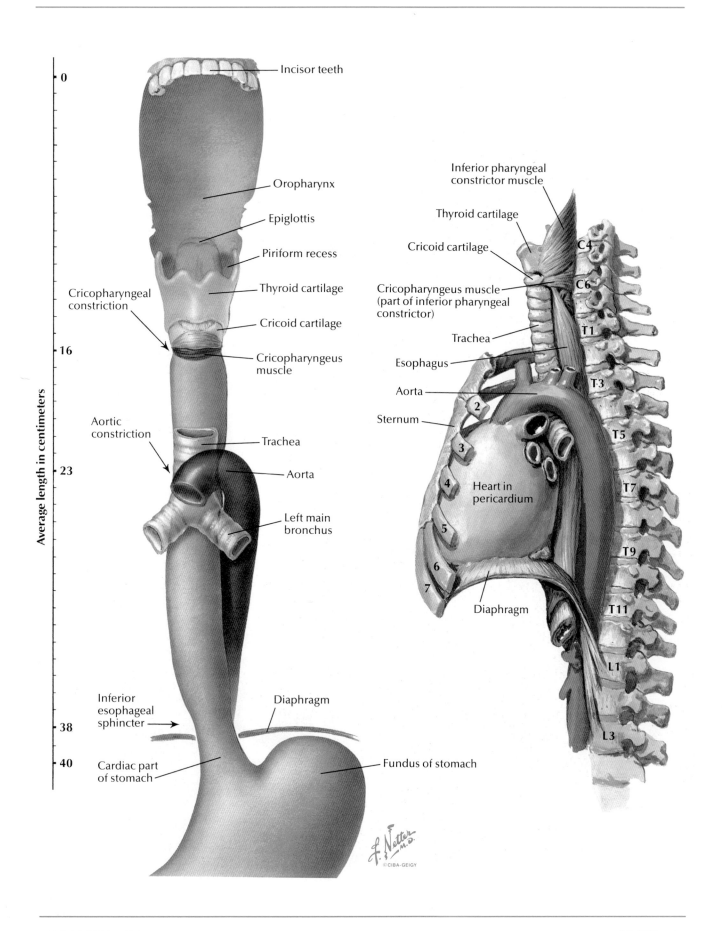

Average length in centimeters

0 — Incisor teeth

Oropharynx

Epiglottis

Piriform recess

Cricopharyngeal constriction — Thyroid cartilage

16 — Cricoid cartilage

Cricopharyngeus muscle

Aortic constriction — Trachea

23 — Aorta

Left main bronchus

Inferior esophageal sphincter — Diaphragm

38 —

40 — Cardiac part of stomach — Fundus of stomach

Inferior pharyngeal constrictor muscle

Thyroid cartilage

Cricoid cartilage — C4

Cricopharyngeus muscle (part of inferior pharyngeal constrictor) — C6

Trachea — T1

Esophagus — T3

Aorta

Sternum

Heart in pericardium — T5

T7

T9

Diaphragm — T11

L1

L3

2, 3, 4, 5, 6, 7

Inferior pharyngeal constrictor muscle

Pharyngeal raphé

Zone of sparse muscle fibers

Cricopharyngeus muscle
(part of inferior pharyngeal
constrictor)

Main longitudinal muscle bundle
passing upward and ventrally to
attach to middle of posterior
surface of cricoid cartilage

Accessory muscle bundle from posterolateral surface of cricoid cartilage

Additional fibers from contralateral
side of cricopharyngeus muscle

Circular muscle layer with
sparse longitudinal fibers
in V-shaped area (of Laimer)

Bare area on ventral surface of esophagus

Lateral mass of longitudinal muscle

Fibroelastic membranes
with sparse muscle fibers

Window cut in longitudinal muscle

Circular muscle layer

Thyroid
cartilage

Cricoid
cartilage

Trachea

Left main
bronchus

Hook

PLATE 222

THORAX

Superior pharyngeal constrictor muscle

Root of tongue

Epiglottis

Middle pharyngeal constrictor muscle

Palatopharyngeus muscle ⎫
Stylopharyngeus muscle ⎭ Longitudinal pharyngeal muscles

Pharyngoepiglottic fold

Aditus of larynx

Thyroid cartilage (superior horn)

Thyrohyoid membrane

Internal branch of superior laryngeal nerve and superior laryngeal artery and vein

Oblique arytenoid muscle

Transverse arytenoid muscle

Thyroid cartilage

Posterior cricoarytenoid muscle

Inferior pharyngeal constrictor muscle

Pharyngeal aponeurosis (*cut away*)

Zone of sparse muscle fibers

Cricopharyngeus muscle (part of inferior pharyngeal constrictor)

Cricoid cartilage (posterior surface)

Tendinous attachment of longitudinal esophageal muscle

Circular esophageal muscle

Esophageal mucosa and submucosa

Circular muscle in V-shaped area (of Laimer)

Right recurrent laryngeal nerve

Longitudinal esophageal muscle

Posterior view with pharynx opened and mucosa removed

Window cut in longitudinal muscle exposes circular muscle layer

f. Netter
©CIBA-GEIGY

Esophagogastric Junction

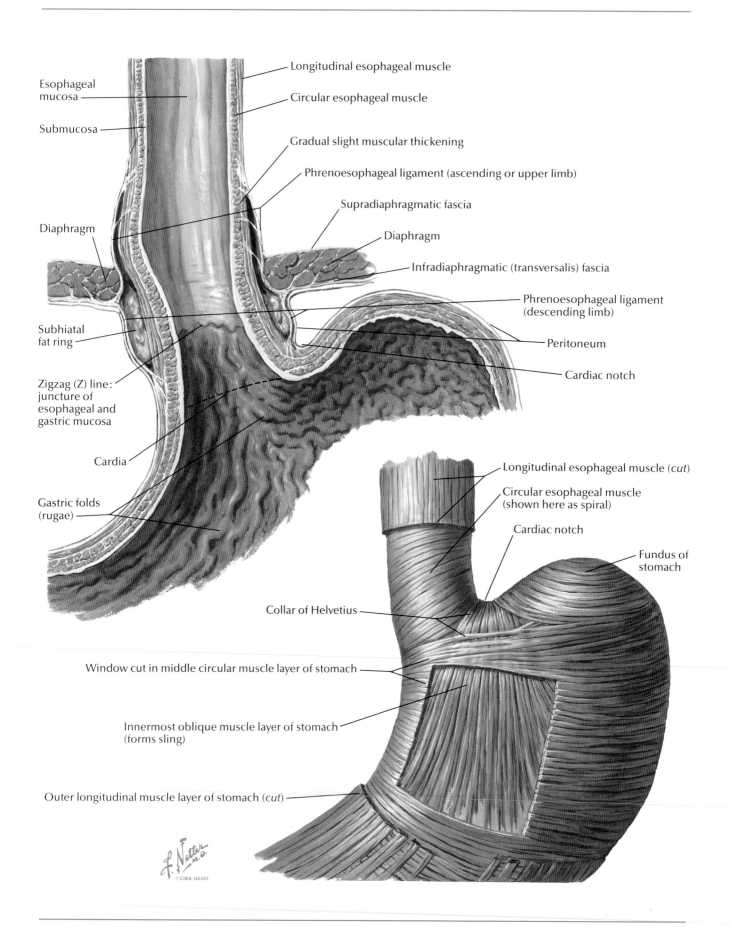

Longitudinal esophageal muscle

Circular esophageal muscle

Esophageal mucosa

Gradual slight muscular thickening

Submucosa

Phrenoesophageal ligament (ascending or upper limb)

Supradiaphragmatic fascia

Diaphragm

Diaphragm

Infradiaphragmatic (transversalis) fascia

Phrenoesophageal ligament (descending limb)

Subhiatal fat ring

Peritoneum

Zigzag (Z) line: juncture of esophageal and gastric mucosa

Cardiac notch

Cardia

Longitudinal esophageal muscle (cut)

Circular esophageal muscle (shown here as spiral)

Cardiac notch

Gastric folds (rugae)

Fundus of stomach

Collar of Helvetius

Window cut in middle circular muscle layer of stomach

Innermost oblique muscle layer of stomach (forms sling)

Outer longitudinal muscle layer of stomach (cut)

PLATE 224

THORAX

Esophageal branch of Inferior thyroid artery

Common carotid artery

Subclavian artery

Esophageal branch of Inferior thyroid artery

Thyrocervical trunk

Subclavian artery

Vertebral artery

Internal thoracic artery

Common carotid artery

Brachiocephalic trunk

Trachea

Arch of aorta

3rd right posterior intercostal artery

Right bronchial artery

Superior left bronchial artery

Esophageal branch of right bronchial artery

Inferior left bronchial artery and esophageal branch

Descending thoracic aorta

Aortic esophageal arteries

Thoracic esophagus

Diaphragm

Stomach

Esophageal branch

Left gastric artery

Celiac trunk

Splenic artery (cut)

Inferior phrenic arteries

Common hepatic artery (cut)

Common variations: esophageal branches may originate from left inferior phrenic artery and/or directly from celiac trunk. Branches to abdominal esophagus may also come from splenic or short gastric arteries

Inferior thyroid vein

Internal jugular vein

External jugular vein

Subclavian vein

Vertebral vein

Right brachiocephalic vein

Superior vena cava

Right highest intercostal vein

Esophagus

6th right intercostal vein

Azygos vein

Junction of hemiazygos and azygos veins

Inferior vena cava (*cut*)

Diaphragm

Liver

Hepatic veins

Inferior vena cava

Portal vein

Right renal vein

Left gastric (coronary) vein

Right gastric vein

Esophageal branches of coronary vein

Inferior thyroid vein

Internal jugular vein

Thoracic duct

Subclavian vein

Left brachio-cephalic vein

Left highest intercostal vein

Esophageal plexus

Accessory hemiazygos vein

Venae comitantes of vagus nerve

Hemiazygos vein

Submucous venous plexus

Left inferior phrenic vein

Short gastric veins

Splenic vein

Left suprarenal vein

Left renal vein

Left gastroepiploic (gastroomental) vein

Superior mesenteric vein

Inferior mesenteric vein

Right gastroepiploic (gastroomental) vein

PLATE 226

THORAX

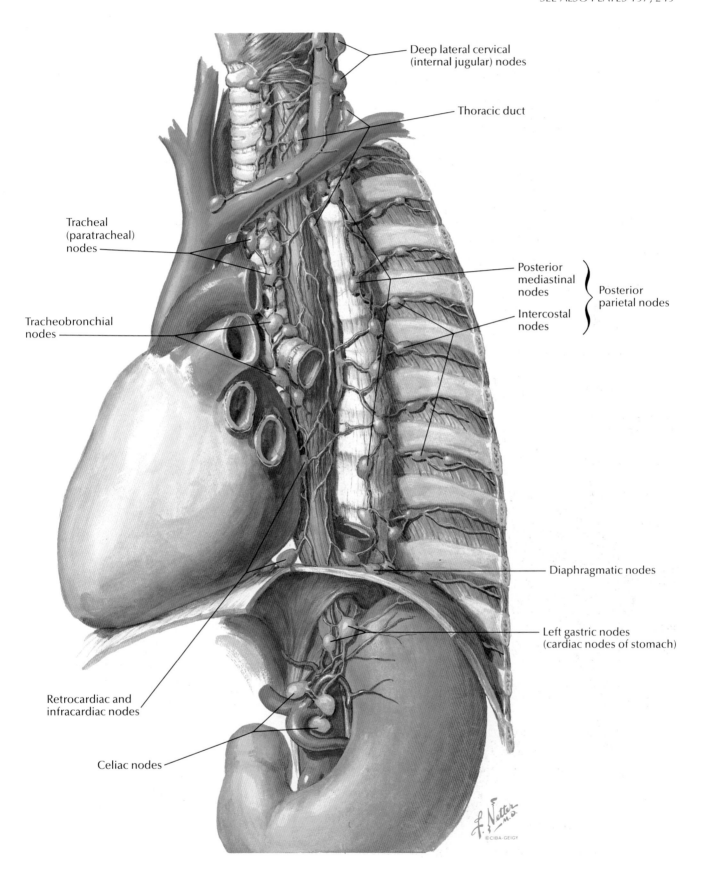

Deep lateral cervical
(internal jugular) nodes

Thoracic duct

Tracheal
(paratracheal)
nodes

Posterior
mediastinal
nodes

Intercostal
nodes

} Posterior
parietal nodes

Tracheobronchial
nodes

Diaphragmatic nodes

Left gastric nodes
(cardiac nodes of stomach)

Retrocardiac and
infracardiac nodes

Celiac nodes

Nerves of Esophagus

SEE ALSO PLATES 152, 198

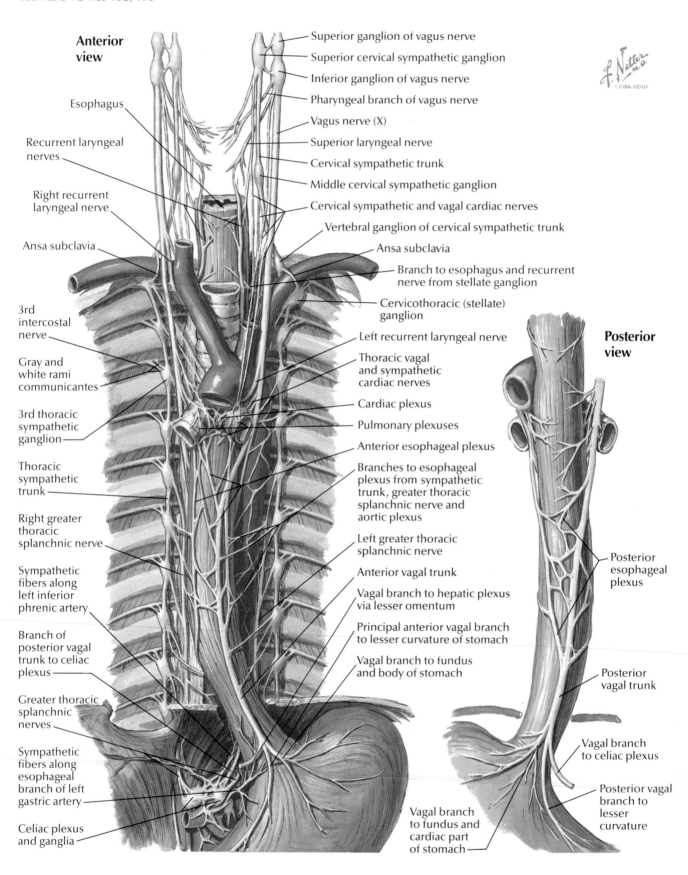

Anterior view

Esophagus

Recurrent laryngeal nerves

Right recurrent laryngeal nerve

Ansa subclavia

3rd intercostal nerve

Gray and white rami communicantes

3rd thoracic sympathetic ganglion

Thoracic sympathetic trunk

Right greater thoracic splanchnic nerve

Sympathetic fibers along left inferior phrenic artery

Branch of posterior vagal trunk to celiac plexus

Greater thoracic splanchnic nerves

Sympathetic fibers along esophageal branch of left gastric artery

Celiac plexus and ganglia

Superior ganglion of vagus nerve

Superior cervical sympathetic ganglion

Inferior ganglion of vagus nerve

Pharyngeal branch of vagus nerve

Vagus nerve (X)

Superior laryngeal nerve

Cervical sympathetic trunk

Middle cervical sympathetic ganglion

Cervical sympathetic and vagal cardiac nerves

Vertebral ganglion of cervical sympathetic trunk

Ansa subclavia

Branch to esophagus and recurrent nerve from stellate ganglion

Cervicothoracic (stellate) ganglion

Left recurrent laryngeal nerve

Thoracic vagal and sympathetic cardiac nerves

Cardiac plexus

Pulmonary plexuses

Anterior esophageal plexus

Branches to esophageal plexus from sympathetic trunk, greater thoracic splanchnic nerve and aortic plexus

Left greater thoracic splanchnic nerve

Anterior vagal trunk

Vagal branch to hepatic plexus via lesser omentum

Principal anterior vagal branch to lesser curvature of stomach

Vagal branch to fundus and body of stomach

Posterior view

Posterior esophageal plexus

Posterior vagal trunk

Vagal branch to celiac plexus

Posterior vagal branch to lesser curvature

Vagal branch to fundus and cardiac part of stomach

PLATE 228

Variations

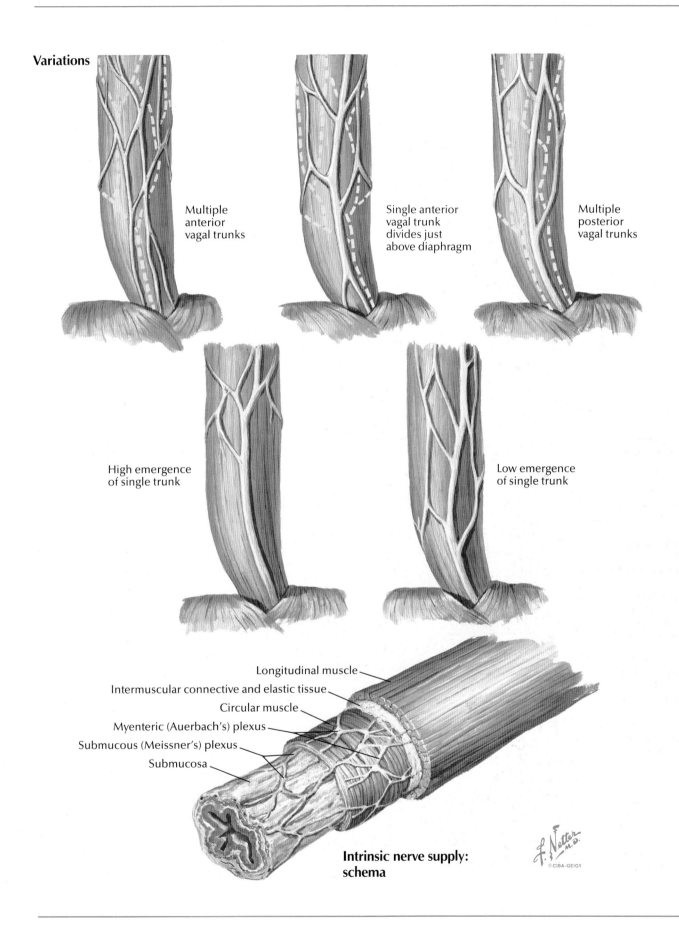

Multiple anterior vagal trunks

Single anterior vagal trunk divides just above diaphragm

Multiple posterior vagal trunks

High emergence of single trunk

Low emergence of single trunk

Longitudinal muscle

Intermuscular connective and elastic tissue

Circular muscle

Myenteric (Auerbach's) plexus

Submucous (Meissner's) plexus

Submucosa

Intrinsic nerve supply: schema

Mediastinum: Cross Section

Superior view

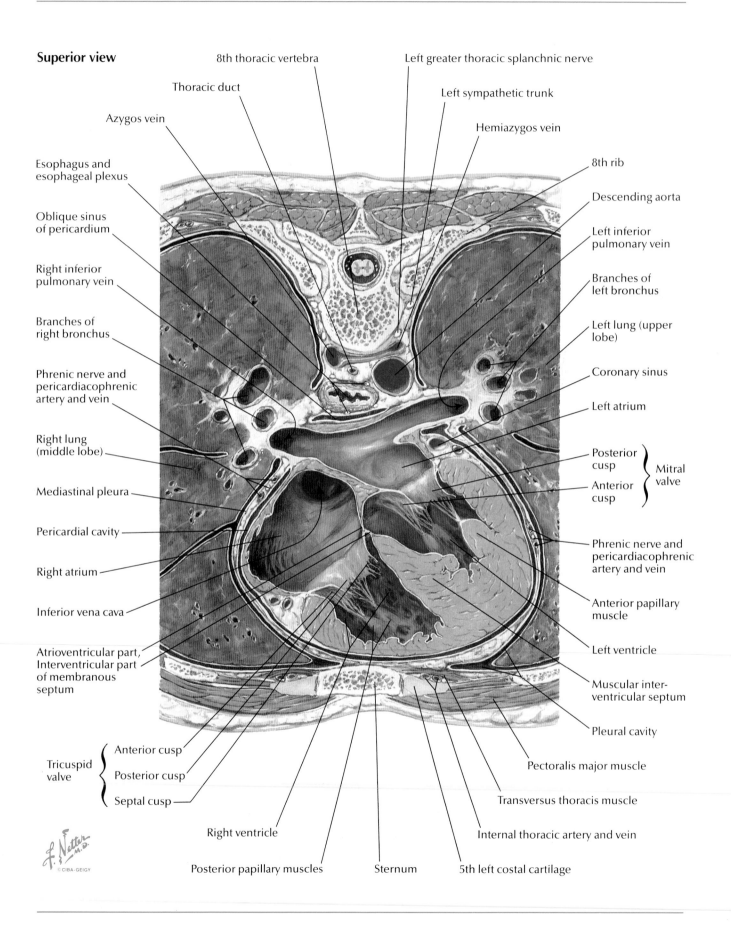

8th thoracic vertebra

Left greater thoracic splanchnic nerve

Thoracic duct

Left sympathetic trunk

Azygos vein

Hemiazygos vein

Esophagus and esophageal plexus

8th rib

Oblique sinus of pericardium

Descending aorta

Right inferior pulmonary vein

Left inferior pulmonary vein

Branches of right bronchus

Branches of left bronchus

Phrenic nerve and pericardiacophrenic artery and vein

Left lung (upper lobe)

Right lung (middle lobe)

Coronary sinus

Mediastinal pleura

Left atrium

Pericardial cavity

Posterior cusp } Mitral valve

Right atrium

Anterior cusp

Inferior vena cava

Phrenic nerve and pericardiacophrenic artery and vein

Atrioventricular part, Interventricular part of membranous septum

Anterior papillary muscle

Left ventricle

Muscular inter-ventricular septum

Pleural cavity

Anterior cusp

Tricuspid valve { Posterior cusp

Septal cusp

Pectoralis major muscle

Transversus thoracis muscle

Internal thoracic artery and vein

Right ventricle

Posterior papillary muscles

Sternum

5th left costal cartilage

PLATE 230

THORAX

Section IV

ABDOMEN

Body of
sternum

Xiphoid
process

12th rib

Transverse processes of lumbar vertebrae

Iliac tuberosity

Iliac crest

Wing (ala) of ilium

Greater
sciatic
notch

Arcuate line

Ischial spine

Lesser
sciatic notch

Greater trochanter
of femur

Pecten pubis
(pectineal line)

Pubic symphysis

Ischial tuberosity

Lesser trochanter
of femur

Costal
cartilages

4
5
6
7
8
9
10

T11
T12
L1
L2
L3
L4
L5

Sacral
promontory

Sacrum

Coccyx

Pubic arch

Iliac
crest

Internal lip
Intermediate
line
External
lip
Tubercle

Anterior superior
iliac spine

Anterior inferior
iliac spine

Iliopubic
eminence

Superior
pubic ramus

Obturator
foramen

Pubic tubercle

Inferior
pubic ramus

Arcuate pubic ligament

Anterior Abdominal Wall: Superficial Dissection

Pectoralis major muscle

Xiphoid process

Rectus sheath

Linea alba

Subcutaneous (superficial) fascia

Thoracoepigastric vein

Camper's (fatty) and Scarpa's (membranous) subcutaneous fascia (*turned back*)

Attachment of Scarpa's fascia to fascia lata

Superficial circumflex iliac vessels

Superficial epigastric vessels

Superficial external pudendal vessels

Fundiform ligament

Superficial (dartos) fascia of penis and scrotum (*cut*)

Deep penile (Buck's) fascia with deep dorsal vein of penis showing through

Serratus anterior muscle

Latissimus dorsi muscle

External abdominal oblique muscle { Muscular part / Aponeurotic part }

Anterior superior iliac spine

Inguinal (Poupart's) ligament

Intercrural fibers

Superficial inguinal ring

External spermatic fascia on spermatic cord

Cribriform fascia in fossa ovalis

Fascia lata

Great saphenous vein

Superficial dorsal vein of penis

PLATE 232

ABDOMEN

Latissimus
dorsi muscle

Serratus
anterior muscle

External abdominal
oblique muscle
(*cut away*)

External
intercostal muscles

External oblique
aponeurosis
(*cut edge*)

Rectus sheath

Internal abdominal
oblique muscle

Anterior superior
iliac spine

Inguinal (Poupart's)
ligament

Cremaster muscle
(lateral origin)

Falx inguinalis
(conjoined tendon)

Reflected
inguinal ligament

Femoral vein
(in femoral sheath)

Fossa ovalis

Cremaster muscle
(medial origin)

Fascia lata

Great saphenous vein

6
7
8
9
10

Pectoralis major
muscles

Anterior layer of
rectus sheath
(*cut edges*)

Linea alba

Rectus abdominis
muscle

External abdominal
oblique muscle
(*cut away*)

Tendinous inscription

Internal abdominal
oblique muscle

Pyramidalis muscle

Falx inguinalis
(conjoined tendon)

Inguinal (Poupart's)
ligament

Anterior superior
iliac spine

External oblique
aponeurosis (*cut and
turned down*)

Pectineal (Cooper's)
ligament

Lacunar (Gimbernat's)
ligament

Reflected inguinal
ligament

Pubic tubercle

Suspensory ligament
of penis

Cremaster muscles
and fascia

Deep penile
(Buck's) fascia

External spermatic
fascia (*cut*)

Superficial (dartos)
fascia of penis
and scrotum (*cut*)

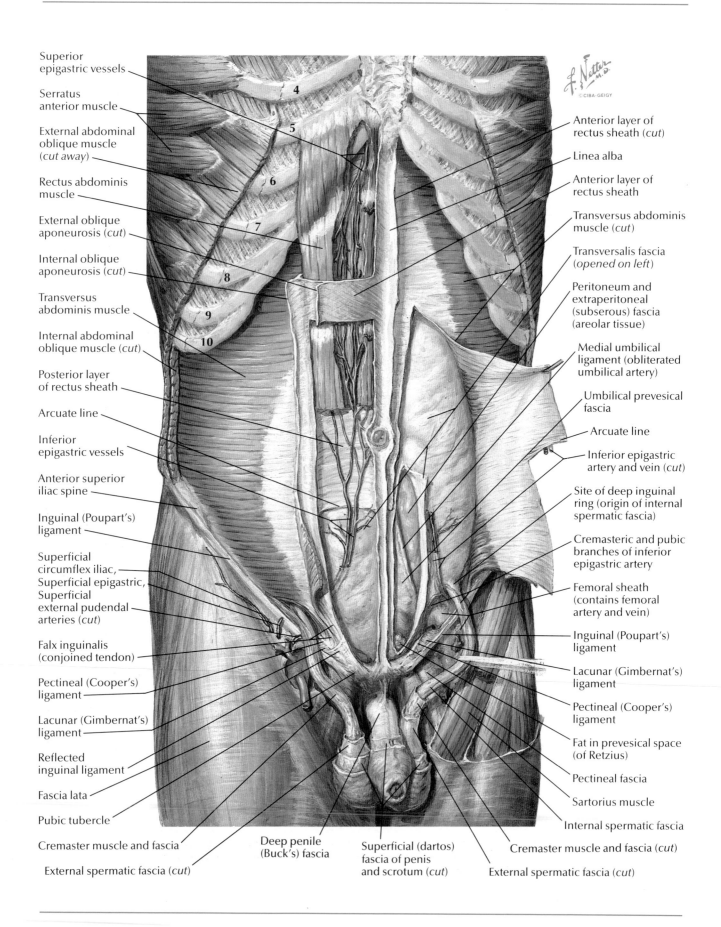

Superior epigastric vessels

Serratus anterior muscle

External abdominal oblique muscle (*cut away*)

Rectus abdominis muscle

External oblique aponeurosis (*cut*)

Internal oblique aponeurosis (*cut*)

Transversus abdominis muscle

Internal abdominal oblique muscle (*cut*)

Posterior layer of rectus sheath

Arcuate line

Inferior epigastric vessels

Anterior superior iliac spine

Inguinal (Poupart's) ligament

Superficial circumflex iliac, Superficial epigastric, Superficial external pudendal arteries (*cut*)

Falx inguinalis (conjoined tendon)

Pectineal (Cooper's) ligament

Lacunar (Gimbernat's) ligament

Reflected inguinal ligament

Fascia lata

Pubic tubercle

Cremaster muscle and fascia

External spermatic fascia (*cut*)

Deep penile (Buck's) fascia

Superficial (dartos) fascia of penis and scrotum (*cut*)

Anterior layer of rectus sheath (*cut*)

Linea alba

Anterior layer of rectus sheath

Transversus abdominis muscle (*cut*)

Transversalis fascia (*opened on left*)

Peritoneum and extraperitoneal (subserous) fascia (areolar tissue)

Medial umbilical ligament (obliterated umbilical artery)

Umbilical prevesical fascia

Arcuate line

Inferior epigastric artery and vein (*cut*)

Site of deep inguinal ring (origin of internal spermatic fascia)

Cremasteric and pubic branches of inferior epigastric artery

Femoral sheath (contains femoral artery and vein)

Inguinal (Poupart's) ligament

Lacunar (Gimbernat's) ligament

Pectineal (Cooper's) ligament

Fat in prevesical space (of Retzius)

Pectineal fascia

Sartorius muscle

Internal spermatic fascia

Cremaster muscle and fascia (*cut*)

External spermatic fascia (*cut*)

PLATE 234

ABDOMEN

Section above arcuate line

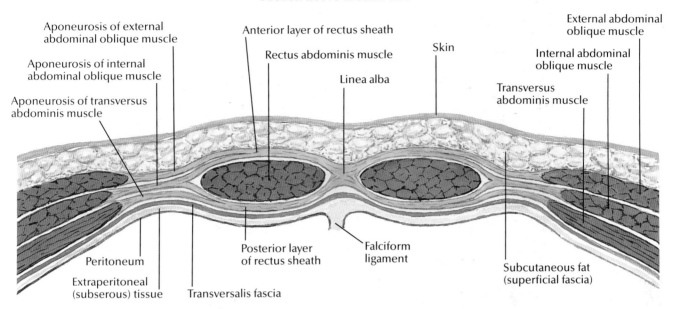

Aponeurosis of external abdominal oblique muscle

Aponeurosis of internal abdominal oblique muscle

Aponeurosis of transversus abdominis muscle

Anterior layer of rectus sheath

Rectus abdominis muscle

Linea alba

Skin

External abdominal oblique muscle

Internal abdominal oblique muscle

Transversus abdominis muscle

Peritoneum

Extraperitoneal (subserous) tissue

Posterior layer of rectus sheath

Transversalis fascia

Falciform ligament

Subcutaneous fat (superficial fascia)

Aponeurosis of internal abdominal oblique muscle splits to form anterior and posterior layers of rectus sheath. Aponeurosis of external abdominal oblique muscle joins anterior layer of sheath; aponeurosis of transversus abdominis muscle joins posterior layer. Anterior and posterior layers of rectus sheath unite medially to form linea alba

Section below arcuate line

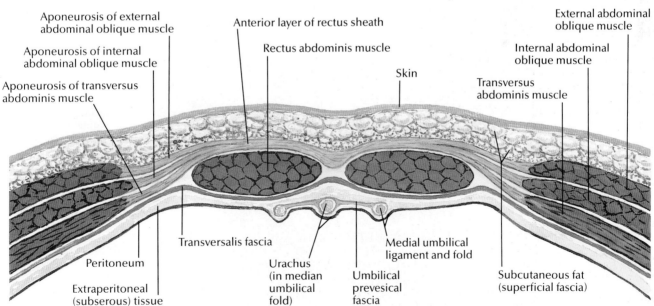

Aponeurosis of external abdominal oblique muscle

Aponeurosis of internal abdominal oblique muscle

Aponeurosis of transversus abdominis muscle

Anterior layer of rectus sheath

Rectus abdominis muscle

Skin

External abdominal oblique muscle

Internal abdominal oblique muscle

Transversus abdominis muscle

Transversalis fascia

Peritoneum

Extraperitoneal (subserous) tissue

Urachus (in median umbilical fold)

Umbilical prevesical fascia

Medial umbilical ligament and fold

Subcutaneous fat (superficial fascia)

Aponeurosis of internal abdominal oblique muscle does not split at this level but passes completely anterior to rectus abdominis muscle and is fused there with both aponeurosis of external abdominal oblique muscle and that of transversus abdominis muscle. Thus posterior wall of rectus sheath is absent below arcuate line and rectus abdominis muscle lies on transversalis fascia

FOR UMBILICAL VESSELS SEE PLATE 217

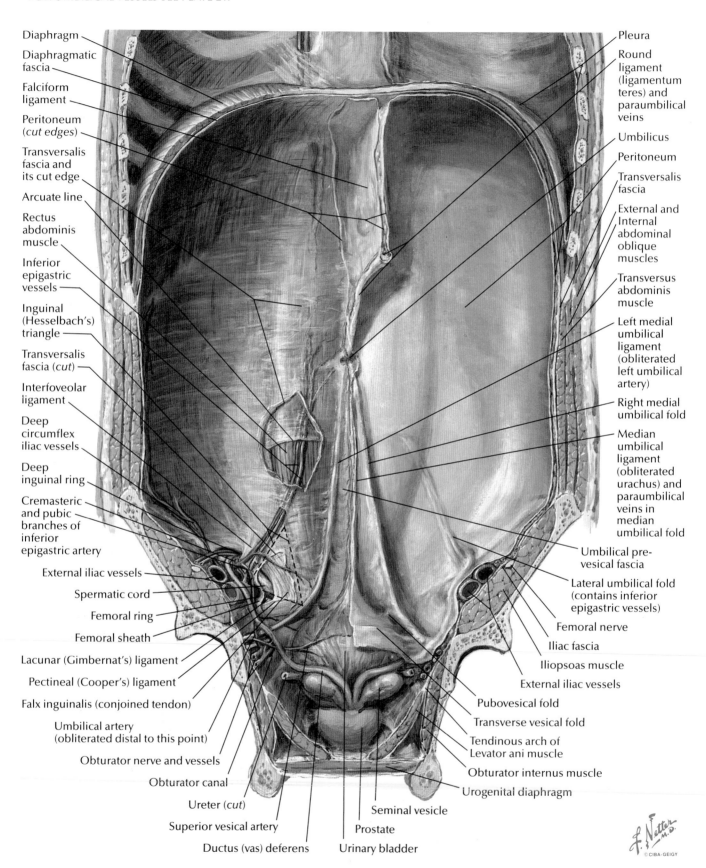

Diaphragm

Diaphragmatic fascia

Falciform ligament

Peritoneum (*cut edges*)

Transversalis fascia and its cut edge

Arcuate line

Rectus abdominis muscle

Inferior epigastric vessels

Inguinal (Hesselbach's) triangle

Transversalis fascia (*cut*)

Interfoveolar ligament

Deep circumflex iliac vessels

Deep inguinal ring

Cremasteric and pubic branches of inferior epigastric artery

External iliac vessels

Spermatic cord

Femoral ring

Femoral sheath

Lacunar (Gimbernat's) ligament

Pectineal (Cooper's) ligament

Falx inguinalis (conjoined tendon)

Umbilical artery (obliterated distal to this point)

Obturator nerve and vessels

Obturator canal

Ureter (*cut*)

Superior vesical artery

Ductus (vas) deferens

Pleura

Round ligament (ligamentum teres) and paraumbilical veins

Umbilicus

Peritoneum

Transversalis fascia

External and Internal abdominal oblique muscles

Transversus abdominis muscle

Left medial umbilical ligament (obliterated left umbilical artery)

Right medial umbilical fold

Median umbilical ligament (obliterated urachus) and paraumbilical veins in median umbilical fold

Umbilical pre-vesical fascia

Lateral umbilical fold (contains inferior epigastric vessels)

Femoral nerve

Iliac fascia

Iliopsoas muscle

External iliac vessels

Pubovesical fold

Transverse vesical fold

Tendinous arch of Levator ani muscle

Obturator internus muscle

Urogenital diaphragm

Seminal vesicle

Prostate

Urinary bladder

PLATE 236

Serratus anterior muscle

Teres major muscle

Infraspinatus fascia

Rhomboideus major muscle

Triangle of auscultation

Lateral cutaneous branch from dorsal ramus of T7

Medial cutaneous branch from dorsal ramus of T7

Trapezius muscle

Latissimus dorsi muscle

External abdominal oblique muscle

Thoracolumbar fascia (posterior layer)

Lateral cutaneous branch of
subcostal nerve (ventral ramus of T12)

Lumbar triangle (of Petit) (inferior lumbar space)

Iliac crest

Lateral cutaneous branch of iliohypogastric nerve (L1)

Superior cluneal nerves (lateral cutaneous
branches from dorsal rami of L1, 2, 3)

Fascia (gluteal aponeurosis) over gluteus medius muscle

Gluteus maximus muscle

Tensor fasciae latae muscle

Latissimus dorsi muscle

Latissimus dorsi muscle (*cut and turned back*)

Serratus posterior inferior muscle

Digitations of origin of latissimus dorsi muscle

Digitations of origin of external abdominal oblique muscle

External abdominal oblique muscle (*cut and turned back*)

Aponeurosis of transversus abdominis muscle
(superior lumbar space)

Internal abdominal oblique muscle

Lateral cutaneous branch of subcostal nerve (ventral ramus of T12)

Lateral cutaneous branch of iliohypogastric nerve (L1)

Iliac crest

Superior cluneal nerves (lateral cutaneous branches
from dorsal rami of L1, 2, 3)

Gluteus maximus muscle

9

10

11

12

Arteries of Anterior Abdominal Wall

Axillary artery

Lateral thoracic artery

Subscapular artery

Serratus anterior muscle

Thoracodorsal artery

Latissimus dorsi muscle

Intercostal arteries

Intercostal muscles { External Internal Innermost

Diaphragm

Anastomoses with lower intercostal, subcostal and lumbar arteries

External, Internal abdominal oblique muscles

Transversus abdominis muscle

Ascending branch of deep circumflex iliac artery

Superficial circumflex iliac artery

Superficial epigastric artery (cut)

Superficial external pudendal artery

Femoral artery

Deep external pudendal artery

Cremasteric, testicular and deferential arteries in spermatic cord

Subclavian artery

Internal thoracic arteries

Pericardiaco-phrenic artery with phrenic nerve

Transversus thoracis muscle

Branch to falciform ligament of liver

Musculophrenic arteries

Superior epigastric arteries

Diaphragm

Transversus abdominis muscle and aponeurosis

Rectus abdominis muscles

Internal abdominal oblique muscle

External abdominal oblique muscle

Posterior layer of rectus sheath

Arcuate line

Inferior epigastric artery

Superficial epigastric artery

Superficial circumflex iliac artery

Femoral artery

Superficial external pudendal artery

Deep external pudendal artery

Dorsal arteries of penis (covered by Buck's fascia)

PLATE 238

ABDOMEN

Subclavian vein

Axillary vein

Cephalic vein

Intercostal tributaries to axillary vein

Lateral thoracic vein

Intercostal veins

Internal thoracic vein

Musculophrenic vein

Superior epigastric veins

Thoracoepigastric vein

Paraumbilical veins in falciform ligament of liver

Inferior epigastric veins

Tributaries to deep circumflex iliac veins

Thoracoepigastric vein (*cut*)

Superficial circumflex iliac vein

Superficial epigastric vein (*cut*)

External pudendal vein

Femoral vein

Great saphenous vein

Pampiniform venous plexus

Deep dorsal vein of penis (under Buck's fascia)

Superficial dorsal vein of penis

External
Internal } Jugular veins
Anterior

Cephalic vein

Axillary vein

Lateral thoracic vein

Areolar venous plexus

Perforating tributaries to internal thoracic vein

Thoracoepigastric vein

Branches to paraumbilical veins

Thoracoepigastric vein

Superficial epigastric vein

Superficial circumflex iliac vein

External pudendal vein

Fossa ovalis

Great saphenous vein

Anterior scrotal veins

Nerves of Anterior Abdominal Wall

SEE ALSO PLATES 163, 237, 250, 468

Supraclavicular nerves (anterior, middle and posterior)

Pectoralis major muscle

Medial brachial cutaneous nerve

Intercostobrachial nerve (T1, 2)

Long thoracic nerve

Latissimus dorsi muscle

Serratus anterior muscle

Lateral cutaneous branches of intercostal nerves (T2–11)

Anterior cutaneous branches of intercostal nerves (T1–11)

Lateral cutaneous branch of subcostal nerve (T12)

Lateral cutaneous branch of iliohypogastric nerve (L1)

Anterior cutaneous branch of subcostal nerve (T12)

Lateral femoral cutaneous nerve

Anterior cutaneous branch of iliohypogastric nerve (L1)

Femoral branches of genitofemoral nerve (L1, 2)

Anterior scrotal branch of ilioinguinal nerve (L1)

Genital branch of genitofemoral nerve (L1, 2)

Serratus anterior muscle

External abdominal oblique muscle (*cut*)

Posterior layer of rectus sheath

Anterior layer of rectus sheath (*cut*)

Rectus abdominis muscle

Transversus abdominis muscle

Internal abdominal oblique muscle and aponeurosis (*cut*)

Anterior branch, Lateral branch of subcostal nerve (T12)

Anterior branch of iliohypogastric nerve (L1)

Ilioinguinal nerve (L1)

External abdominal oblique aponeurosis (*cut*)

Anterior cutaneous branch of iliohypogastric nerve (L1)

Ilioinguinal nerve (L1)

Spermatic cord

PLATE 240

ABDOMEN

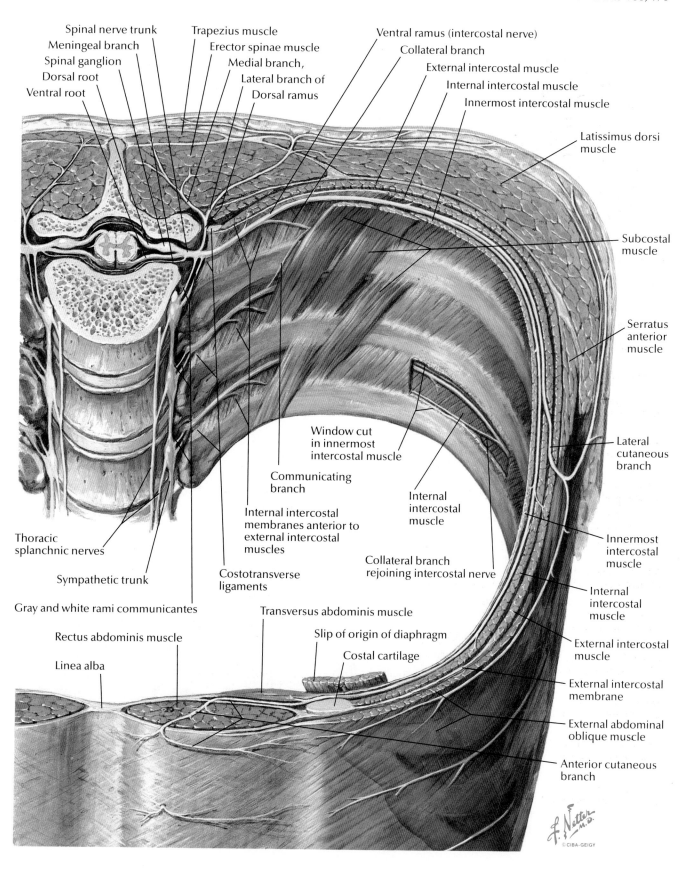

Spinal nerve trunk
Meningeal branch
Spinal ganglion
Dorsal root
Ventral root

Trapezius muscle
Erector spinae muscle
Medial branch,
Lateral branch of
Dorsal ramus

Ventral ramus (intercostal nerve)
Collateral branch
External intercostal muscle
Internal intercostal muscle
Innermost intercostal muscle

Latissimus dorsi muscle

Subcostal muscle

Serratus anterior muscle

Window cut in innermost intercostal muscle

Communicating branch

Internal intercostal membranes anterior to external intercostal muscles

Internal intercostal muscle

Lateral cutaneous branch

Thoracic splanchnic nerves

Costotransverse ligaments

Collateral branch rejoining intercostal nerve

Innermost intercostal muscle

Sympathetic trunk

Internal intercostal muscle

Gray and white rami communicantes

Transversus abdominis muscle

External intercostal muscle

Rectus abdominis muscle

Slip of origin of diaphragm

External intercostal membrane

Linea alba

Costal cartilage

External abdominal oblique muscle

Anterior cutaneous branch

External abdominal oblique muscle

External abdominal oblique aponeurosis

Rectus sheath (anterior layer)

Linea alba

Anterior superior iliac spine

Inguinal (Poupart's) ligament

Superficial epigastric vessels

Intercrural fibers

Superficial inguinal ring

Spermatic cord (*cut*)

Cribriform fascia over fossa ovalis

Pubic tubercle

Suspensory ligament of penis

Great saphenous vein

Superficial circumflex iliac vessels

Fascia lata

Skin and subcutaneous fascia removed

External abdominal oblique muscle

Internal abdominal oblique muscle

Rectus sheath (anterior layer)

External abdominal oblique aponeurosis (*cut and reflected*)

Inguinal (Poupart's) ligament

Deep inguinal ring

Cremaster muscle (lateral origin)

Falx inguinalis (conjoined tendon)

Cremaster muscle (medial origin)

Femoral vein

Great saphenous vein

Fossa ovalis

External abdominal oblique aponeurosis reflected and cribriform fascia removed

PLATE 242

ABDOMEN

External abdominal oblique muscle and Aponeurosis

Anterior superior iliac spine

Internal abdominal oblique muscle

Transversus abdominis muscle

Cremaster muscle (lateral origin)

Inferior epigastric vessels (covered by transversalis fascia)

Inguinal (Poupart's) ligament

Lacunar (Gimbernat's) ligament

Pectineal (Cooper's) ligament

Cremaster muscle (medial origin)

Superficial inguinal ring
Lateral crus
Medial crus

Pubic crest

Linea alba

Rectus sheath (anterior layer)

Transversalis fascia (site of direct inguinal hernia)

Falx inguinalis (conjoined tendon)

Reflected inguinal ligament

Intercrural fibers

External spermatic fascia on spermatic cord exiting
Superficial inguinal ring

Fundiform ligament of penis

Anterior view

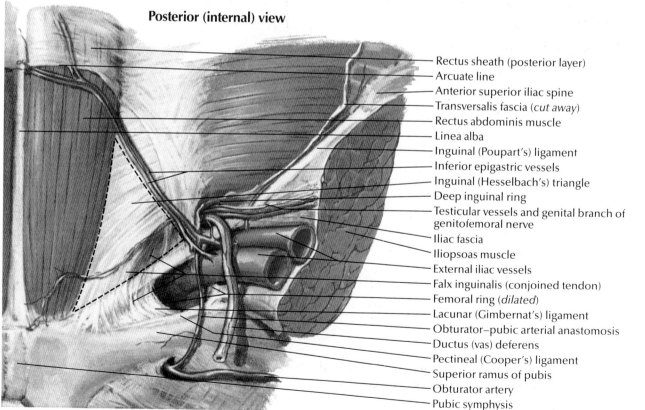

Posterior (internal) view

Rectus sheath (posterior layer)
Arcuate line
Anterior superior iliac spine
Transversalis fascia (*cut away*)
Rectus abdominis muscle
Linea alba
Inguinal (Poupart's) ligament
Inferior epigastric vessels
Inguinal (Hesselbach's) triangle
Deep inguinal ring
Testicular vessels and genital branch of genitofemoral nerve
Iliac fascia
Iliopsoas muscle
External iliac vessels
Falx inguinalis (conjoined tendon)
Femoral ring (*dilated*)
Lacunar (Gimbernat's) ligament
Obturator–pubic arterial anastomosis
Ductus (vas) deferens
Pectineal (Cooper's) ligament
Superior ramus of pubis
Obturator artery
Pubic symphysis

BODY WALL

PLATE 243

Transversalis fascia (*cut edge*)

Umbilical prevesical fascia (*cut edge*)

Extraperitoneal (subserous) areolar tissue

Parietal peritoneum

Median umbilical ligament (urachus)

Medial umbilical ligament (obliterated umbilical artery)

Inferior epigastric vessels

Iliac fascia

Deep circumflex iliac vessels

Testicular vessels

Cremasteric artery

Ductus (vas) deferens

External iliac vessels

Pubic vessels (obturator anastomotic)

External abdominal oblique aponeurosis (*cut*)

Internal spermatic fascia on spermatic cord

Femoral nerve (beneath fascia)

Femoral vessels in femoral sheath

Pectineal fascia

Falciform margin of fossa ovalis (*cut and reflected*)

Urinary bladder

Pectineal (Cooper's) ligament

Lacunar (Gimbernat's) ligament

Inguinal (Poupart's) ligament

Transversalis fascia forms anterior wall of femoral sheath (posterior wall formed by pectineal fascia)

Ureter

Genitofemoral nerve

Lateral femoral cutaneous nerve

Iliac fascia

Genital branch of genitofemoral nerve

Femoral branch of genitofemoral nerve

Testicular vessels

External iliac vessels

Inferior epigastric vessels

Ductus (vas) deferens and cremasteric artery

Pectineal (Cooper's) ligament

Femoral ring

Transversalis fascia forms anterior wall of femoral sheath

Lacunar (Gimbernat's) ligament

Inguinal (Poupart's) ligament

Lymph node in femoral canal

Femoral sheath (*cut open*)

Pectineal fascia

PLATE 244

ABDOMEN

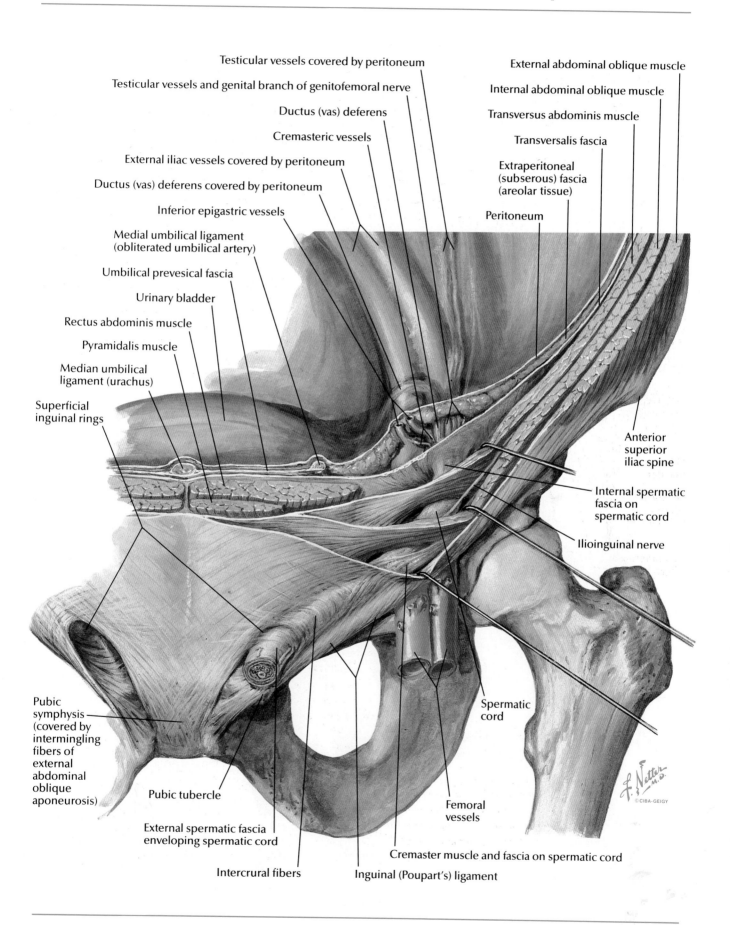

Testicular vessels covered by peritoneum

Testicular vessels and genital branch of genitofemoral nerve

Ductus (vas) deferens

Cremasteric vessels

External iliac vessels covered by peritoneum

Ductus (vas) deferens covered by peritoneum

Inferior epigastric vessels

Medial umbilical ligament (obliterated umbilical artery)

Umbilical prevesical fascia

Urinary bladder

Rectus abdominis muscle

Pyramidalis muscle

Median umbilical ligament (urachus)

Superficial inguinal rings

Pubic symphysis (covered by intermingling fibers of external abdominal oblique aponeurosis)

Pubic tubercle

External spermatic fascia enveloping spermatic cord

Intercrural fibers

Inguinal (Poupart's) ligament

External abdominal oblique muscle

Internal abdominal oblique muscle

Transversus abdominis muscle

Transversalis fascia

Extraperitoneal (subserous) fascia (areolar tissue)

Peritoneum

Anterior superior iliac spine

Internal spermatic fascia on spermatic cord

Ilioinguinal nerve

Spermatic cord

Femoral vessels

Cremaster muscle and fascia on spermatic cord

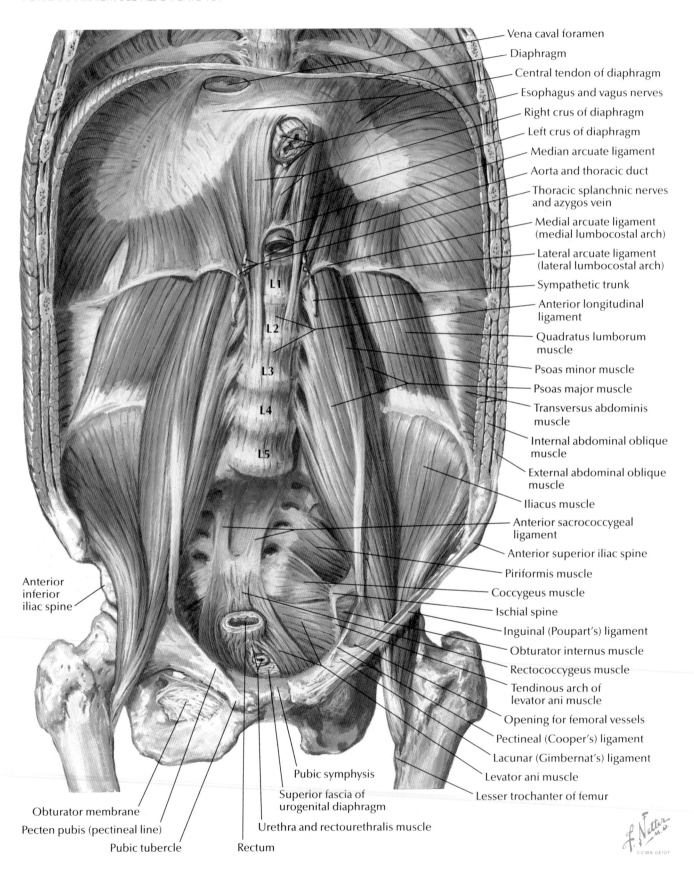

Vena caval foramen

Diaphragm

Central tendon of diaphragm

Esophagus and vagus nerves

Right crus of diaphragm

Left crus of diaphragm

Median arcuate ligament

Aorta and thoracic duct

Thoracic splanchnic nerves and azygos vein

Medial arcuate ligament (medial lumbocostal arch)

Lateral arcuate ligament (lateral lumbocostal arch)

Sympathetic trunk

Anterior longitudinal ligament

Quadratus lumborum muscle

Psoas minor muscle

Psoas major muscle

Transversus abdominis muscle

Internal abdominal oblique muscle

External abdominal oblique muscle

Iliacus muscle

Anterior sacrococcygeal ligament

Anterior superior iliac spine

Piriformis muscle

Coccygeus muscle

Ischial spine

Inguinal (Poupart's) ligament

Obturator internus muscle

Rectococcygeus muscle

Tendinous arch of levator ani muscle

Opening for femoral vessels

Pectineal (Cooper's) ligament

Lacunar (Gimbernat's) ligament

Levator ani muscle

Lesser trochanter of femur

L1

L2

L3

L4

L5

Anterior inferior iliac spine

Obturator membrane

Pecten pubis (pectineal line)

Pubic tubercle

Rectum

Pubic symphysis

Superior fascia of urogenital diaphragm

Urethra and rectourethralis muscle

PLATE 246

ABDOMEN

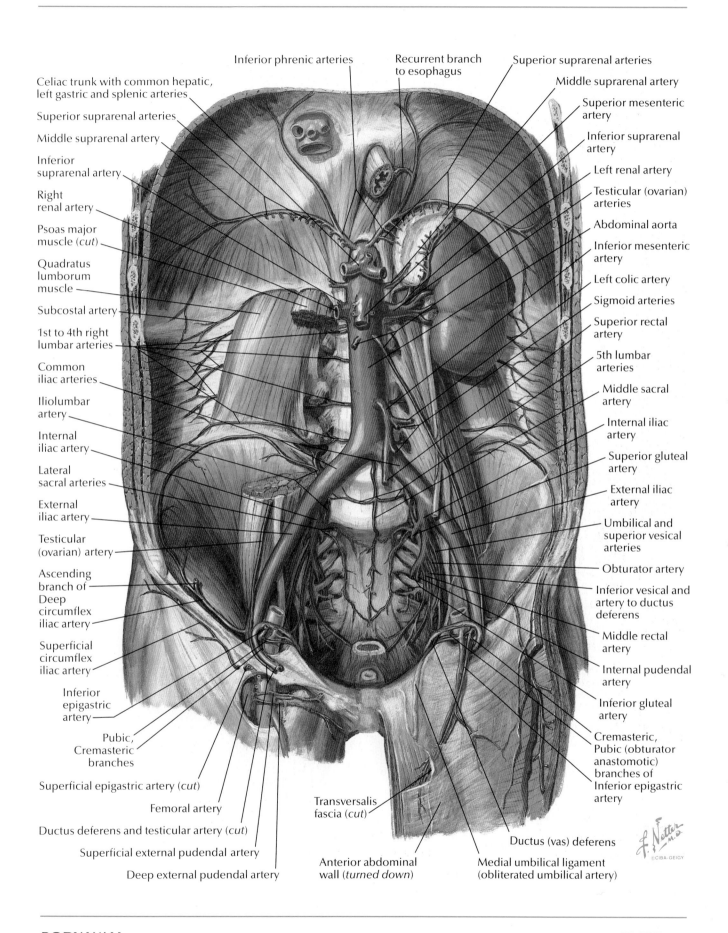

Inferior phrenic arteries

Recurrent branch to esophagus

Superior suprarenal arteries

Celiac trunk with common hepatic, left gastric and splenic arteries

Middle suprarenal artery

Superior suprarenal arteries

Superior mesenteric artery

Middle suprarenal artery

Inferior suprarenal artery

Inferior suprarenal artery

Left renal artery

Right renal artery

Testicular (ovarian) arteries

Psoas major muscle (cut)

Abdominal aorta

Inferior mesenteric artery

Quadratus lumborum muscle

Left colic artery

Subcostal artery

Sigmoid arteries

Superior rectal artery

1st to 4th right lumbar arteries

5th lumbar arteries

Common iliac arteries

Middle sacral artery

Iliolumbar artery

Internal iliac artery

Internal iliac artery

Superior gluteal artery

Lateral sacral arteries

External iliac artery

External iliac artery

Umbilical and superior vesical arteries

Testicular (ovarian) artery

Obturator artery

Ascending branch of Deep circumflex iliac artery

Inferior vesical and artery to ductus deferens

Superficial circumflex iliac artery

Middle rectal artery

Internal pudendal artery

Inferior epigastric artery

Inferior gluteal artery

Pubic, Cremasteric branches

Cremasteric, Pubic (obturator anastomotic) branches of Inferior epigastric artery

Superficial epigastric artery (cut)

Femoral artery

Transversalis fascia (cut)

Ductus (vas) deferens

Ductus deferens and testicular artery (cut)

Superficial external pudendal artery

Anterior abdominal wall (turned down)

Medial umbilical ligament (obliterated umbilical artery)

Deep external pudendal artery

Veins of Posterior Abdominal Wall

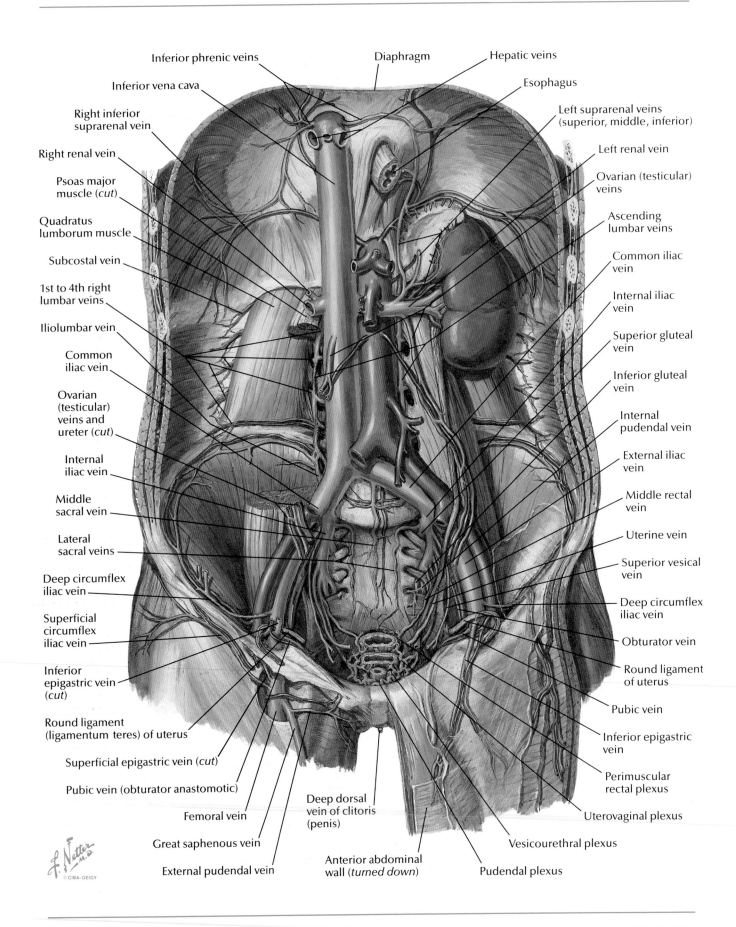

Inferior phrenic veins

Diaphragm

Hepatic veins

Inferior vena cava

Esophagus

Right inferior suprarenal vein

Left suprarenal veins (superior, middle, inferior)

Right renal vein

Left renal vein

Psoas major muscle (cut)

Ovarian (testicular) veins

Quadratus lumborum muscle

Ascending lumbar veins

Subcostal vein

Common iliac vein

1st to 4th right lumbar veins

Internal iliac vein

Iliolumbar vein

Superior gluteal vein

Common iliac vein

Inferior gluteal vein

Ovarian (testicular) veins and ureter (cut)

Internal pudendal vein

Internal iliac vein

External iliac vein

Middle sacral vein

Middle rectal vein

Lateral sacral veins

Uterine vein

Deep circumflex iliac vein

Superior vesical vein

Superficial circumflex iliac vein

Deep circumflex iliac vein

Obturator vein

Inferior epigastric vein (cut)

Round ligament of uterus

Round ligament (ligamentum teres) of uterus

Pubic vein

Superficial epigastric vein (cut)

Inferior epigastric vein

Pubic vein (obturator anastomotic)

Perimuscular rectal plexus

Femoral vein

Deep dorsal vein of clitoris (penis)

Uterovaginal plexus

Great saphenous vein

Vesicourethral plexus

External pudendal vein

Anterior abdominal wall (turned down)

Pudendal plexus

PLATE 248

ABDOMEN

Lymph Vessels and Nodes of Posterior Abdominal Wall

SEE ALSO PLATE 382

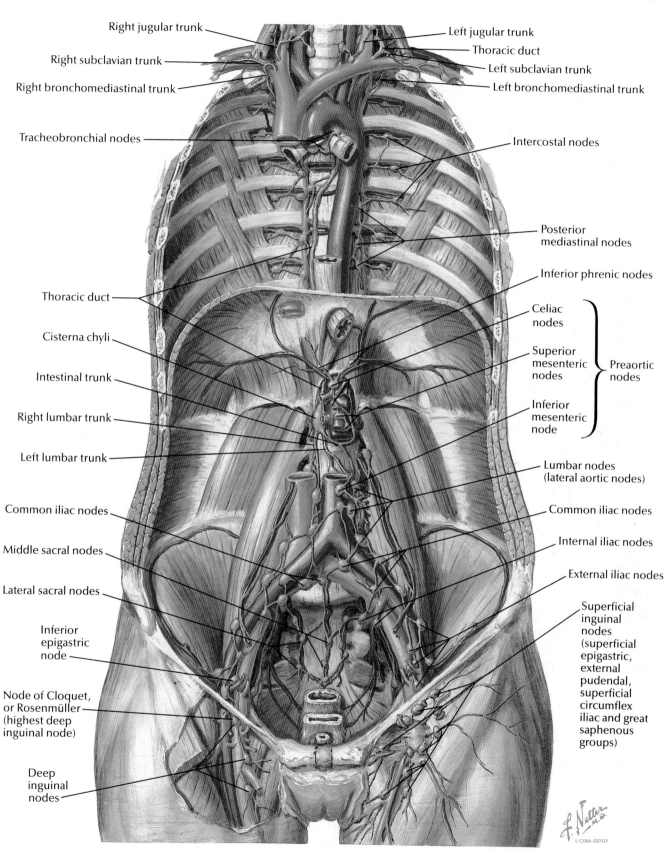

Right jugular trunk

Right subclavian trunk

Right bronchomediastinal trunk

Tracheobronchial nodes

Thoracic duct

Cisterna chyli

Intestinal trunk

Right lumbar trunk

Left lumbar trunk

Common iliac nodes

Middle sacral nodes

Lateral sacral nodes

Inferior epigastric node

Node of Cloquet, or Rosenmüller (highest deep inguinal node)

Deep inguinal nodes

Left jugular trunk

Thoracic duct

Left subclavian trunk

Left bronchomediastinal trunk

Intercostal nodes

Posterior mediastinal nodes

Inferior phrenic nodes

Celiac nodes

Superior mesenteric nodes

Inferior mesenteric node

Preaortic nodes

Lumbar nodes (lateral aortic nodes)

Common iliac nodes

Internal iliac nodes

External iliac nodes

Superficial inguinal nodes (superficial epigastric, external pudendal, superficial circumflex iliac and great saphenous groups)

BODY WALL

PLATE 249

Nerves of Posterior Abdominal Wall

Thoracic splanchnic nerves (greater, lesser and least)

Sympathetic trunks

Subcostal nerve (T12)

Iliohypogastric nerve

Ilioinguinal nerve

Genitofemoral nerve

Transversus abdominis muscle (cut)

Subcostal nerve (T12) and its Lateral cutaneous branch

Intermesenteric (aortic) plexus

Gray and white rami communicantes

Gray rami communicantes

Lateral femoral cutaneous nerve

Femoral nerve

Anterior cutaneous branches of femoral nerve

Celiac, superior mesenteric and aorticorenal ganglia

Vena caval foramen

Thoracic splanchnic nerves (greater, lesser and least)

Iliohypogastric nerve

Ilioinguinal nerve

Muscular branches from lumbar plexus

Subcostal nerve (T12)

Psoas major muscle (cut)

Quadratus lumborum muscle

Iliohypogastric nerve

Ilioinguinal nerve

Genitofemoral nerve

Lateral femoral cutaneous nerve

Femoral branch, Genital branch of genitofemoral nerve

Lumbosacral trunks

Obturator nerves

Accessory obturator nerve

Femoral nerve

Sacral plexus

Pelvic splanchnic nerves

Pudendal nerve

Nerves to coccygeus and levator ani muscles

Obturator nerve

Dorsal nerve of penis (clitoris)

Anterior cutaneous branch of iliohypogastric nerve

Anterior scrotal (labial) branches of ilioinguinal nerve

Genital branch

Femoral branches

} of genitofemoral nerve

PLATE 250

ABDOMEN

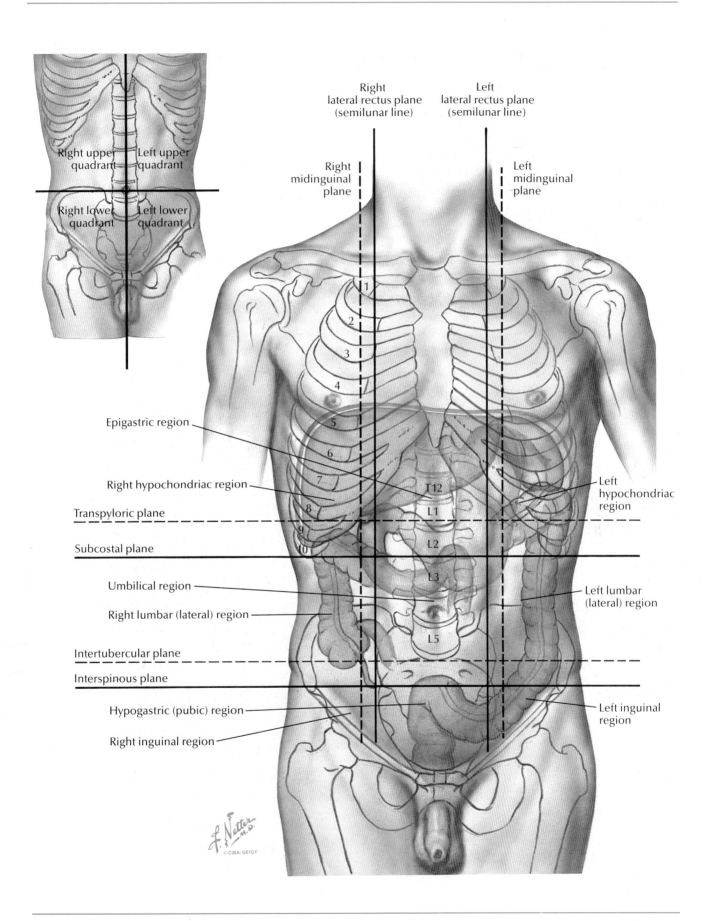

Right upper quadrant

Left upper quadrant

Right lower quadrant

Left lower quadrant

Right
lateral rectus plane
(semilunar line)

Left
lateral rectus plane
(semilunar line)

Right
midinguinal
plane

Left
midinguinal
plane

Epigastric region

Right hypochondriac region

Transpyloric plane

Subcostal plane

Umbilical region

Right lumbar (lateral) region

Intertubercular plane

Interspinous plane

Hypogastric (pubic) region

Right inguinal region

Left
hypochondriac
region

Left lumbar
(lateral) region

Left inguinal
region

T12

L1

L2

L3

L5

1
2
3
4
5
6
7
8
9
10

Greater Omentum and Abdominal Viscera

SEE ALSO PLATES 258, 332, 333

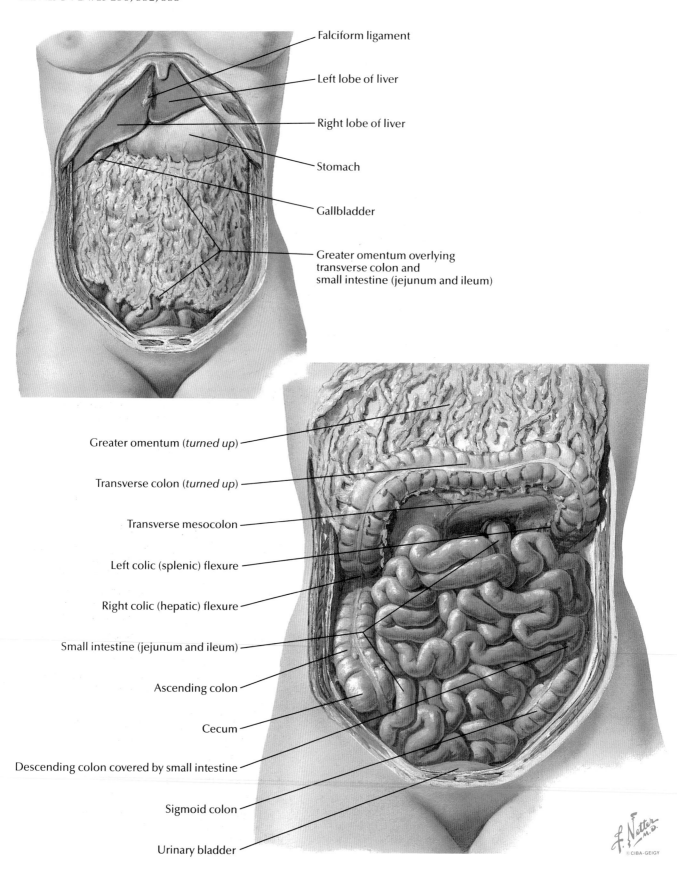

Falciform ligament

Left lobe of liver

Right lobe of liver

Stomach

Gallbladder

Greater omentum overlying transverse colon and small intestine (jejunum and ileum)

Greater omentum (*turned up*)

Transverse colon (*turned up*)

Transverse mesocolon

Left colic (splenic) flexure

Right colic (hepatic) flexure

Small intestine (jejunum and ileum)

Ascending colon

Cecum

Descending colon covered by small intestine

Sigmoid colon

Urinary bladder

PLATE 252

ABDOMEN

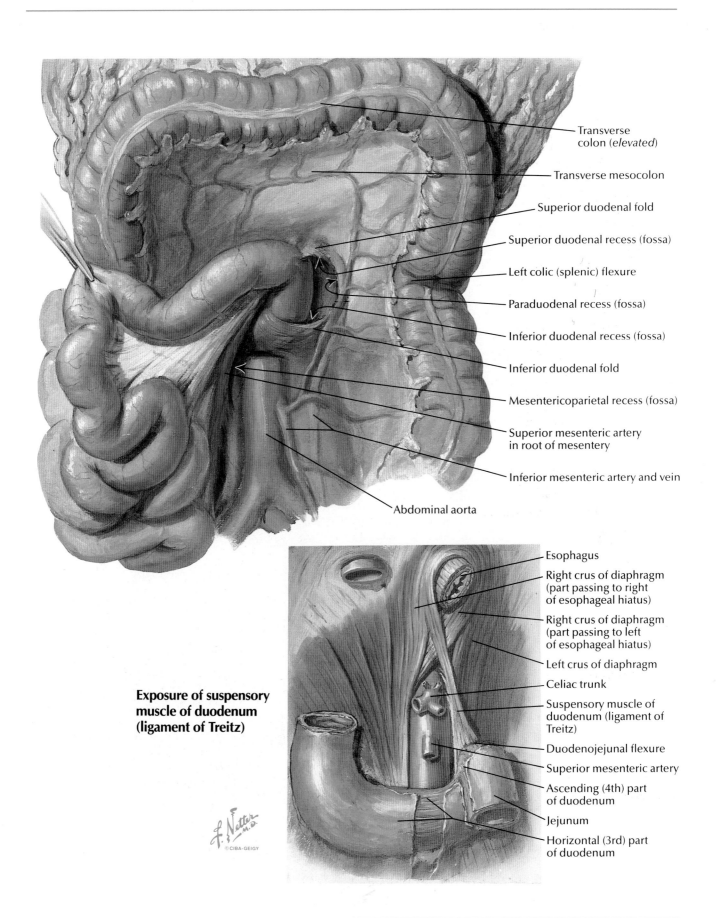

Transverse colon (*elevated*)

Transverse mesocolon

Superior duodenal fold

Superior duodenal recess (fossa)

Left colic (splenic) flexure

Paraduodenal recess (fossa)

Inferior duodenal recess (fossa)

Inferior duodenal fold

Mesentericoparietal recess (fossa)

Superior mesenteric artery in root of mesentery

Inferior mesenteric artery and vein

Abdominal aorta

Esophagus

Right crus of diaphragm (part passing to right of esophageal hiatus)

Right crus of diaphragm (part passing to left of esophageal hiatus)

Left crus of diaphragm

Celiac trunk

Suspensory muscle of duodenum (ligament of Treitz)

Duodenojejunal flexure

Superior mesenteric artery

Ascending (4th) part of duodenum

Jejunum

Horizontal (3rd) part of duodenum

Exposure of suspensory muscle of duodenum (ligament of Treitz)

©CIBA-GEIGY

Mesenteric Relations of Intestines (continued)

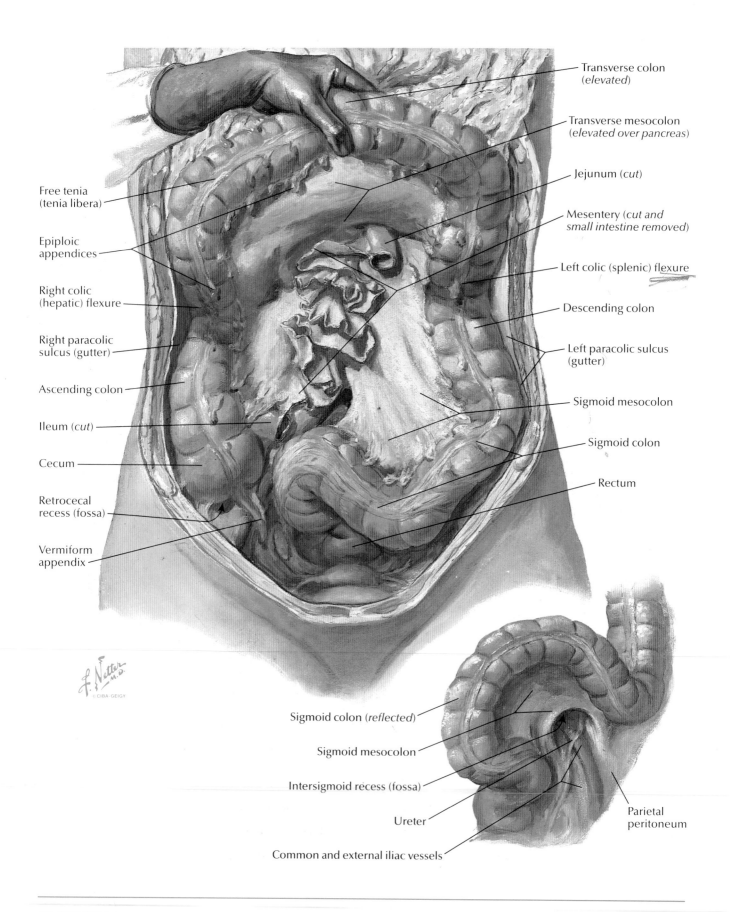

Transverse colon (*elevated*)

Transverse mesocolon (*elevated over pancreas*)

Jejunum (*cut*)

Mesentery (*cut and small intestine removed*)

Left colic (splenic) flexure

Descending colon

Left paracolic sulcus (gutter)

Sigmoid mesocolon

Sigmoid colon

Rectum

Free tenia (tenia libera)

Epiploic appendices

Right colic (hepatic) flexure

Right paracolic sulcus (gutter)

Ascending colon

Ileum (*cut*)

Cecum

Retrocecal recess (fossa)

Vermiform appendix

Sigmoid colon (*reflected*)

Sigmoid mesocolon

Intersigmoid recess (fossa)

Ureter

Common and external iliac vessels

Parietal peritoneum

PLATE 254

ABDOMEN

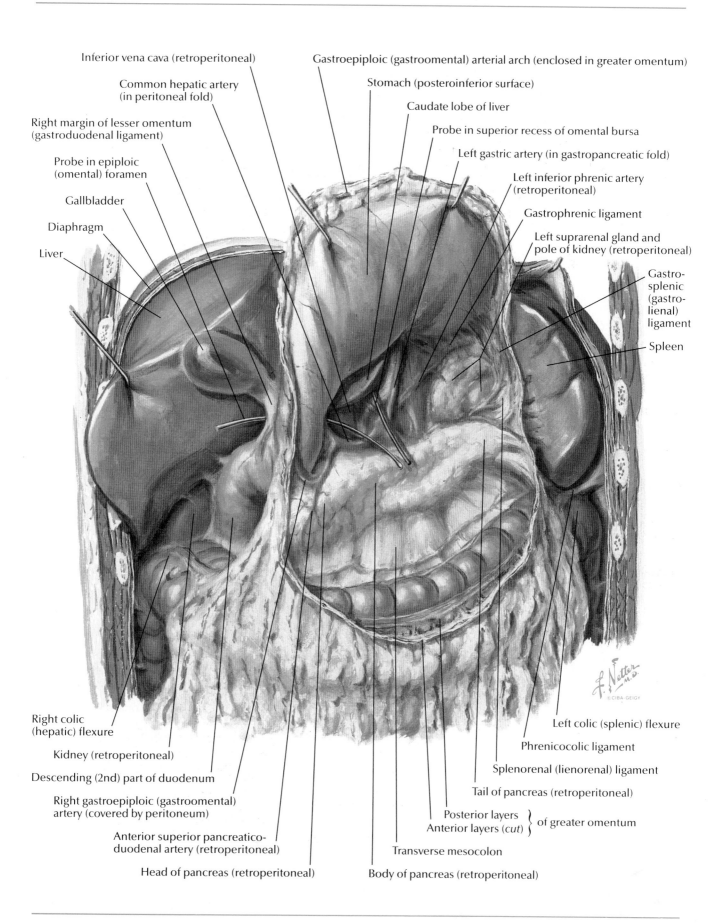

Inferior vena cava (retroperitoneal)

Common hepatic artery (in peritoneal fold)

Right margin of lesser omentum (gastroduodenal ligament)

Probe in epiploic (omental) foramen

Gallbladder

Diaphragm

Liver

Gastroepiploic (gastroomental) arterial arch (enclosed in greater omentum)

Stomach (posteroinferior surface)

Caudate lobe of liver

Probe in superior recess of omental bursa

Left gastric artery (in gastropancreatic fold)

Left inferior phrenic artery (retroperitoneal)

Gastrophrenic ligament

Left suprarenal gland and pole of kidney (retroperitoneal)

Gastro-splenic (gastro-lienal) ligament

Spleen

Right colic (hepatic) flexure

Kidney (retroperitoneal)

Descending (2nd) part of duodenum

Right gastroepiploic (gastroomental) artery (covered by peritoneum)

Anterior superior pancreatico-duodenal artery (retroperitoneal)

Head of pancreas (retroperitoneal)

Left colic (splenic) flexure

Phrenicocolic ligament

Splenorenal (lienorenal) ligament

Tail of pancreas (retroperitoneal)

Posterior layers } of greater omentum
Anterior layers (*cut*)

Transverse mesocolon

Body of pancreas (retroperitoneal)

Omental Bursa: Cross Section

SEE ALSO PLATE 331

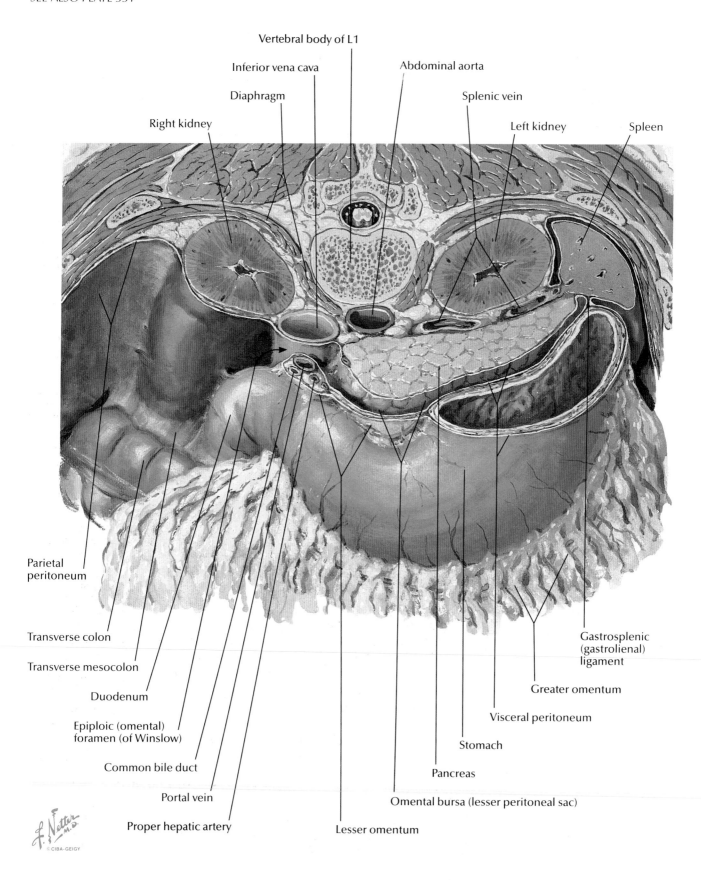

Vertebral body of L1

Inferior vena cava

Diaphragm

Right kidney

Abdominal aorta

Splenic vein

Left kidney

Spleen

Parietal peritoneum

Transverse colon

Transverse mesocolon

Duodenum

Epiploic (omental) foramen (of Winslow)

Common bile duct

Portal vein

Proper hepatic artery

Lesser omentum

Pancreas

Stomach

Omental bursa (lesser peritoneal sac)

Visceral peritoneum

Greater omentum

Gastrosplenic (gastrolienal) ligament

PLATE 256

Inferior vena cava

Common bile duct and proper hepatic artery

Coronary ligament of liver

Right suprarenal gland

Hepatic veins

Abdominal aorta and celiac trunk

Falciform ligament of liver

Superior recess of omental bursa (lesser sac)

Attachment of lesser omentum and left gastric artery

Esophagus

Epiploic (omental) foramen behind right free margin of lesser omentum

Right triangular ligament of liver

Attachment of greater omentum and right gastroepiploic (gastro-omental) vessels

Duodenum

Right kidney

Parietal peritoneum

Transversalis fascia

Root of mesentery

Site of ascending colon

Common iliac artery (retroperitoneal)

External iliac artery (retroperitoneal)

Testicular vessels (retroperitoneal)

Ureters (retroperitoneal)

Site of deep inguinal ring

Median umbilical fold (contains urachus)

Left triangular ligament of liver

Gastrophrenic ligament and left inferior phrenic vessels

Gastrosplenic ligament and short gastric vessels

Splenorenal (lienorenal) ligament and splenic vessels

Phrenicocolic ligament

Pancreas and splenic artery (retroperitoneal)

Attachment of transverse mesocolon

Superior mesenteric vessels

Site of descending colon

Attachment of sigmoid mesocolon and sigmoid vessels

Superior rectal vessels

Sacrogenital fold (ligament)

Lateral umbilical fold (contains inferior epigastric vessels)

Medial umbilical fold (contains obliterated umbilical artery)

Rectum

Urinary bladder

Stomach In Situ

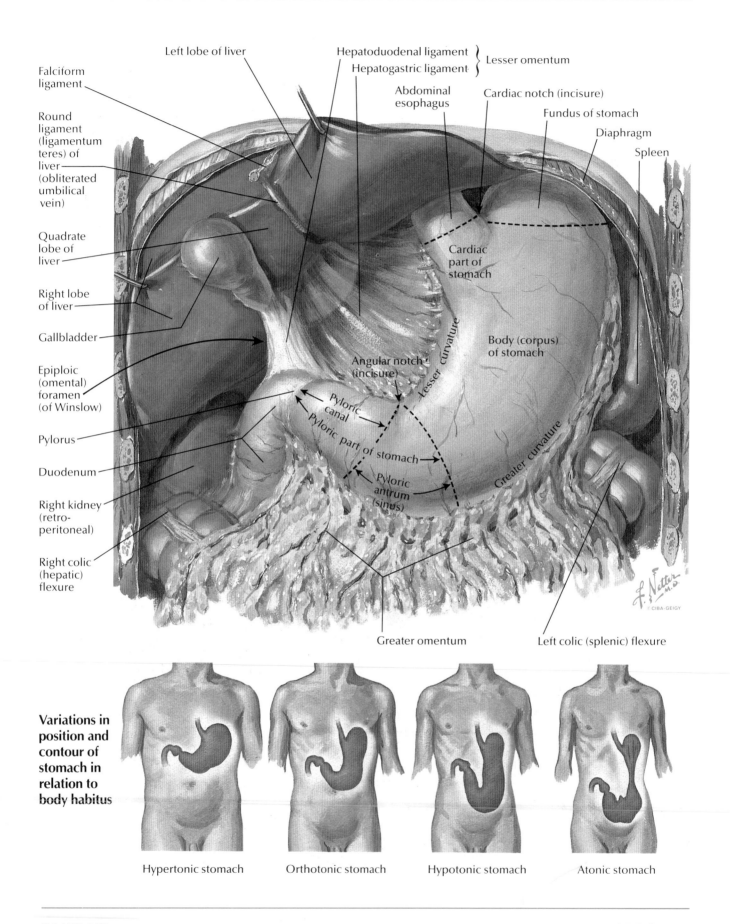

Falciform ligament

Round ligament (ligamentum teres) of liver (obliterated umbilical vein)

Quadrate lobe of liver

Right lobe of liver

Gallbladder

Epiploic (omental) foramen (of Winslow)

Pylorus

Duodenum

Right kidney (retroperitoneal)

Right colic (hepatic) flexure

Left lobe of liver

Hepatoduodenal ligament

Hepatogastric ligament

Lesser omentum

Abdominal esophagus

Cardiac notch (incisure)

Fundus of stomach

Diaphragm

Spleen

Cardiac part of stomach

Body (corpus) of stomach

Lesser curvature

Angular notch (incisure)

Pyloric canal

Pyloric part of stomach

Pyloric antrum (sinus)

Greater curvature

Greater omentum

Left colic (splenic) flexure

Variations in position and contour of stomach in relation to body habitus

Hypertonic stomach

Orthotonic stomach

Hypotonic stomach

Atonic stomach

PLATE 258

ABDOMEN

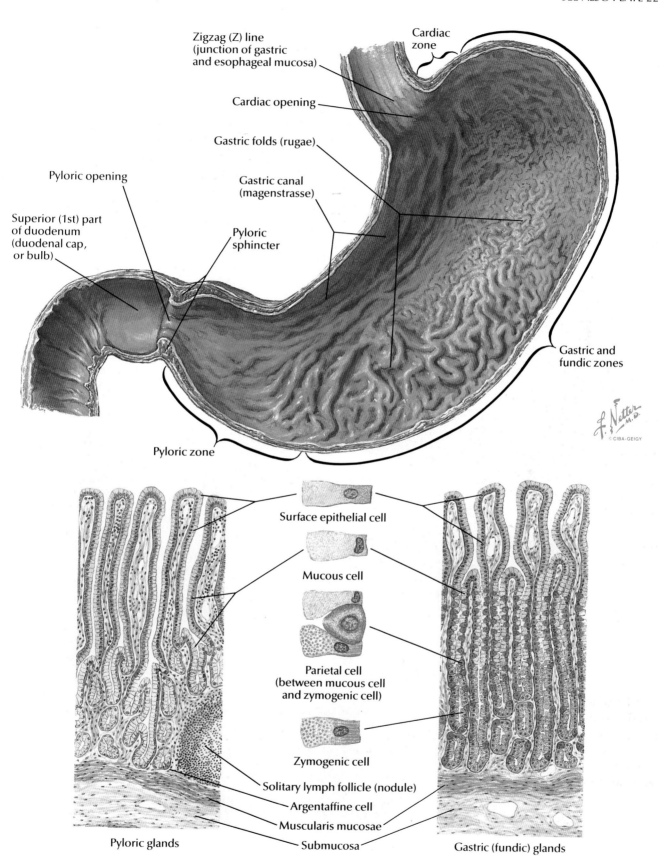

Zigzag (Z) line (junction of gastric and esophageal mucosa)

Cardiac zone

Cardiac opening

Gastric folds (rugae)

Pyloric opening

Gastric canal (magenstrasse)

Superior (1st) part of duodenum (duodenal cap, or bulb)

Pyloric sphincter

Gastric and fundic zones

Pyloric zone

Surface epithelial cell

Mucous cell

Parietal cell (between mucous cell and zymogenic cell)

Zymogenic cell

Solitary lymph follicle (nodule)

Argentaffine cell

Muscularis mucosae

Submucosa

Pyloric glands

Gastric (fundic) glands

Musculature of Stomach

Longitudinal muscle of esophagus

Outer longitudinal muscle layer of stomach (concentrated chiefly at lesser and greater curvatures and at pyloric area)

Middle circular muscle layer of stomach

Collar of Helvetius (middle circular and innermost oblique fibers blend here)

Longitudinal muscle of duodenum

Outer longitudinal muscle layer (*cut away*)

Section through pyloric sphincter (composed chiefly of thickened circular muscle)

Middle circular muscle layer

Innermost oblique muscle layer

Circular muscle of duodenum

Longitudinal muscle of duodenum (*cut away*)

Windows cut in middle circular muscle layer

PLATE 260

ABDOMEN

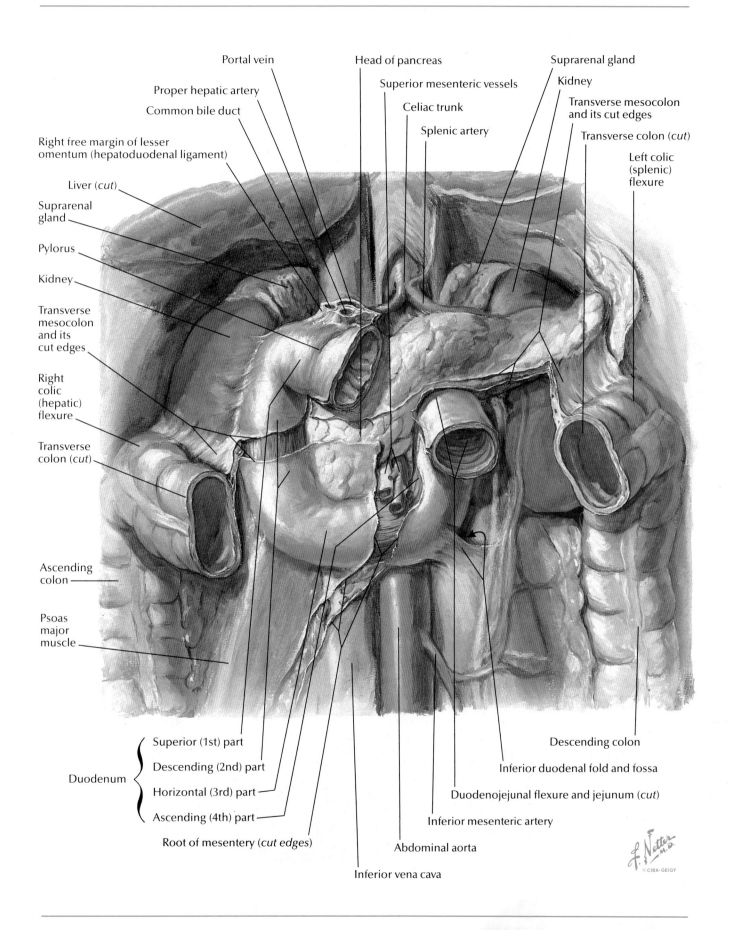

Portal vein

Proper hepatic artery

Common bile duct

Head of pancreas

Superior mesenteric vessels

Celiac trunk

Splenic artery

Suprarenal gland

Kidney

Transverse mesocolon and its cut edges

Transverse colon (*cut*)

Left colic (splenic) flexure

Right free margin of lesser omentum (hepatoduodenal ligament)

Liver (*cut*)

Suprarenal gland

Pylorus

Kidney

Transverse mesocolon and its cut edges

Right colic (hepatic) flexure

Transverse colon (*cut*)

Ascending colon

Psoas major muscle

Descending colon

Inferior duodenal fold and fossa

Duodenojejunal flexure and jejunum (*cut*)

Inferior mesenteric artery

Abdominal aorta

Inferior vena cava

Root of mesentery (*cut edges*)

Duodenum {
Superior (1st) part

Descending (2nd) part

Horizontal (3rd) part

Ascending (4th) part
}

Mucosa and Musculature of Duodenum

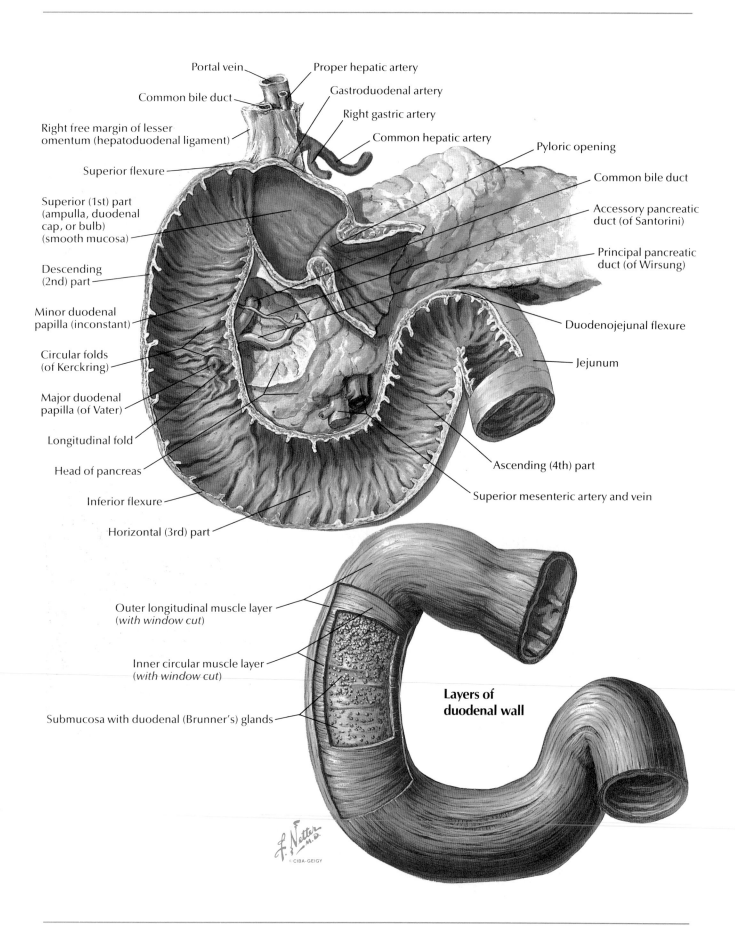

Portal vein

Proper hepatic artery

Common bile duct

Gastroduodenal artery

Right gastric artery

Right free margin of lesser omentum (hepatoduodenal ligament)

Common hepatic artery

Pyloric opening

Superior flexure

Common bile duct

Superior (1st) part (ampulla, duodenal cap, or bulb) (smooth mucosa)

Accessory pancreatic duct (of Santorini)

Principal pancreatic duct (of Wirsung)

Descending (2nd) part

Minor duodenal papilla (inconstant)

Duodenojejunal flexure

Circular folds (of Kerckring)

Jejunum

Major duodenal papilla (of Vater)

Longitudinal fold

Head of pancreas

Ascending (4th) part

Inferior flexure

Superior mesenteric artery and vein

Horizontal (3rd) part

Outer longitudinal muscle layer (with window cut)

Inner circular muscle layer (with window cut)

Layers of duodenal wall

Submucosa with duodenal (Brunner's) glands

PLATE 262

ABDOMEN

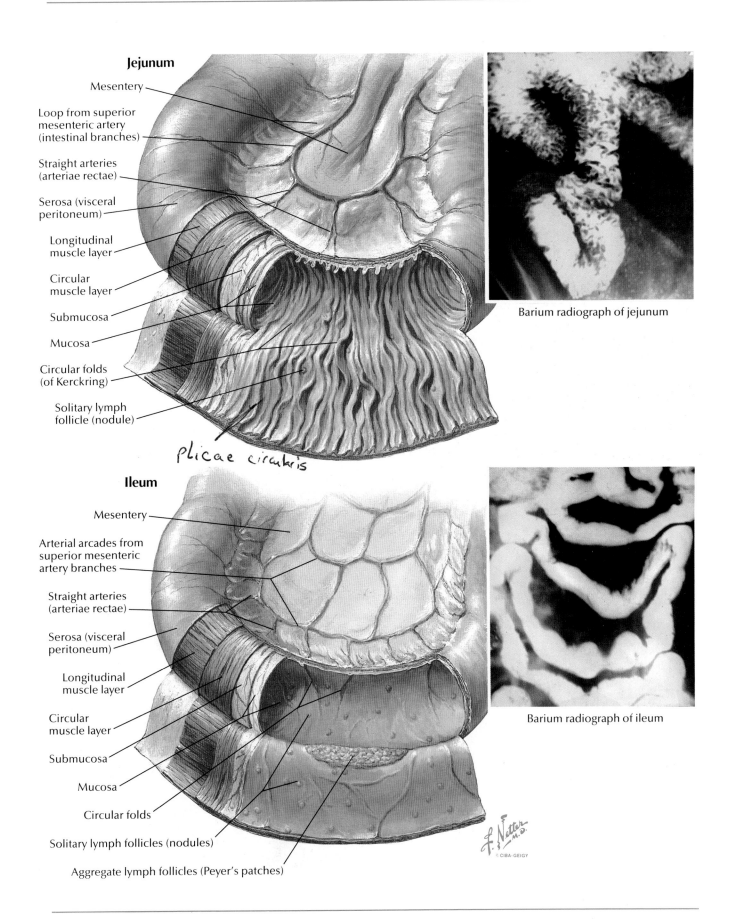

Jejunum

Mesentery

Loop from superior mesenteric artery (intestinal branches)

Straight arteries (arteriae rectae)

Serosa (visceral peritoneum)

Longitudinal muscle layer

Circular muscle layer

Submucosa

Mucosa

Circular folds (of Kerckring)

Solitary lymph follicle (nodule)

plicae circularis

Barium radiograph of jejunum

Ileum

Mesentery

Arterial arcades from superior mesenteric artery branches

Straight arteries (arteriae rectae)

Serosa (visceral peritoneum)

Longitudinal muscle layer

Circular muscle layer

Submucosa

Mucosa

Circular folds

Solitary lymph follicles (nodules)

Aggregate lymph follicles (Peyer's patches)

Barium radiograph of ileum

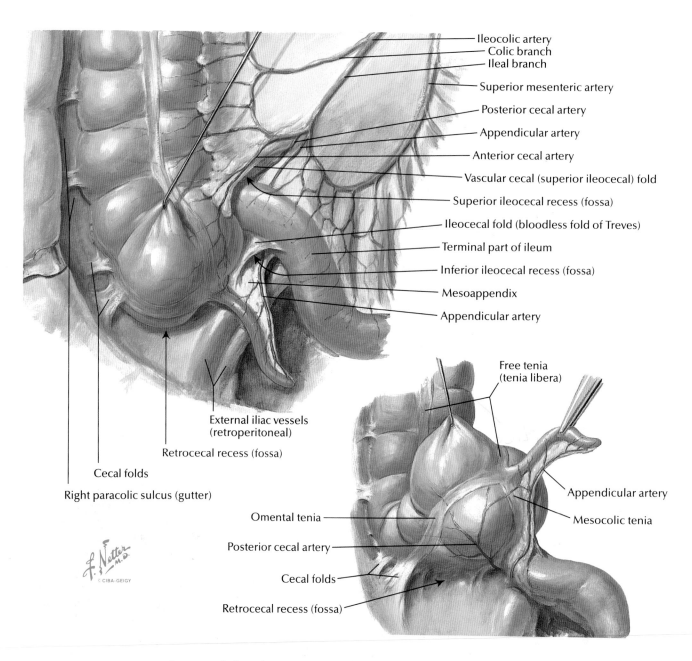

Ileocolic artery

Colic branch

Ileal branch

Superior mesenteric artery

Posterior cecal artery

Appendicular artery

Anterior cecal artery

Vascular cecal (superior ileocecal) fold

Superior ileocecal recess (fossa)

Ileocecal fold (bloodless fold of Treves)

Terminal part of ileum

Inferior ileocecal recess (fossa)

Mesoappendix

Appendicular artery

External iliac vessels (retroperitoneal)

Retrocecal recess (fossa)

Cecal folds

Right paracolic sulcus (gutter)

Free tenia (tenia libera)

Appendicular artery

Mesocolic tenia

Omental tenia

Posterior cecal artery

Cecal folds

Retrocecal recess (fossa)

Some variations in posterior peritoneal attachment of cecum

Attached area — Lines of posterior peritoneal reflection

Attached area — Lines of posterior peritoneal reflection

Attached area — Lines of posterior peritoneal reflection

Attached area — Lines of posterior peritoneal reflection

PLATE 264

ABDOMEN

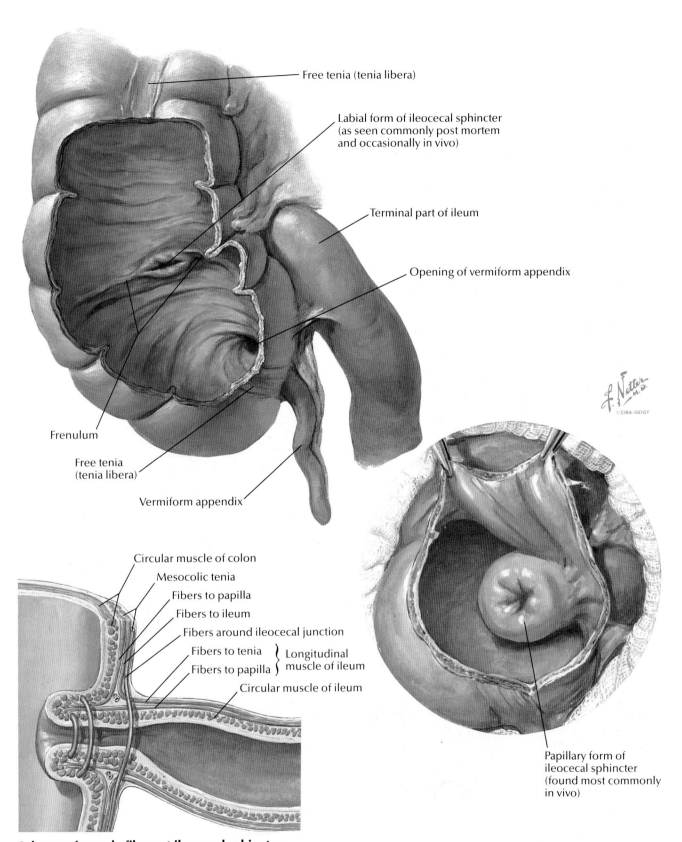

Free tenia (tenia libera)

Labial form of ileocecal sphincter (as seen commonly post mortem and occasionally in vivo)

Terminal part of ileum

Opening of vermiform appendix

Frenulum

Free tenia (tenia libera)

Vermiform appendix

Circular muscle of colon
Mesocolic tenia
Fibers to papilla
Fibers to ileum
Fibers around ileocecal junction
Fibers to tenia } Longitudinal
Fibers to papilla } muscle of ileum
Circular muscle of ileum

Schema of muscle fibers at ileocecal sphincter

Papillary form of ileocecal sphincter (found most commonly in vivo)

Vermiform Appendix

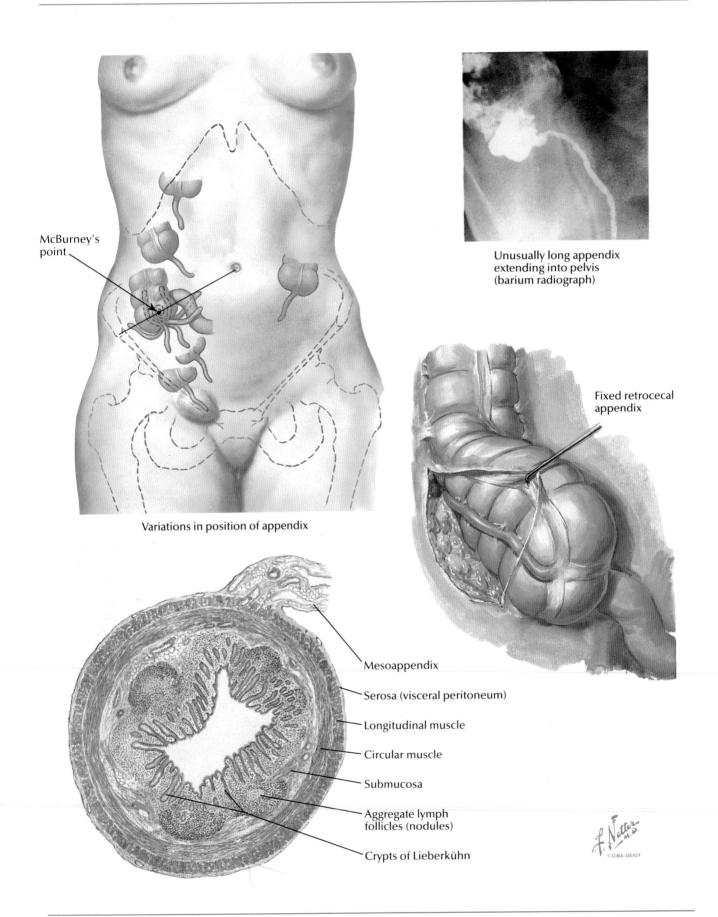

McBurney's point

Variations in position of appendix

Unusually long appendix extending into pelvis (barium radiograph)

Fixed retrocecal appendix

Mesoappendix

Serosa (visceral peritoneum)

Longitudinal muscle

Circular muscle

Submucosa

Aggregate lymph follicles (nodules)

Crypts of Lieberkühn

PLATE 266

ABDOMEN

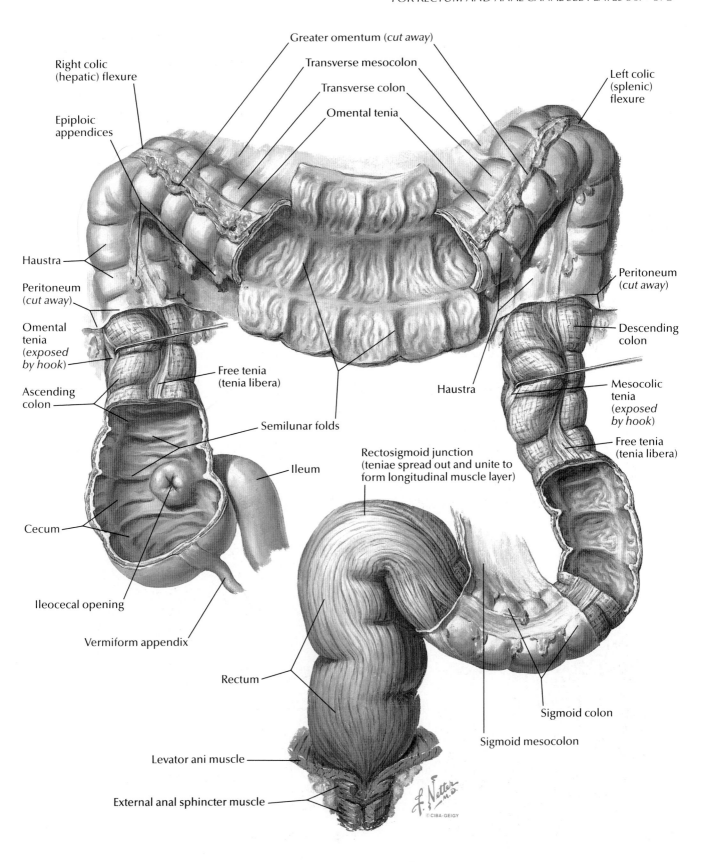

Greater omentum (*cut away*)

Transverse mesocolon

Transverse colon

Omental tenia

Right colic (hepatic) flexure

Left colic (splenic) flexure

Epiploic appendices

Haustra

Peritoneum (*cut away*)

Peritoneum (*cut away*)

Omental tenia (*exposed by hook*)

Descending colon

Ascending colon

Free tenia (tenia libera)

Haustra

Mesocolic tenia (*exposed by hook*)

Semilunar folds

Free tenia (tenia libera)

Ileum

Rectosigmoid junction (teniae spread out and unite to form longitudinal muscle layer)

Cecum

Ileocecal opening

Vermiform appendix

Rectum

Sigmoid colon

Sigmoid mesocolon

Levator ani muscle

External anal sphincter muscle

F. Netter M.D.

© CIBA-GEIGY

Sigmoid Colon: Variations in Position

FOR RECTUM SEE PLATES 341, 342, 367, 368, 369, 370

Typical

Short, straight, obliquely into pelvis

Looping to right side

Ascending high into abdomen

PLATE 268

ABDOMEN

Midinguinal plane

Transpyloric plane

Diaphragm

Liver covered by diaphragm, pleura and lung (percussion dullness)

Liver covered by diaphragm and pleura (percussion flatness)

Liver covered by diaphragm (percussion flatness or intestinal resonance)

Gallbladder

Liver

Diaphragm

Liver covered by diaphragm, pleura and lung (percussion dullness)

Liver covered by diaphragm and pleura (percussion flatness)

Liver covered by diaphragm, pleura and lung (percussion dullness)

Liver covered by diaphragm and pleura (percussion flatness)

Diaphragm

Gallbladder

Inferior margin of liver

Surfaces and Bed of Liver

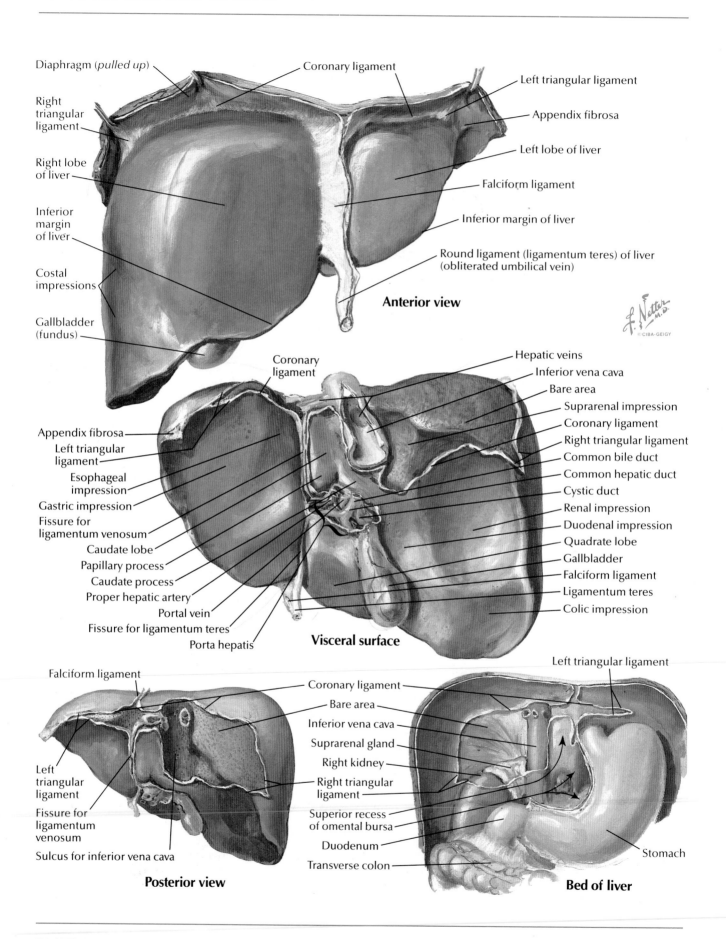

Diaphragm (*pulled up*)

Coronary ligament

Left triangular ligament

Appendix fibrosa

Right triangular ligament

Left lobe of liver

Right lobe of liver

Falciform ligament

Inferior margin of liver

Inferior margin of liver

Costal impressions

Round ligament (ligamentum teres) of liver (obliterated umbilical vein)

Gallbladder (fundus)

Anterior view

Coronary ligament

Hepatic veins

Inferior vena cava

Bare area

Suprarenal impression

Coronary ligament

Right triangular ligament

Common bile duct

Common hepatic duct

Cystic duct

Renal impression

Duodenal impression

Quadrate lobe

Gallbladder

Falciform ligament

Ligamentum teres

Colic impression

Appendix fibrosa

Left triangular ligament

Esophageal impression

Gastric impression

Fissure for ligamentum venosum

Caudate lobe

Papillary process

Caudate process

Proper hepatic artery

Portal vein

Fissure for ligamentum teres

Porta hepatis

Visceral surface

Falciform ligament

Coronary ligament

Left triangular ligament

Bare area

Inferior vena cava

Suprarenal gland

Right kidney

Right triangular ligament

Left triangular ligament

Fissure for ligamentum venosum

Superior recess of omental bursa

Sulcus for inferior vena cava

Duodenum

Transverse colon

Stomach

Posterior view

Bed of liver

PLATE 270

ABDOMEN

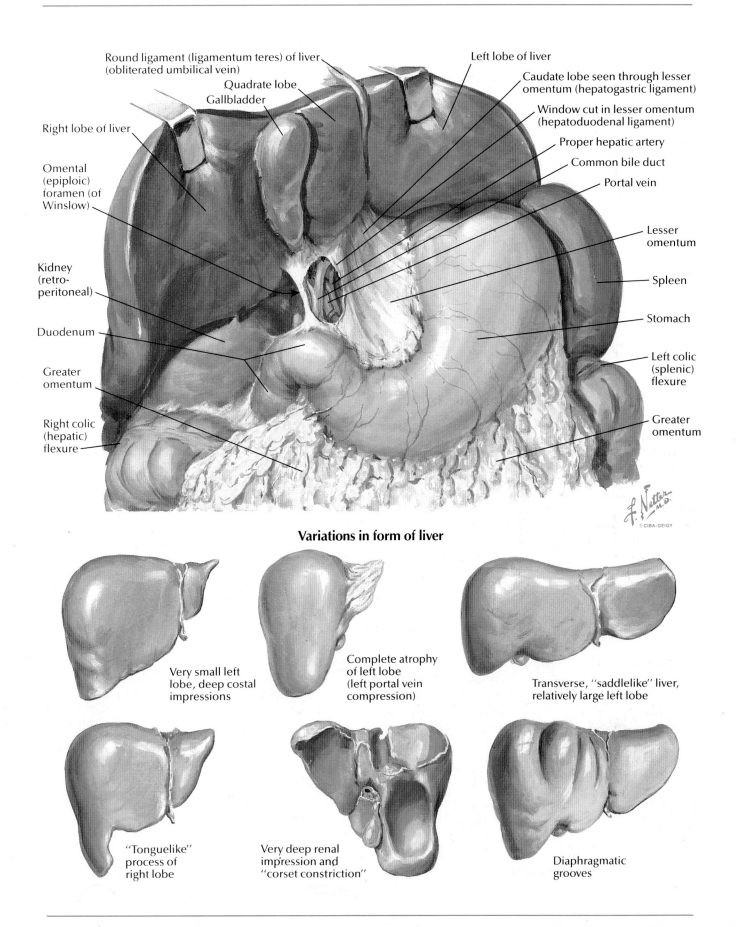

Round ligament (ligamentum teres) of liver (obliterated umbilical vein)

Quadrate lobe

Gallbladder

Right lobe of liver

Omental (epiploic) foramen (of Winslow)

Kidney (retroperitoneal)

Duodenum

Greater omentum

Right colic (hepatic) flexure

Left lobe of liver

Caudate lobe seen through lesser omentum (hepatogastric ligament)

Window cut in lesser omentum (hepatoduodenal ligament)

Proper hepatic artery

Common bile duct

Portal vein

Lesser omentum

Spleen

Stomach

Left colic (splenic) flexure

Greater omentum

Variations in form of liver

Very small left lobe, deep costal impressions

Complete atrophy of left lobe (left portal vein compression)

Transverse, "saddlelike" liver, relatively large left lobe

"Tonguelike" process of right lobe

Very deep renal impression and "corset constriction"

Diaphragmatic grooves

Liver Segments and Lobules: Vessel and Duct Distribution

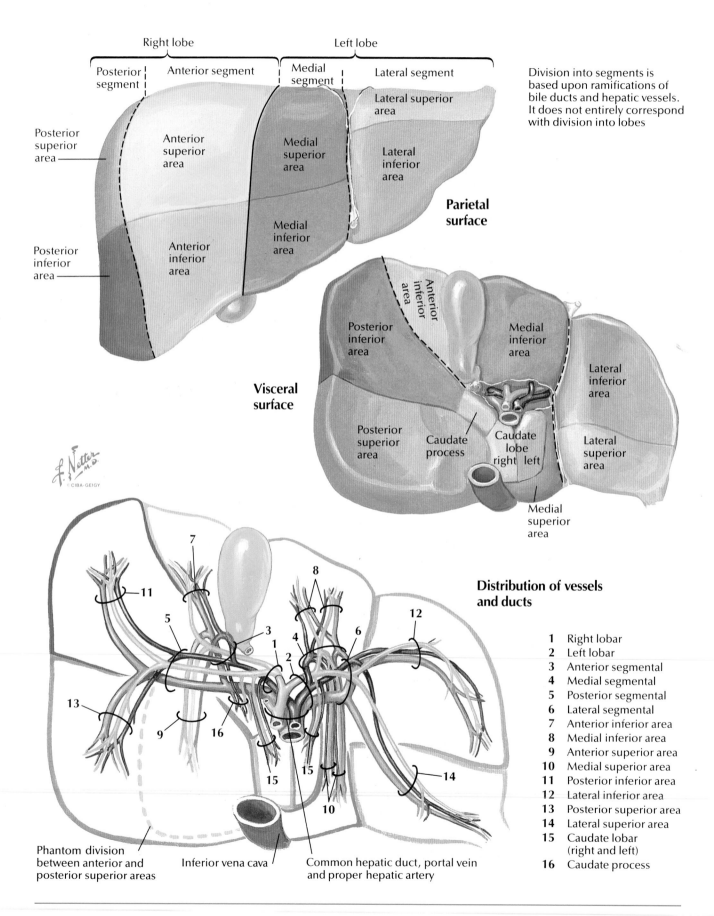

Division into segments is based upon ramifications of bile ducts and hepatic vessels. It does not entirely correspond with division into lobes

Right lobe — Left lobe

Posterior segment — Anterior segment — Medial segment — Lateral segment

Posterior superior area

Posterior inferior area

Anterior superior area

Anterior inferior area

Medial superior area

Medial inferior area

Lateral superior area

Lateral inferior area

Parietal surface

Visceral surface

Anterior inferior area

Posterior inferior area

Posterior superior area

Caudate process

Caudate lobe right left

Medial inferior area

Lateral inferior area

Lateral superior area

Medial superior area

Distribution of vessels and ducts

1 Right lobar
2 Left lobar
3 Anterior segmental
4 Medial segmental
5 Posterior segmental
6 Lateral segmental
7 Anterior inferior area
8 Medial inferior area
9 Anterior superior area
10 Medial superior area
11 Posterior inferior area
12 Lateral inferior area
13 Posterior superior area
14 Lateral superior area
15 Caudate lobar (right and left)
16 Caudate process

Phantom division between anterior and posterior superior areas

Inferior vena cava

Common hepatic duct, portal vein and proper hepatic artery

PLATE 272

ABDOMEN

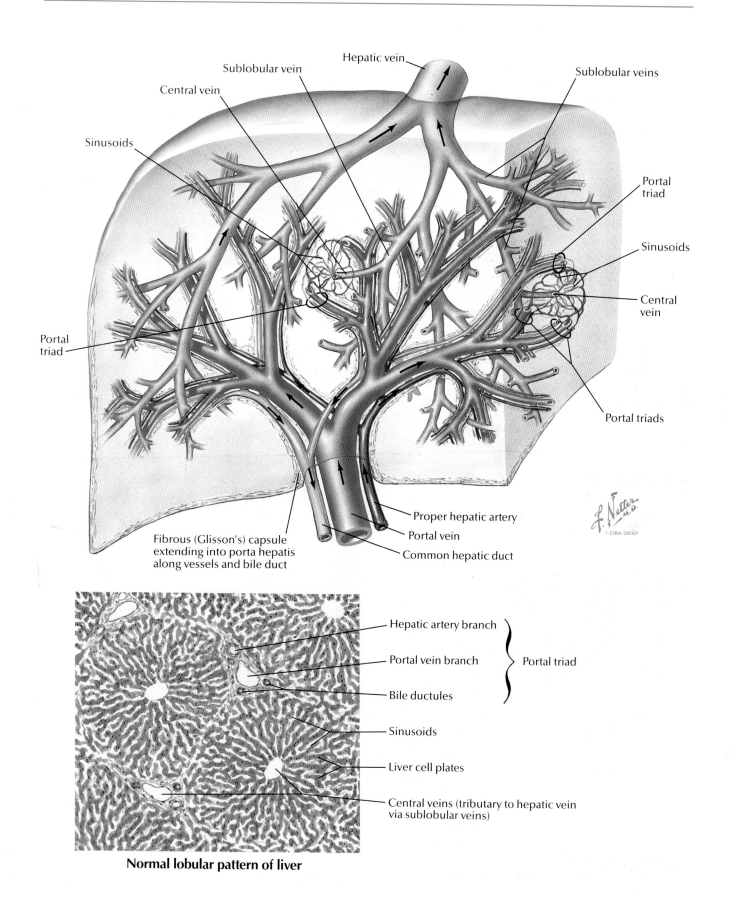

Hepatic vein

Sublobular vein

Central vein

Sinusoids

Portal triad

Fibrous (Glisson's) capsule extending into porta hepatis along vessels and bile duct

Sublobular veins

Portal triad

Sinusoids

Central vein

Portal triads

Proper hepatic artery

Portal vein

Common hepatic duct

Hepatic artery branch

Portal vein branch   } Portal triad

Bile ductules

Sinusoids

Liver cell plates

Central veins (tributary to hepatic vein via sublobular veins)

Normal lobular pattern of liver

Liver Structure: Schema

Connective tissue

Lymph vessel

Limiting plate
of portal space

Central vein

Periportal
space (of Mall)

Sublobular vein (tributary to hepatic vein)

Central vein

Perisinusoidal spaces (of Disse)

Sinusoids

Central vein

Periportal
bile ductule
(canal of Hering)

Branch of
portal vein

Bile duct

Branch of
hepatic artery

Portal arteriole

Periportal arteriole

Intralobular arteriole

Intralobular bile ductule (cholangiole)

Central vein

Periportal bile ductule (canal of Hering)

Inlet venule

Distributing vein

PLATE 274

ABDOMEN

Branch of portal vein

Bile ducts

Periportal bile ductules (canals of Hering)

Limiting plate of portal space

Bile canaliculi

Sinusoid

Intralobular bile ductules (cholangioles)

Note: in above illustration, bile canaliculi appear as structures with walls of their own. However, as shown in histologic section at right, boundaries of canaliculi are actually a specialization of surface membranes of adjoining liver parenchymal cells

Branch of portal vein

Bile ducts

Bile ductules

Bile canaliculi

Branch of hepatic artery

Low-power section of liver

Right and left hepatic ducts

Common hepatic duct

Cystic artery

Cystic duct

Portal vein

Liver

Common bile duct

Gallbladder

Superior (1st) part of duodenum

Transverse colon (cut)

Head of pancreas

Right and left hepatic arteries

Proper hepatic artery

Anterior layer of lesser omentum (cut edge)

Right gastric artery

Common hepatic artery

Gastroduodenal artery

Stomach

Hepatic ducts

Right   Left

Cystic duct

Spiral part   Smooth part

Neck

Infundibulum (Hartmann's pouch)

Body (corpus)

Gallbladder

Fundus

Common hepatic duct

Gland openings

Common bile duct

Descending (2nd) part of duodenum

Ampulla (of Vater)

Major duodenal papilla (of Vater)

Pancreatic duct

PLATE 276

ABDOMEN

Variations in cystic duct

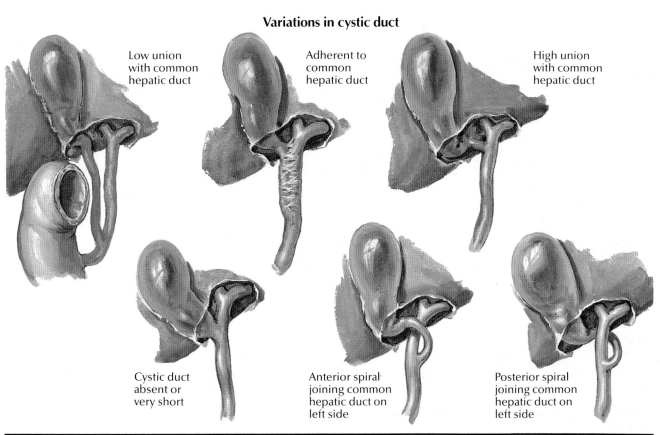

Low union with common hepatic duct

Adherent to common hepatic duct

High union with common hepatic duct

Cystic duct absent or very short

Anterior spiral joining common hepatic duct on left side

Posterior spiral joining common hepatic duct on left side

Accessory (aberrant) hepatic ducts

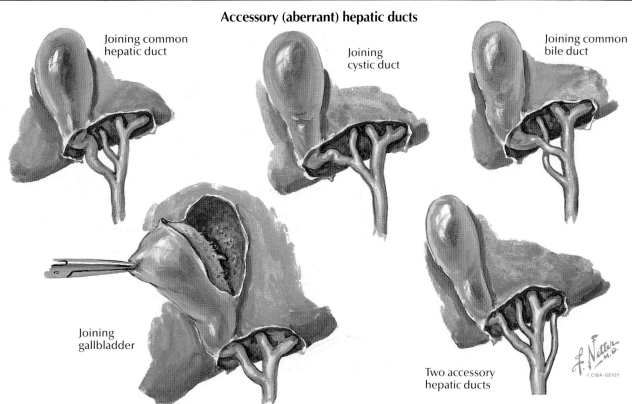

Joining common hepatic duct

Joining cystic duct

Joining common bile duct

Joining gallbladder

Two accessory hepatic ducts

Choledochoduodenal Junction

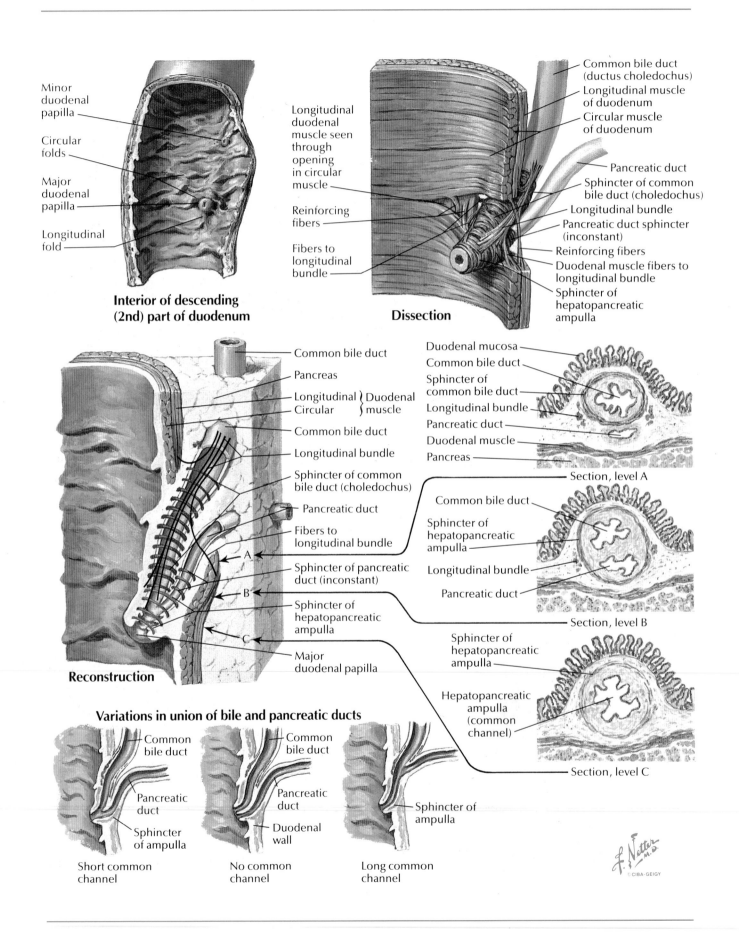

Minor duodenal papilla

Circular folds

Major duodenal papilla

Longitudinal fold

Interior of descending (2nd) part of duodenum

Longitudinal duodenal muscle seen through opening in circular muscle

Reinforcing fibers

Fibers to longitudinal bundle

Dissection

Common bile duct (ductus choledochus)

Longitudinal muscle of duodenum

Circular muscle of duodenum

Pancreatic duct

Sphincter of common bile duct (choledochus)

Longitudinal bundle

Pancreatic duct sphincter (inconstant)

Reinforcing fibers

Duodenal muscle fibers to longitudinal bundle

Sphincter of hepatopancreatic ampulla

Common bile duct

Pancreas

Longitudinal } Duodenal
Circular } muscle

Common bile duct

Longitudinal bundle

Sphincter of common bile duct (choledochus)

Pancreatic duct

Fibers to longitudinal bundle

A

Sphincter of pancreatic duct (inconstant)

B

Sphincter of hepatopancreatic ampulla

C

Major duodenal papilla

Reconstruction

Duodenal mucosa

Common bile duct

Sphincter of common bile duct

Longitudinal bundle

Pancreatic duct

Duodenal muscle

Pancreas

Section, level A

Common bile duct

Sphincter of hepatopancreatic ampulla

Longitudinal bundle

Pancreatic duct

Section, level B

Sphincter of hepatopancreatic ampulla

Hepatopancreatic ampulla (common channel)

Section, level C

Variations in union of bile and pancreatic ducts

Common bile duct

Pancreatic duct

Sphincter of ampulla

Short common channel

Common bile duct

Pancreatic duct

Duodenal wall

No common channel

Sphincter of ampulla

Long common channel

PLATE 278

ABDOMEN

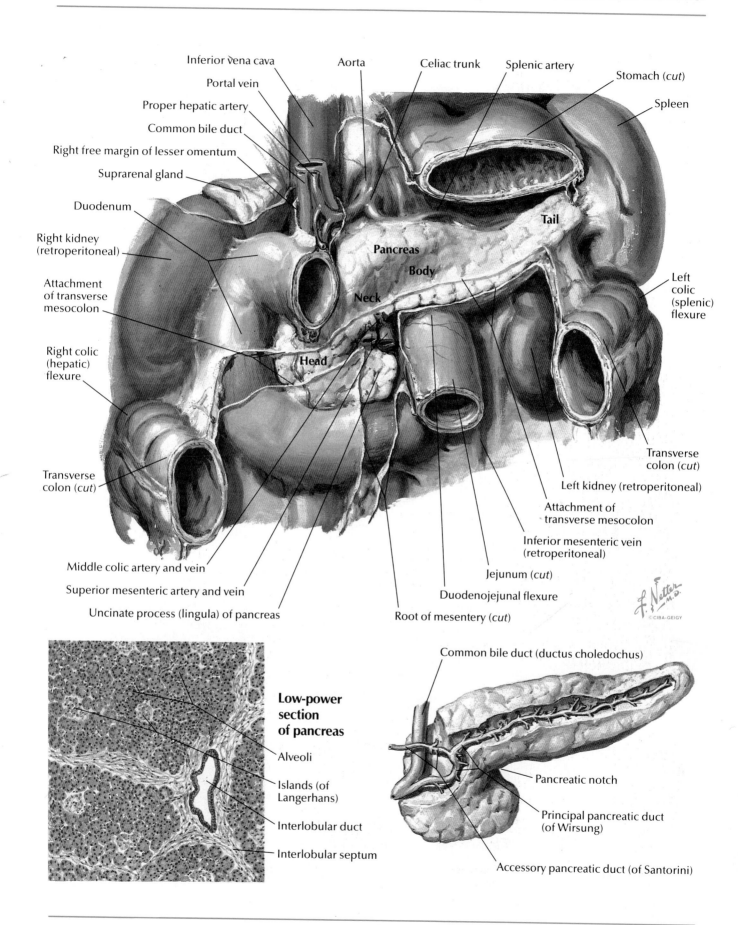

Inferior vena cava

Portal vein

Proper hepatic artery

Common bile duct

Right free margin of lesser omentum

Suprarenal gland

Duodenum

Right kidney (retroperitoneal)

Attachment of transverse mesocolon

Right colic (hepatic) flexure

Transverse colon (*cut*)

Middle colic artery and vein

Superior mesenteric artery and vein

Uncinate process (lingula) of pancreas

Aorta

Celiac trunk

Splenic artery

Stomach (*cut*)

Spleen

Tail

Pancreas

Body

Neck

Head

Left colic (splenic) flexure

Transverse colon (*cut*)

Left kidney (retroperitoneal)

Attachment of transverse mesocolon

Inferior mesenteric vein (retroperitoneal)

Jejunum (*cut*)

Duodenojejunal flexure

Root of mesentery (*cut*)

Low-power section of pancreas

Alveoli

Islands (of Langerhans)

Interlobular duct

Interlobular septum

Common bile duct (ductus choledochus)

Pancreatic notch

Principal pancreatic duct (of Wirsung)

Accessory pancreatic duct (of Santorini)

Variations in Pancreatic Ducts

Accessory duct (of Santorini) abnormally large

Minor duodenal papilla

Major duodenal papilla

Principal duct (of Wirsung) abnormally small

Reversal in relative size of ducts

Double accessory duct (of Santorini)

Anastomosis between ducts

Crossing of ducts

Double crossing of ducts

No communication between ducts

Double principal duct (of Wirsung)

Tortuosity of ducts

Absence of accessory duct (of Santorini)

PLATE 280

ABDOMEN

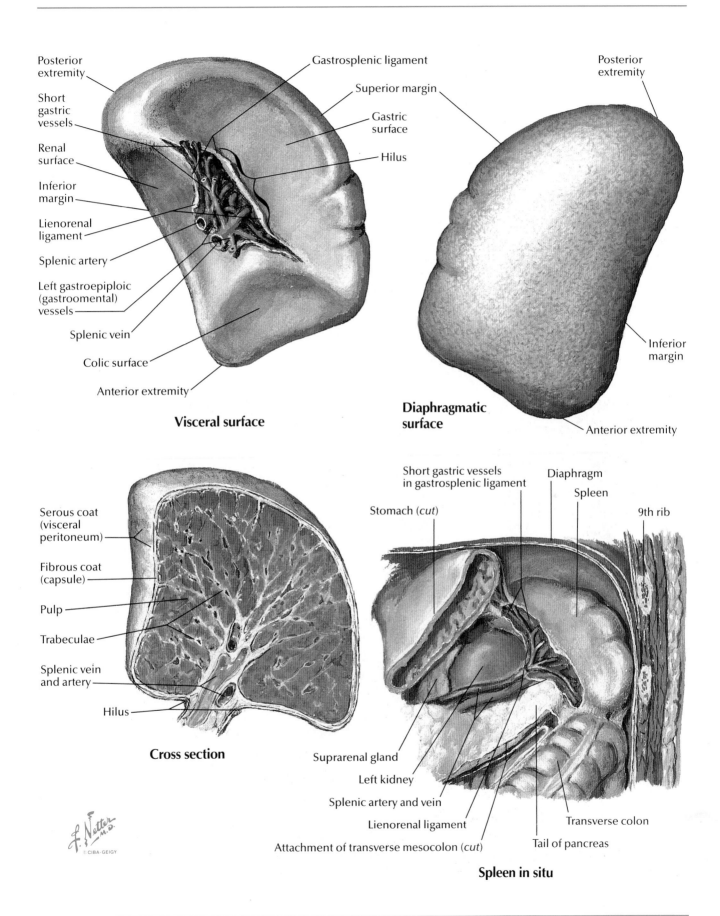

Posterior extremity

Short gastric vessels

Renal surface

Inferior margin

Lienorenal ligament

Splenic artery

Left gastroepiploic (gastroomental) vessels

Splenic vein

Colic surface

Anterior extremity

Gastrosplenic ligament

Superior margin

Gastric surface

Hilus

Visceral surface

Posterior extremity

Inferior margin

Anterior extremity

Diaphragmatic surface

Serous coat (visceral peritoneum)

Fibrous coat (capsule)

Pulp

Trabeculae

Splenic vein and artery

Hilus

Cross section

Short gastric vessels in gastrosplenic ligament

Diaphragm

Spleen

9th rib

Stomach (*cut*)

Suprarenal gland

Left kidney

Splenic artery and vein

Lienorenal ligament

Attachment of transverse mesocolon (*cut*)

Transverse colon

Tail of pancreas

Spleen in situ

Arteries of Stomach, Liver and Spleen

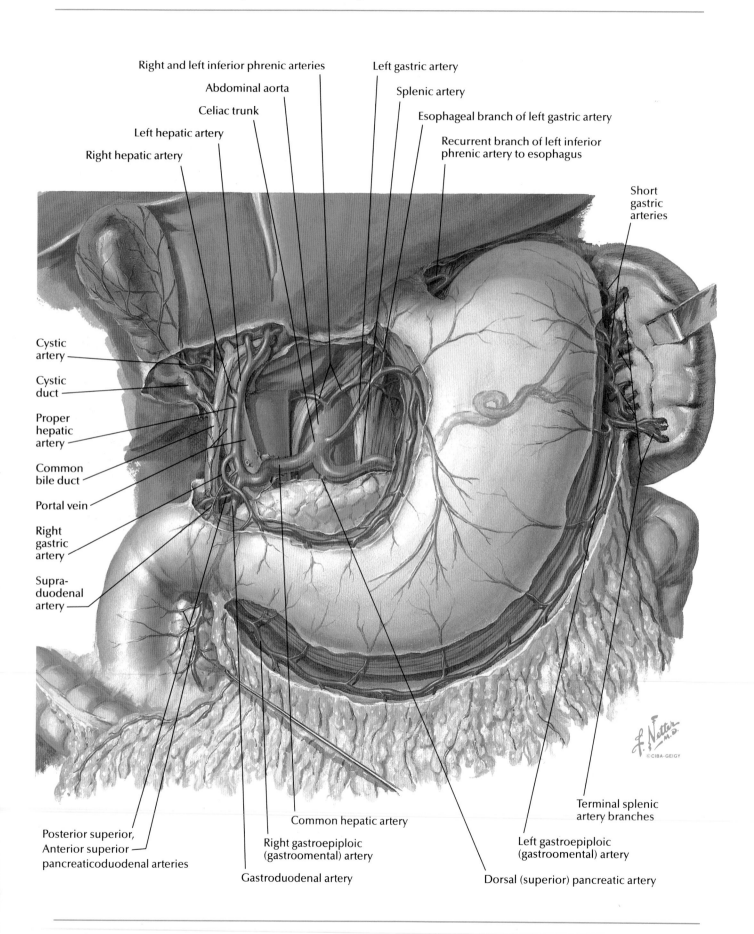

Right and left inferior phrenic arteries

Abdominal aorta

Celiac trunk

Left hepatic artery

Right hepatic artery

Left gastric artery

Splenic artery

Esophageal branch of left gastric artery

Recurrent branch of left inferior phrenic artery to esophagus

Short gastric arteries

Cystic artery

Cystic duct

Proper hepatic artery

Common bile duct

Portal vein

Right gastric artery

Supra-duodenal artery

Posterior superior, Anterior superior pancreaticoduodenal arteries

Right gastroepiploic (gastroomental) artery

Gastroduodenal artery

Common hepatic artery

Terminal splenic artery branches

Left gastroepiploic (gastroomental) artery

Dorsal (superior) pancreatic artery

PLATE 282

ABDOMEN

Arteries of Stomach, Duodenum, Pancreas and Spleen

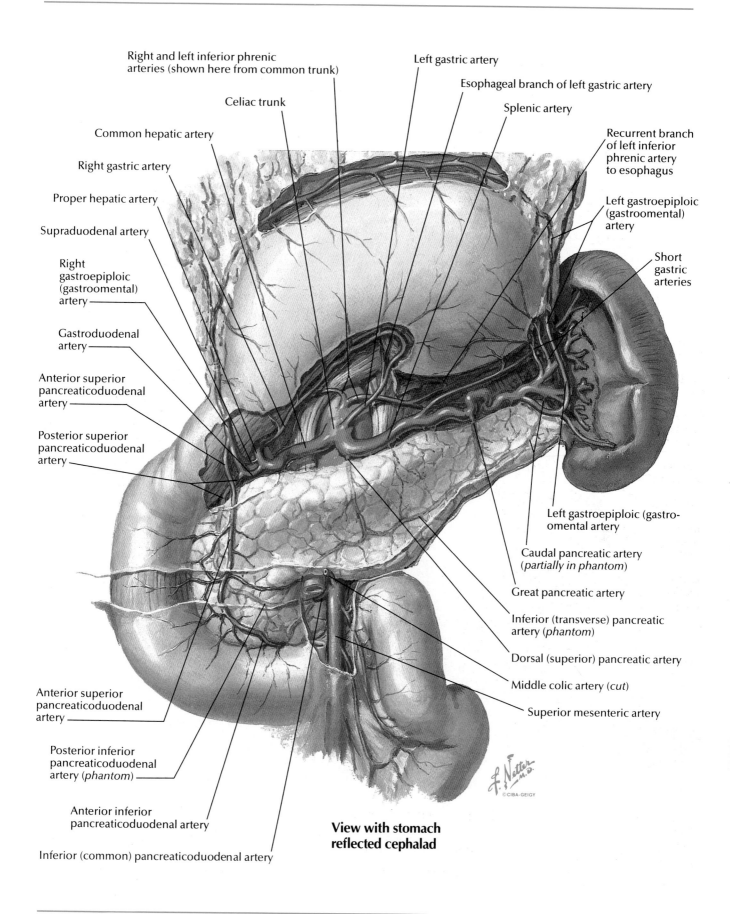

Right and left inferior phrenic arteries (shown here from common trunk)

Celiac trunk

Common hepatic artery

Right gastric artery

Proper hepatic artery

Supraduodenal artery

Right gastroepiploic (gastroomental) artery

Gastroduodenal artery

Anterior superior pancreaticoduodenal artery

Posterior superior pancreaticoduodenal artery

Anterior superior pancreaticoduodenal artery

Posterior inferior pancreaticoduodenal artery (phantom)

Anterior inferior pancreaticoduodenal artery

Inferior (common) pancreaticoduodenal artery

Left gastric artery

Esophageal branch of left gastric artery

Splenic artery

Recurrent branch of left inferior phrenic artery to esophagus

Left gastroepiploic (gastroomental) artery

Short gastric arteries

Left gastroepiploic (gastro-omental artery

Caudal pancreatic artery (partially in phantom)

Great pancreatic artery

Inferior (transverse) pancreatic artery (phantom)

Dorsal (superior) pancreatic artery

Middle colic artery (cut)

Superior mesenteric artery

View with stomach reflected cephalad

Arteries of Liver, Pancreas, Duodenum and Spleen

Intermediate hepatic artery

Proper hepatic artery

Right hepatic artery

Cystic artery

Gallbladder

Left hepatic artery

Portal vein

Common hepatic artery

Left gastric artery

Right and left inferior phrenic arteries (shown here from common stem)

Celiac trunk

Abdominal aorta

Short gastric arteries

Cystic triangle (of Calot)

Cystic duct

Common hepatic duct

Common bile duct

Right gastric artery

Supraduodenal artery

Gastroduodenal artery

Posterior superior pancreaticoduodenal artery (*phantom*)

Anterior superior pancreaticoduodenal artery

Right gastroepiploic (gastroomental) artery

Left gastroepiploic (gastroomental) artery

Caudal pancreatic artery

Great pancreatic artery

Splenic artery

Dorsal (superior) pancreatic artery

Inferior (transverse) pancreatic artery

Anastomotic branch

Middle colic artery (*cut*)

Superior mesenteric artery

Inferior (common) pancreaticoduodenal artery

Posterior inferior pancreaticoduodenal artery

Anterior inferior pancreaticoduodenal artery

PLATE 284

ABDOMEN

Duodenum and head of pancreas reflected to left

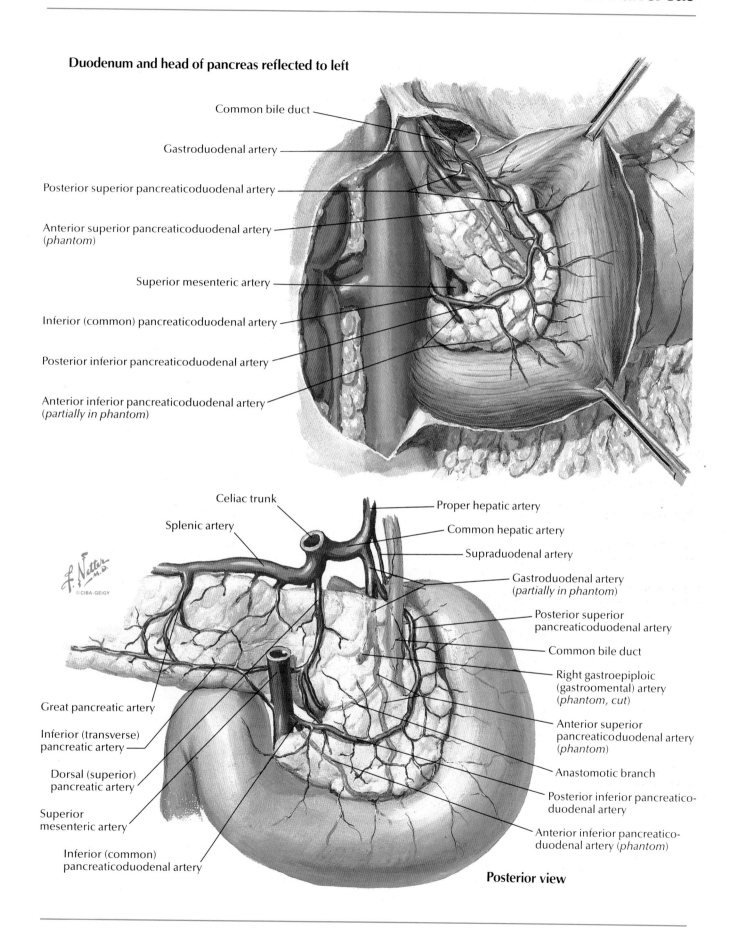

Common bile duct

Gastroduodenal artery

Posterior superior pancreaticoduodenal artery

Anterior superior pancreaticoduodenal artery (*phantom*)

Superior mesenteric artery

Inferior (common) pancreaticoduodenal artery

Posterior inferior pancreaticoduodenal artery

Anterior inferior pancreaticoduodenal artery (*partially in phantom*)

Celiac trunk

Splenic artery

Proper hepatic artery

Common hepatic artery

Supraduodenal artery

Gastroduodenal artery (*partially in phantom*)

Posterior superior pancreaticoduodenal artery

Common bile duct

Right gastroepiploic (gastroomental) artery (*phantom, cut*)

Anterior superior pancreaticoduodenal artery (*phantom*)

Anastomotic branch

Posterior inferior pancreatico-duodenal artery

Anterior inferior pancreatico-duodenal artery (*phantom*)

Great pancreatic artery

Inferior (transverse) pancreatic artery

Dorsal (superior) pancreatic artery

Superior mesenteric artery

Inferior (common) pancreaticoduodenal artery

Posterior view

Arteries of Small Intestine

Common hepatic artery

Right gastric artery

Supraduodenal artery

Gastroduodenal artery

Posterior superior pancreaticoduodenal artery

Right gastroepiploic (gastroomental) artery

Anterior superior pancreaticoduodenal artery

Inferior pancreatico-duodenal arteries
{ Common
  Posterior
  Anterior }

Anastomosis (inferior pancreatico-duodenal to 1st jejunal artery)

Right colic artery

Ileocolic artery

Colic branch

Ileal branch

Superior mesenteric artery

Anterior cecal artery

Posterior cecal artery

Appendicular artery

Right and left inferior phrenic arteries

Left gastric artery

Celiac trunk

Splenic artery and vein

Short gastric arteries

Dorsal (superior) pancreatic artery

Inferior (transverse) pancreatic artery

Superior mesenteric artery and vein

Left gastroepiploic (gastroomental) artery

Middle colic artery (cut)

Intestinal (jejunal and ileal) arteries

Anastomotic loops

Straight arteries (arteriae rectae)

PLATE 286

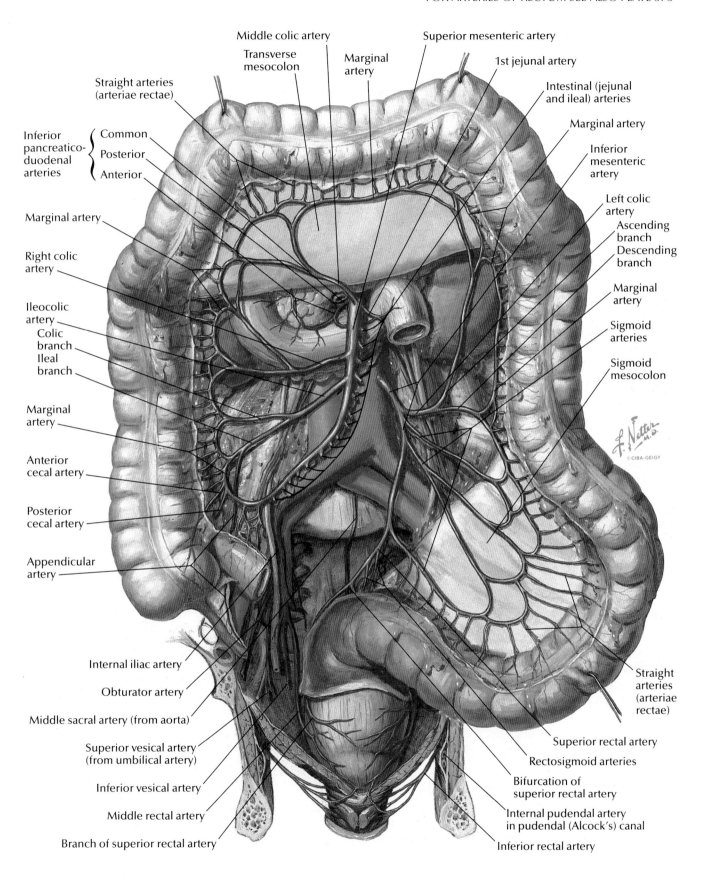

Middle colic artery

Transverse mesocolon

Marginal artery

Superior mesenteric artery

1st jejunal artery

Intestinal (jejunal and ileal) arteries

Marginal artery

Inferior mesenteric artery

Left colic artery

Ascending branch

Descending branch

Marginal artery

Sigmoid arteries

Sigmoid mesocolon

Straight arteries (arteriae rectae)

Inferior pancreatico-duodenal arteries
{ Common
Posterior
Anterior

Marginal artery

Right colic artery

Ileocolic artery

Colic branch

Ileal branch

Marginal artery

Anterior cecal artery

Posterior cecal artery

Appendicular artery

Internal iliac artery

Obturator artery

Middle sacral artery (from aorta)

Superior vesical artery (from umbilical artery)

Inferior vesical artery

Middle rectal artery

Branch of superior rectal artery

Straight arteries (arteriae rectae)

Superior rectal artery

Rectosigmoid arteries

Bifurcation of superior rectal artery

Internal pudendal artery in pudendal (Alcock's) canal

Inferior rectal artery

Variations in Celiac Trunk

Common origin of celiac trunk and superior mesenteric artery

Celiacomesenteric trunk

Splenic artery takes origin from superior mesenteric (note replaced left hepatic artery from left gastric)

Hepatogastric trunk

Lienomesenteric trunk

Splenic and hepatic arteries take origin from superior mesenteric

Gastrophrenic trunk

Hepatolieno-mesenteric trunk

Replaced hepatic artery takes origin from superior mesenteric (note inferior pancreaticoduodenal artery from 1st jejunal)

Lienogastric trunk

Hepato-mesenteric trunk

Replaced right hepatic artery takes origin from superior mesenteric; inferior pancreaticoduodenal and 1st jejunal arteries from replaced right hepatic

Incomplete celiac trunk

Hepatomesenteric trunk

Accessory right hepatic artery takes origin from superior mesenteric

Complete celiac trunk

Hepato-mesenteric trunk

Accessory right hepatic artery takes origin from superior mesenteric; inferior pancreaticoduodenal arteries from accessory right hepatic; 1st jejunal artery from anterior inferior pancreaticoduodenal

Complete celiac trunk

Hepatomesenteric trunk

(Note accessory left gastric artery from left hepatic)

Right gastroepiploic (gastroomental) artery takes origin from superior mesenteric (note accessory left hepatic artery from left gastric)

PLATE 288

Replaced common hepatic artery may originate from superior mesenteric artery

Left gastric artery

Splenic artery

Gastroduodenal artery

Proximal bifurcation of common hepatic artery

Right and left hepatic arteries may originate directly from celiac trunk

Replaced right hepatic artery may originate from superior mesenteric artery

Replaced left hepatic artery may originate from left gastric artery

Accessory right hepatic artery may originate from superior mesenteric artery

Accessory left hepatic artery may originate from left gastric artery

Accessory left hepatic artery may originate from right hepatic artery

Right hepatic artery may cross anterior to common hepatic duct instead of posterior

Variations in Cystic Artery

May originate from normal right hepatic outside cystic triangle

Intermediate hepatic artery

Left hepatic artery

Cystic artery

Right hepatic artery

Proper hepatic artery

Right gastric artery

Left gastric artery

Celiac trunk

Splenic artery

Common hepatic artery

Gastroduodenal artery

May originate from intermediate (or left) hepatic

May cross anterior to hepatic duct

May originate from proper hepatic

May originate from gastroduodenal

May cross anterior to common bile duct

May originate from celiac trunk (or from aorta)

Aorta

May originate in cystic triangle from aberrant right hepatic (from superior mesenteric)

Superior mesenteric artery

May originate outside cystic triangle from aberrant right hepatic

May cross anterior to hepatic duct

Double cystic artery; both from normal right hepatic in cystic triangle

Double cystic artery; both from normal right hepatic, one inside and one outside cystic triangle

Double cystic artery; both from aberrant right hepatic, one inside and one outside cystic triangle

Double cystic artery; posterior from right hepatic, anterior from gastroduodenal

PLATE 290

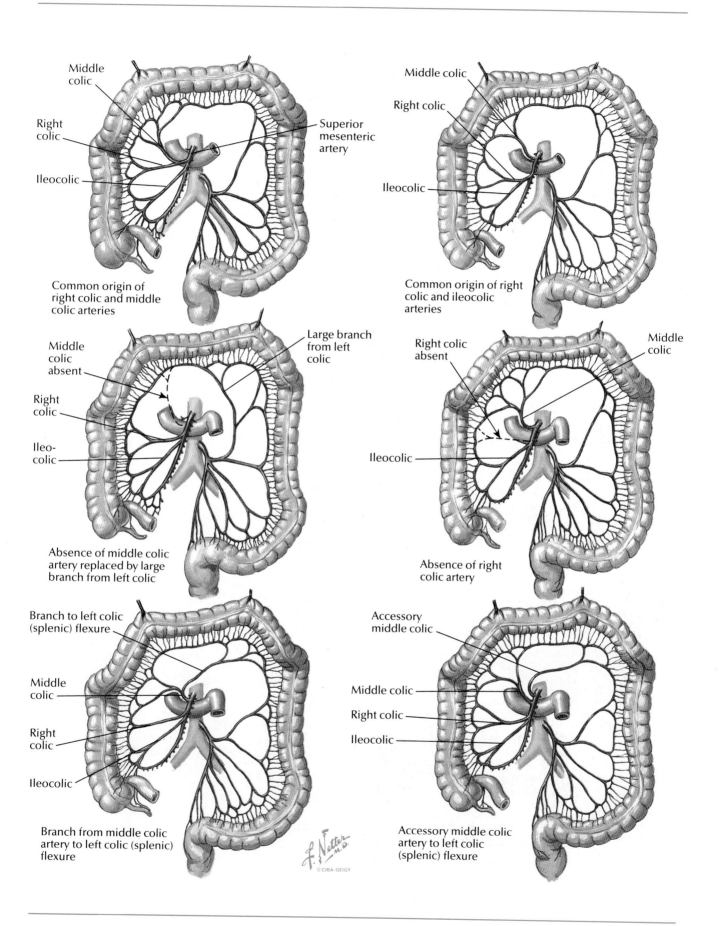

Middle colic

Right colic

Ileocolic

Superior mesenteric artery

Common origin of right colic and middle colic arteries

Middle colic

Right colic

Ileocolic

Common origin of right colic and ileocolic arteries

Middle colic absent

Large branch from left colic

Right colic

Ileo-colic

Absence of middle colic artery replaced by large branch from left colic

Right colic absent

Middle colic

Ileocolic

Absence of right colic artery

Branch to left colic (splenic) flexure

Middle colic

Right colic

Ileocolic

Branch from middle colic artery to left colic (splenic) flexure

Accessory middle colic

Middle colic

Right colic

Ileocolic

Accessory middle colic artery to left colic (splenic) flexure

Variations in Colic Arteries (continued)

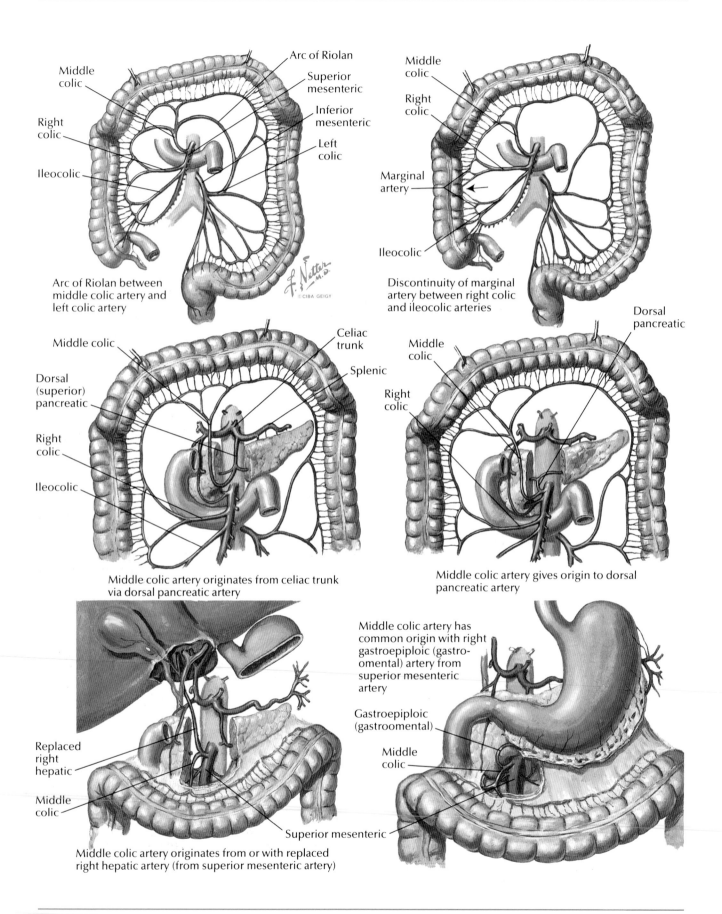

Arc of Riolan between middle colic artery and left colic artery

Discontinuity of marginal artery between right colic and ileocolic arteries

Middle colic artery originates from celiac trunk via dorsal pancreatic artery

Middle colic artery gives origin to dorsal pancreatic artery

Middle colic artery originates from or with replaced right hepatic artery (from superior mesenteric artery)

Middle colic artery has common origin with right gastroepiploic (gastroomental) artery from superior mesenteric artery

PLATE 292

ABDOMEN

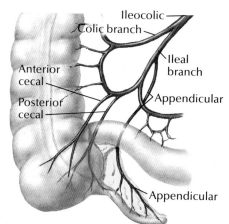

Anterior cecal and posterior cecal arteries originate from arcade between colic and ileal branches of ileocolic; appendicular artery from ileal branch

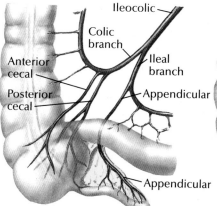

Anterior cecal and posterior cecal arteries originate from colic branch; appendicular artery from ileal branch of ileocolic artery

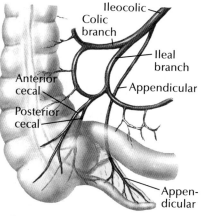

Anterior cecal and posterior cecal arteries have common origin from arcade; appendicular artery from ileocolic artery proper

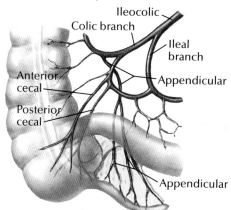

Anterior cecal and posterior cecal arteries originate from arcade between colic and ileal branches of ileocolic artery; appendicular artery from colic branch bifurcates high

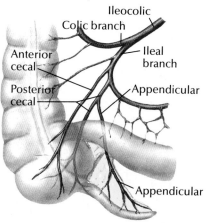

Anterior cecal and posterior cecal arteries originate from ileal branch of ileocolic artery; appendicular artery from posterior cecal artery

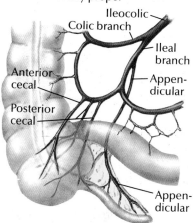

Anterior cecal and two posterior cecal arteries originate from arcade; appendicular artery from ileal branch of ileocolic artery

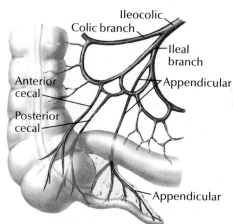

Multiple arcades between ileal branch and colic branch of ileocolic artery; anterior cecal and posterior cecal arteries originate from these arcades; appendicular artery from ileal branch of ileocolic artery

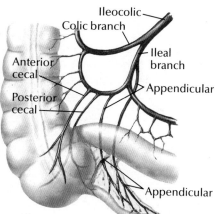

Anterior cecal and posterior cecal arteries originate from arcade between colic and ileal branches of ileocolic artery; two appendicular arteries, one from arcade, one from ileal branch of ileocolic artery

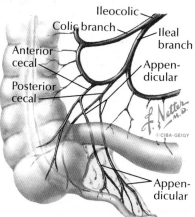

Anterior cecal and posterior cecal arteries originate from arcade; two appendicular arteries, one from anterior cecal, other from posterior cecal artery

Veins of Stomach, Duodenum and Pancreas

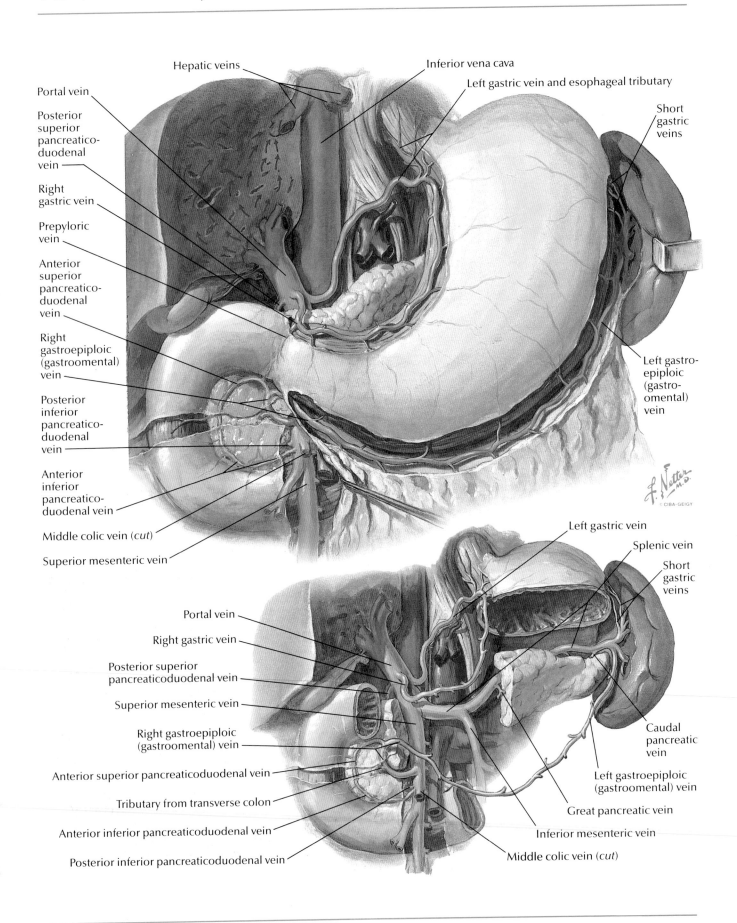

Hepatic veins

Inferior vena cava

Left gastric vein and esophageal tributary

Portal vein

Posterior superior pancreaticoduodenal vein

Right gastric vein

Prepyloric vein

Anterior superior pancreaticoduodenal vein

Right gastroepiploic (gastroomental) vein

Posterior inferior pancreaticoduodenal vein

Anterior inferior pancreaticoduodenal vein

Middle colic vein (cut)

Superior mesenteric vein

Short gastric veins

Left gastroepiploic (gastroomental) vein

Portal vein

Right gastric vein

Posterior superior pancreaticoduodenal vein

Superior mesenteric vein

Right gastroepiploic (gastroomental) vein

Anterior superior pancreaticoduodenal vein

Tributary from transverse colon

Anterior inferior pancreaticoduodenal vein

Posterior inferior pancreaticoduodenal vein

Left gastric vein

Splenic vein

Short gastric veins

Caudal pancreatic vein

Left gastroepiploic (gastroomental) vein

Great pancreatic vein

Inferior mesenteric vein

Middle colic vein (cut)

PLATE 294

ABDOMEN

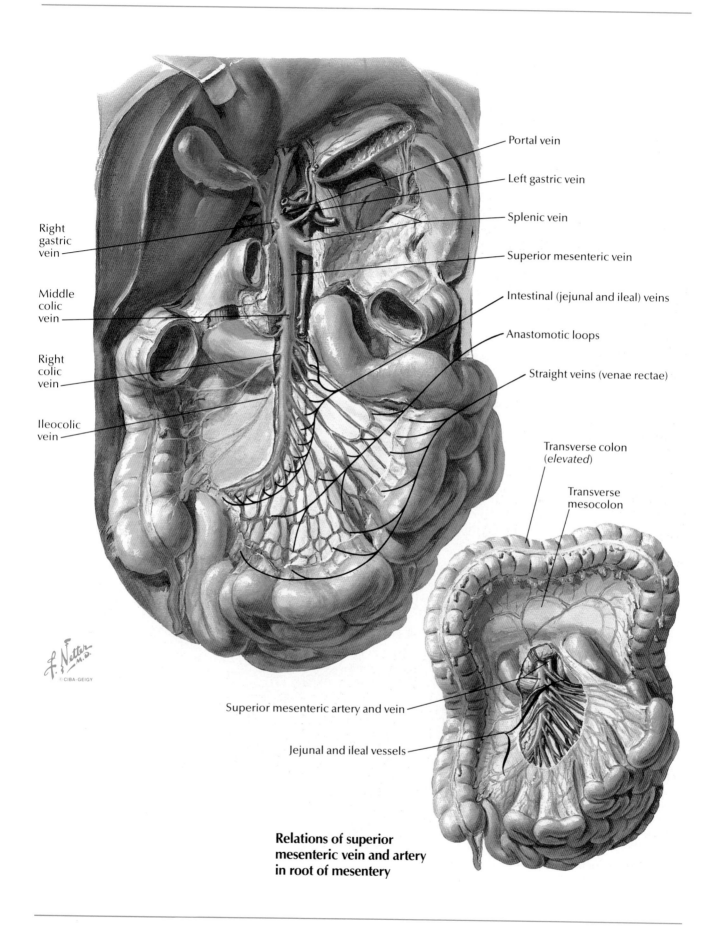

Portal vein

Left gastric vein

Splenic vein

Superior mesenteric vein

Intestinal (jejunal and ileal) veins

Anastomotic loops

Straight veins (venae rectae)

Transverse colon
(*elevated*)

Transverse
mesocolon

Right
gastric
vein

Middle
colic
vein

Right
colic
vein

Ileocolic
vein

Superior mesenteric artery and vein

Jejunal and ileal vessels

**Relations of superior
mesenteric vein and artery
in root of mesentery**

Veins of Small and Large Intestines

FOR VEINS OF RECTUM SEE ALSO PLATE 374

Portal vein

Right gastric vein (*cut*)

Posterior superior pancreatico-duodenal vein

Prepyloric vein

Superior mesenteric vein

Right gastro-epiploic (gastro-omental) vein

Anterior superior pancreaticoduodenal vein

Tributary from colon (*cut*)

Posterior inferior pancreaticoduodenal vein

Anterior inferior pancreaticoduodenal vein

Middle colic vein (*cut*)

Right colic vein

Ileocolic vein

Anterior cecal vein

Posterior cecal vein

Appendicular vein

Right testicular (ovarian) vessels

External iliac vessels

Internal iliac vein

Superior gluteal vein

Obturator vein

Right inferior gluteal vein

Right internal pudendal vein

Right vesical, prostatic and deferential (vesical, uterine and vaginal) veins

Right middle rectal vein

Right inferior rectal vein (to internal pudendal vein)

Left gastric vein

Short gastric veins

Splenic vein

Great pancreatic vein

Left gastroepiploic (gastroomental) vein

Dorsal (superior) pancreatic vein

Inferior mesenteric vein

Intestinal (jejunal and ileal) veins

Left colic vein

Left testicular (ovarian) vessels

Inferior mesenteric vein

Sigmoid veins

Middle sacral vein

Superior rectal vein

Rectosigmoid vein

Tributaries of left and right superior rectal veins

Perimuscular rectal plexus

Left middle rectal vein

Left internal pudendal vein in pudendal (Alcock's) canal

External rectal plexus

PLATE 296

ABDOMEN

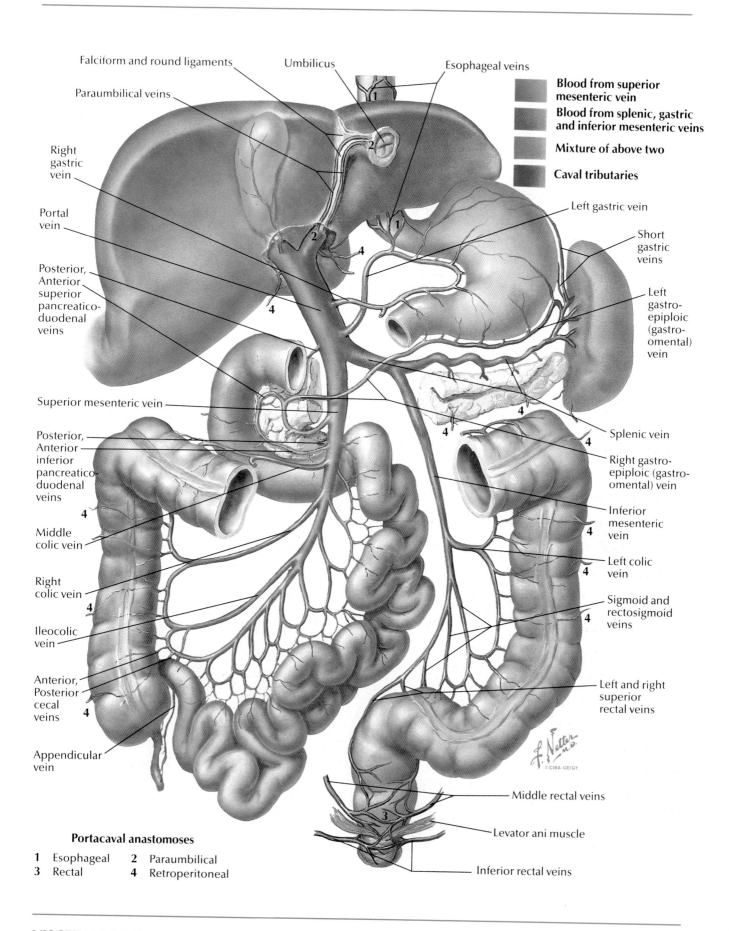

Falciform and round ligaments

Umbilicus

Esophageal veins

Blood from superior mesenteric vein

Blood from splenic, gastric and inferior mesenteric veins

Mixture of above two

Caval tributaries

Paraumbilical veins

Right gastric vein

Left gastric vein

Short gastric veins

Portal vein

Posterior, Anterior superior pancreatico-duodenal veins

Left gastro-epiploic (gastro-omental) vein

Superior mesenteric vein

Splenic vein

Posterior, Anterior inferior pancreatico-duodenal veins

Right gastro-epiploic (gastro-omental) vein

Middle colic vein

Inferior mesenteric vein

Right colic vein

Left colic vein

Ileocolic vein

Sigmoid and rectosigmoid veins

Anterior, Posterior cecal veins

Left and right superior rectal veins

Appendicular vein

Middle rectal veins

Levator ani muscle

Inferior rectal veins

Portacaval anastomoses

| 1 | Esophageal | 2 | Paraumbilical |
| 3 | Rectal | 4 | Retroperitoneal |

Variations and Anomalies of Portal Vein

Cystic vein

Portal vein

Right gastric vein

Esophageal vein

Left gastric vein

Short gastric veins

Splenic vein

0.45 cm

1.09 cm

Posterior superior pancreaticoduodenal vein

Superior mesenteric vein

Right gastroepiploic (gastroomental) vein

Inferior pancreatico-duodenal veins

Middle colic vein

Right colic vein

Ileocolic vein

Jejunal and ileal veins

Pancreatic veins

Left gastroepiploic (gastroomental) vein

Inferior mesenteric vein

Left colic vein

Typical arrangement

Left gastric vein often enters junction of splenic and superior mesenteric veins

Portal vein

Superior mesenteric vein

Left gastric vein

Splenic vein

Left gastric vein may enter splenic vein (24% of cases)

Portal vein

Right gastric vein

Splenic vein

Left gastric vein

Inferior mesenteric vein may enter junction of splenic and superior mesenteric veins

Portal vein

Splenic vein

Superior mesenteric vein

Inferior mesenteric vein

Inferior mesenteric vein may enter superior mesenteric vein

Portal vein

High intestinal veins

Splenic vein

Superior mesenteric vein

Inferior mesenteric vein

Anomalies

Portal vein anterior to head of pancreas and 1st part of duodenum

Portal vein may enter inferior vena cava (hepatic arteries enlarged)

Pulmonary vein may enter portal vein

Congenital stricture of portal vein

PLATE 298

ABDOMEN

Celiac nodes

Hepatic nodes

Right superior pancreatic node

Supra-pyloric nodes

Infra-pyloric nodes

Cardiac ring of nodes

Left gastric nodes

Splenic nodes

Left gastro-epiploic (gastro-omental) node

Right gastroepiploic (gastromental) nodes

To cisterna chyli

Zones and pathways of gastric lymph drainage (zones not sharply demarcated)

Right gastroepiploic (gastromental) nodes

Suprapyloric, retropyloric and infrapyloric nodes

Right superior pancreatic node

Left gastric nodes

Cardiac node

Left gastro-epiploic (gastro-omental) node

Splenic nodes

Left superior pancreatic nodes

Celiac nodes

Superior mesenteric nodes

Lymph Vessels and Nodes of Small Intestine

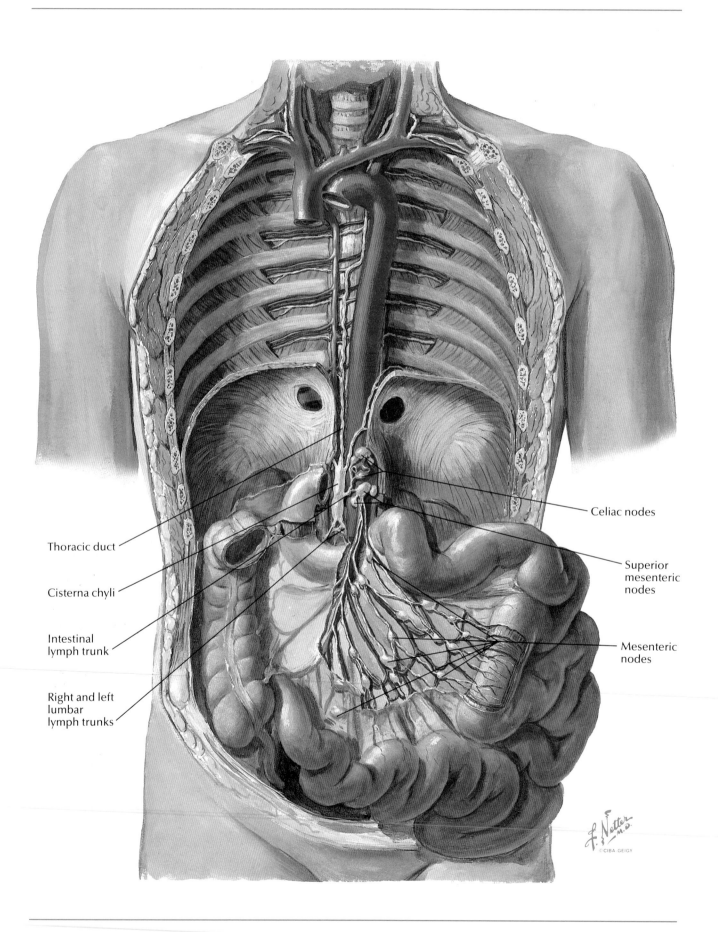

Thoracic duct

Cisterna chyli

Intestinal
lymph trunk

Right and left
lumbar
lymph trunks

Celiac nodes

Superior
mesenteric
nodes

Mesenteric
nodes

PLATE 300

ABDOMEN

Lymph Vessels and Nodes of Large Intestine

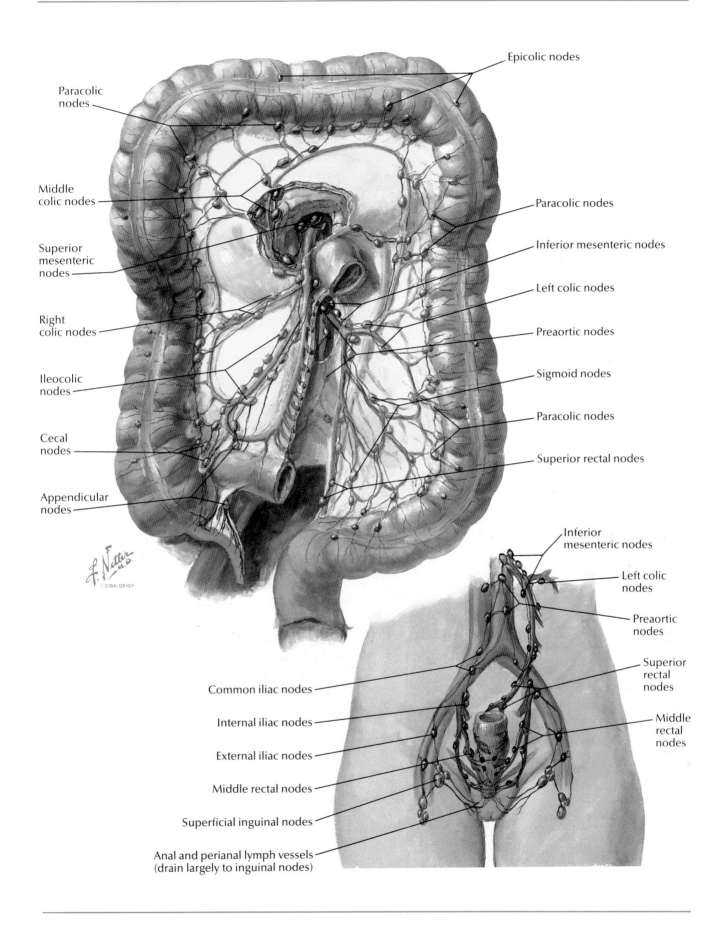

Epicolic nodes

Paracolic nodes

Middle colic nodes

Superior mesenteric nodes

Right colic nodes

Ileocolic nodes

Cecal nodes

Appendicular nodes

Paracolic nodes

Inferior mesenteric nodes

Left colic nodes

Preaortic nodes

Sigmoid nodes

Paracolic nodes

Superior rectal nodes

Inferior mesenteric nodes

Left colic nodes

Preaortic nodes

Superior rectal nodes

Middle rectal nodes

Common iliac nodes

Internal iliac nodes

External iliac nodes

Middle rectal nodes

Superficial inguinal nodes

Anal and perianal lymph vessels (drain largely to inguinal nodes)

Lymph Vessels and Nodes of Liver

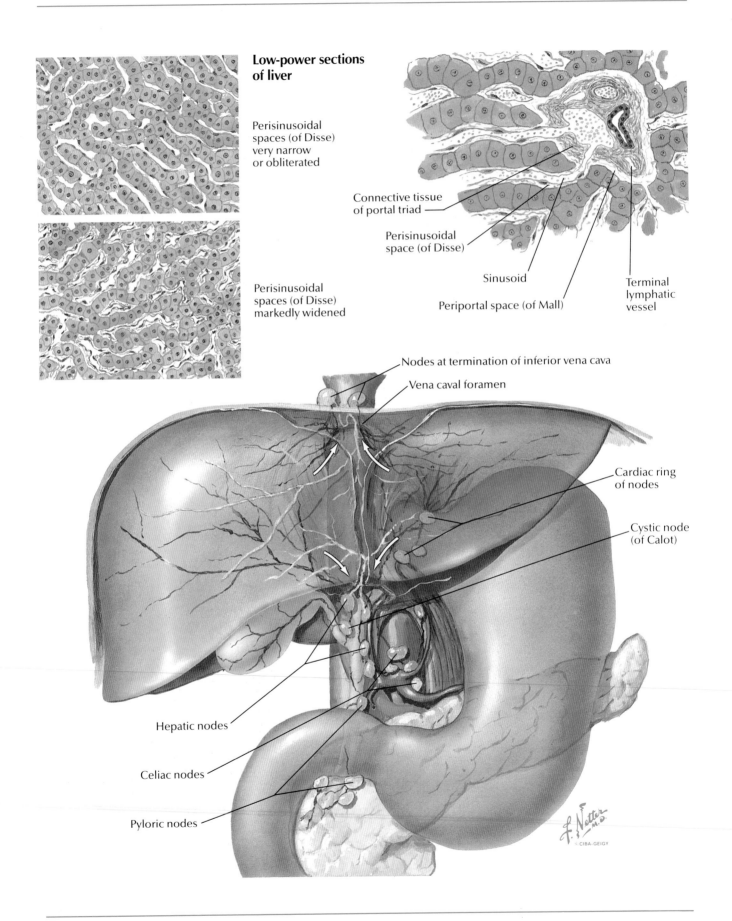

Low-power sections of liver

Perisinusoidal spaces (of Disse) very narrow or obliterated

Perisinusoidal spaces (of Disse) markedly widened

Connective tissue of portal triad

Perisinusoidal space (of Disse)

Sinusoid

Periportal space (of Mall)

Terminal lymphatic vessel

Nodes at termination of inferior vena cava

Vena caval foramen

Cardiac ring of nodes

Cystic node (of Calot)

Hepatic nodes

Celiac nodes

Pyloric nodes

PLATE 302

ABDOMEN

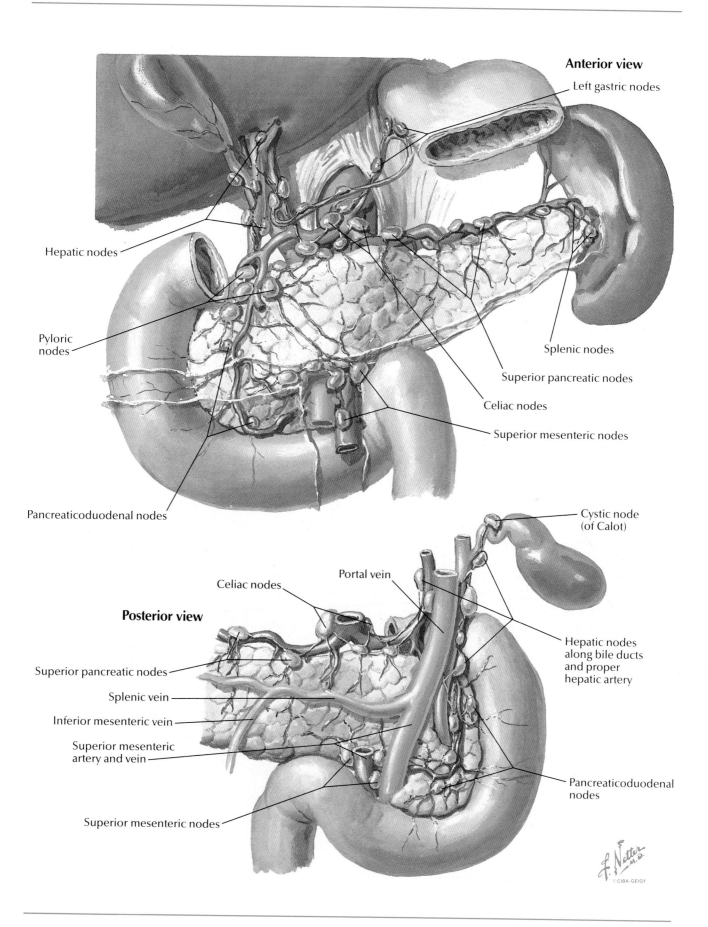

Anterior view

Left gastric nodes

Hepatic nodes

Pyloric nodes

Splenic nodes

Superior pancreatic nodes

Celiac nodes

Superior mesenteric nodes

Pancreaticoduodenal nodes

Cystic node (of Calot)

Portal vein

Celiac nodes

Posterior view

Hepatic nodes along bile ducts and proper hepatic artery

Superior pancreatic nodes

Splenic vein

Inferior mesenteric vein

Superior mesenteric artery and vein

Pancreaticoduodenal nodes

Superior mesenteric nodes

Autonomic Nerves and Ganglia of Abdomen

SEE ALSO PLATE 152

Right sympathetic trunk

Thoracic duct

Right greater and lesser thoracic splanchnic nerves

Right phrenic nerve

Inferior phrenic arteries and plexuses

Right greater and lesser thoracic splanchnic nerves

Right suprarenal plexus

Right aortico-renal ganglion

Right least thoracic splanchnic nerve

Right renal artery and plexus

Right sympathetic trunk

White and gray rami communicantes

Cisterna chyli

Gray ramus communicans

3rd lumbar sympathetic ganglion

2nd and 3rd lumbar splanchnic nerves

Right ureter and plexus

Right testicular (ovarian) artery and plexus

4th lumbar splanchnic nerve

1st sacral sympathetic ganglion

Gray rami communicantes

Anterior, Posterior vagal trunks

Left gastric artery and plexus

Celiac ganglia

Left greater thoracic splanchnic nerve

Left lesser thoracic splanchnic nerve

Splenic artery and plexus

Common hepatic artery and plexus

Superior mesenteric ganglion and plexus

Left aorticorenal ganglion

Left sympathetic trunk

Intermesenteric (aortic) plexus

Inferior mesenteric ganglion

Left colic artery and plexus

Inferior mesenteric artery and plexus

Left common iliac artery and plexus

Superior rectal artery and plexus

Superior hypogastric plexus

Internal and external iliac arteries and plexuses

Right and left hypogastric nerves to inferior hypo-gastric (pelvic) plexus

Left sacral plexus

Pelvic splanchnic nerves

PLATE 304

ABDOMEN

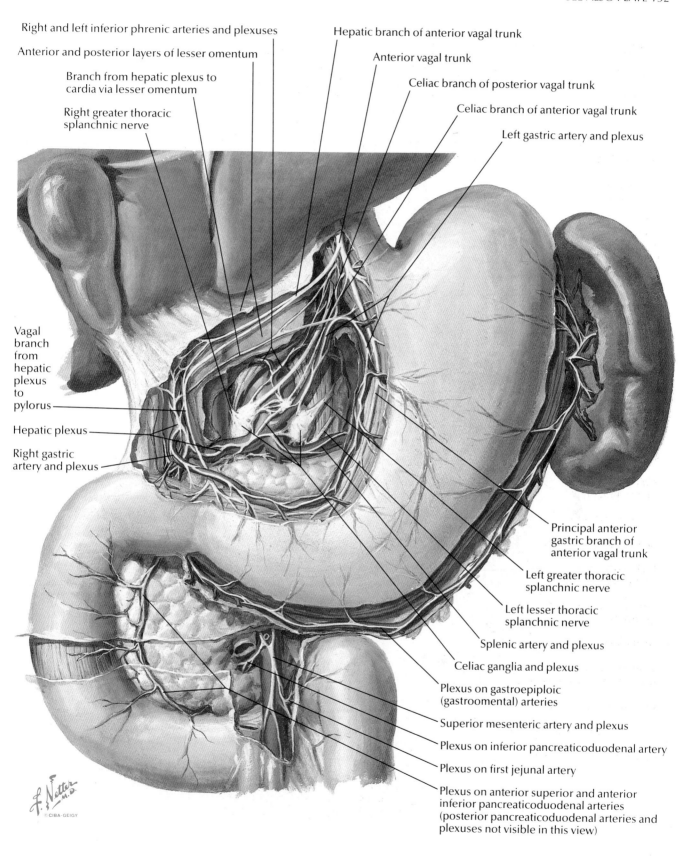

Right and left inferior phrenic arteries and plexuses

Anterior and posterior layers of lesser omentum

Branch from hepatic plexus to cardia via lesser omentum

Right greater thoracic splanchnic nerve

Hepatic branch of anterior vagal trunk

Anterior vagal trunk

Celiac branch of posterior vagal trunk

Celiac branch of anterior vagal trunk

Left gastric artery and plexus

Vagal branch from hepatic plexus to pylorus

Hepatic plexus

Right gastric artery and plexus

Principal anterior gastric branch of anterior vagal trunk

Left greater thoracic splanchnic nerve

Left lesser thoracic splanchnic nerve

Splenic artery and plexus

Celiac ganglia and plexus

Plexus on gastroepiploic (gastroomental) arteries

Superior mesenteric artery and plexus

Plexus on inferior pancreaticoduodenal artery

Plexus on first jejunal artery

Plexus on anterior superior and anterior inferior pancreaticoduodenal arteries (posterior pancreaticoduodenal arteries and plexuses not visible in this view)

Nerves of Stomach and Duodenum (continued)

SEE ALSO PLATE 152

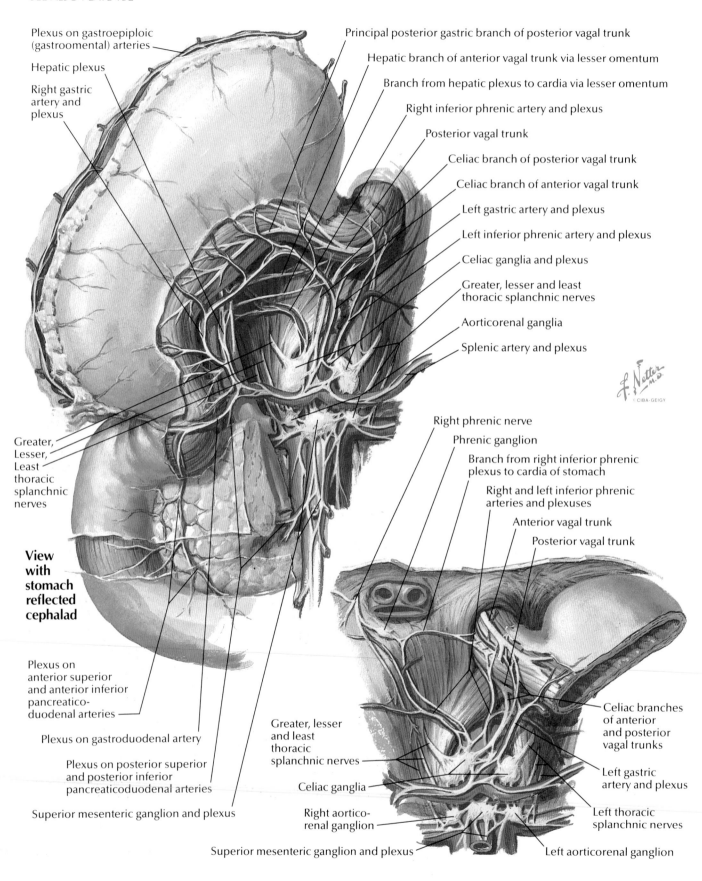

Plexus on gastroepiploic (gastroomental) arteries

Hepatic plexus

Right gastric artery and plexus

Principal posterior gastric branch of posterior vagal trunk

Hepatic branch of anterior vagal trunk via lesser omentum

Branch from hepatic plexus to cardia via lesser omentum

Right inferior phrenic artery and plexus

Posterior vagal trunk

Celiac branch of posterior vagal trunk

Celiac branch of anterior vagal trunk

Left gastric artery and plexus

Left inferior phrenic artery and plexus

Celiac ganglia and plexus

Greater, lesser and least thoracic splanchnic nerves

Aorticorenal ganglia

Splenic artery and plexus

Greater, Lesser, Least thoracic splanchnic nerves

Right phrenic nerve

Phrenic ganglion

Branch from right inferior phrenic plexus to cardia of stomach

Right and left inferior phrenic arteries and plexuses

Anterior vagal trunk

Posterior vagal trunk

View with stomach reflected cephalad

Plexus on anterior superior and anterior inferior pancreaticoduodenal arteries

Plexus on gastroduodenal artery

Plexus on posterior superior and posterior inferior pancreaticoduodenal arteries

Superior mesenteric ganglion and plexus

Greater, lesser and least thoracic splanchnic nerves

Celiac ganglia

Right aorticorenal ganglion

Superior mesenteric ganglion and plexus

Celiac branches of anterior and posterior vagal trunks

Left gastric artery and plexus

Left thoracic splanchnic nerves

Left aorticorenal ganglion

PLATE 306

ABDOMEN

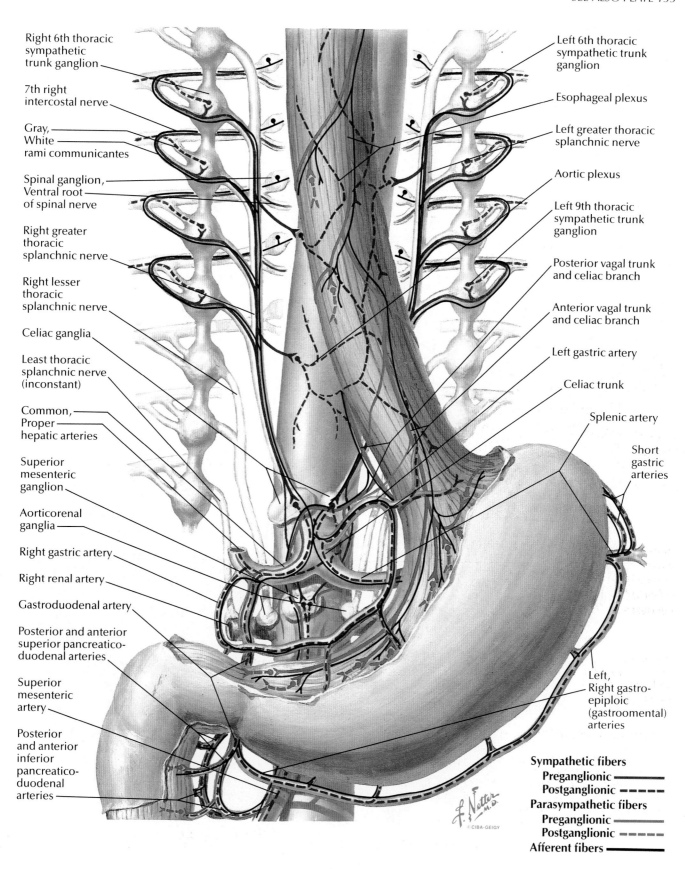

Right 6th thoracic sympathetic trunk ganglion

7th right intercostal nerve

Gray, White rami communicantes

Spinal ganglion, Ventral root of spinal nerve

Right greater thoracic splanchnic nerve

Right lesser thoracic splanchnic nerve

Celiac ganglia

Least thoracic splanchnic nerve (inconstant)

Common, Proper hepatic arteries

Superior mesenteric ganglion

Aorticorenal ganglia

Right gastric artery

Right renal artery

Gastroduodenal artery

Posterior and anterior superior pancreatico-duodenal arteries

Superior mesenteric artery

Posterior and anterior inferior pancreatico-duodenal arteries

Left 6th thoracic sympathetic trunk ganglion

Esophageal plexus

Left greater thoracic splanchnic nerve

Aortic plexus

Left 9th thoracic sympathetic trunk ganglion

Posterior vagal trunk and celiac branch

Anterior vagal trunk and celiac branch

Left gastric artery

Celiac trunk

Splenic artery

Short gastric arteries

Left, Right gastro-epiploic (gastroomental) arteries

Sympathetic fibers
Preganglionic
Postganglionic
Parasympathetic fibers
Preganglionic
Postganglionic
Afferent fibers

Nerves of Small Intestine

SEE ALSO PLATE 152

Recurrent branch of left inferior phrenic artery and plexus to esophagus

Anterior vagal trunk

Posterior vagal trunk

Hepatic branch of anterior vagal trunk in lesser omentum

Celiac branches of anterior and posterior vagal trunks

Inferior phrenic arteries and plexuses

Left gastric artery and plexus

Hepatic plexus

Greater thoracic splanchnic nerves

Right gastric artery and plexus (*cut*)

Celiac ganglia and plexus

Gastroduodenal artery and plexus

Lesser thoracic splanchnic nerves

Least thoracic splanchnic nerves

Aorticorenal ganglia

Superior mesenteric ganglion

Intermesenteric (aortic) plexus

Inferior pancreaticoduodenal arteries and plexuses

Superior mesenteric artery and plexus

Middle colic artery and plexus (*cut*)

Right colic artery and plexus

Ileocolic artery and plexus

Superior mesenteric artery and plexus

Peritoneum (*cut edge*)

Mesenteric branches

Mesoappendix contains appendicular artery and nerve plexus

PLATE 308

ABDOMEN

Anterior vagal trunk and hepatic branch

Posterior vagal trunk

Celiac branches of anterior and posterior vagal trunks

Right inferior phrenic artery and plexus

Right greater thoracic splanchnic nerve

Celiac ganglia and plexus

Right lesser and least thoracic splanchnic nerves

Right aortico-renal ganglion

Superior mesenteric ganglion

Middle colic artery and plexus

Inferior pancreatico-duodenal arteries and plexuses

Right colic artery and plexus

Ileocolic artery and plexus

Cecal and appendicular arteries and plexuses

Right internal iliac artery and plexus (cut)

Sacral sympathetic trunk

Right sacral plexus

Sacral splanchnic nerves (nervi erigentes)

Middle rectal artery and plexus

Right inferior hypogastric (pelvic) plexus

Vesical plexus

Rectal plexus

Urinary bladder

Marginal artery and plexus

Esophagus

Left inferior phrenic artery and plexus

Left gastric artery and plexus

Left greater thoracic splanchnic nerve

Left suprarenal plexus

Left lesser and least thoracic splanchnic nerves

Left aorticorenal ganglion

Left renal artery and plexus

Left lumbar sympathetic trunk

1st left lumbar splanchnic nerve

Intermesenteric (aortic) plexus

Left colic artery and plexus

Inferior mesenteric ganglion, artery and plexus

Sigmoid arteries and plexuses

Superior hypogastric plexus

Superior rectal artery and plexus

Right and left hypogastric nerves

Rectosigmoid artery and plexus

Nerves from inferior hypogastric plexuses to sigmoid colon, descending colon and splenic flexure

F. Netter M.D.

©CIBA-GEIGY

Thalamus

Hypothalamus
(red = sympathetic part,
blue = parasympathetic part)

Abdominal aorta

Celiac gan

C
tr

Dorsal vagal nucleus

Vagus nerve (X)

Medulla
oblongata

Sympathetic trunk

Spinal ganglia

Rami
communicantes { White
{ Gray

Thoracic
splanchnic
nerves { Greater
Lesser
Least

Superic
mesent
ganglio

T9

T10

T11

Aorticore
ganglion

T12

Intermeser
(aortic) ple

L1

Inferior
mesente
ganglion

Thoracolumbar
spinal cord

L2

L3

Lumbar
splanchnic
nerves

Superior
hypogas
plexus

L4

L5

S1

Hypogas
nerves

S2

Sacral
splanchnic
nerves

Inferior
hypogastr
(pelvic) ple

Sacral
spinal cord

S3

S4

Pelvic splanchnic nerves (nervi erigentes)

Pudendal nerve

PLATE 310

ABDOMEN

Sympathetic efferents	
Parasympathetic efferents	
Somatic efferents	
Afferents and CNS connections	
Indefinite paths	

Superior mesenteric artery and plexus

T12, L1

T9 (8)

T9, 10

L1, 2

Inferior mesenteric and left colic arteries and plexuses

T10–12

T10 (11)

T10–12

Superior rectal artery and nerves

L1, 2

Rectal plexus

Inferior rectal nerve

Levator ani muscle

External anal sphincter muscle

Chief segmental sources of sympathetic fibers innervating different regions of intestinal tract are indicated. Numerous afferent fibers are carried centripetally through approximately same sympathetic splanchnic nerves that transmit preganglionic fibers

Autonomic Reflex Pathways: Schema

Sympathetic trunk

Dorsal root

Thoracic part of spinal cord

Spinal ganglion

Sympathetic trunk ganglion

Spinal nerve to vessels and glands of skin

Ventral root

White ramus communicans

Recurrent meningeal branch to spinal meninges and spinal perivascular plexuses

Stretch (distention)

Gray ramus communicans

Thoracic splanchnic nerve

Sympathetic trunk ganglion

Pain

Vagus nerve (X)

Celiac ganglion

Enteric plexuses

Sympathetic trunk ganglion

Superior mesenteric ganglion

| Sympathetic fibers | Preganglionic ——— | Parasympathetic fibers | Preganglionic ——— | Afferent fibers ——— |
| | Postganglionic ----- | | Postganglionic ----- | Antidromic conduction ——— |

PLATE 311

ABDOMEN

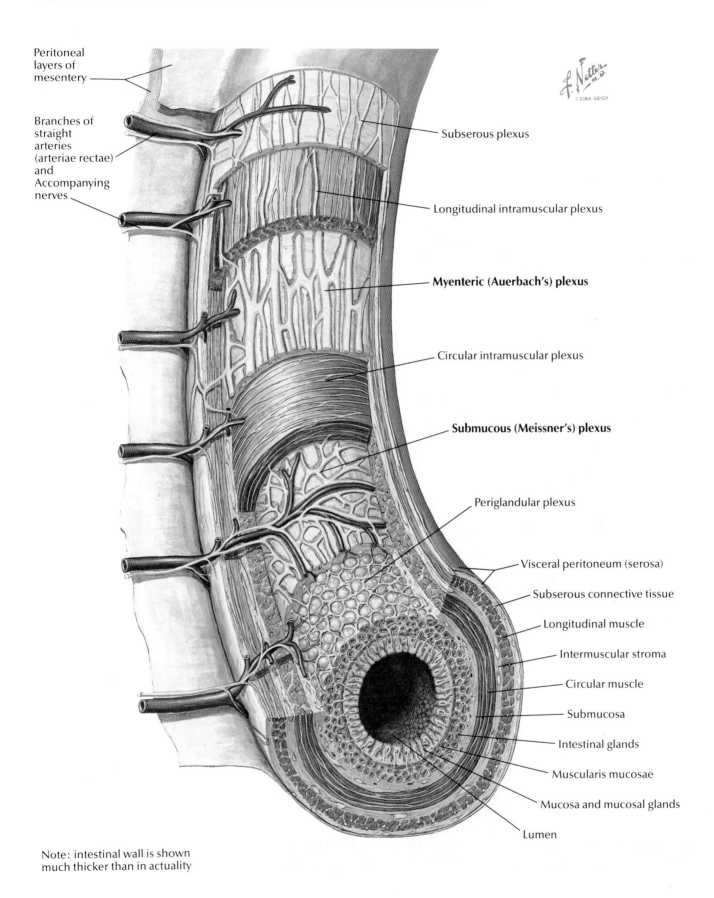

Peritoneal layers of mesentery

Branches of straight arteries (arteriae rectae) and Accompanying nerves

Subserous plexus

Longitudinal intramuscular plexus

Myenteric (Auerbach's) plexus

Circular intramuscular plexus

Submucous (Meissner's) plexus

Periglandular plexus

Visceral peritoneum (serosa)

Subserous connective tissue

Longitudinal muscle

Intermuscular stroma

Circular muscle

Submucosa

Intestinal glands

Muscularis mucosae

Mucosa and mucosal glands

Lumen

Note: intestinal wall is shown much thicker than in actuality

Innervation of Liver and Biliary Tract: Schema

SEE ALSO PLATE 153

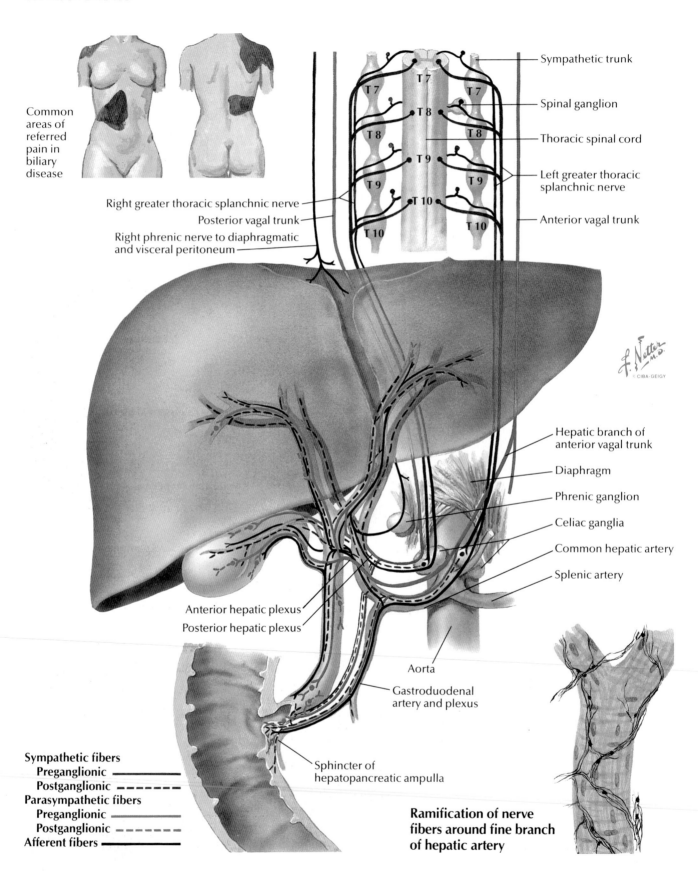

Common areas of referred pain in biliary disease

Sympathetic trunk

T 7

Spinal ganglion

Thoracic spinal cord

Left greater thoracic splanchnic nerve

Right greater thoracic splanchnic nerve

Posterior vagal trunk

Right phrenic nerve to diaphragmatic and visceral peritoneum

Anterior vagal trunk

T 7 · T 8 · T 9 · T 10

Hepatic branch of anterior vagal trunk

Diaphragm

Phrenic ganglion

Celiac ganglia

Common hepatic artery

Splenic artery

Anterior hepatic plexus

Posterior hepatic plexus

Aorta

Gastroduodenal artery and plexus

Sphincter of hepatopancreatic ampulla

Sympathetic fibers
Preganglionic ————
Postganglionic – – – –
Parasympathetic fibers
Preganglionic ————
Postganglionic – – – –
Afferent fibers ————

Ramification of nerve fibers around fine branch of hepatic artery

PLATE 313

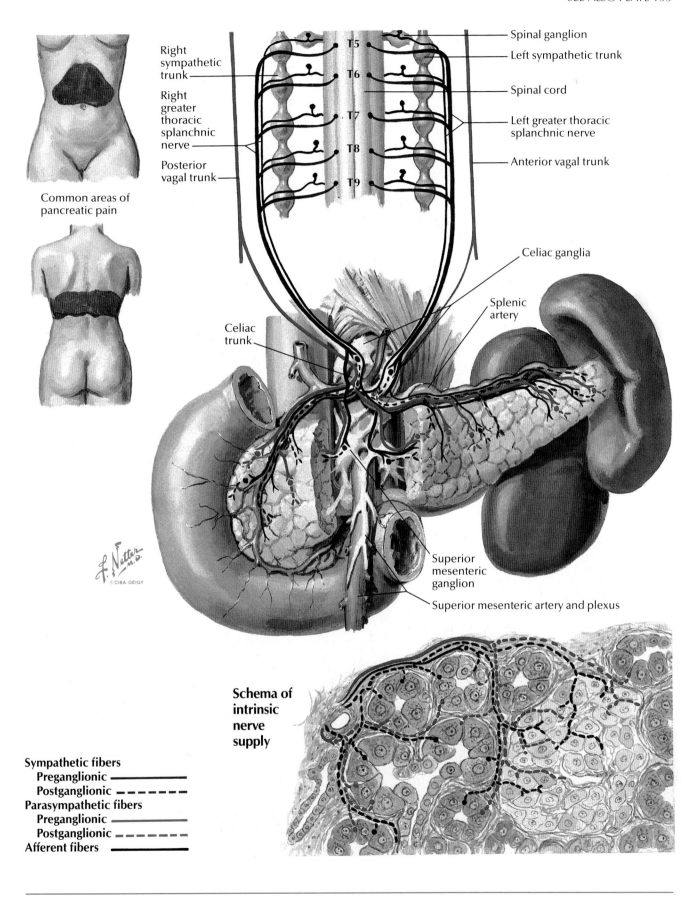

Common areas of pancreatic pain

Right sympathetic trunk

Right greater thoracic splanchnic nerve

Posterior vagal trunk

Celiac trunk

T5
T6
T7
T8
T9

Spinal ganglion

Left sympathetic trunk

Spinal cord

Left greater thoracic splanchnic nerve

Anterior vagal trunk

Celiac ganglia

Splenic artery

Superior mesenteric ganglion

Superior mesenteric artery and plexus

Schema of intrinsic nerve supply

Sympathetic fibers
  Preganglionic ————
  Postganglionic – – – –
Parasympathetic fibers
  Preganglionic ————
  Postganglionic – – – –
Afferent fibers ————

Diaphragm

Right suprarenal gland

Right kidney

Right renal artery and vein

Right subcostal nerve

Transversus abdominis muscle

Quadratus lumborum muscle

Iliac crest

Psoas major muscle

Iliacus muscle

Right ureter

Right common iliac artery

Right external iliac artery

Right internal iliac artery

Urinary bladder

Esophagus

Left suprarenal gland

Celiac trunk

Left kidney

Left renal artery and vein

Superior mesenteric artery (cut)

Subcostal nerve

Abdominal aorta

Iliohypogastric nerve

Ilioinguinal nerve

Lateral femoral cutaneous nerve

Genitofemoral nerve

Left testicular (ovarian) artery and vein

Inferior mesenteric artery (cut)

Peritoneum (cut)

Sigmoid mesocolon (cut)

Rectum

Esophagus

Inferior vena cava

Area for bare area of liver

Right suprarenal gland

Peritoneum (cut)

Area for liver

Duodenum

Peritoneum (cut)

Area for colon

Area for small intestine

Gastrophrenic ligament

Gastrosplenic ligament

Left suprarenal gland

Splenorenal ligament

Area for stomach

Area for spleen

Tail of pancreas

Transverse mesocolon

Area for small intestine

Area for descending colon

Anterior relations of kidneys

PLATE 315

ABDOMEN

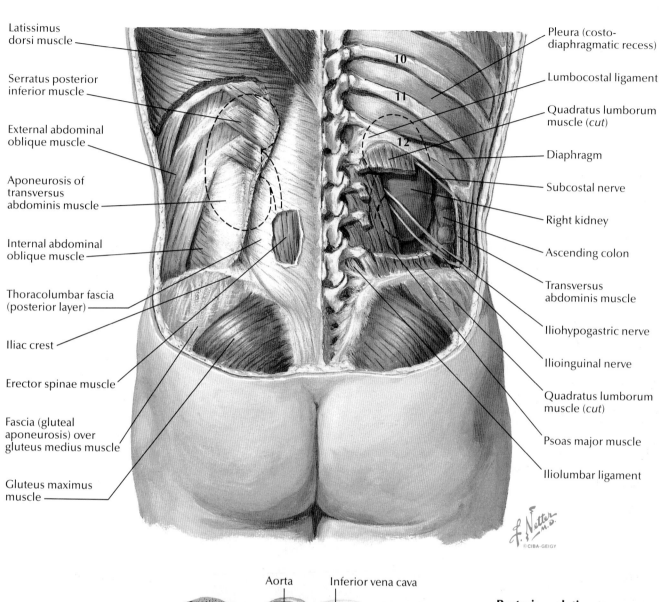

Latissimus dorsi muscle

Serratus posterior inferior muscle

External abdominal oblique muscle

Aponeurosis of transversus abdominis muscle

Internal abdominal oblique muscle

Thoracolumbar fascia (posterior layer)

Iliac crest

Erector spinae muscle

Fascia (gluteal aponeurosis) over gluteus medius muscle

Gluteus maximus muscle

Pleura (costo-diaphragmatic recess)

Lumbocostal ligament

Quadratus lumborum muscle (cut)

Diaphragm

Subcostal nerve

Right kidney

Ascending colon

Transversus abdominis muscle

Iliohypogastric nerve

Ilioinguinal nerve

Quadratus lumborum muscle (cut)

Psoas major muscle

Iliolumbar ligament

10

11

12

Aorta

Inferior vena cava

Posterior relations of kidneys

Projection of 11th rib

Area for diaphragm

Projection of 12th rib

Area for aponeurosis of transversus abdominis muscle

Area for quadratus lumborum muscle

Area for psoas major muscle

Area for diaphragm

Projection of 12th rib

Area for aponeurosis of transversus abdominis muscle

Area for quadratus lumborum muscle

Area for psoas major muscle

Gross Structure of Kidney

Superior extremity

**Anterior surface
of right kidney**

Fibrous capsule
(*cut and peeled back*)

Medial margin

Lateral margin

Hilus

Renal artery

Renal vein

Renal pelvis

Stellate veins visible
through capsule

Medial margin

Ureter

Inferior extremity

**Suprarenal gland
and lobulated
kidney of infant**

Cortex

Fibrous capsule

Minor calyces

Blood vessels
entering renal
parenchyma

Medulla (pyramid)

Papilla of pyramid

Renal sinus

Major calyces

Renal column
(of Bertin)

Renal pelvis

Fat in renal sinus

Medullary rays

Minor calyces

Base of pyramid

Ureter

**Right kidney sectioned in
several planes, exposing
parenchyma and renal pelvis**

PLATE 317

ABDOMEN

Inferior vena cava

Esophagus

Right and left inferior phrenic arteries

Left inferior phrenic vein

Celiac trunk

Left superior suprarenal arteries

Right superior suprarenal arteries

Left middle suprarenal artery

Right middle suprarenal artery

Left suprarenal vein

Right suprarenal vein

Left inferior suprarenal artery

Right inferior suprarenal artery

Ureteric branch of left renal artery

Left renal artery and vein

Left testicular (ovarian) artery and vein

Ureteric branch of right renal artery

Left 2nd lumbar vein and communication to ascending lumbar and/or hemiazygos veins

Right renal artery and vein

Right testicular (ovarian) artery and vein

Inferior vena cava

Inferior mesenteric artery

Abdominal aorta

Superior mesenteric artery *(cut)*

Intrarenal Arteries and Kidney Segments

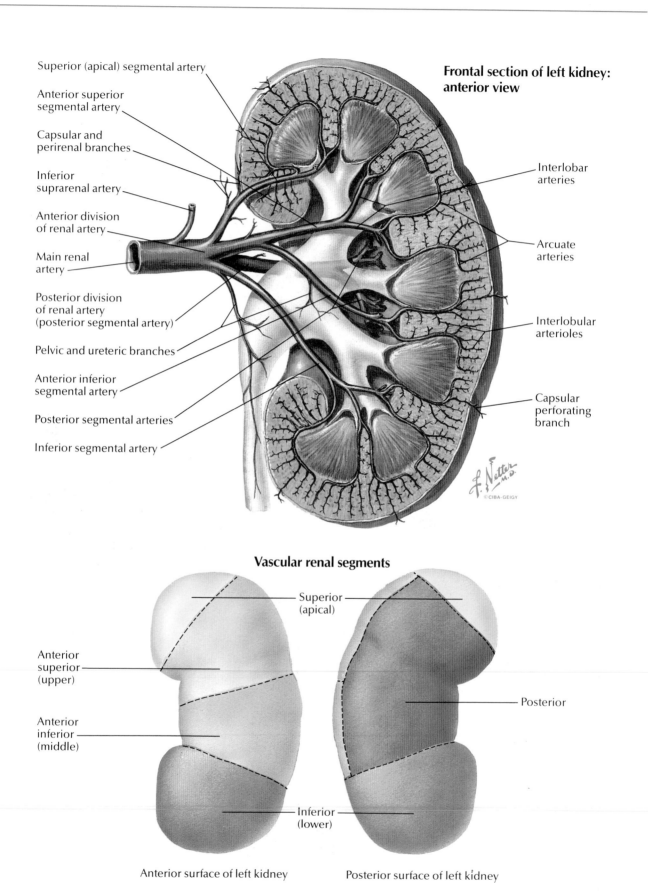

Superior (apical) segmental artery

Anterior superior segmental artery

Capsular and perirenal branches

Inferior suprarenal artery

Anterior division of renal artery

Main renal artery

Posterior division of renal artery (posterior segmental artery)

Pelvic and ureteric branches

Anterior inferior segmental artery

Posterior segmental arteries

Inferior segmental artery

Frontal section of left kidney: anterior view

Interlobar arteries

Arcuate arteries

Interlobular arterioles

Capsular perforating branch

Vascular renal segments

Superior (apical)

Anterior superior (upper)

Anterior inferior (middle)

Posterior

Inferior (lower)

Anterior surface of left kidney

Posterior surface of left kidney

PLATE 319

ABDOMEN

Proximal
subdivision
of renal
artery

A Low accessory right renal artery
may pass in front of inferior
vena cava instead of behind it

B Inferior phrenic artery with
suprarenal arteries may arise
from renal artery

Double renal vein
may form ring
around aorta

Multiple renal veins

Persistent left
inferior vena cava
may join left renal vein

Nephron and Collecting Tubule: Schema

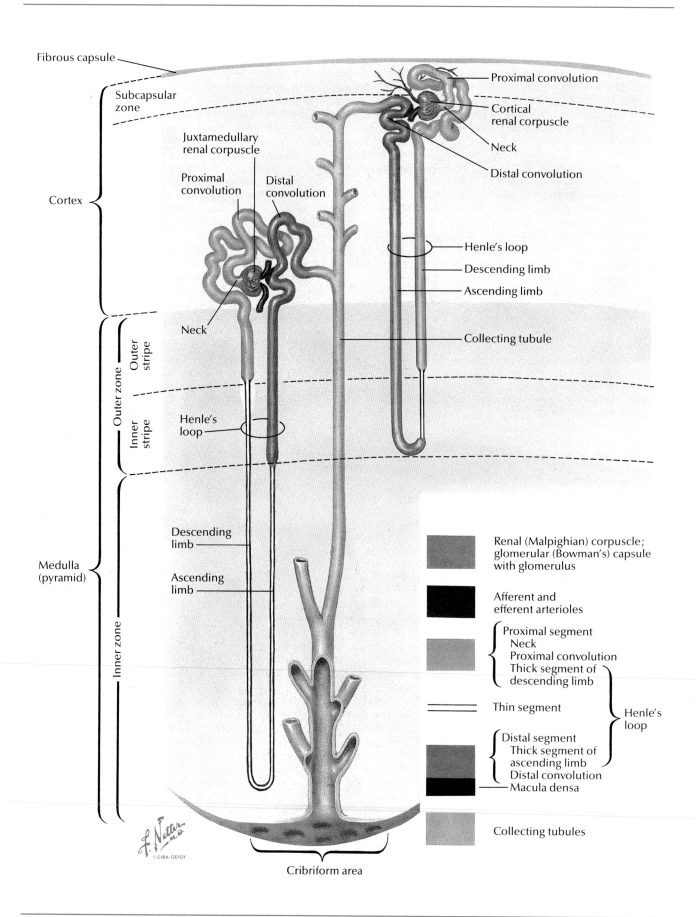

Fibrous capsule

Subcapsular zone

Proximal convolution

Cortical renal corpuscle

Neck

Distal convolution

Juxtamedullary renal corpuscle

Cortex

Proximal convolution

Distal convolution

Henle's loop

Descending limb

Ascending limb

Neck

Outer stripe

Outer zone

Inner stripe

Collecting tubule

Henle's loop

Medulla (pyramid)

Inner zone

Descending limb

Ascending limb

Renal (Malpighian) corpuscle; glomerular (Bowman's) capsule with glomerulus

Afferent and efferent arterioles

Proximal segment
Neck
Proximal convolution
Thick segment of descending limb

Thin segment

Henle's loop

Distal segment
Thick segment of ascending limb
Distal convolution
Macula densa

Collecting tubules

Cribriform area

PLATE 321

ABDOMEN

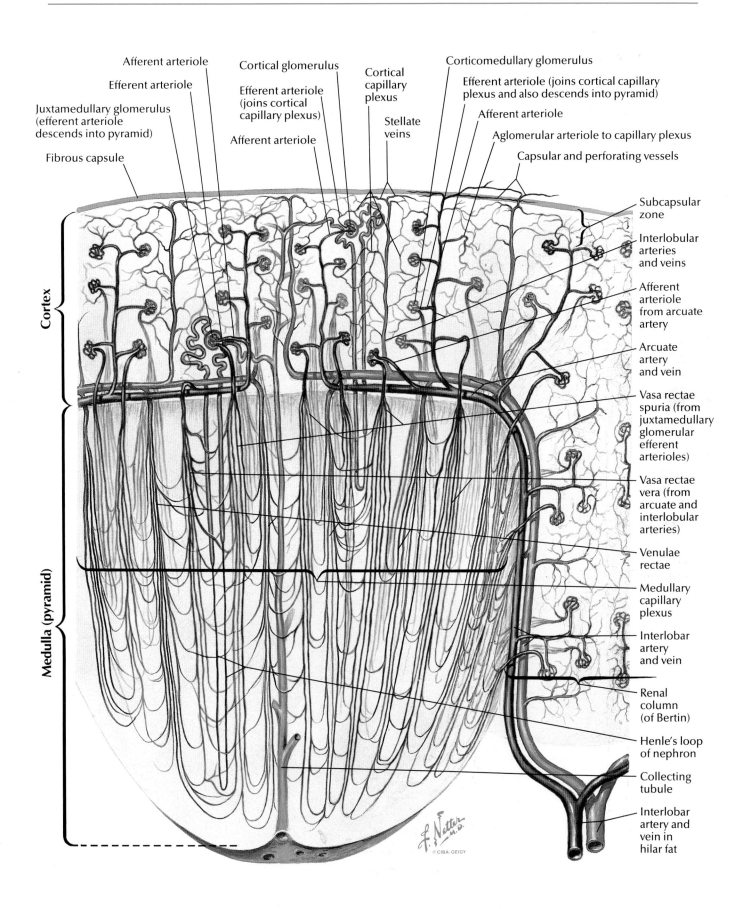

Afferent arteriole

Efferent arteriole

Juxtamedullary glomerulus (efferent arteriole descends into pyramid)

Fibrous capsule

Cortical glomerulus

Efferent arteriole (joins cortical capillary plexus)

Afferent arteriole

Cortical capillary plexus

Stellate veins

Corticomedullary glomerulus

Efferent arteriole (joins cortical capillary plexus and also descends into pyramid)

Afferent arteriole

Aglomerular arteriole to capillary plexus

Capsular and perforating vessels

Cortex

Medulla (pyramid)

Subcapsular zone

Interlobular arteries and veins

Afferent arteriole from arcuate artery

Arcuate artery and vein

Vasa rectae spuria (from juxtamedullary glomerular efferent arterioles)

Vasa rectae vera (from arcuate and interlobular arteries)

Venulae rectae

Medullary capillary plexus

Interlobar artery and vein

Renal column (of Bertin)

Henle's loop of nephron

Collecting tubule

Interlobar artery and vein in hilar fat

F. Netter M.D.

©CIBA-GEIGY

Ureters

SEE ALSO PLATES 343, 344, 348

Ureters in male: anterior view

Right kidney

Duodenum

Superior mesenteric artery

Right colic artery

Right ureter

Ileocolic artery

Testicular vessels

Common iliac artery

Internal iliac artery

External iliac artery

Middle rectal artery

Diagonal course of ureter through bladder wall

Left kidney

Left ureter

Inferior mesenteric artery

Left colic artery

Sigmoid arteries

Superior rectal artery (*cut*)

Genitofemoral nerve

Obturator artery and nerve

Superior vesical artery

Inferior vesical and deferential artery

Obliterated umbilical artery

Ductus deferens

Urinary bladder

Urinary bladder

Medial umbilical ligament (obliterated umbilical artery)

Round ligament (ligamentum teres)

Superior vesical artery

Uterine artery

Obturator artery and nerve

Inferior vesical and vaginal artery

External iliac artery

Ovarian vessels

Internal iliac artery

Common iliac artery

Root of mesentery

Broad ligament

Uterosacral (sacrogenital) fold

Ureter (retroperitoneal)

Intersigmoid recess

Sigmoid mesocolon

Ureters in female: superior view

PLATE 323

ABDOMEN

Abdominal aorta

Superior mesenteric artery

Inferior suprarenal artery

Renal artery and vein

Ureteric branch from renal artery

Ovarian (testicular) artery

Ureter

Psoas major muscle

Inferior mesenteric artery (*cut*)

Ureteric branch from aorta

Ureteric branches from ovarian and common iliac arteries

Common iliac artery

Internal iliac artery

Superior gluteal artery

Inferior gluteal and internal pudendal arteries

Middle rectal artery

Uterine artery

Obturator artery

Vaginal artery

Inferior vesical artery and ureteric branch

Superior vesical arteries

Inferior epigastric artery

Ureteric branch from superior vesical artery

Lymph Vessels and Nodes of Kidneys and Urinary Bladder

SEE ALSO PLATES 381, 383

Subcapsular lymphatic plexus

Cortical lymph vessels along interlobular arteries

Lymph vessels along arcuate arteries

Lymph vessels along interlobar arteries

Medullary lymph vessels

Note: arrows indicate direction of flow

Lumbar lymph trunks to cisterna chyli and thoracic duct

Lateral aortic (lumbar) nodes

Common iliac nodes

Promontory (middle sacral) node

Internal iliac nodes

External iliac nodes

Lymph vessels from dorsal part and trigone of bladder

Lymph vessels from superior and anterior parts of bladder

Lateral and anterior paravesical nodes

PLATE 325

Anterior vagal trunk

Posterior vagal trunk

Greater thoracic splanchnic nerve

Celiac ganglia and plexus

Lesser thoracic splanchnic nerve

Superior mesenteric ganglion

Least thoracic splanchnic nerve

Aorticorenal ganglion

Renal plexus and ganglion

2nd lumbar splanchnic nerve

Renal and upper ureteric branches
from intermesenteric plexus

Intermesenteric (aortic) plexus

Testicular (ovarian) artery and plexus

Inferior mesenteric ganglion

Sympathetic trunk and ganglion

Middle ureteric branch

Superior hypogastric plexus

Sacral splanchnic nerves
(branches from sacral sympathetic
trunk to hypogastric plexus)

Gray ramus communicans

Hypogastric nerves

Sacral plexus

Pudendal nerve

Pelvic splanchnic nerves
(nervi erigentes)

Inferior hypogastric (pelvic) plexus
with periureteric loops and
branches to lower ureter

Rectal plexus

Vesical plexus

Prostatic plexus

Innervation of Kidneys and Upper Ureters: Schema

SEE ALSO PLATES 153, 392

Spinal ganglion

Gray ramus communicans

Ventral ramus of T10
(intercostal nerve)

White ramus communicans

Sympathetic trunk ganglia

1st lumbar splanchnic nerve

Renal artery,
plexus and
ganglion

Solitary tract nucleus

Dorsal vagal nucleus

Medulla oblongata

Vagus nerve (X)

Descending fibers

Ascending fibers

Spinal cord (T10–L1)

Lesser thoracic
splanchnic nerve

Least thoracic
splanchnic nerve

Celiac plexus

Superior mesenteric
ganglion

Aorticorenal ganglion

Intermesenteric plexus

Superior hypogastric
plexus

Hypogastric nerve

Inferior hypogastric
(pelvic) plexus

T10
T11
T12
L1

S2
S3
S4

Sacral plexus

Pelvic
splanchnic
nerves

Sympathetic fibers
  Preganglionic
  Postganglionic
Parasympathetic fibers
  Preganglionic
  Postganglionic
Afferent fibers

PLATE 327

ABDOMEN

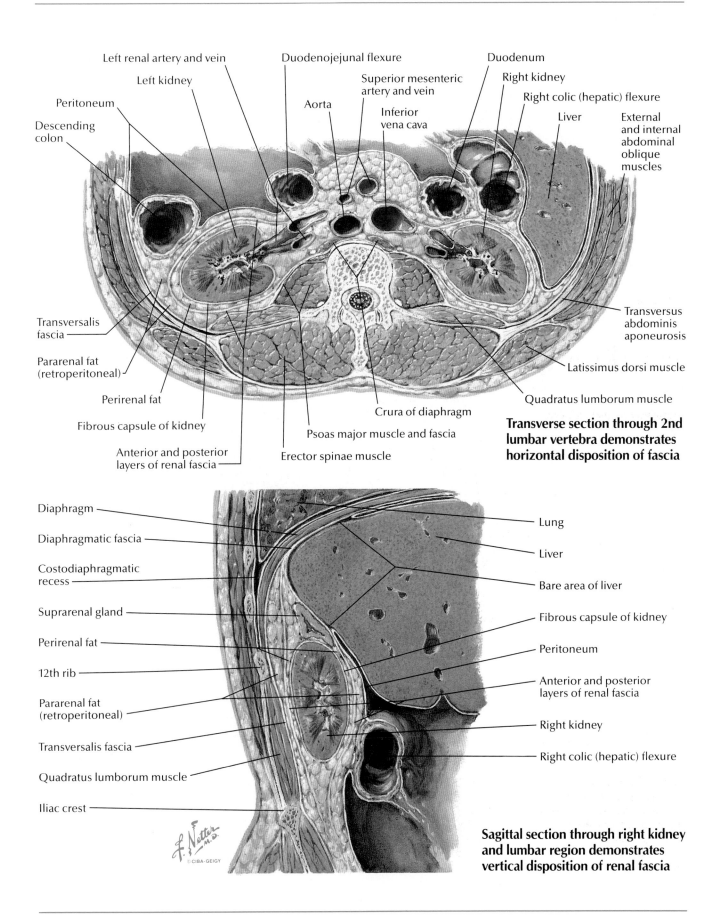

Left renal artery and vein

Left kidney

Duodenojejunal flexure

Duodenum

Right kidney

Superior mesenteric artery and vein

Right colic (hepatic) flexure

Peritoneum

Aorta

Liver

Inferior vena cava

External and internal abdominal oblique muscles

Descending colon

Transversus abdominis aponeurosis

Transversalis fascia

Latissimus dorsi muscle

Pararenal fat (retroperitoneal)

Quadratus lumborum muscle

Perirenal fat

Crura of diaphragm

Transverse section through 2nd lumbar vertebra demonstrates horizontal disposition of fascia

Fibrous capsule of kidney

Psoas major muscle and fascia

Anterior and posterior layers of renal fascia

Erector spinae muscle

Diaphragm

Lung

Diaphragmatic fascia

Liver

Costodiaphragmatic recess

Bare area of liver

Suprarenal gland

Fibrous capsule of kidney

Perirenal fat

Peritoneum

12th rib

Anterior and posterior layers of renal fascia

Pararenal fat (retroperitoneal)

Right kidney

Transversalis fascia

Right colic (hepatic) flexure

Quadratus lumborum muscle

Iliac crest

Sagittal section through right kidney and lumbar region demonstrates vertical disposition of renal fascia

Arteries and Veins of Suprarenal Glands In Situ

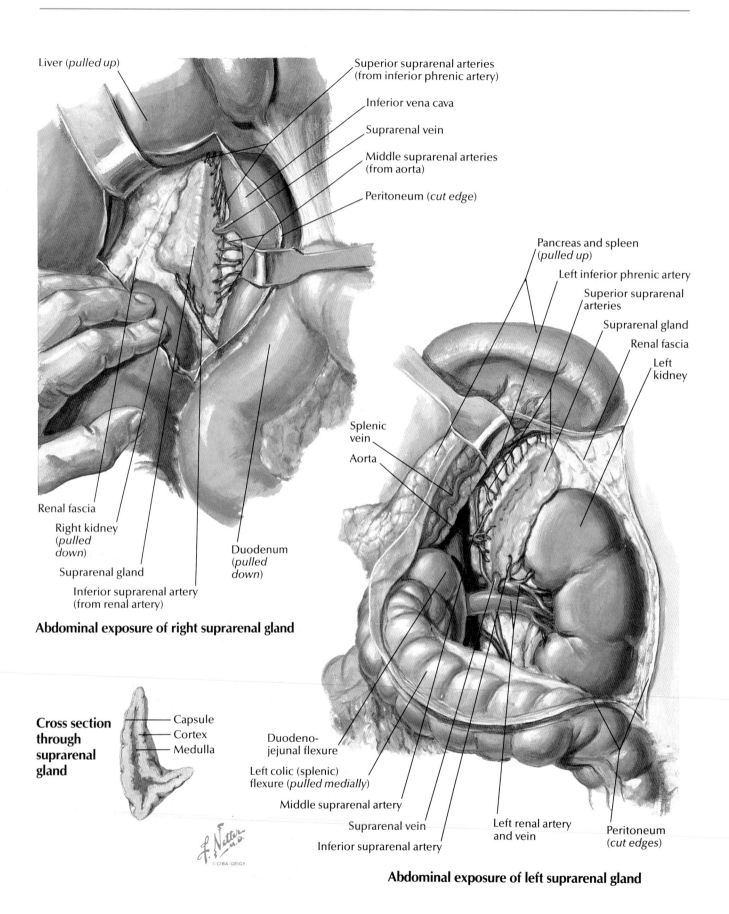

Liver (*pulled up*)

Superior suprarenal arteries (from inferior phrenic artery)

Inferior vena cava

Suprarenal vein

Middle suprarenal arteries (from aorta)

Peritoneum (*cut edge*)

Pancreas and spleen (*pulled up*)

Left inferior phrenic artery

Superior suprarenal arteries

Suprarenal gland

Renal fascia

Left kidney

Splenic vein

Aorta

Renal fascia

Right kidney (*pulled down*)

Suprarenal gland

Inferior suprarenal artery (from renal artery)

Duodenum (*pulled down*)

Abdominal exposure of right suprarenal gland

Cross section through suprarenal gland

Capsule

Cortex

Medulla

Duodeno-jejunal flexure

Left colic (splenic) flexure (*pulled medially*)

Middle suprarenal artery

Suprarenal vein

Inferior suprarenal artery

Left renal artery and vein

Peritoneum (*cut edges*)

Abdominal exposure of left suprarenal gland

PLATE 329

ABDOMEN

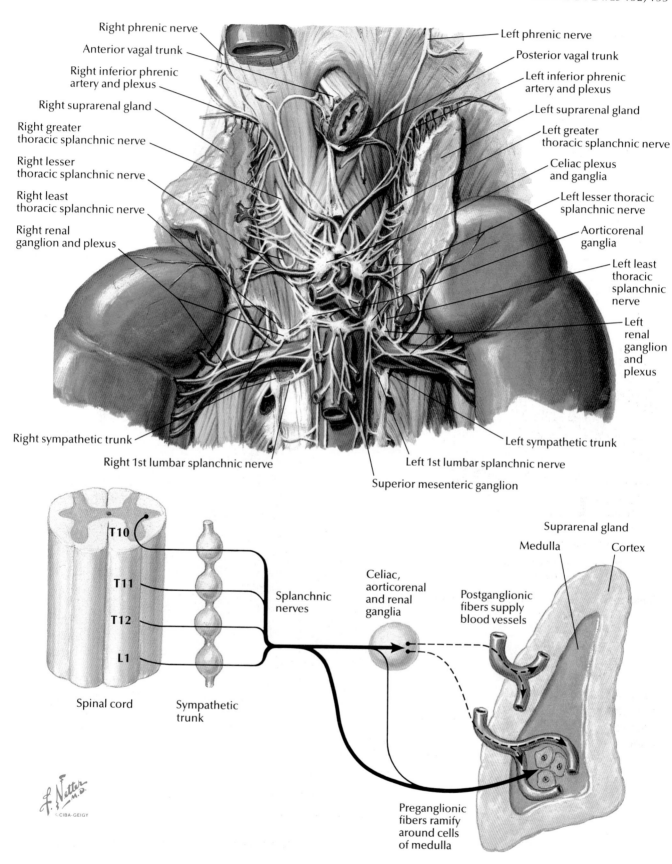

Right phrenic nerve

Anterior vagal trunk

Right inferior phrenic artery and plexus

Right suprarenal gland

Right greater thoracic splanchnic nerve

Right lesser thoracic splanchnic nerve

Right least thoracic splanchnic nerve

Right renal ganglion and plexus

Right sympathetic trunk

Right 1st lumbar splanchnic nerve

Left phrenic nerve

Posterior vagal trunk

Left inferior phrenic artery and plexus

Left suprarenal gland

Left greater thoracic splanchnic nerve

Celiac plexus and ganglia

Left lesser thoracic splanchnic nerve

Aorticorenal ganglia

Left least thoracic splanchnic nerve

Left renal ganglion and plexus

Left sympathetic trunk

Left 1st lumbar splanchnic nerve

Superior mesenteric ganglion

T10

T11

T12

L1

Splanchnic nerves

Spinal cord

Sympathetic trunk

Celiac, aorticorenal and renal ganglia

Postganglionic fibers supply blood vessels

Suprarenal gland

Medulla

Cortex

Preganglionic fibers ramify around cells of medulla

Abdominal Wall and Viscera: Cross Section at T12

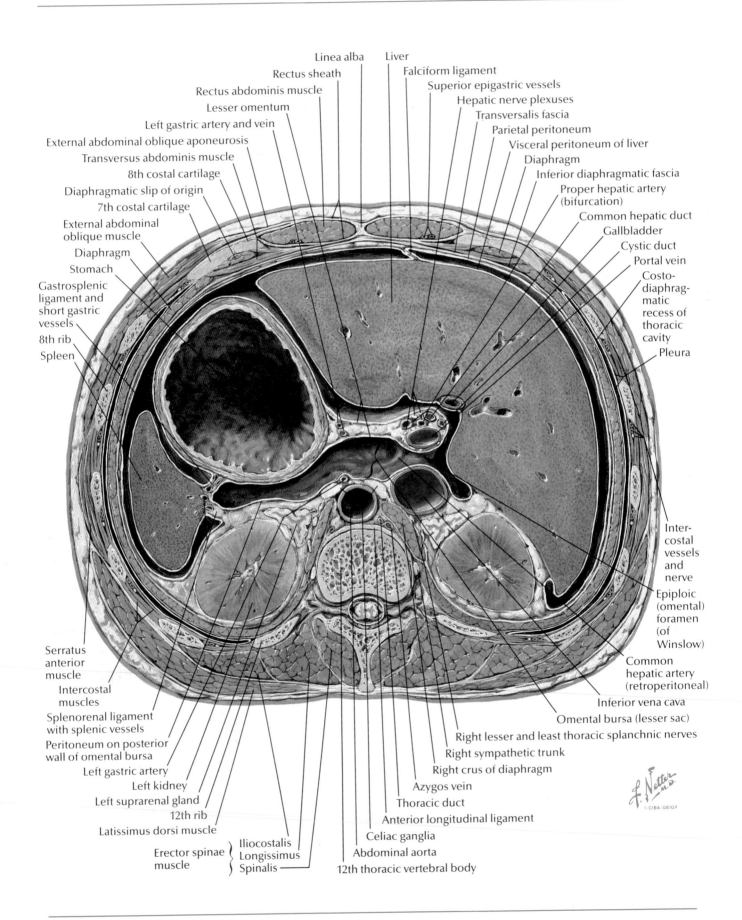

Linea alba
Rectus sheath
Rectus abdominis muscle
Lesser omentum
Left gastric artery and vein
External abdominal oblique aponeurosis
Transversus abdominis muscle
8th costal cartilage
Diaphragmatic slip of origin
7th costal cartilage
External abdominal oblique muscle
Diaphragm
Stomach
Gastrosplenic ligament and short gastric vessels
8th rib
Spleen

Liver
Falciform ligament
Superior epigastric vessels
Hepatic nerve plexuses
Transversalis fascia
Parietal peritoneum
Visceral peritoneum of liver
Diaphragm
Inferior diaphragmatic fascia
Proper hepatic artery (bifurcation)
Common hepatic duct
Gallbladder
Cystic duct
Portal vein
Costo-diaphragmatic recess of thoracic cavity
Pleura

Serratus anterior muscle
Intercostal muscles
Splenorenal ligament with splenic vessels
Peritoneum on posterior wall of omental bursa
Left gastric artery
Left kidney
Left suprarenal gland
12th rib
Latissimus dorsi muscle
Erector spinae muscle { Iliocostalis Longissimus Spinalis

Inter-costal vessels and nerve
Epiploic (omental) foramen (of Winslow)
Common hepatic artery (retroperitoneal)
Inferior vena cava
Omental bursa (lesser sac)
Right lesser and least thoracic splanchnic nerves
Right sympathetic trunk
Right crus of diaphragm
Azygos vein
Thoracic duct
Anterior longitudinal ligament
Celiac ganglia
Abdominal aorta
12th thoracic vertebral body

PLATE 331

ABDOMEN

Abdominal Wall and Viscera: Cross Section Between L2 and L3

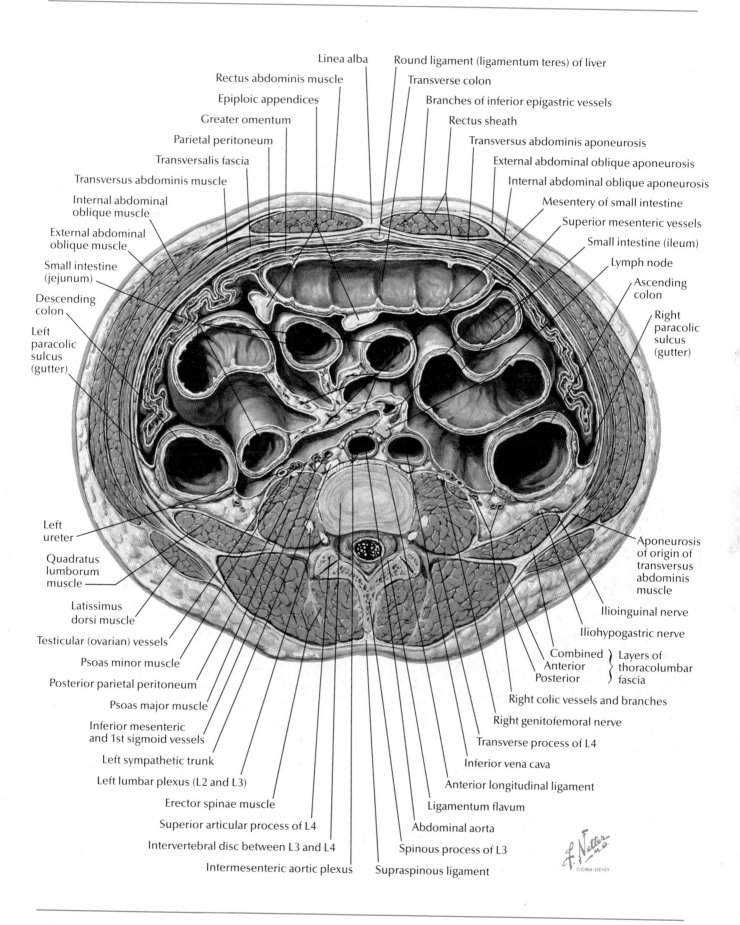

Linea alba

Rectus abdominis muscle

Epiploic appendices

Greater omentum

Parietal peritoneum

Transversalis fascia

Transversus abdominis muscle

Internal abdominal oblique muscle

External abdominal oblique muscle

Small intestine (jejunum)

Descending colon

Left paracolic sulcus (gutter)

Left ureter

Quadratus lumborum muscle

Latissimus dorsi muscle

Testicular (ovarian) vessels

Psoas minor muscle

Posterior parietal peritoneum

Psoas major muscle

Inferior mesenteric and 1st sigmoid vessels

Left sympathetic trunk

Left lumbar plexus (L2 and L3)

Erector spinae muscle

Superior articular process of L4

Intervertebral disc between L3 and L4

Intermesenteric aortic plexus

Round ligament (ligamentum teres) of liver

Transverse colon

Branches of inferior epigastric vessels

Rectus sheath

Transversus abdominis aponeurosis

External abdominal oblique aponeurosis

Internal abdominal oblique aponeurosis

Mesentery of small intestine

Superior mesenteric vessels

Small intestine (ileum)

Lymph node

Ascending colon

Right paracolic sulcus (gutter)

Aponeurosis of origin of transversus abdominis muscle

Ilioinguinal nerve

Iliohypogastric nerve

Combined Anterior Posterior } Layers of thoracolumbar fascia

Right colic vessels and branches

Right genitofemoral nerve

Transverse process of L4

Inferior vena cava

Anterior longitudinal ligament

Ligamentum flavum

Abdominal aorta

Spinous process of L3

Supraspinous ligament

f. Netter M.D.
©CIBA-GEIGY

KIDNEYS AND SUPRARENAL GLANDS

PLATE 332

Sternum

Diaphragm

Inferior diaphragmatic fascia and Parietal peritoneum

Liver

Lesser omentum

Portal vein and proper hepatic artery in right margin of lesser omentum

Omental bursa (lesser peritoneal sac)

Stomach

Middle colic artery

Transverse mesocolon

Parietal peritoneum (of anterior abdominal wall)

Transverse colon

Greater omentum

Small intestine

Rectus abdominis muscle

Rectus sheath

Arcuate line

Transversalis fascia

Umbilical prevesical fascia

Urachus (median umbilical ligament)

Camper's fascia

Scarpa's fascia

Urinary bladder

Fundiform ligament of penis

Pubic bone

Suspensory ligament of penis

Retropubic (prevesical) space (of Retzius)

Deep (Buck's) fascia of penis

Superficial (dartos) fascia of penis and scrotum

Tunica vaginalis testis

Testis

Superior and inferior fascia of urogenital diaphragm contains membranous urethral sphincter and deep transverse perineal muscles

Coronary ligament enclosing bare area of liver

Esophagus

Superior recess of omental bursa (lesser sac)

Diaphragm

Left gastric artery

Epiploic (omental) foramen (of Winslow)

Celiac trunk

Splenic vessels

Renal vessels

Pancreas

Superior mesenteric artery

Horizontal (3rd) part of duodenum

Inferior mesenteric artery

Abdominal aorta

Parietal peritoneum (of posterior abdominal wall)

Mesentery of small intestine

Anterior longitudinal ligament

Vesical fascia

Rectal fascia

Presacral fascia

Rectovesical recess

Rectum

Rectovesical (Denonvilliers') fascia

Levator ani muscle

Prostate

Deep
Superficial
Subcutaneous } External anal sphincter muscle

Bulbospongiosus muscle

Superficial perineal (Colles') fascia

T10

T11

T12

L1

L2

L3

L4

L5

S1

S2

PLATE 333

ABDOMEN

Section V

PELVIS AND PERINEUM

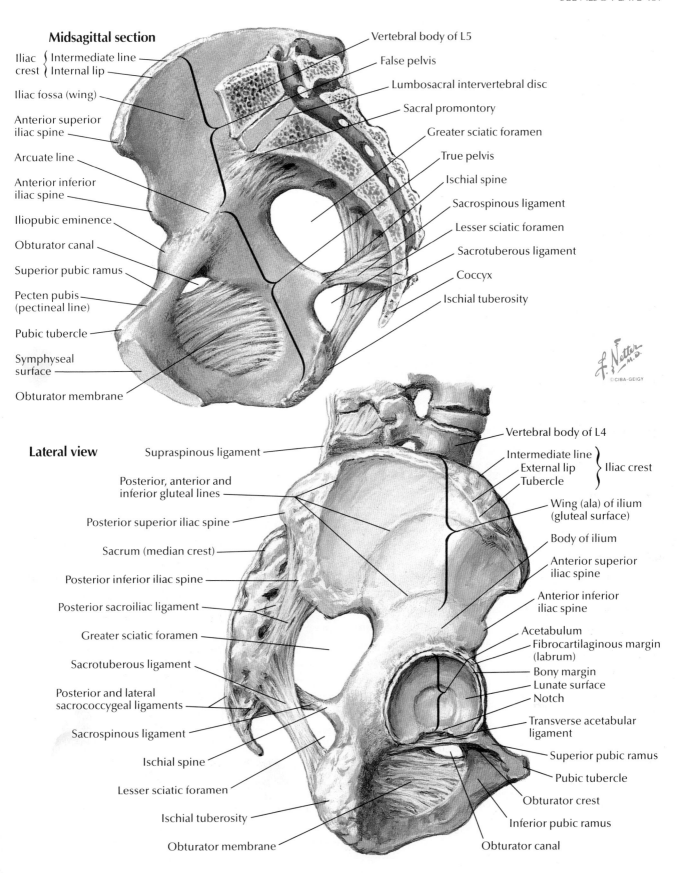

Midsagittal section

Iliac crest { Intermediate line
Iliac crest { Internal lip

Iliac fossa (wing)

Anterior superior iliac spine

Arcuate line

Anterior inferior iliac spine

Iliopubic eminence

Obturator canal

Superior pubic ramus

Pecten pubis (pectineal line)

Pubic tubercle

Symphyseal surface

Obturator membrane

Vertebral body of L5

False pelvis

Lumbosacral intervertebral disc

Sacral promontory

Greater sciatic foramen

True pelvis

Ischial spine

Sacrospinous ligament

Lesser sciatic foramen

Sacrotuberous ligament

Coccyx

Ischial tuberosity

Lateral view

Supraspinous ligament

Posterior, anterior and inferior gluteal lines

Posterior superior iliac spine

Sacrum (median crest)

Posterior inferior iliac spine

Posterior sacroiliac ligament

Greater sciatic foramen

Sacrotuberous ligament

Posterior and lateral sacrococcygeal ligaments

Sacrospinous ligament

Ischial spine

Lesser sciatic foramen

Ischial tuberosity

Obturator membrane

Vertebral body of L4

Intermediate line } Iliac crest
External lip
Tubercle

Wing (ala) of ilium (gluteal surface)

Body of ilium

Anterior superior iliac spine

Anterior inferior iliac spine

Acetabulum

Fibrocartilaginous margin (labrum)

Bony margin

Lunate surface

Notch

Transverse acetabular ligament

Superior pubic ramus

Pubic tubercle

Obturator crest

Inferior pubic ramus

Obturator canal

Bones and Ligaments of Pelvis (continued)

SEE ALSO PLATE 145

Iliolumbar ligament

Iliac crest

Supraspinous ligament

Posterior superior iliac spine

Posterior sacroiliac ligaments

Tubercle of iliac crest

Posterior (dorsal) sacral foramina

Anterior superior iliac spine

Greater sciatic foramen

Sacrospinous ligament

Sacrotuberous ligament

Lesser sciatic foramen

Acetabular margin (limbus)

Ischial tuberosity

Tendon of long head of biceps femoris muscle

Deep } Posterior
Superficial } sacrococcygeal ligaments

Iliac crest

Lateral sacrococcygeal ligament

Posterior view

Anterior longitudinal ligament

Iliac fossa

Iliolumbar ligament

Iliac crest {
External lip
Tubercle
Intermediate line
Internal lip

Anterior sacroiliac ligament

Sacral promontory

Greater sciatic foramen

Sacrotuberous ligament

Anterior superior iliac spine

Sacrospinous ligament

Anterior inferior iliac spine

Ischial spine

Arcuate line

Lesser sciatic foramen

Iliopubic eminence

Superior pubic ramus

Linea terminalis

Iliopectineal line

Pecten pubis (pectineal line)

Obturator foramen

Pubic tubercle

Inferior pubic ramus

Anterior sacral (pelvic) foramina

Coccyx

Anterior sacrococcygeal ligaments

Pubic symphysis

Anterior view

PLATE 335

PELVIS AND PERINEUM

Female pelvis: anterior view

- Sacroiliac joint
- Sacral promontory
- Conjugate (~11 cm) ⎫
- Transverse (~13 cm) ⎬ Diameters of pelvic inlet
- Oblique (~12.5 cm) ⎭
- Ischial spine
- Iliopubic eminence
- Pubic symphysis
- Ischial tuberosity

Male pelvis: anterior view

All measurements slightly shorter in relation to body size than in female
Pelvic inlet oriented more antero-posteriorly than in female where it tends to be transversely oval
Pubic symphysis deeper (taller)
Pubic arch (subpubic angle) narrower
Ischial tuberosities less far apart
Iliac wings less flared

Female pelvis: inferior view

Transverse diameter of pelvic outlet (~11 cm)

Pubic symphysis

Anteroposterior diameter of pelvic outlet (varies 9.5–11.5 cm because of mobility of coccyx)

Ischial tuberosity

Ischial spine

Tip of coccyx

Female: sagittal section

Sacral promontory

Plane of inlet

Conjugate diameter of inlet (~11 cm)

Plane of outlet

Anteroposterior diameter of outlet (9.5–11.5 cm)

Pubic symphysis

Pelvic Diaphragm: Female

SEE ALSO PLATES 246, 347, 349, 368

Superior view

Pubic symphysis

Inguinal (Poupart's) ligament

Arcuate pubic ligament

Deep dorsal vein of clitoris

Transverse perineal ligament

Superior fascia of urogenital diaphragm

Urethra

Vagina

Obturator canal

Fascia over obturator internus muscle

Pubococcygeus and puborectalis part of levator ani muscle

Tendinous arch of levator ani muscle

Rectum

Iliococcygeus part of levator ani muscle

Ischial spine

Levator plate (median raphé) of levator ani muscle

Coccygeus muscle

Piriformis muscle

Coccyx

Anterior sacro-coccygeal ligament

Sacral promontory

Medial view

Arcuate line of ilium

Obturator internus muscle and fascia (*cut*)

Tendinous arch of levator ani muscle

Obturator canal

Iliococcygeus part of levator ani muscle

Rectum

Pubococcygeus part of levator ani muscle

Vagina

Urethra

Transverse perineal ligament

Superior and inferior fascia of urogenital diaphragm

Superficial transverse perineal muscle

Piriformis muscle

Ischial spine

Coccygeus muscle

Left levator ani muscle (*cut*)

External anal sphincter muscle

PLATE 337

PELVIS AND PERINEUM

FOR UROGENITAL DIAPHRAGM SEE PLATE 356

Inferior view

Pubic symphysis

Arcuate pubic ligament

Deep dorsal
vein of clitoris

Inferior pubic ramus

Urethra

Vagina

Rectum

Ischial spine

Coccygeus muscle

Piriformis muscle (*cut*)

Sacrospinous ligament (*cut*)

Sacrotuberous ligament (*cut*)

Sacrum

Musculofascial extensions to urethra

Musculofascial extensions to vagina

Interdigitating fibers of perineum

Puborectalis part of levator ani muscle

Pubococcygeus part of levator ani muscle

Tendinous arch of levator ani muscle

Obturator internus muscle

Iliococcygeus part of
levator ani muscle

Ischial tuberosity

Ischial spine

Obturator internus
tendon

Sacrospinous ligament

Sacrotuberous ligament

Piriformis muscle

Levator plate (median raphé)
of levator ani muscle

Anococcygeal ligament (attachment of
external anal sphincter muscle)

Tip of coccyx

Lateral view

Sacrum (median crest)

Sacrotuberous ligament (*cut*)

4th posterior (dorsal) sacral foramen

Coccygeus muscle

Sacrospinous ligament (*cut*)

Coccyx

Anococcygeal ligament
(attachment of external
anal sphincter muscle)

Piriformis muscle

Greater sciatic foramen

Ischial spine

Iliococcygeus part of levator ani muscle

Tendinous arch of levator ani muscle

Pubococcygeus part of levator ani muscle

Puborectalis part of
levator ani muscle

Pubic bone
(*cut surface*)

Deep dorsal vein
of clitoris

Urethra

Vagina

Rectum

Pelvic Diaphragm: Male

SEE ALSO PLATES 246, 347, 368

**Superior view
(*viscera removed*)**

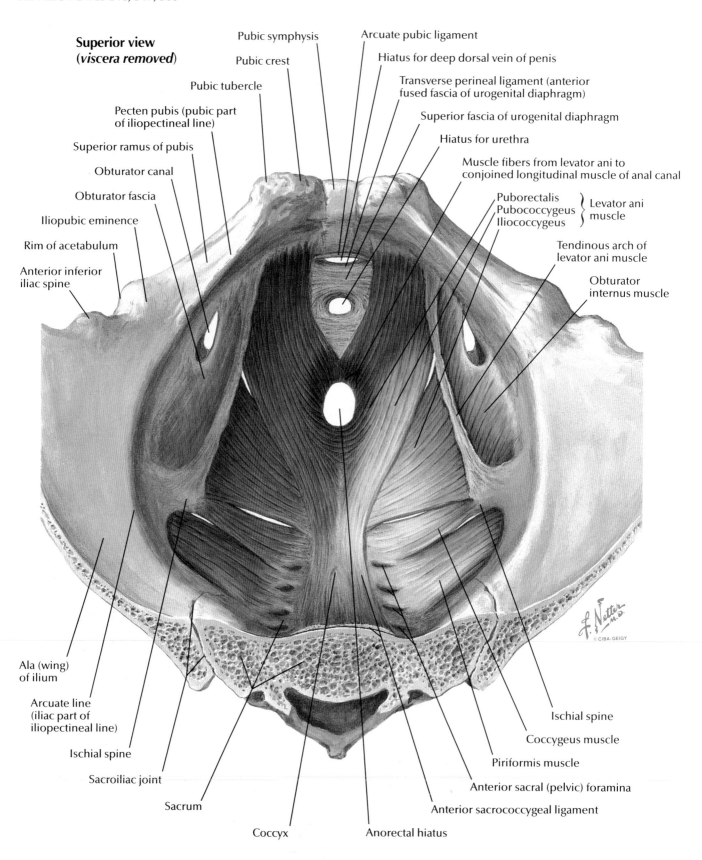

Pubic symphysis

Arcuate pubic ligament

Pubic crest

Hiatus for deep dorsal vein of penis

Pubic tubercle

Transverse perineal ligament (anterior fused fascia of urogenital diaphragm)

Pecten pubis (pubic part of iliopectineal line)

Superior fascia of urogenital diaphragm

Superior ramus of pubis

Hiatus for urethra

Obturator canal

Muscle fibers from levator ani to conjoined longitudinal muscle of anal canal

Obturator fascia

Puborectalis
Pubococcygeus } Levator ani muscle
Iliococcygeus

Iliopubic eminence

Rim of acetabulum

Tendinous arch of levator ani muscle

Anterior inferior iliac spine

Obturator internus muscle

Ala (wing) of ilium

Arcuate line (iliac part of iliopectineal line)

Ischial spine

Sacroiliac joint

Sacrum

Coccyx

Anorectal hiatus

Anterior sacrococcygeal ligament

Anterior sacral (pelvic) foramina

Piriformis muscle

Coccygeus muscle

Ischial spine

PLATE 339

FOR UROGENITAL DIAPHRAGM SEE PLATE 361

Inferior view

Deep dorsal veins of penis

Fat in retropubic (prevesical) space

Prostate

Urethra

Rectovesical (Denonvilliers') fascia

Medial border (pillar) of levator ani muscle

Urogenital diaphragm (cut away)

Ischiopubic ramus

Pubic symphysis

Arcuate pubic ligament

Pubic tubercle

Fibromuscular extensions of levator ani muscle to prostate

Rectourethralis muscle

Prerectal muscle fibers (of Luschka) from levator ani muscle

Muscle fibers from levator ani to conjoined longitudinal muscle of anal canal

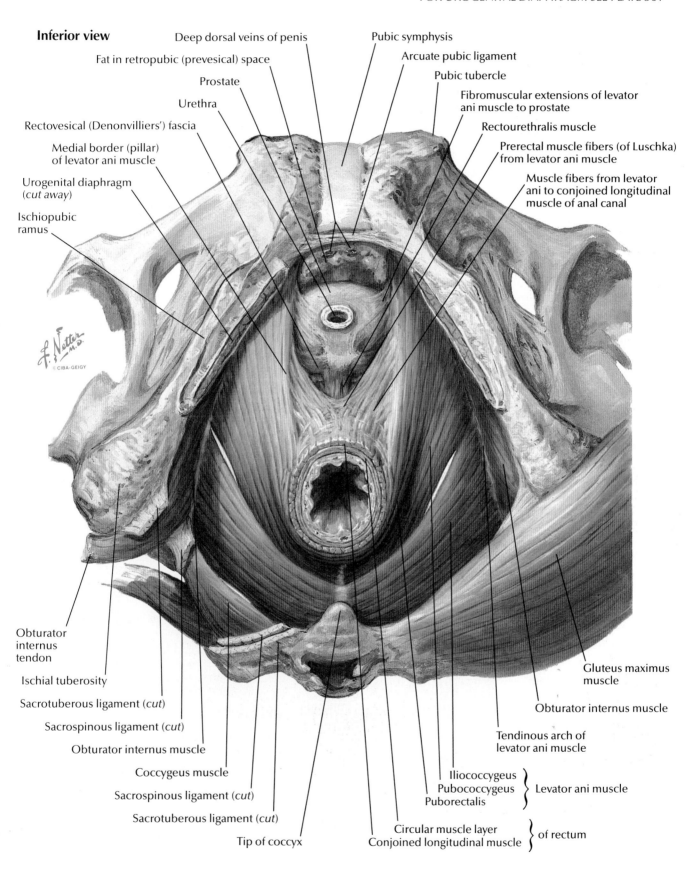

Obturator internus tendon

Ischial tuberosity

Sacrotuberous ligament (cut)

Sacrospinous ligament (cut)

Obturator internus muscle

Coccygeus muscle

Sacrospinous ligament (cut)

Sacrotuberous ligament (cut)

Tip of coccyx

Gluteus maximus muscle

Obturator internus muscle

Tendinous arch of levator ani muscle

Iliococcygeus ⎫
Pubococcygeus ⎬ Levator ani muscle
Puborectalis ⎭

Circular muscle layer ⎫ of rectum
Conjoined longitudinal muscle ⎭

Pelvic Viscera and Perineum: Female

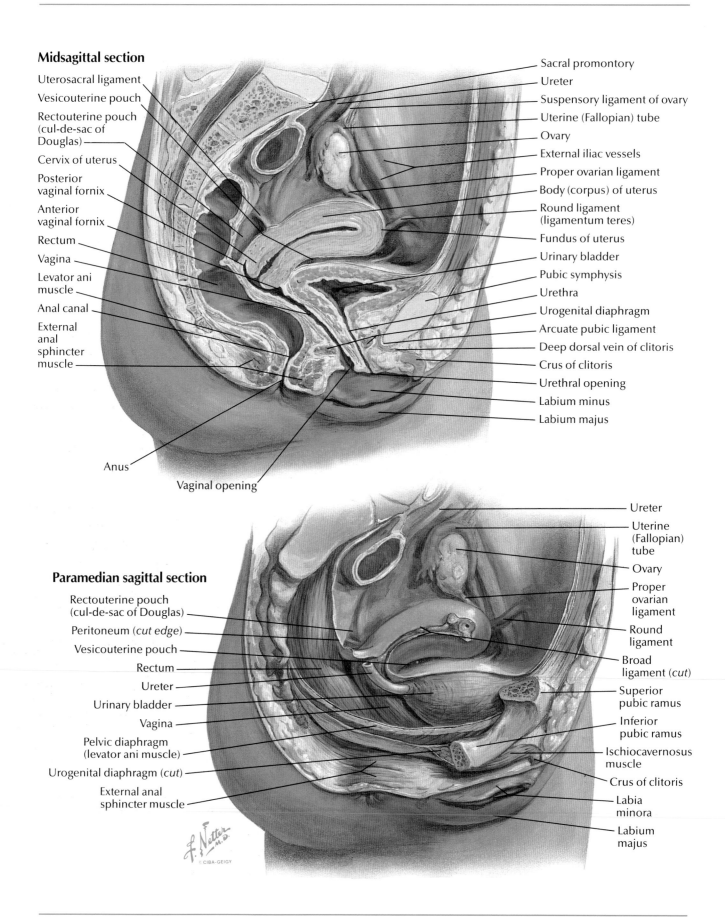

Midsagittal section

Uterosacral ligament
Vesicouterine pouch
Rectouterine pouch (cul-de-sac of Douglas)
Cervix of uterus
Posterior vaginal fornix
Anterior vaginal fornix
Rectum
Vagina
Levator ani muscle
Anal canal
External anal sphincter muscle
Anus
Vaginal opening

Sacral promontory
Ureter
Suspensory ligament of ovary
Uterine (Fallopian) tube
Ovary
External iliac vessels
Proper ovarian ligament
Body (corpus) of uterus
Round ligament (ligamentum teres)
Fundus of uterus
Urinary bladder
Pubic symphysis
Urethra
Urogenital diaphragm
Arcuate pubic ligament
Deep dorsal vein of clitoris
Crus of clitoris
Urethral opening
Labium minus
Labium majus

Paramedian sagittal section

Rectouterine pouch (cul-de-sac of Douglas)
Peritoneum (cut edge)
Vesicouterine pouch
Rectum
Ureter
Urinary bladder
Vagina
Pelvic diaphragm (levator ani muscle)
Urogenital diaphragm (cut)
External anal sphincter muscle

Ureter
Uterine (Fallopian) tube
Ovary
Proper ovarian ligament
Round ligament
Broad ligament (cut)
Superior pubic ramus
Inferior pubic ramus
Ischiocavernosus muscle
Crus of clitoris
Labia minora
Labium majus

PLATE 341

PELVIS AND PERINEUM

Paramedian sagittal section

- External iliac vessels
- Peritoneum
- Rectus abdominis muscle
- Anterior rectus sheath
- Transversalis fascia
- Umbilical prevesical fascia
- Subcutaneous fascia { Camper's / Scarpa's }
- Superior pubic ramus (*cut*)
- Fundiform ligament
- Suspensory ligament of penis
- Areolar tissue and vesical venous plexus in retro-pubic (prevesical) space
- Deep dorsal vein of penis
- Corpus cavernosum
- Deep (Buck's) fascia of penis
- Corpus spongiosum
- Superficial (dartos) fascia of penis and scrotum
- Scrotal septum
- Ischiocavernosus muscle
- Testis

- Ductus (vas) deferens
- Urinary bladder and fascia
- Ureter (*cut*)
- Seminal vesicle
- Rectovesical recess
- Rectum
- Rectovesical (Denonvilliers') fascia
- Prostate (covered by fascia)
- Ischiopubic ramus (*cut*)
- Pelvic diaphragm (levator ani muscle)
- Urogenital diaphragm
- Central tendon of perineum
- Deep / Superficial / Subcutaneous } External anal sphincter muscle
- Investing (Gallaudet's) fascia
- Superficial perineal (Colles') fascia (inferior fascia of superficial perineal space)
- Superficial (dartos) fascia of scrotum
- External spermatic fascia

Midsagittal section

- Urachus
- Urinary bladder { Fundus / Apex / Body / Trigone / Neck }
- Pubic symphysis
- Fundiform ligament
- Suspensory ligament of penis
- Arcuate pubic ligament
- Transverse perineal ligament (anterior fused fascia of urogenital diaphragm)
- Superficial perineal space
- Corpus cavernosum
- Corpus spongiosum
- Superficial (dartos) fascia of penis and scrotum
- Deep (Buck's) fascia of penis
- Prepuce
- Glans of penis and external urethral meatus

- Rectovesical recess (space)
- Rectum
- Vesical fascia
- Seminal vesicle
- Prostate and fascia
- Rectovesical (Denonvilliers') fascia
- Urogenital diaphragm
- Bulbourethral (Cowper's) gland
- Central tendon of perineum
- Bulbospongiosus muscle
- Investing (Gallaudet's) fascia
- Superficial perineal (Colles') fascia
- Buck's fascia
- Scrotal septum
- Navicular fossa

Pelvic Contents: Female

Superior view

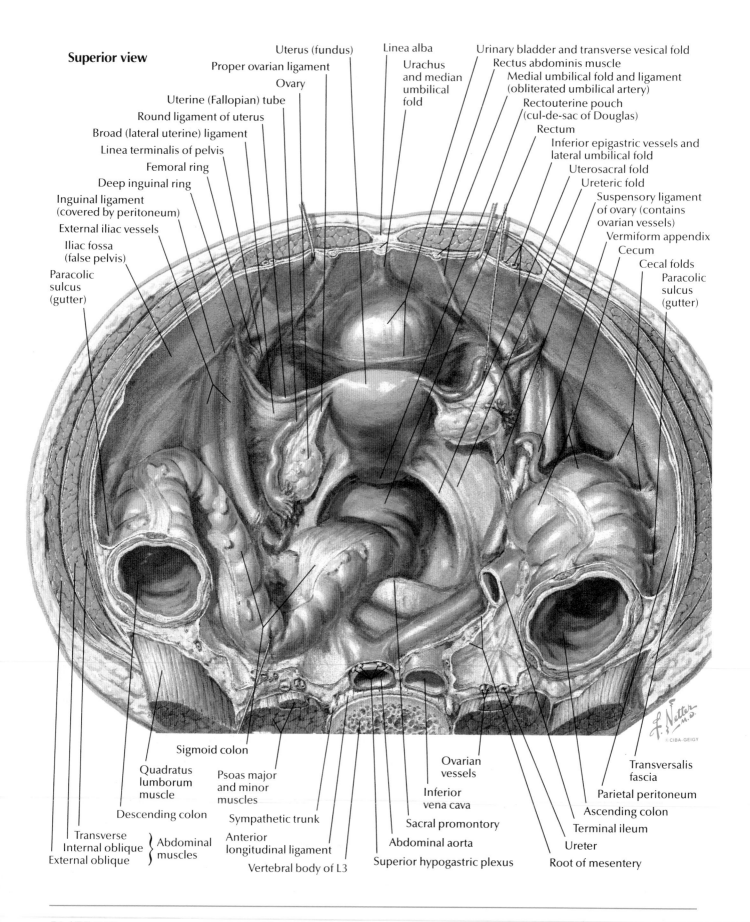

Uterus (fundus)

Proper ovarian ligament

Ovary

Uterine (Fallopian) tube

Round ligament of uterus

Broad (lateral uterine) ligament

Linea terminalis of pelvis

Femoral ring

Deep inguinal ring

Inguinal ligament (covered by peritoneum)

External iliac vessels

Iliac fossa (false pelvis)

Paracolic sulcus (gutter)

Linea alba

Urachus and median umbilical fold

Urinary bladder and transverse vesical fold

Rectus abdominis muscle

Medial umbilical fold and ligament (obliterated umbilical artery)

Rectouterine pouch (cul-de-sac of Douglas)

Rectum

Inferior epigastric vessels and lateral umbilical fold

Uterosacral fold

Ureteric fold

Suspensory ligament of ovary (contains ovarian vessels)

Vermiform appendix

Cecum

Cecal folds

Paracolic sulcus (gutter)

Sigmoid colon

Quadratus lumborum muscle

Psoas major and minor muscles

Descending colon

Transverse

Internal oblique

External oblique

} Abdominal muscles

Anterior longitudinal ligament

Vertebral body of L3

Sympathetic trunk

Ovarian vessels

Inferior vena cava

Sacral promontory

Abdominal aorta

Superior hypogastric plexus

Transversalis fascia

Parietal peritoneum

Ascending colon

Terminal ileum

Ureter

Root of mesentery

PLATE 343

PELVIS AND PERINEUM

Superior view

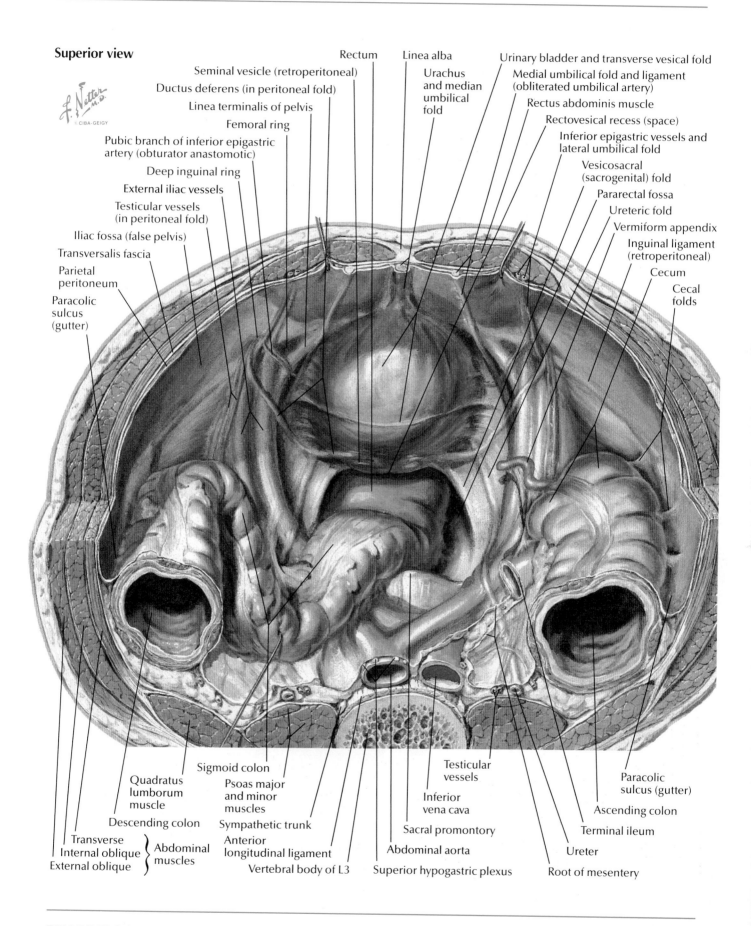

Rectum

Linea alba

Seminal vesicle (retroperitoneal)

Ductus deferens (in peritoneal fold)

Linea terminalis of pelvis

Femoral ring

Pubic branch of inferior epigastric artery (obturator anastomotic)

Deep inguinal ring

External iliac vessels

Testicular vessels (in peritoneal fold)

Iliac fossa (false pelvis)

Transversalis fascia

Parietal peritoneum

Paracolic sulcus (gutter)

Urachus and median umbilical fold

Urinary bladder and transverse vesical fold

Medial umbilical fold and ligament (obliterated umbilical artery)

Rectus abdominis muscle

Rectovesical recess (space)

Inferior epigastric vessels and lateral umbilical fold

Vesicosacral (sacrogenital) fold

Pararectal fossa

Ureteric fold

Vermiform appendix

Inguinal ligament (retroperitoneal)

Cecum

Cecal folds

Quadratus lumborum muscle

Sigmoid colon

Psoas major and minor muscles

Descending colon

Sympathetic trunk

Transverse
Internal oblique } Abdominal muscles
External oblique

Anterior longitudinal ligament

Vertebral body of L3

Testicular vessels

Inferior vena cava

Sacral promontory

Abdominal aorta

Superior hypogastric plexus

Paracolic sulcus (gutter)

Ascending colon

Terminal ileum

Ureter

Root of mesentery

Endopelvic Fascia and Spaces

Female: superior view

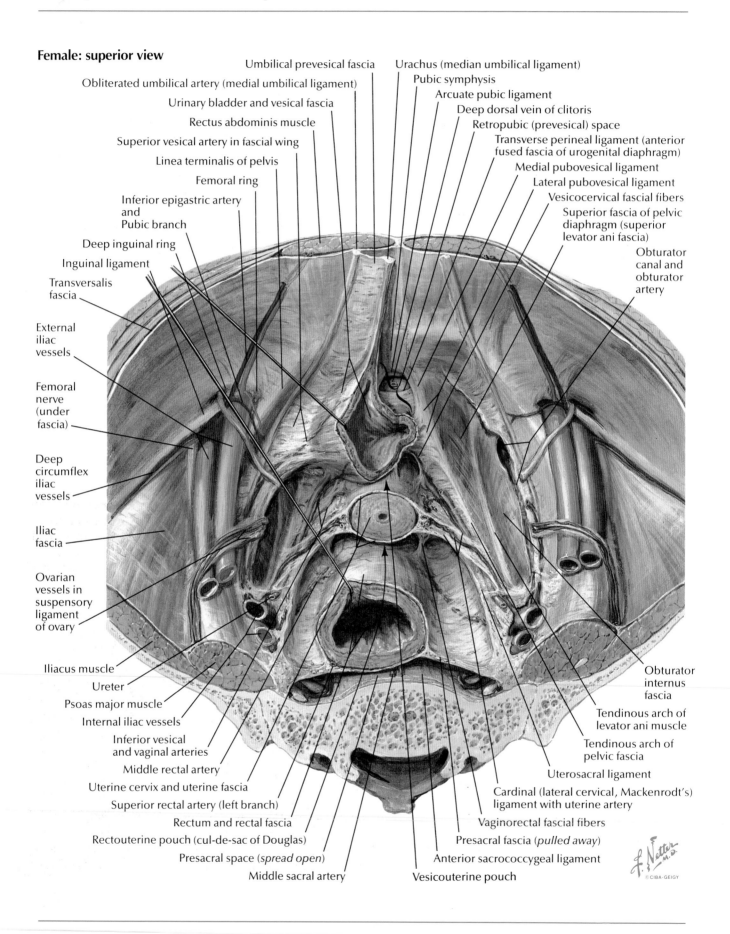

Umbilical prevesical fascia

Obliterated umbilical artery (medial umbilical ligament)

Urinary bladder and vesical fascia

Rectus abdominis muscle

Superior vesical artery in fascial wing

Linea terminalis of pelvis

Femoral ring

Inferior epigastric artery and Pubic branch

Deep inguinal ring

Inguinal ligament

Transversalis fascia

External iliac vessels

Femoral nerve (under fascia)

Deep circumflex iliac vessels

Iliac fascia

Ovarian vessels in suspensory ligament of ovary

Iliacus muscle

Ureter

Psoas major muscle

Internal iliac vessels

Inferior vesical and vaginal arteries

Middle rectal artery

Uterine cervix and uterine fascia

Superior rectal artery (left branch)

Rectum and rectal fascia

Rectouterine pouch (cul-de-sac of Douglas)

Presacral space (spread open)

Middle sacral artery

Urachus (median umbilical ligament)

Pubic symphysis

Arcuate pubic ligament

Deep dorsal vein of clitoris

Retropubic (prevesical) space

Transverse perineal ligament (anterior fused fascia of urogenital diaphragm)

Medial pubovesical ligament

Lateral pubovesical ligament

Vesicocervical fascial fibers

Superior fascia of pelvic diaphragm (superior levator ani fascia)

Obturator canal and obturator artery

Obturator internus fascia

Tendinous arch of levator ani muscle

Tendinous arch of pelvic fascia

Uterosacral ligament

Cardinal (lateral cervical, Mackenrodt's) ligament with uterine artery

Vaginorectal fascial fibers

Presacral fascia (pulled away)

Anterior sacrococcygeal ligament

Vesicouterine pouch

PLATE 345

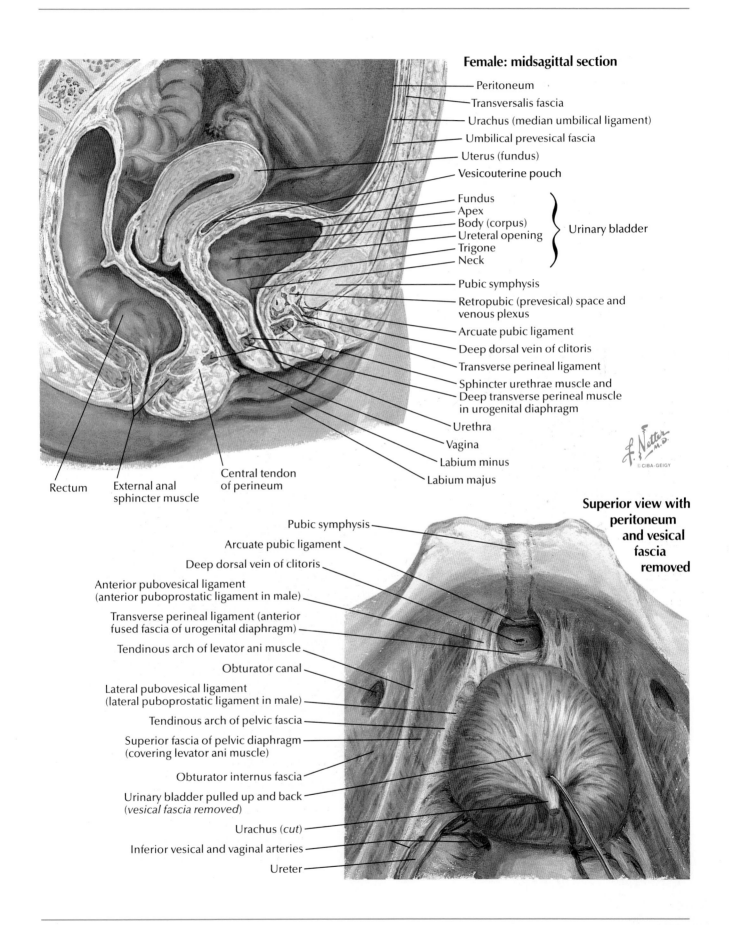

Female: midsagittal section

Peritoneum

Transversalis fascia

Urachus (median umbilical ligament)

Umbilical prevesical fascia

Uterus (fundus)

Vesicouterine pouch

Fundus
Apex
Body (corpus)
Ureteral opening } Urinary bladder
Trigone
Neck

Pubic symphysis

Retropubic (prevesical) space and venous plexus

Arcuate pubic ligament

Deep dorsal vein of clitoris

Transverse perineal ligament

Sphincter urethrae muscle and
Deep transverse perineal muscle in urogenital diaphragm

Urethra

Vagina

Labium minus

Labium majus

Rectum

External anal sphincter muscle

Central tendon of perineum

Superior view with peritoneum and vesical fascia removed

Pubic symphysis

Arcuate pubic ligament

Deep dorsal vein of clitoris

Anterior pubovesical ligament (anterior puboprostatic ligament in male)

Transverse perineal ligament (anterior fused fascia of urogenital diaphragm)

Tendinous arch of levator ani muscle

Obturator canal

Lateral pubovesical ligament (lateral puboprostatic ligament in male)

Tendinous arch of pelvic fascia

Superior fascia of pelvic diaphragm (covering levator ani muscle)

Obturator internus fascia

Urinary bladder pulled up and back (vesical fascia removed)

Urachus (cut)

Inferior vesical and vaginal arteries

Ureter

Urinary Bladder: Female and Male

SEE ALSO PLATES 325, 341, 342, 346, 375, 377, 378, 392

Female: frontal section

- Peritoneum
- Fundus of bladder
- Body of bladder
- Interureteric fold
- Opening of left ureter
- Trigone of bladder
- Neck of bladder
- Paravesical space and venous plexus
- Tendinous arch of levator ani muscle
- Levator ani muscle
- Obturator internus muscle
- Vesical fascia
- Uvula of bladder
- Tendinous arch of pelvic fascia
- Lateral pubovesical ligament
- Urethra
- Inferior pubic ramus
- Sphincter urethrae muscle in urogenital diaphragm
- Crus of clitoris and ischiocavernosus muscle
- Corpus spongiosum and bulbospongiosus muscle
- Investing (Gallaudet's) fascia
- Superficial perineal (Colles') fascia

End of round ligament

Vagina

Male: frontal section

- Peritoneum

- Fundus of bladder
- Body of bladder
- Ductus (vas) deferens
- Interureteric fold
- Opening of right ureter
- Trigone of bladder
- Neck of bladder
- Tendinous arch of levator ani muscle
- Paravesical space and venous plexus
- Levator ani muscle
- Obturator internus muscle
- Uvula of bladder
- Prostatic fascia
- Tendinous arch of pelvic fascia
- Lateral puboprostatic ligament
- Prostate and prostatic urethra
- Seminal colliculus (verumontanum)
- Sphincter urethrae muscle in urogenital diaphragm
- Urethral bulb
- Corpus spongiosum and bulbospongiosus muscle
- Investing (Gallaudet's) fascia

- Inferior pubic ramus
- Crus of penis and ischiocavernosus muscle
- Superficial perineal (Colles') fascia

PLATE 347

PELVIS AND PERINEUM

Superior view with peritoneum intact

Median umbilical fold (urachus)

Urinary bladder

Fundus of uterus

Deep inguinal ring

Round ligament (ligamentum teres)

Body (corpus) of uterus

Broad ligament

Proper ovarian ligament

Mesovarium

Cervix of uterus

Ovary

Rectouterine pouch (cul-de-sac of Douglas)

Uterosacral fold

Uterine (Fallopian) tube

External iliac vessels

Suspensory ligament of ovary (contains ovarian vessels)

Ureteric fold

Sigmoid colon

Sacral promontory

Middle sacral vessels

Abdominal aorta

Urinary bladder

Vesical fascia (*cut edge*)

Obturator fascia

Obturator canal

Obturator artery

Superior fascia of pelvic diaphragm

Uterine cervix and uterovaginal fascia

Uterine vessels

Cardinal (Mackenrodt's) ligament

Rectouterine pouch

Rectal fascia (*cut edge*)

Uterosacral ligament

External iliac vessels

Ureter

Sacral promontory

Superior view with peritoneum and uterus removed

Uterus, Vagina and Supporting Structures

SEE ALSO PLATES 375, 377, 379, 381, 387, 389, 390

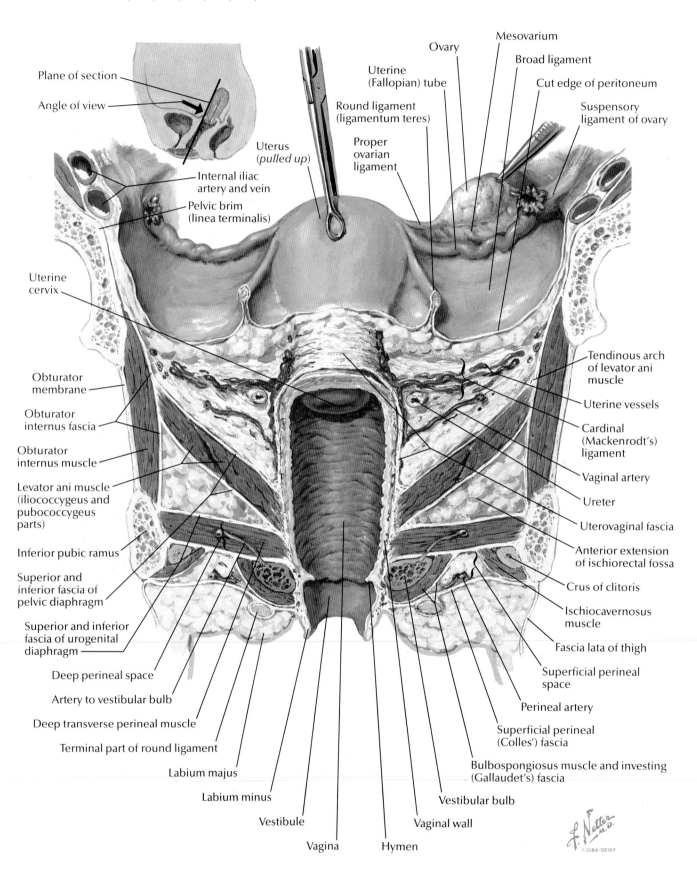

Plane of section

Angle of view

Ovary

Mesovarium

Broad ligament

Uterine (Fallopian) tube

Cut edge of peritoneum

Round ligament (ligamentum teres)

Suspensory ligament of ovary

Uterus (*pulled up*)

Proper ovarian ligament

Internal iliac artery and vein

Pelvic brim (linea terminalis)

Uterine cervix

Obturator membrane

Obturator internus fascia

Obturator internus muscle

Levator ani muscle (iliococcygeus and pubococcygeus parts)

Inferior pubic ramus

Superior and inferior fascia of pelvic diaphragm

Superior and inferior fascia of urogenital diaphragm

Deep perineal space

Artery to vestibular bulb

Deep transverse perineal muscle

Terminal part of round ligament

Labium majus

Labium minus

Vestibule

Vagina

Hymen

Vaginal wall

Vestibular bulb

Bulbospongiosus muscle and investing (Gallaudet's) fascia

Superficial perineal (Colles') fascia

Perineal artery

Superficial perineal space

Fascia lata of thigh

Ischiocavernosus muscle

Crus of clitoris

Anterior extension of ischiorectal fossa

Uterovaginal fascia

Ureter

Vaginal artery

Cardinal (Mackenrodt's) ligament

Uterine vessels

Tendinous arch of levator ani muscle

PLATE 349

Uterus and Adnexa

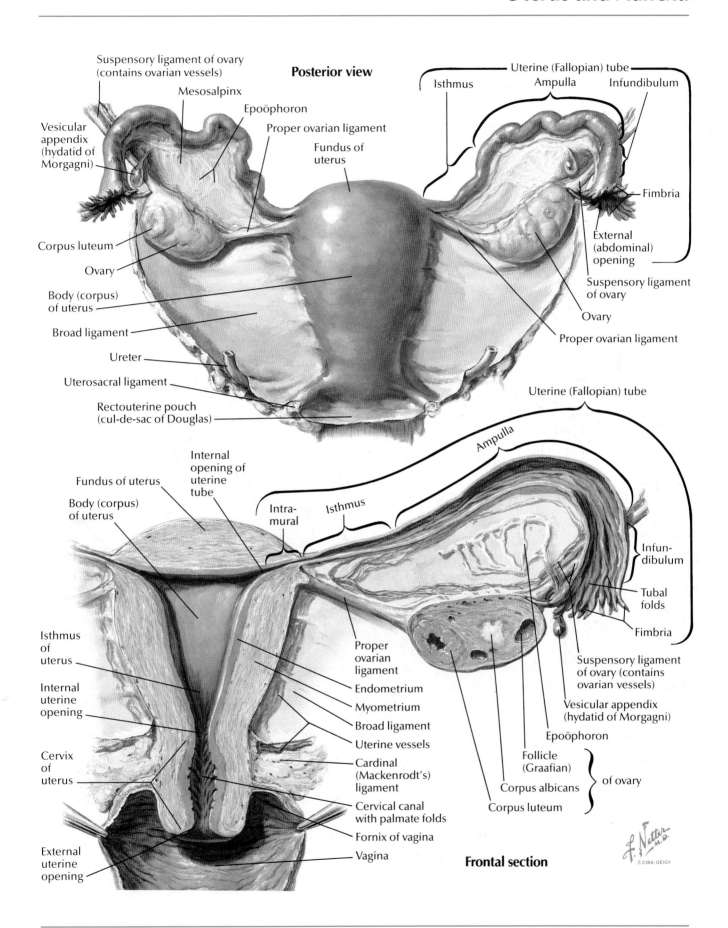

Posterior view

Suspensory ligament of ovary (contains ovarian vessels)

Mesosalpinx

Epoöphoron

Proper ovarian ligament

Fundus of uterus

Vesicular appendix (hydatid of Morgagni)

Corpus luteum

Ovary

Body (corpus) of uterus

Broad ligament

Ureter

Uterosacral ligament

Rectouterine pouch (cul-de-sac of Douglas)

Uterine (Fallopian) tube

Isthmus

Ampulla

Infundibulum

Fimbria

External (abdominal) opening

Suspensory ligament of ovary

Ovary

Proper ovarian ligament

Internal opening of uterine tube

Fundus of uterus

Body (corpus) of uterus

Intra-mural

Isthmus

Ampulla

Uterine (Fallopian) tube

Infundibulum

Tubal folds

Fimbria

Suspensory ligament of ovary (contains ovarian vessels)

Vesicular appendix (hydatid of Morgagni)

Epoöphoron

Follicle (Graafian)

Corpus albicans

Corpus luteum

of ovary

Isthmus of uterus

Internal uterine opening

Cervix of uterus

External uterine opening

Proper ovarian ligament

Endometrium

Myometrium

Broad ligament

Uterine vessels

Cardinal (Mackenrodt's) ligament

Cervical canal with palmate folds

Fornix of vagina

Vagina

Frontal section

Uterus: Age Changes and Muscle Pattern

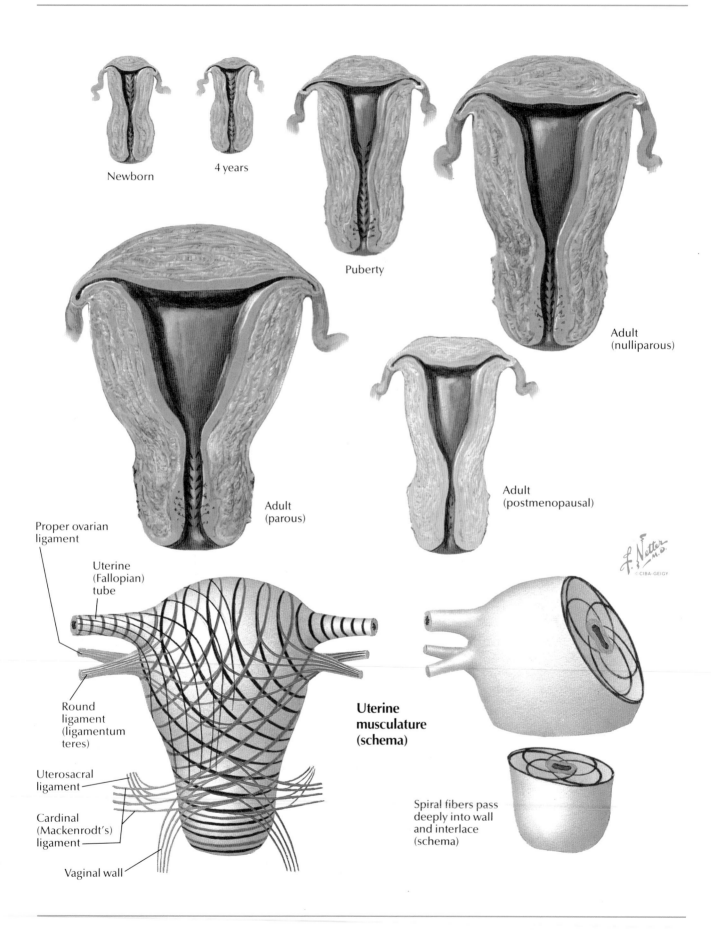

Newborn

4 years

Puberty

Adult
(nulliparous)

Adult
(parous)

Adult
(postmenopausal)

Proper ovarian
ligament

Uterine
(Fallopian)
tube

Round
ligament
(ligamentum
teres)

Uterosacral
ligament

Cardinal
(Mackenrodt's)
ligament

Vaginal wall

Uterine
musculature
(schema)

Spiral fibers pass
deeply into wall
and interlace
(schema)

PLATE 351

PELVIS AND PERINEUM

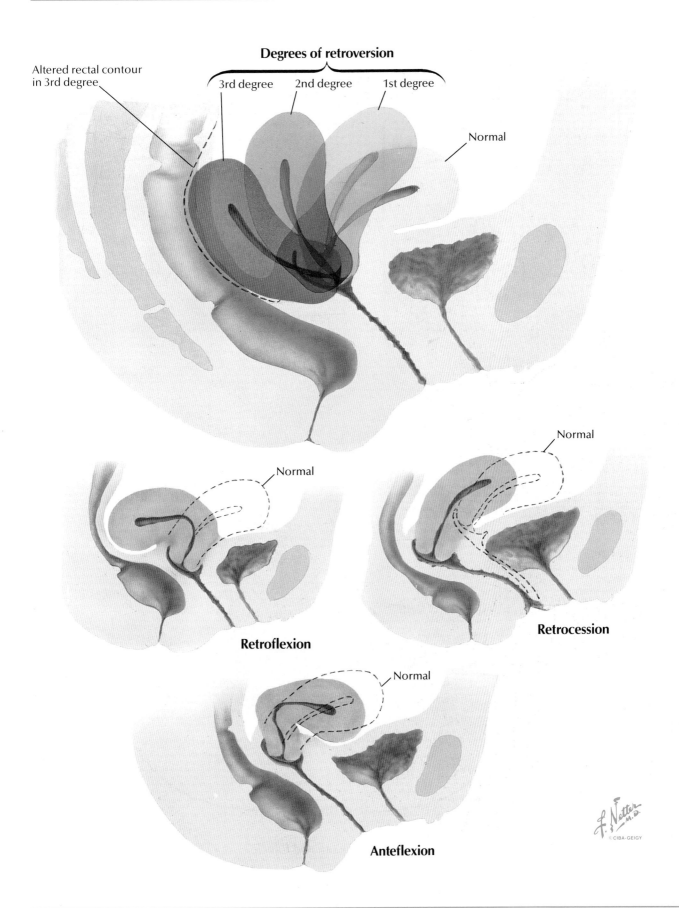

Degrees of retroversion

Altered rectal contour in 3rd degree

3rd degree   2nd degree   1st degree

Normal

Retroflexion

Retrocession

Normal

Anteflexion

Ovary, Ova and Follicles

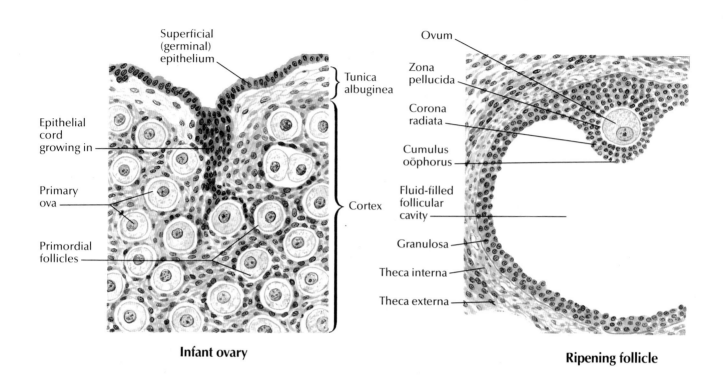

Infant ovary

Superficial (germinal) epithelium

Tunica albuginea

Epithelial cord growing in

Primary ova

Primordial follicles

Cortex

Ripening follicle

Ovum

Zona pellucida

Corona radiata

Cumulus oöphorus

Fluid-filled follicular cavity

Granulosa

Theca interna

Theca externa

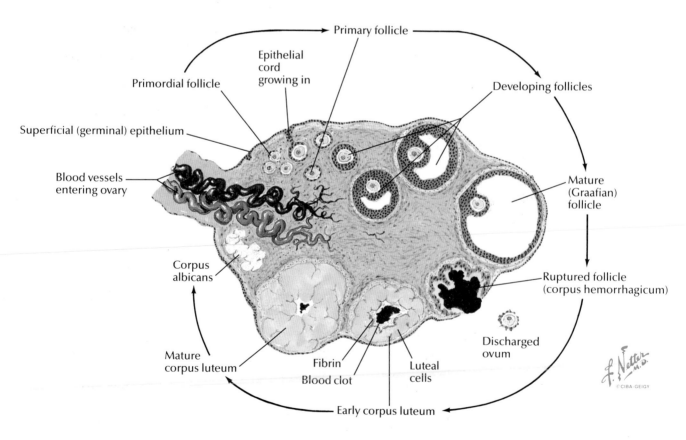

Primary follicle

Epithelial cord growing in

Primordial follicle

Developing follicles

Superficial (germinal) epithelium

Blood vessels entering ovary

Mature (Graafian) follicle

Corpus albicans

Ruptured follicle (corpus hemorrhagicum)

Mature corpus luteum

Fibrin

Blood clot

Luteal cells

Discharged ovum

Early corpus luteum

Stages of ovum and follicle

PLATE 353

PELVIS AND PERINEUM

SEE ALSO PLATES 379, 381, 382, 388

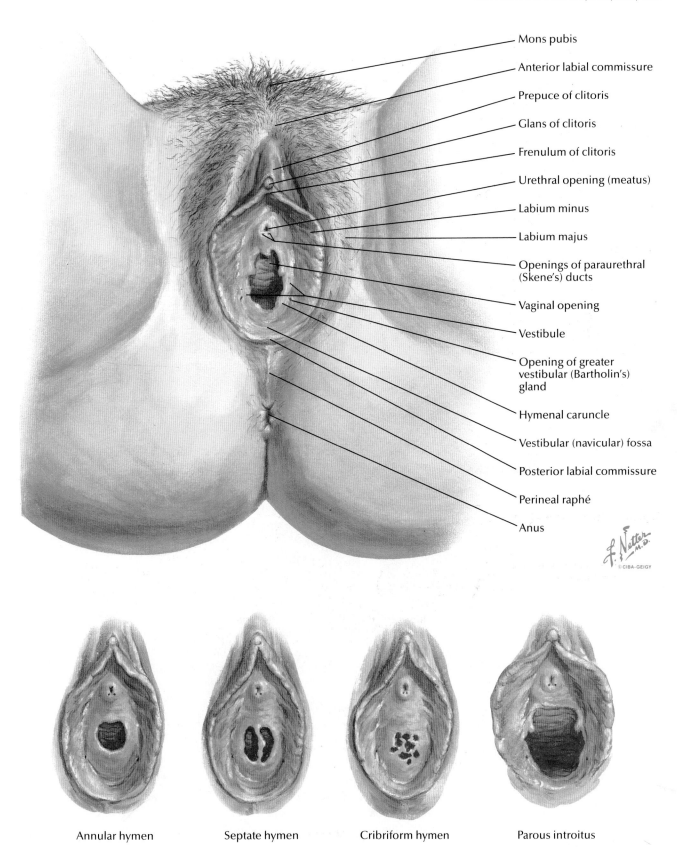

Mons pubis

Anterior labial commissure

Prepuce of clitoris

Glans of clitoris

Frenulum of clitoris

Urethral opening (meatus)

Labium minus

Labium majus

Openings of paraurethral (Skene's) ducts

Vaginal opening

Vestibule

Opening of greater vestibular (Bartholin's) gland

Hymenal caruncle

Vestibular (navicular) fossa

Posterior labial commissure

Perineal raphé

Anus

Annular hymen   Septate hymen   Cribriform hymen   Parous introitus

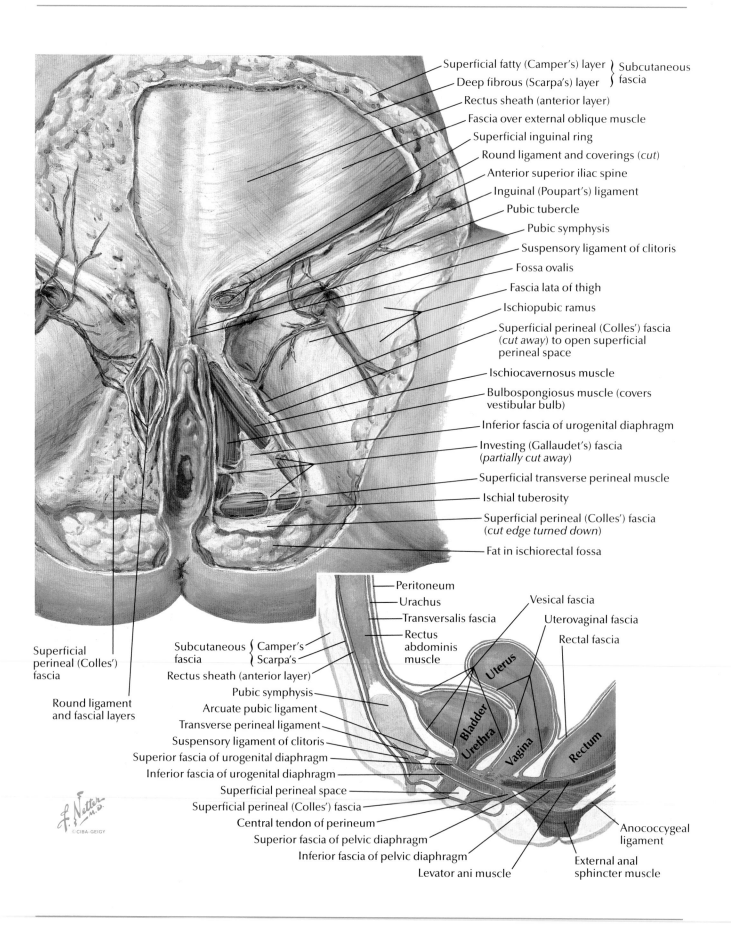

Superficial fatty (Camper's) layer ⎫ Subcutaneous
Deep fibrous (Scarpa's) layer ⎭ fascia
Rectus sheath (anterior layer)
Fascia over external oblique muscle
Superficial inguinal ring
Round ligament and coverings (*cut*)
Anterior superior iliac spine
Inguinal (Poupart's) ligament
Pubic tubercle
Pubic symphysis
Suspensory ligament of clitoris
Fossa ovalis
Fascia lata of thigh
Ischiopubic ramus
Superficial perineal (Colles') fascia (*cut away*) to open superficial perineal space
Ischiocavernosus muscle
Bulbospongiosus muscle (covers vestibular bulb)
Inferior fascia of urogenital diaphragm
Investing (Gallaudet's) fascia (*partially cut away*)
Superficial transverse perineal muscle
Ischial tuberosity
Superficial perineal (Colles') fascia (*cut edge turned down*)
Fat in ischiorectal fossa

Superficial perineal (Colles') fascia
Round ligament and fascial layers

Subcutaneous ⎧ Camper's
fascia ⎩ Scarpa's
Rectus sheath (anterior layer)
Pubic symphysis
Arcuate pubic ligament
Transverse perineal ligament
Suspensory ligament of clitoris
Superior fascia of urogenital diaphragm
Inferior fascia of urogenital diaphragm
Superficial perineal space
Superficial perineal (Colles') fascia
Central tendon of perineum
Superior fascia of pelvic diaphragm
Inferior fascia of pelvic diaphragm
Levator ani muscle

Peritoneum
Urachus
Transversalis fascia
Rectus abdominis muscle
Vesical fascia
Uterovaginal fascia
Rectal fascia
Uterus
Bladder
Urethra
Vagina
Rectum
Anococcygeal ligament
External anal sphincter muscle

PLATE 355

PELVIS AND PERINEUM

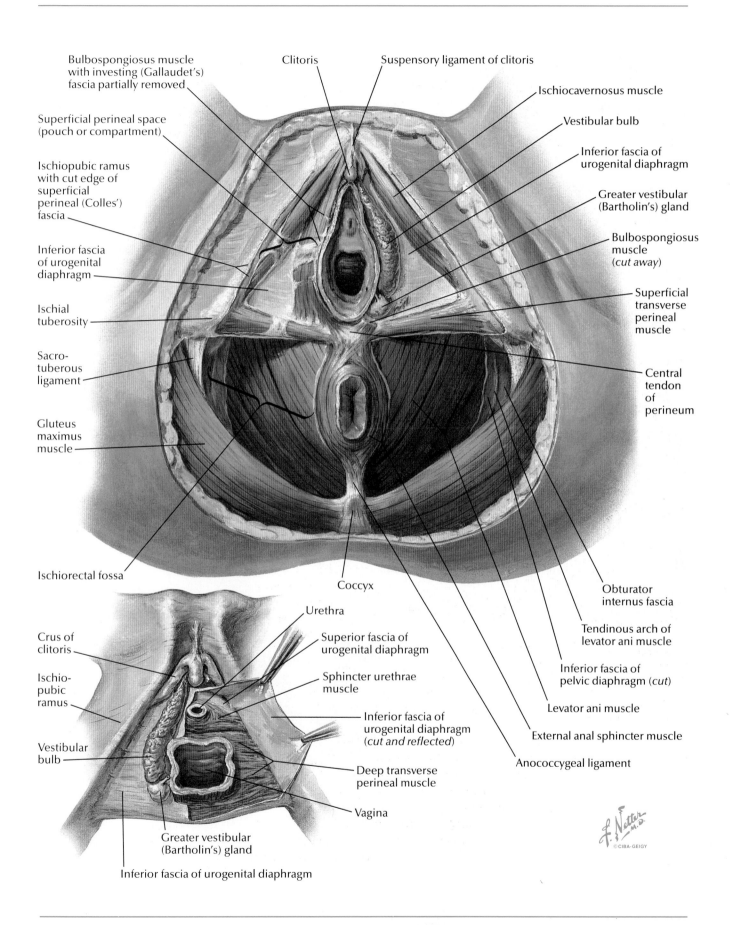

Bulbospongiosus muscle with investing (Gallaudet's) fascia partially removed

Clitoris

Suspensory ligament of clitoris

Superficial perineal space (pouch or compartment)

Ischiocavernosus muscle

Vestibular bulb

Ischiopubic ramus with cut edge of superficial perineal (Colles') fascia

Inferior fascia of urogenital diaphragm

Greater vestibular (Bartholin's) gland

Inferior fascia of urogenital diaphragm

Bulbospongiosus muscle (*cut away*)

Ischial tuberosity

Superficial transverse perineal muscle

Sacro-tuberous ligament

Central tendon of perineum

Gluteus maximus muscle

Ischiorectal fossa

Coccyx

Obturator internus fascia

Crus of clitoris

Urethra

Superior fascia of urogenital diaphragm

Tendinous arch of levator ani muscle

Ischio-pubic ramus

Sphincter urethrae muscle

Inferior fascia of pelvic diaphragm (*cut*)

Inferior fascia of urogenital diaphragm (*cut and reflected*)

Levator ani muscle

External anal sphincter muscle

Vestibular bulb

Deep transverse perineal muscle

Anococcygeal ligament

Vagina

Greater vestibular (Bartholin's) gland

Inferior fascia of urogenital diaphragm

Urethra: Female

SEE ALSO PLATES 341, 346

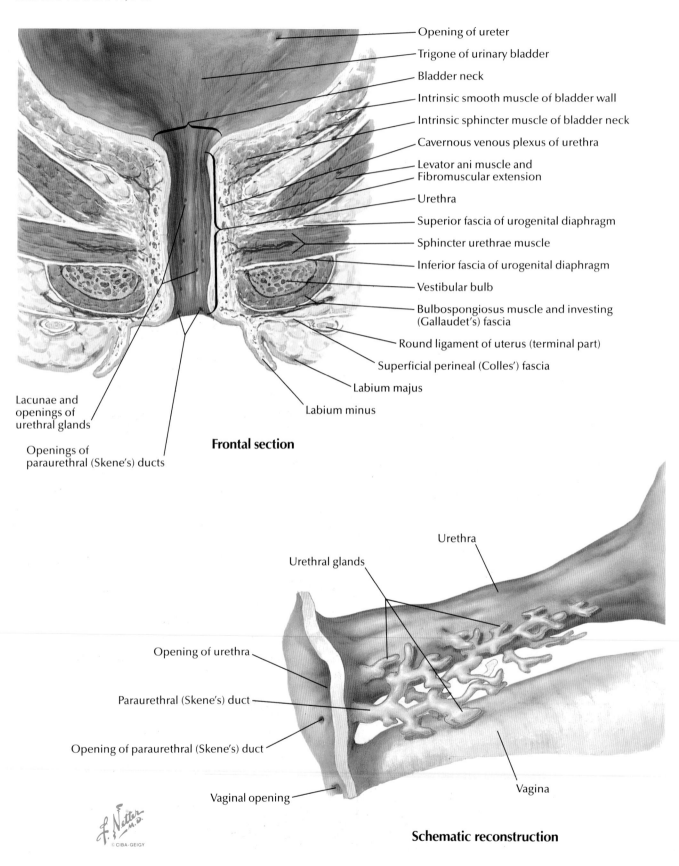

Opening of ureter

Trigone of urinary bladder

Bladder neck

Intrinsic smooth muscle of bladder wall

Intrinsic sphincter muscle of bladder neck

Cavernous venous plexus of urethra

Levator ani muscle and
Fibromuscular extension

Urethra

Superior fascia of urogenital diaphragm

Sphincter urethrae muscle

Inferior fascia of urogenital diaphragm

Vestibular bulb

Bulbospongiosus muscle and investing
(Gallaudet's) fascia

Round ligament of uterus (terminal part)

Superficial perineal (Colles') fascia

Labium majus

Labium minus

Lacunae and
openings of
urethral glands

Openings of
paraurethral (Skene's) ducts

Frontal section

Urethra

Urethral glands

Opening of urethra

Paraurethral (Skene's) duct

Opening of paraurethral (Skene's) duct

Vaginal opening

Vagina

Schematic reconstruction

PLATE 357

PELVIS AND PERINEUM

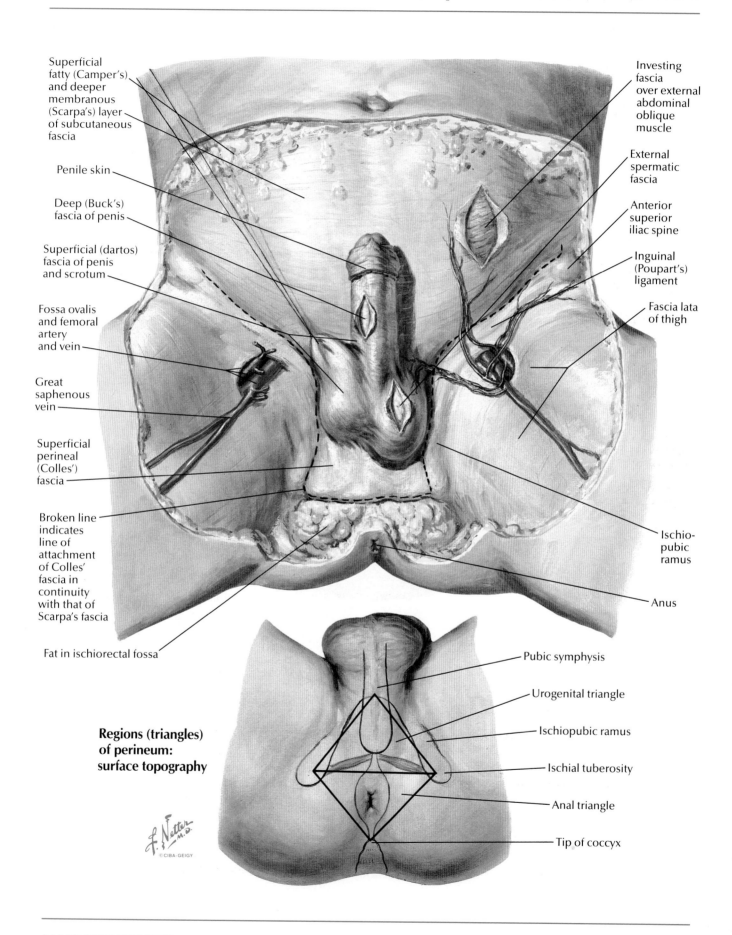

Superficial fatty (Camper's) and deeper membranous (Scarpa's) layer of subcutaneous fascia

Penile skin

Deep (Buck's) fascia of penis

Superficial (dartos) fascia of penis and scrotum

Fossa ovalis and femoral artery and vein

Great saphenous vein

Superficial perineal (Colles') fascia

Broken line indicates line of attachment of Colles' fascia in continuity with that of Scarpa's fascia

Fat in ischiorectal fossa

Investing fascia over external abdominal oblique muscle

External spermatic fascia

Anterior superior iliac spine

Inguinal (Poupart's) ligament

Fascia lata of thigh

Ischio-pubic ramus

Anus

Regions (triangles) of perineum: surface topography

Pubic symphysis

Urogenital triangle

Ischiopubic ramus

Ischial tuberosity

Anal triangle

Tip of coccyx

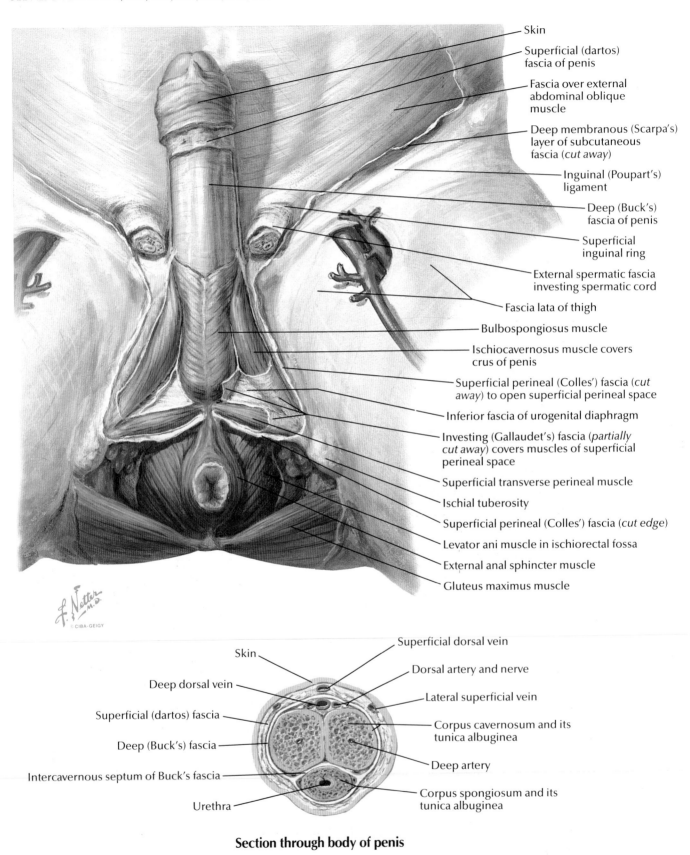

Skin

Superficial (dartos) fascia of penis

Fascia over external abdominal oblique muscle

Deep membranous (Scarpa's) layer of subcutaneous fascia (*cut away*)

Inguinal (Poupart's) ligament

Deep (Buck's) fascia of penis

Superficial inguinal ring

External spermatic fascia investing spermatic cord

Fascia lata of thigh

Bulbospongiosus muscle

Ischiocavernosus muscle covers crus of penis

Superficial perineal (Colles') fascia (*cut away*) to open superficial perineal space

Inferior fascia of urogenital diaphragm

Investing (Gallaudet's) fascia (*partially cut away*) covers muscles of superficial perineal space

Superficial transverse perineal muscle

Ischial tuberosity

Superficial perineal (Colles') fascia (*cut edge*)

Levator ani muscle in ischiorectal fossa

External anal sphincter muscle

Gluteus maximus muscle

Skin

Superficial dorsal vein

Deep dorsal vein

Dorsal artery and nerve

Superficial (dartos) fascia

Lateral superficial vein

Deep (Buck's) fascia

Corpus cavernosum and its tunica albuginea

Intercavernous septum of Buck's fascia

Deep artery

Urethra

Corpus spongiosum and its tunica albuginea

Section through body of penis

PLATE 359

PELVIS AND PERINEUM

External urethral opening (meatus)

Glans of penis

Corona of glans

Frenulum

Neck of glans

Skin

Opening of preputial (Tyson's) gland

Superficial (dartos) fascia of penis

Deep (Buck's) fascia of penis

External spermatic fascia investing spermatic cord (*cut*)

Superficial perineal (Colles') fascia (*cut away*) to open superficial perineal space

Ischiopubic ramus

Investing (Gallaudet's) fascia (*cut away*) over muscles of superficial perineal space

Ischiocavernosus muscle (*cut away*)

Superficial transverse perineal muscle

Anus

Glans of penis

Corpora cavernosa of penis

Intercavernous septum of deep (Buck's) fascia

Corpus spongiosum

Pubic tubercle

Superior pubic ramus

Ischiopubic ramus

Bulb of corpus spongiosum

Crus of penis

Inferior fascia of urogenital diaphragm

Ischial tuberosity

Ischial tuberosity

Gluteus maximus muscle

Levator ani muscle in ischiorectal fossa

External anal sphincter muscle

Inferior fascia of urogenital diaphragm

Central tendon of perineum

Tip of coccyx

Central tendon of perineum

External anal sphincter muscle

Urogenital Diaphragm: Male

Pubic symphysis

Superior pubic ramus

Arcuate pubic ligament

Deep dorsal vein of penis

Ischiopubic ramus

Urethra

Inferior fascia of urogenital diaphragm

Central tendon of perineum

External anal sphincter muscle

Pubic bone

Transverse perineal ligament (anterior fused fascia of urogenital diaphragm)

Dorsal artery and nerve of penis

Deep artery of penis

Urethral artery

Bulbourethral duct

Artery of urethral bulb

Investing (Gallaudet's) fascia over ischiocavernosus, bulbospongiosus and superficial transverse perineal muscles (*cut away*)

Superficial perineal (Colles') fascia (*cut away*)

Posterior fused fascia of urogenital diaphragm

Superficial transverse perineal muscle (*cut and reflected*)

Ischial tuberosity

Dorsal artery and nerve of penis

Deep artery of penis

Urethral artery

Bulbourethral (Cowper's) gland

Artery of urethral bulb

Inferior fascia of urogenital diaphragm (*cut edge*)

Intradiaphragmatic part of internal pudendal artery (artery of penis) and dorsal nerve of penis

Internal pudendal artery and perineal branch

Sphincter muscle of membranous urethra

Urethra

Deep transverse perineal muscle

Levator ani muscle

Superior and inferior fascia of urogenital diaphragm

Muscles of urogenital diaphragm

Investing (Gallaudet's) fascia

Corpus cavernosum (crus of penis) and deep (Buck's) fascia of penis

Ischiocavernosus muscle

Superficial perineal (Colles') fascia (closes superficial perineal space)

Urinary bladder

Prostate

Obturator internus muscle

Ischiopubic ramus

Corpus cavernosum (crus of penis) and deep (Buck's) fascia of penis

Ischiocavernosus muscle

Corpus spongiosum and deep (Buck's) fascia of penis

Bulbospongiosus muscle

Frontal section through perineum and urethral bulb: schema

PLATE 361

PELVIS AND PERINEUM

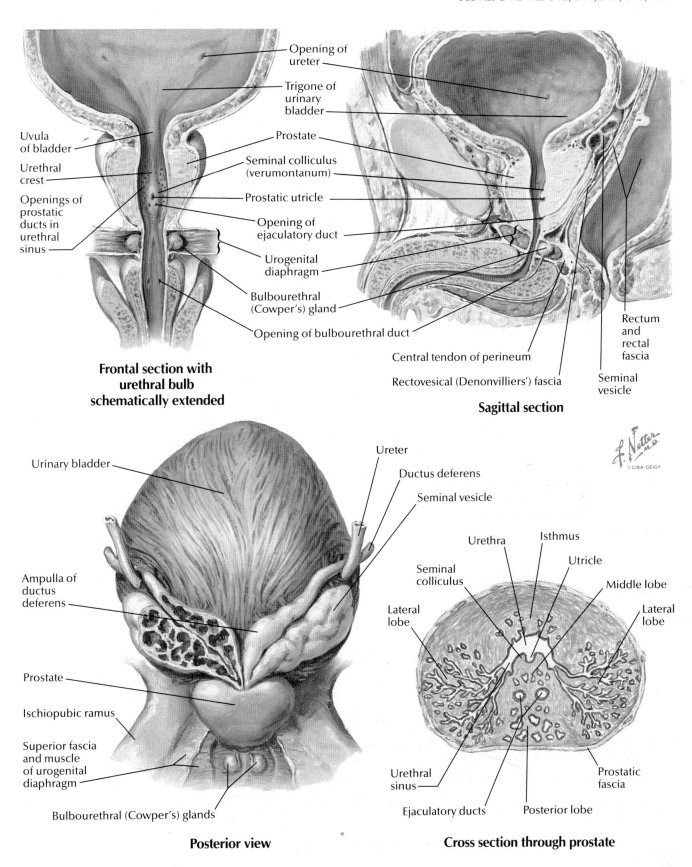

Opening of ureter

Trigone of urinary bladder

Prostate

Seminal colliculus (verumontanum)

Prostatic utricle

Opening of ejaculatory duct

Urogenital diaphragm

Bulbourethral (Cowper's) gland

Opening of bulbourethral duct

Uvula of bladder

Urethral crest

Openings of prostatic ducts in urethral sinus

Frontal section with urethral bulb schematically extended

Central tendon of perineum

Rectovesical (Denonvilliers') fascia

Rectum and rectal fascia

Seminal vesicle

Sagittal section

Urinary bladder

Ureter

Ductus deferens

Seminal vesicle

Ampulla of ductus deferens

Prostate

Ischiopubic ramus

Superior fascia and muscle of urogenital diaphragm

Bulbourethral (Cowper's) glands

Posterior view

Urethra

Isthmus

Utricle

Middle lobe

Lateral lobe

Seminal colliculus

Lateral lobe

Urethral sinus

Ejaculatory ducts

Posterior lobe

Prostatic fascia

Cross section through prostate

Urethra: Male

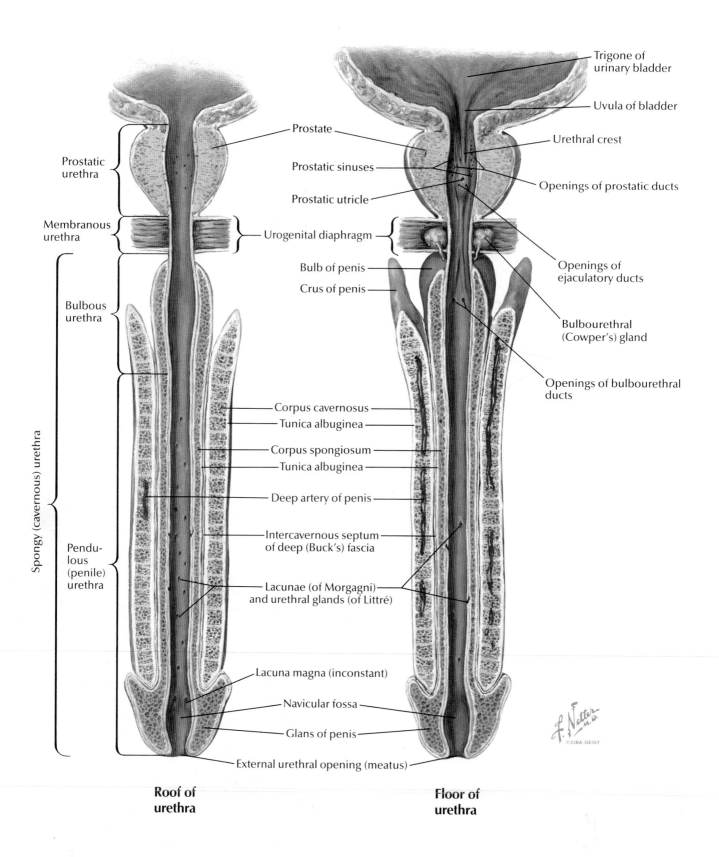

Trigone of
urinary bladder

Uvula of bladder

Prostate

Prostatic urethra

Prostatic sinuses

Prostatic utricle

Urethral crest

Openings of prostatic ducts

Membranous urethra

Urogenital diaphragm

Openings of
ejaculatory ducts

Bulb of penis

Crus of penis

Bulbourethral
(Cowper's) gland

Bulbous urethra

Openings of bulbourethral
ducts

Corpus cavernosus

Tunica albuginea

Corpus spongiosum

Tunica albuginea

Spongy (cavernous) urethra

Deep artery of penis

Intercavernous septum
of deep (Buck's) fascia

Pendu-lous
(penile)
urethra

Lacunae (of Morgagni)
and urethral glands (of Littré)

Lacuna magna (inconstant)

Navicular fossa

Glans of penis

External urethral opening (meatus)

Roof of
urethra

Floor of
urethra

PLATE 363

PELVIS AND PERINEUM

Suprarenal gland

Suspensory (diaphragmatic) ligament

Gonads

Mesonephric (Wolffian) duct

Gubernaculum

Urinary bladder

**8 weeks
(22.5-mm crown rump)**

Suprarenal gland

Kidney

Suspensory (diaphragmatic) ligament (atrophic)

Testes

Epididymis

Gubernaculum

Deep inguinal ring

Urinary bladder

**11 weeks
(43-mm crown rump)**

Testis

Epididymis

Gubernaculum

Deep inguinal ring

**4 lunar months
(107-mm crown rump)**

Superficial inguinal ring

Ductus deferens

Scrotal sac (*cut open*)

Epididymis

Testis

Gubernaculum

**8 lunar months
(26-cm crown rump)**

Scrotum and Contents

Penile skin

Superficial penile (dartos) fascia

Deep penile (Buck's) fascia

Testicular artery

Ductus deferens

Artery of ductus deferens

Genital branch of genitofemoral nerve

Pampiniform venous plexus

Epididymis

Appendix epididymidis

Appendix testis

Testis (covered by visceral layer of tunica vaginalis)

Parietal layer of tunica vaginalis

Superficial inguinal ring

External spermatic fascia

Cremaster muscle and fascia

Scrotal septum

Superficial scrotal (dartos) fascia

Scrotal skin

Superficial scrotal (dartos) fascia

External spermatic fascia

Cremaster muscle and fascia

Internal spermatic fascia

Parietal layer of tunica vaginalis

Epididymis

Testis (covered by visceral layer of tunica vaginalis)

Scrotal skin

PLATE 365

PELVIS AND PERINEUM

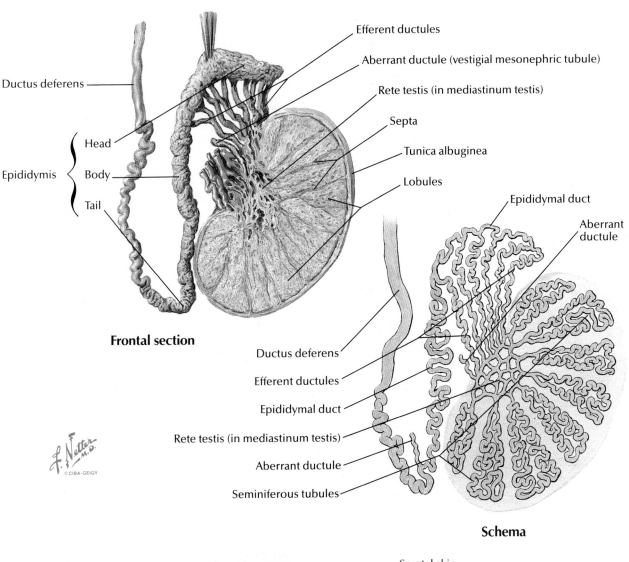

Efferent ductules

Aberrant ductule (vestigial mesonephric tubule)

Rete testis (in mediastinum testis)

Septa

Tunica albuginea

Lobules

Ductus deferens

Head

Epididymis

Body

Tail

Frontal section

Epididymal duct

Aberrant ductule

Ductus deferens

Efferent ductules

Epididymal duct

Rete testis (in mediastinum testis)

Aberrant ductule

Seminiferous tubules

Schema

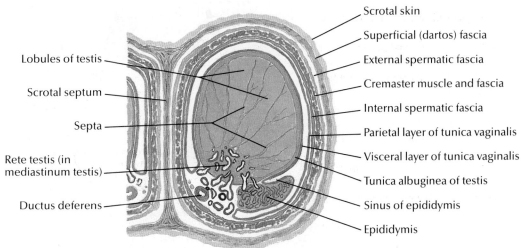

Scrotal skin

Superficial (dartos) fascia

External spermatic fascia

Cremaster muscle and fascia

Internal spermatic fascia

Parietal layer of tunica vaginalis

Visceral layer of tunica vaginalis

Tunica albuginea of testis

Sinus of epididymis

Epididymis

Lobules of testis

Scrotal septum

Septa

Rete testis (in mediastinum testis)

Ductus deferens

Cross section through scrotum and testis

Rectum In Situ: Female and Male

Male

Sigmoid colon

Sigmoid mesocolon

Rectosigmoid junction

Peritoneal reflection

Rectovesical recess

Rectum and rectal fascia

Levator ani muscle (pelvic diaphragm)

Coccyx

Puborectalis part of levator ani muscle

External anal sphincter muscle
- Deep
- Superficial
- Subcutaneous

Free tenia (tenia libera)

Ductus (vas) deferens (cut)

Ureter (cut)

Urinary bladder

Seminal vesicle

Rectovesical (Denonvilliers') fascia

Prostate

Ischiocavernosus muscle and investing (Gallaudet's) fascia (partially cut away)

Urogenital diaphragm

Superficial transverse perineal muscle and investing fascia

Central tendon of perineum

Superficial perineal (Colles') fascia

Female

Sigmoid mesocolon

Rectosigmoid junction

Peritoneal reflection

Rectal fascia and rectum

Rectouterine pouch (cul-de-sac of Douglas)

Coccyx

Levator ani muscle (pelvic diaphragm)

Puborectalis part of levator ani muscle

External anal sphincter muscle
Deep
Superficial
Subcutaneous

Sigmoid colon

Free tenia (tenia libera)

Uterus

Vesicouterine pouch

Ureter (cut)

Vagina and vaginal fascia

Urinary bladder and vesical fascia

Ischiocavernosus muscle and investing (Gallaudet's) fascia

Urogenital diaphragm

Superficial perineal (Colles') fascia

Superficial transverse perineal muscle and investing (Gallaudet's) fascia

Central tendon of perineum

PLATE 367

PELVIS AND PERINEUM

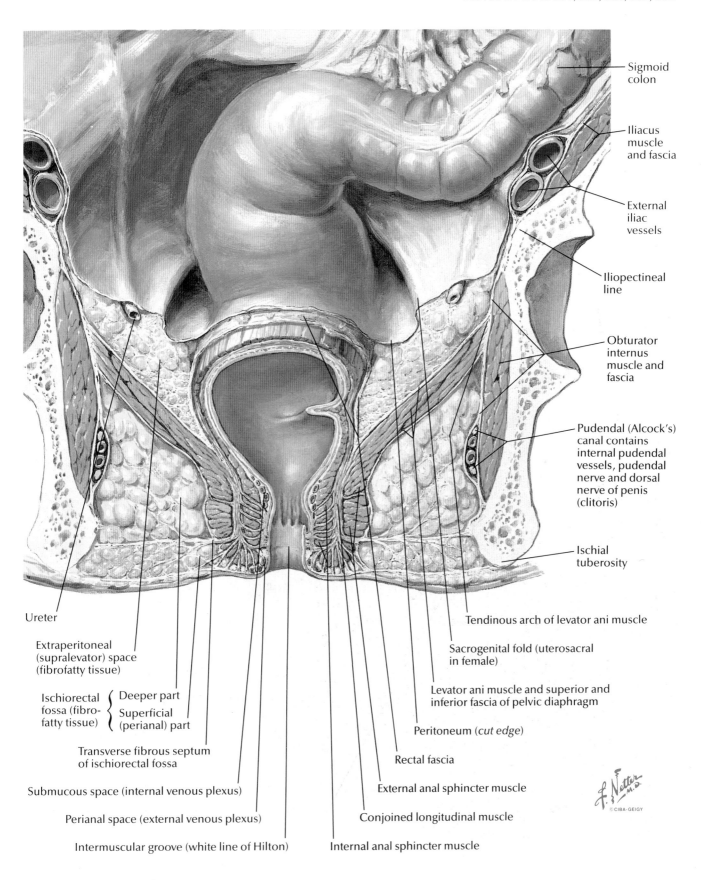

Sigmoid colon

Iliacus muscle and fascia

External iliac vessels

Iliopectineal line

Obturator internus muscle and fascia

Pudendal (Alcock's) canal contains internal pudendal vessels, pudendal nerve and dorsal nerve of penis (clitoris)

Ischial tuberosity

Tendinous arch of levator ani muscle

Sacrogenital fold (uterosacral in female)

Levator ani muscle and superior and inferior fascia of pelvic diaphragm

Peritoneum (*cut edge*)

Rectal fascia

External anal sphincter muscle

Conjoined longitudinal muscle

Internal anal sphincter muscle

Ureter

Extraperitoneal (supralevator) space (fibrofatty tissue)

Ischiorectal fossa (fibro-fatty tissue) { Deeper part / Superficial (perianal) part

Transverse fibrous septum of ischiorectal fossa

Submucous space (internal venous plexus)

Perianal space (external venous plexus)

Intermuscular groove (white line of Hilton)

Rectum and Anal Canal

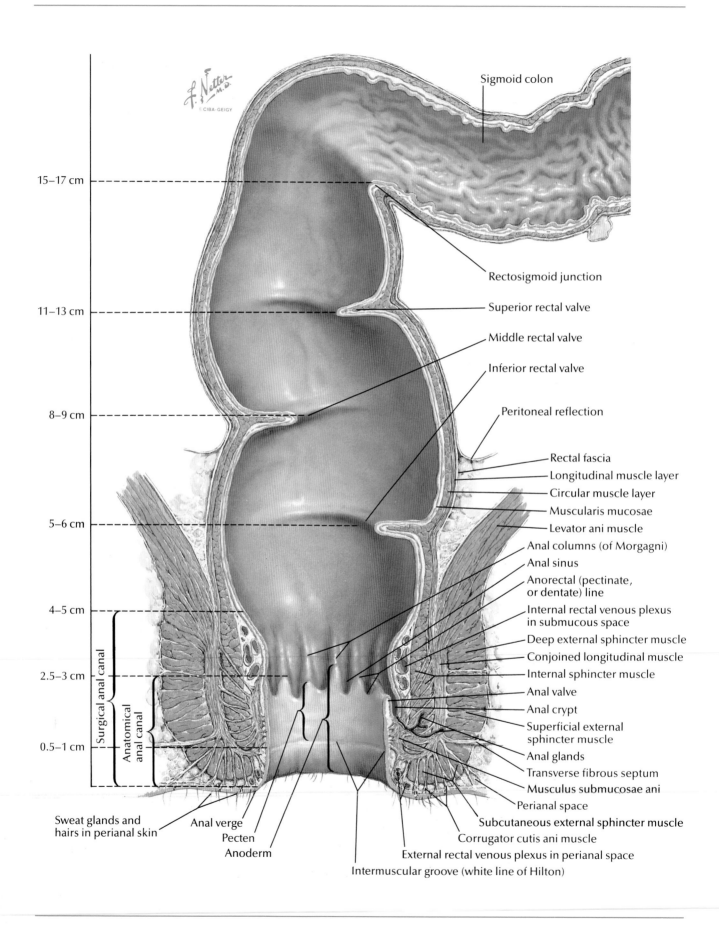

Sigmoid colon

Rectosigmoid junction

Superior rectal valve

Middle rectal valve

Inferior rectal valve

Peritoneal reflection

Rectal fascia

Longitudinal muscle layer

Circular muscle layer

Muscularis mucosae

Levator ani muscle

Anal columns (of Morgagni)

Anal sinus

Anorectal (pectinate, or dentate) line

Internal rectal venous plexus in submucous space

Deep external sphincter muscle

Conjoined longitudinal muscle

Internal sphincter muscle

Anal valve

Anal crypt

Superficial external sphincter muscle

Anal glands

Transverse fibrous septum

Musculus submucosae ani

Perianal space

Subcutaneous external sphincter muscle

Corrugator cutis ani muscle

External rectal venous plexus in perianal space

Intermuscular groove (white line of Hilton)

Sweat glands and hairs in perianal skin

Anal verge

Pecten

Anoderm

Surgical anal canal

Anatomical anal canal

15–17 cm

11–13 cm

8–9 cm

5–6 cm

4–5 cm

2.5–3 cm

0.5–1 cm

PLATE 369

PELVIS AND PERINEUM

Anterior view

Rectosigmoid junction

Sigmoid colon

Free tenia (tenia libera)

Fibers of tenia spread out to form longitudinal muscle layer of rectum

Fibers from longitudinal muscle join circular muscle layer

Window cut in longitudinal muscle layer to expose underlying Circular muscle layer

Levator ani muscle

Deep
Superficial
Subcutaneous
} External anal sphincter muscle

Fibrous septum

Corrugator cutis ani muscle

Perianal skin

Frontal section

Superior fascia of pelvic diaphragm
Inferior fascia of pelvic diaphragm
Levator ani muscle
Rectal fascia
Longitudinal muscle of rectum
Circular muscle of rectum
Muscularis mucosae of rectum
Deep external anal sphincter muscle
Internal rectal venous plexus
Conjoined longitudinal muscle
Superficial external anal sphincter muscle
Internal anal sphincter muscle
Musculus submucosae ani
Transverse fibrous septum of ischiorectal fossa
Subcutaneous external anal sphincter muscle
Corrugator cutis ani muscle

External rectal venous plexus

Intermuscular groove (white line of Hilton)

External Anal Sphincter Muscle: Perineal Views

Male

Superficial scrotal (dartos) fascia

Scrotal septum

Deep (Buck's) fascia of penis

Bulbospongiosus muscle with investing (Gallaudet's) fascia removed

Ischiocavernosus muscle with investing (Gallaudet's) fascia removed

Inferior fascia of urogenital diaphragm

Ischiopubic ramus

Central tendon of perineum

Superficial transverse perineal muscle with investing (Gallaudet's) fascia removed

Subcutaneous ⎫
Superficial ⎬ External anal sphincter muscle
Deep ⎭

Superficial perineal (Colles') fascia (*cut edges*)

Transverse fibrous septum of ischiorectal fossa (*cut*)

Ischial tuberosity

Sacrotuberous ligament

Pubococcygeus ⎫
Puborectalis ⎬ Levator ani muscle
Iliococcygeus ⎭

Anococcygeal ligament (posterior extensions of superficial external anal sphincter muscle)

Gluteus maximus muscle

Tip of coccyx

Female

Clitoris

Urethral opening

Vagina

Ischiopubic ramus

Anus

Superficial perineal (Colles') fascia (*cut edge*)

Ischiocavernosus muscle with investing (Gallaudet's) fascia removed

Bulbospongiosus muscle with investing (Gallaudet's) fascia removed

Fibers from superficial external sphincter muscle to ischiopubic ramus

Inferior fascia of urogenital diaphragm

Superficial transverse perineal muscle with investing (Gallaudet's) fascia removed

Superficial perineal (Colles') fascia (*cut edge*)

Central tendon of perineum

Crossed fibers from superficial and deep external sphincters to superficial transverse perineal muscle

External anal sphincter muscle ⎰ Deep
⎱ Superficial
  Subcutaneous

Levator ani muscle ⎰ Pubococcygeus
⎱ Puborectalis
  Iliococcygeus

Gluteus maximus muscle

Anococcygeal ligament (posterior extensions of superficial external anal sphincter muscle)

PLATE 371

PELVIS AND PERINEUM

Sagittal section

Peritoneum

Vesical fascia

Rectal fascia

Rectal fascia

Presacral fascia

Presacral space

Retropubic (prevesical) space (of Retzius)

Recto-vesical space { Retrovesical — Prerectal — Retroprostatic

Urogenital diaphragm

External anal sphincter muscle { Deep — Superficial — Subcutaneous

Deep (Buck's) fascia of penis

Superficial perineal (Colles') fascia

Rectovesical (Denonvilliers') fascia

Levator ani muscle and fascia of pelvic diaphragm

Deep postanal space

Anococcygeal ligament

Superficial postanal space (part of perianal space)

Submucous space

Perianal space

Bulbospongiosus muscle and investing (Gallaudet's) fascia

Superficial perineal space (pouch or compartment)

Urogenital diaphragm and Superficial transverse perineal muscle (*cut away*) to expose Anterior extension of ischiorectal fossa

Preanal communication (inconstant) between right and left ischiorectal fossae

Pus in ischiorectal fossa

Posterior communication between right and left ischiorectal fossae via deep postanal space deep to anococcygeal ligament

Gluteus maximus muscle and Sacrotuberous ligament (*cut away*) to expose Posterior extension of ischiorectal fossa

Perineal view

RECTUM

PLATE 372

Arteries of Rectum and Anal Canal

Posterior view

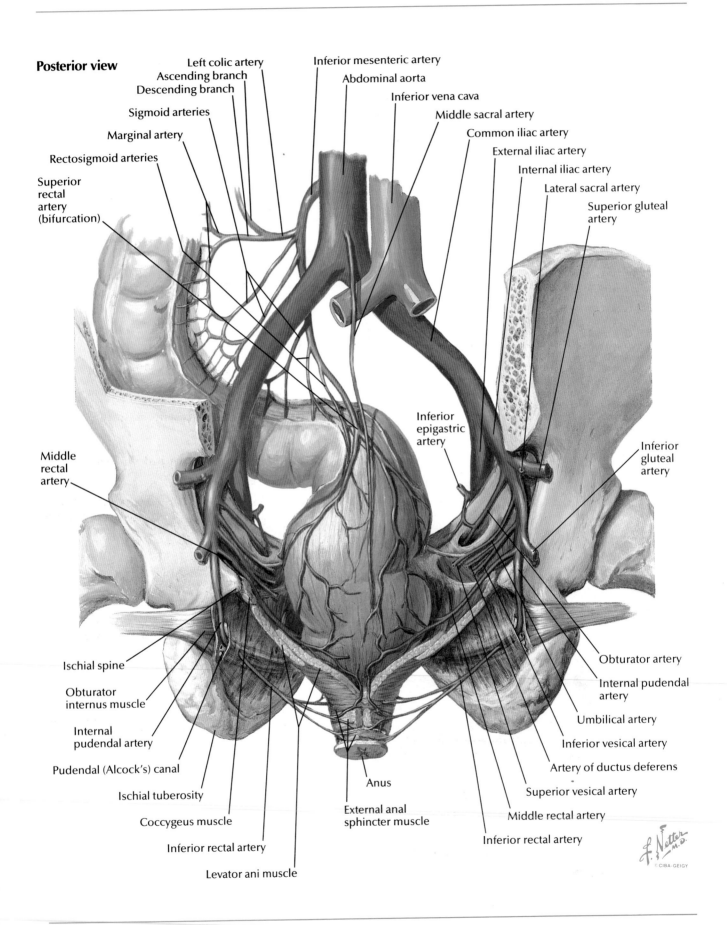

Left colic artery
Ascending branch
Descending branch
Sigmoid arteries
Marginal artery
Rectosigmoid arteries
Superior rectal artery (bifurcation)
Inferior mesenteric artery
Abdominal aorta
Inferior vena cava
Middle sacral artery
Common iliac artery
External iliac artery
Internal iliac artery
Lateral sacral artery
Superior gluteal artery
Inferior epigastric artery
Inferior gluteal artery
Middle rectal artery
Ischial spine
Obturator internus muscle
Internal pudendal artery
Pudendal (Alcock's) canal
Ischial tuberosity
Coccygeus muscle
Inferior rectal artery
Levator ani muscle
Anus
External anal sphincter muscle
Inferior rectal artery
Middle rectal artery
Superior vesical artery
Artery of ductus deferens
Inferior vesical artery
Umbilical artery
Internal pudendal artery
Obturator artery

PLATE 373

PELVIS AND PERINEUM

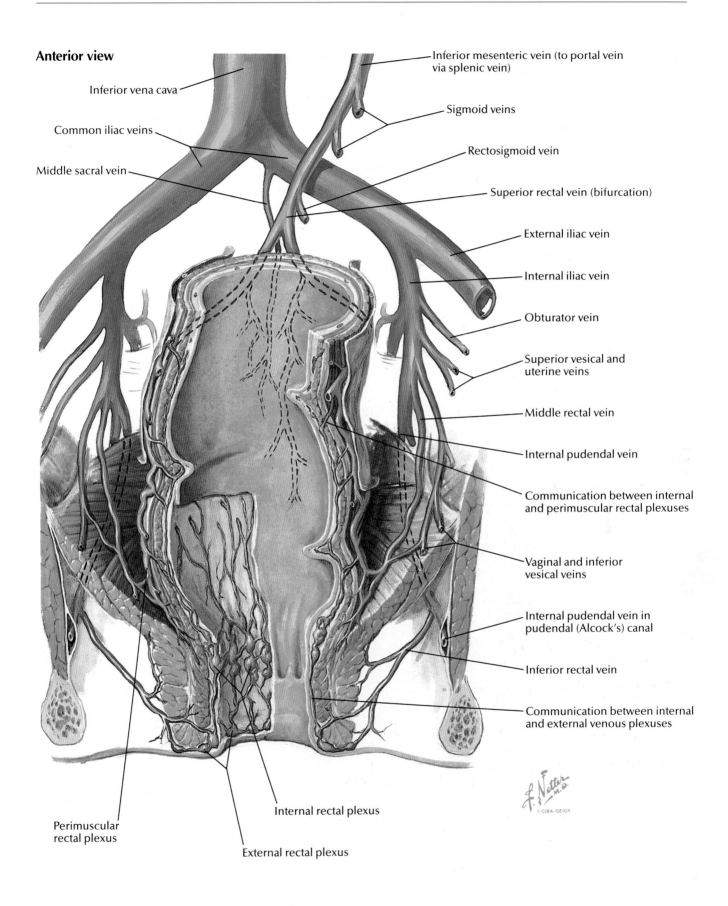

Anterior view

Inferior vena cava

Common iliac veins

Middle sacral vein

Inferior mesenteric vein (to portal vein via splenic vein)

Sigmoid veins

Rectosigmoid vein

Superior rectal vein (bifurcation)

External iliac vein

Internal iliac vein

Obturator vein

Superior vesical and uterine veins

Middle rectal vein

Internal pudendal vein

Communication between internal and perimuscular rectal plexuses

Vaginal and inferior vesical veins

Internal pudendal vein in pudendal (Alcock's) canal

Inferior rectal vein

Communication between internal and external venous plexuses

Internal rectal plexus

Perimuscular rectal plexus

External rectal plexus

Anterior view

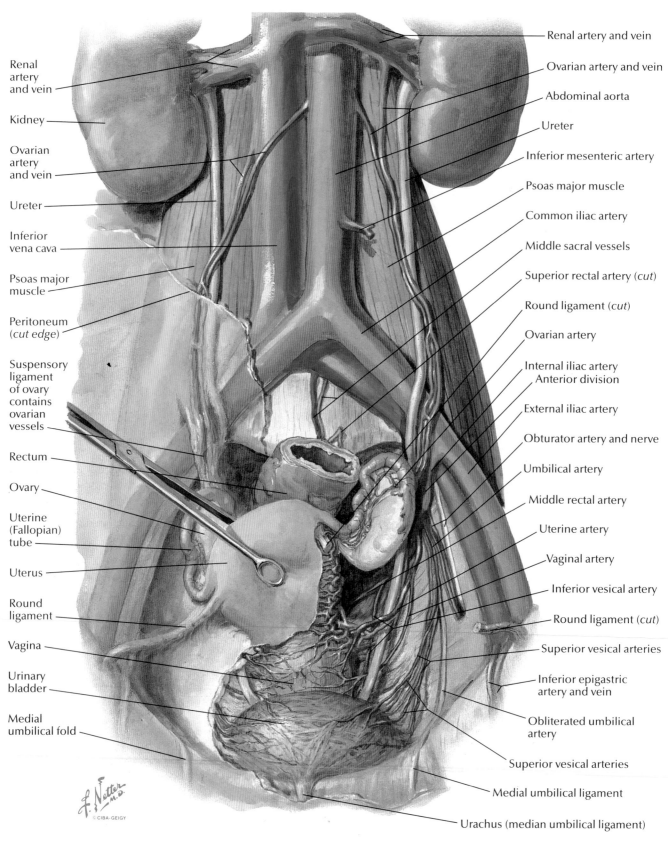

Renal artery and vein — Ovarian artery and vein — Abdominal aorta — Ureter — Inferior mesenteric artery — Psoas major muscle — Common iliac artery — Middle sacral vessels — Superior rectal artery (cut) — Round ligament (cut) — Ovarian artery — Internal iliac artery Anterior division — External iliac artery — Obturator artery and nerve — Umbilical artery — Middle rectal artery — Uterine artery — Vaginal artery — Inferior vesical artery — Round ligament (cut) — Superior vesical arteries — Inferior epigastric artery and vein — Obliterated umbilical artery — Superior vesical arteries — Medial umbilical ligament — Urachus (median umbilical ligament)

Renal artery and vein — Kidney — Ovarian artery and vein — Ureter — Inferior vena cava — Psoas major muscle — Peritoneum (cut edge) — Suspensory ligament of ovary contains ovarian vessels — Rectum — Ovary — Uterine (Fallopian) tube — Uterus — Round ligament — Vagina — Urinary bladder — Medial umbilical fold

PLATE 375

PELVIS AND PERINEUM

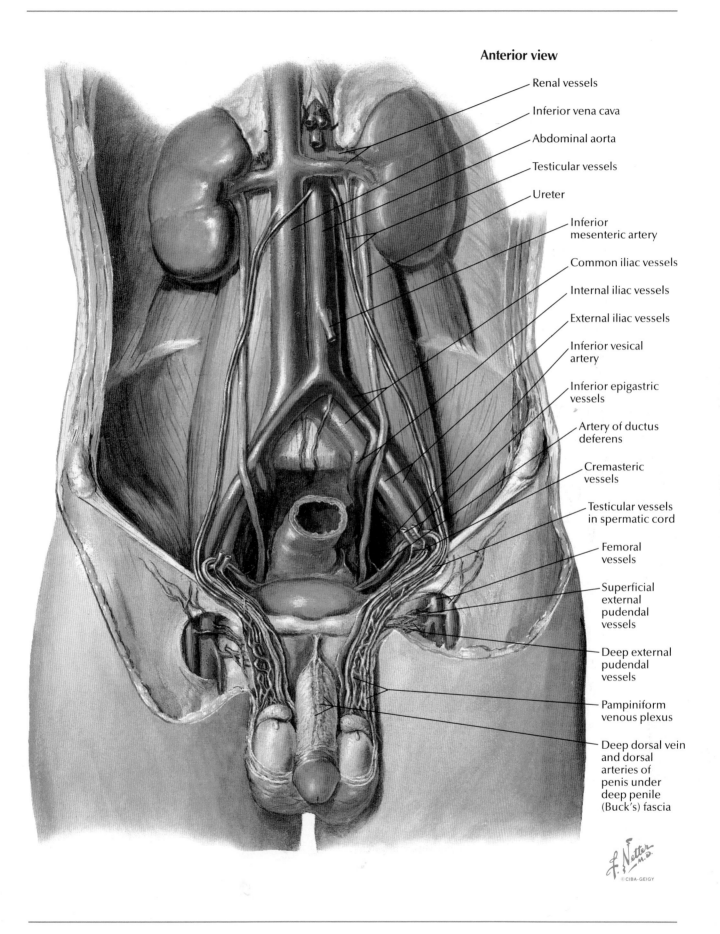

Anterior view

Renal vessels

Inferior vena cava

Abdominal aorta

Testicular vessels

Ureter

Inferior mesenteric artery

Common iliac vessels

Internal iliac vessels

External iliac vessels

Inferior vesical artery

Inferior epigastric vessels

Artery of ductus deferens

Cremasteric vessels

Testicular vessels in spermatic cord

Femoral vessels

Superficial external pudendal vessels

Deep external pudendal vessels

Pampiniform venous plexus

Deep dorsal vein and dorsal arteries of penis under deep penile (Buck's) fascia

Arteries and Veins of Pelvis: Female

Middle sacral artery

Iliolumbar artery

Lateral sacral arteries

Superior gluteal artery

Piriformis muscle

Inferior gluteal artery

Internal pudendal artery

Coccygeus muscle

Sacrotuberous ligament

Obturator internus fascia

Internal pudendal artery in pudendal (Alcock's) canal

Levator ani muscle (*cut edge*)

Abdominal aorta

Right ⎱ Common iliac
Left ⎰ arteries

Internal iliac artery
 Posterior division
 Anterior division

External iliac artery

Obturator artery

Umbilical artery

Middle rectal artery

Uterine artery

Vaginal artery

Inferior vesical artery

Superior vesical arteries

Obliterated umbilical artery (medial umbilical ligament)

Pubic symphysis

Sagittal section

Right paramedian section: lateral view

Abdominal aorta

Inferior vena cava

Right common iliac artery

Left common iliac artery

Ureters

External iliac artery (*cut*)

Internal iliac artery
 Posterior division
 Anterior division

Superior gluteal artery

Obturator artery

Umbilical artery

Piriformis muscle

Internal pudendal artery

Inferior gluteal artery

Coccygeus muscle

Middle rectal artery

Uterine artery

Vaginal artery

Inferior vesical artery

Internal pudendal artery

Inferior rectal artery

Superior vesical arteries

Obliterated umbilical artery

Obturator canal

Obturator internus muscle

Levator ani muscle

PLATE 377

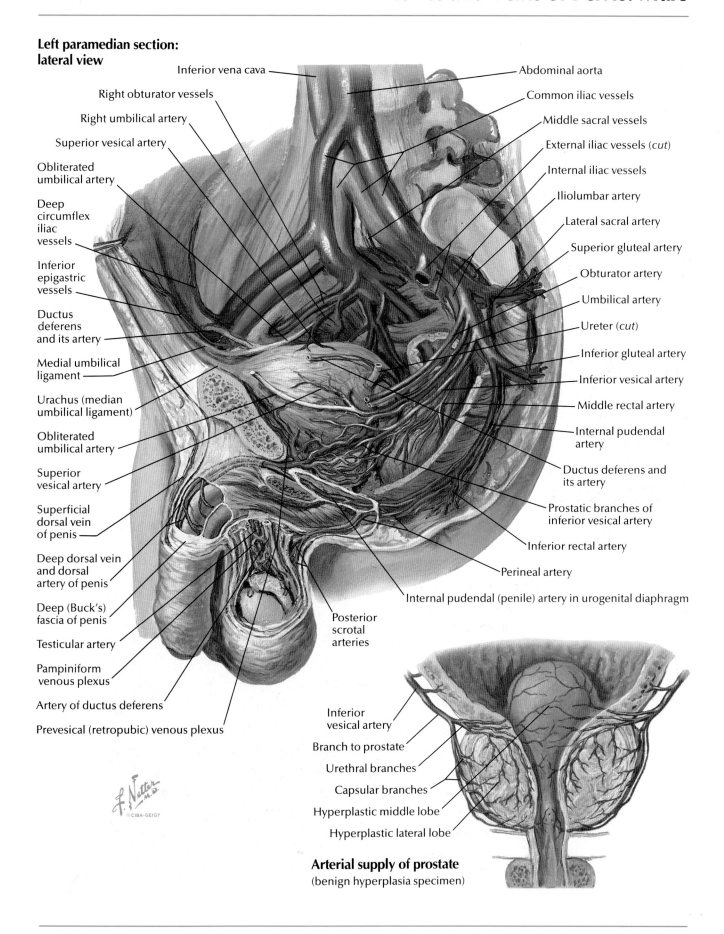

Left paramedian section: lateral view

Inferior vena cava

Right obturator vessels

Right umbilical artery

Superior vesical artery

Obliterated umbilical artery

Deep circumflex iliac vessels

Inferior epigastric vessels

Ductus deferens and its artery

Medial umbilical ligament

Urachus (median umbilical ligament)

Obliterated umbilical artery

Superior vesical artery

Superficial dorsal vein of penis

Deep dorsal vein and dorsal artery of penis

Deep (Buck's) fascia of penis

Testicular artery

Pampiniform venous plexus

Artery of ductus deferens

Prevesical (retropubic) venous plexus

Abdominal aorta

Common iliac vessels

Middle sacral vessels

External iliac vessels (*cut*)

Internal iliac vessels

Iliolumbar artery

Lateral sacral artery

Superior gluteal artery

Obturator artery

Umbilical artery

Ureter (*cut*)

Inferior gluteal artery

Inferior vesical artery

Middle rectal artery

Internal pudendal artery

Ductus deferens and its artery

Prostatic branches of inferior vesical artery

Inferior rectal artery

Perineal artery

Internal pudendal (penile) artery in urogenital diaphragm

Posterior scrotal arteries

Inferior vesical artery

Branch to prostate

Urethral branches

Capsular branches

Hyperplastic middle lobe

Hyperplastic lateral lobe

Arterial supply of prostate
(benign hyperplasia specimen)

Arteries and Veins of Perineum and Uterus

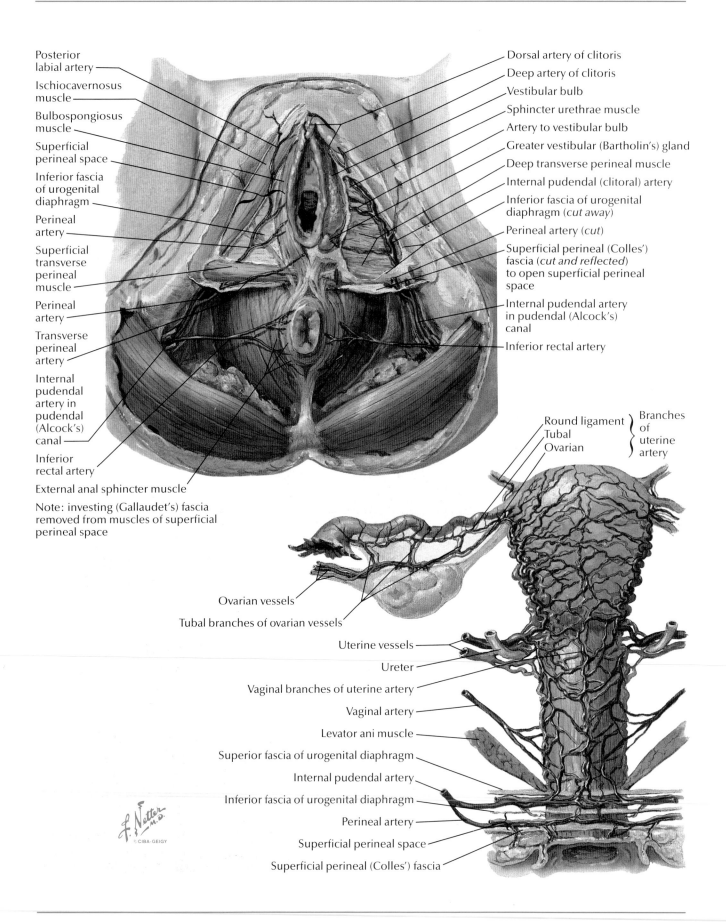

Posterior labial artery

Ischiocavernosus muscle

Bulbospongiosus muscle

Superficial perineal space

Inferior fascia of urogenital diaphragm

Perineal artery

Superficial transverse perineal muscle

Perineal artery

Transverse perineal artery

Internal pudendal artery in pudendal (Alcock's) canal

Inferior rectal artery

External anal sphincter muscle

Note: investing (Gallaudet's) fascia removed from muscles of superficial perineal space

Dorsal artery of clitoris

Deep artery of clitoris

Vestibular bulb

Sphincter urethrae muscle

Artery to vestibular bulb

Greater vestibular (Bartholin's) gland

Deep transverse perineal muscle

Internal pudendal (clitoral) artery

Inferior fascia of urogenital diaphragm (*cut away*)

Perineal artery (*cut*)

Superficial perineal (Colles') fascia (*cut and reflected*) to open superficial perineal space

Internal pudendal artery in pudendal (Alcock's) canal

Inferior rectal artery

Round ligament ⎫
Tubal   ⎬ Branches of uterine artery
Ovarian   ⎭

Ovarian vessels

Tubal branches of ovarian vessels

Uterine vessels

Ureter

Vaginal branches of uterine artery

Vaginal artery

Levator ani muscle

Superior fascia of urogenital diaphragm

Internal pudendal artery

Inferior fascia of urogenital diaphragm

Perineal artery

Superficial perineal space

Superficial perineal (Colles') fascia

PLATE 379

PELVIS AND PERINEUM

External spermatic fascia over testis and spermatic cord

Bulbospongiosus muscle

Ischiocavernosus muscle

Inferior fascia of urogenital diaphragm

Central tendon of perineum

Superficial transverse perineal muscle

Transverse perineal artery

Superficial perineal (Colles') fascia (cut edge)

Pudendal (Alcock's) canal

Note: investing (Gallaudet's) fascia removed from muscles of superficial perineal space

Superficial scrotal (dartos) fascia

Scrotal septum

Posterior scrotal arteries

Deep (Buck's) fascia of penis

Superficial perineal (Colles') fascia (cut edge)

Superficial perineal space (opened)

Perineal artery and vein

Posterior fused fascia of urogenital diaphragm

Internal pudendal artery enters urogenital diaphragm

Superficial transverse perineal muscle and transverse perineal artery (cut and reflected)

Internal pudendal vessels and pudendal nerve (cut) in pudendal (Alcock's) canal (opened up)

Inferior rectal artery

Inferior fascia of pelvic diaphragm (roof of ischiorectal fossa)

Deep artery of penis

Deep dorsal vein of penis

Dorsal artery and nerve of penis

Transverse perineal ligament (anterior fused fascia of urogenital diaphragm)

Deep artery of penis

Dorsal artery of penis

Urethral artery

Inferior fascia of urogenital diaphragm (cut edge)

Artery of bulb of penis

Internal pudendal artery

Perineal artery (cut)

Internal pudendal vessels in pudendal (Alcock's) canal

Superficial perineal (Colles') fascia (cut edge)

Lymph Vessels and Nodes of Pelvis and Genitalia: Female

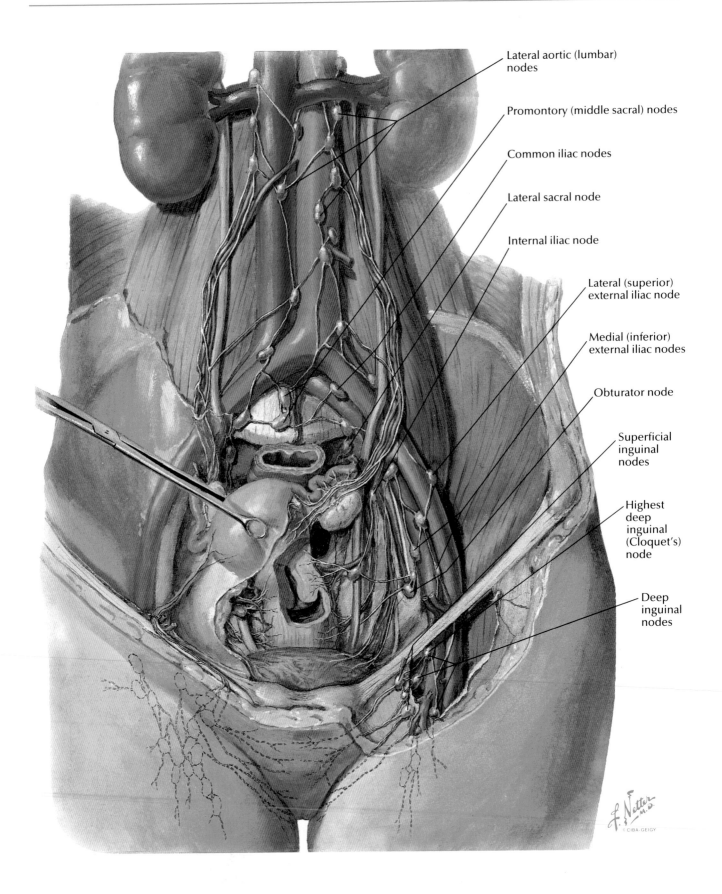

Lateral aortic (lumbar) nodes

Promontory (middle sacral) nodes

Common iliac nodes

Lateral sacral node

Internal iliac node

Lateral (superior) external iliac node

Medial (inferior) external iliac nodes

Obturator node

Superficial inguinal nodes

Highest deep inguinal (Cloquet's) node

Deep inguinal nodes

PLATE 381

PELVIS AND PERINEUM

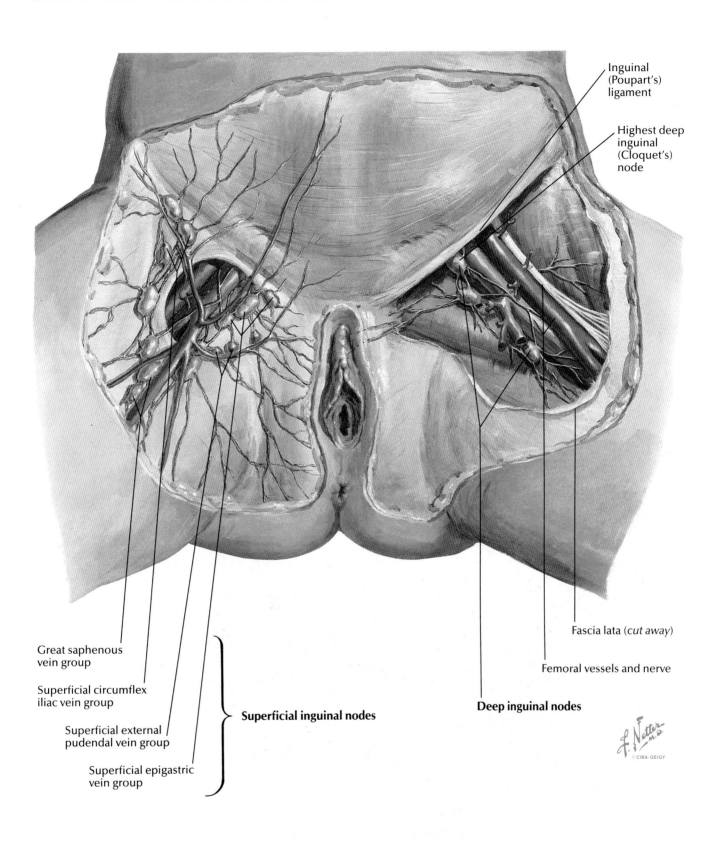

Inguinal (Poupart's) ligament

Highest deep inguinal (Cloquet's) node

Fascia lata (*cut away*)

Femoral vessels and nerve

Deep inguinal nodes

Great saphenous vein group

Superficial circumflex iliac vein group

Superficial external pudendal vein group

Superficial epigastric vein group

Superficial inguinal nodes

Lymph Vessels and Nodes of Pelvis and Genitalia: Male

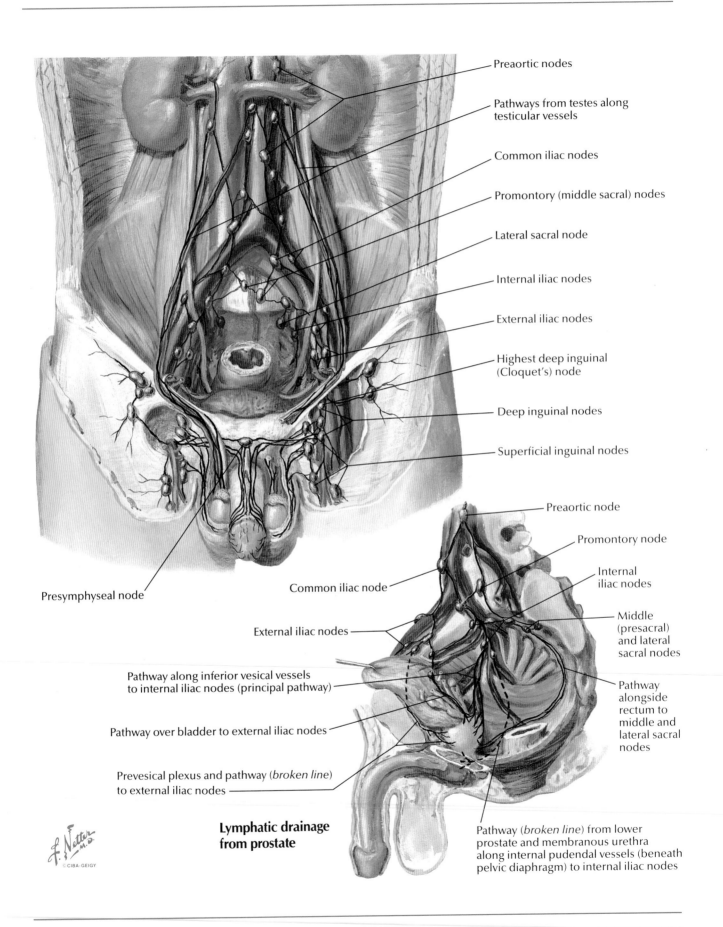

Preaortic nodes

Pathways from testes along testicular vessels

Common iliac nodes

Promontory (middle sacral) nodes

Lateral sacral node

Internal iliac nodes

External iliac nodes

Highest deep inguinal (Cloquet's) node

Deep inguinal nodes

Superficial inguinal nodes

Presymphyseal node

Preaortic node

Promontory node

Internal iliac nodes

Middle (presacral) and lateral sacral nodes

Common iliac node

External iliac nodes

Pathway alongside rectum to middle and lateral sacral nodes

Pathway along inferior vesical vessels to internal iliac nodes (principal pathway)

Pathway over bladder to external iliac nodes

Prevesical plexus and pathway (*broken line*) to external iliac nodes

Lymphatic drainage from prostate

Pathway (*broken line*) from lower prostate and membranous urethra along internal pudendal vessels (beneath pelvic diaphragm) to internal iliac nodes

PLATE 383

PELVIS AND PERINEUM

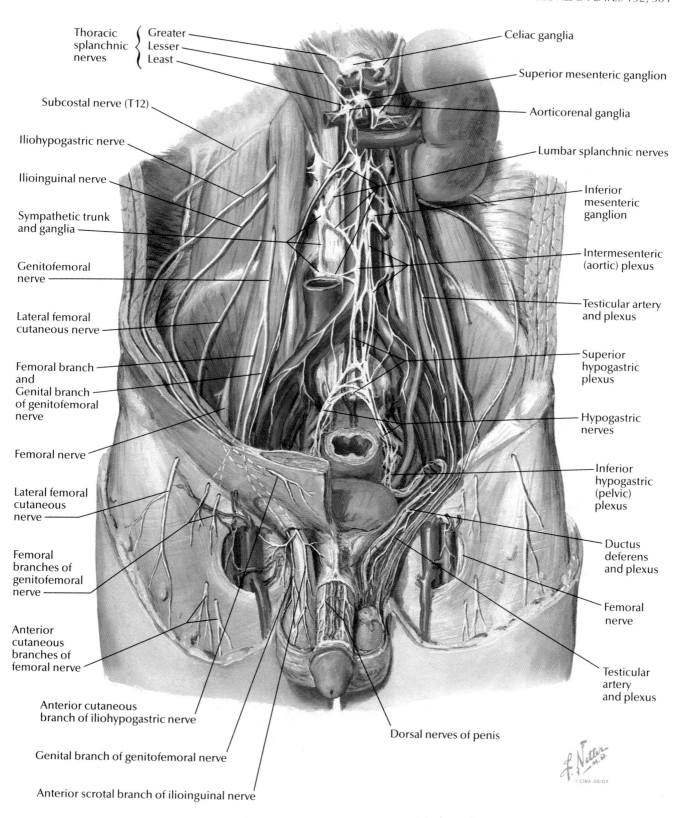

Thoracic splanchnic nerves { Greater — Lesser — Least }

Subcostal nerve (T12)

Iliohypogastric nerve

Ilioinguinal nerve

Sympathetic trunk and ganglia

Genitofemoral nerve

Lateral femoral cutaneous nerve

Femoral branch and Genital branch of genitofemoral nerve

Femoral nerve

Lateral femoral cutaneous nerve

Femoral branches of genitofemoral nerve

Anterior cutaneous branches of femoral nerve

Anterior cutaneous branch of iliohypogastric nerve

Genital branch of genitofemoral nerve

Anterior scrotal branch of ilioinguinal nerve

Celiac ganglia

Superior mesenteric ganglion

Aorticorenal ganglia

Lumbar splanchnic nerves

Inferior mesenteric ganglion

Intermesenteric (aortic) plexus

Testicular artery and plexus

Superior hypogastric plexus

Hypogastric nerves

Inferior hypogastric (pelvic) plexus

Ductus deferens and plexus

Femoral nerve

Testicular artery and plexus

Dorsal nerves of penis

Anterior vagal trunk

Posterior vagal trunk
and
Celiac branch

Inferior phrenic arteries and plexuses

Left gastric artery and plexus

Celiac ganglia, plexus and trunk

Left aorticorenal ganglion

Superior mesenteric ganglion

Superior mesenteric artery and plexus

Intermesenteric (aortic) plexus

Inferior mesenteric ganglion,
artery and plexus

Ureter and ureteric plexus

Superior hypogastric plexus

Superior rectal artery and plexus

Hypogastric nerves

Nerve from pelvic plexus
to sigmoid and descending
colon (parasympathetic)

Sacral splanchnic nerves
(sympathetic)

Inferior hypogastric
(pelvic) plexus

Obturator nerve
and artery

Ductus deferens
and plexus

Vesical plexus

Rectal plexus

Prostatic plexus

Cavernous nerves
Greater
Lesser

10th thoracic nerve (ventral ramus)

White and gray rami communicantes

Greater ⎫
Lesser ⎬ Thoracic splanchnic nerves
Least ⎭

Diaphragm

Left renal artery
and plexus

1st lumbar nerve
(ventral ramus)

Gray ⎫ Rami
White ⎬ communicantes

1st, 2nd, 3rd lumbar splanchnic nerves

Gray rami communicantes

Sympathetic trunk and ganglia

5th lumbar splanchnic nerve

5th lumbar nerve (ventral ramus)

Lumbosacral trunk

Gray rami communicantes

1st sacral nerve
(ventral ramus)

Pelvic splanchnic
nerves
(nervi erigentes)
(parasympathetic)

Sacral plexus

Piriformis muscle

Gluteus maximus
muscle and sacro-
tuberous ligament

Coccygeus muscle and
sacrospinous ligament

Pudendal nerve

Levator ani muscle

Inferior rectal nerve

Perineal nerve

Dorsal nerve of penis

Posterior scrotal nerves

PLATE 385

PELVIS AND PERINEUM

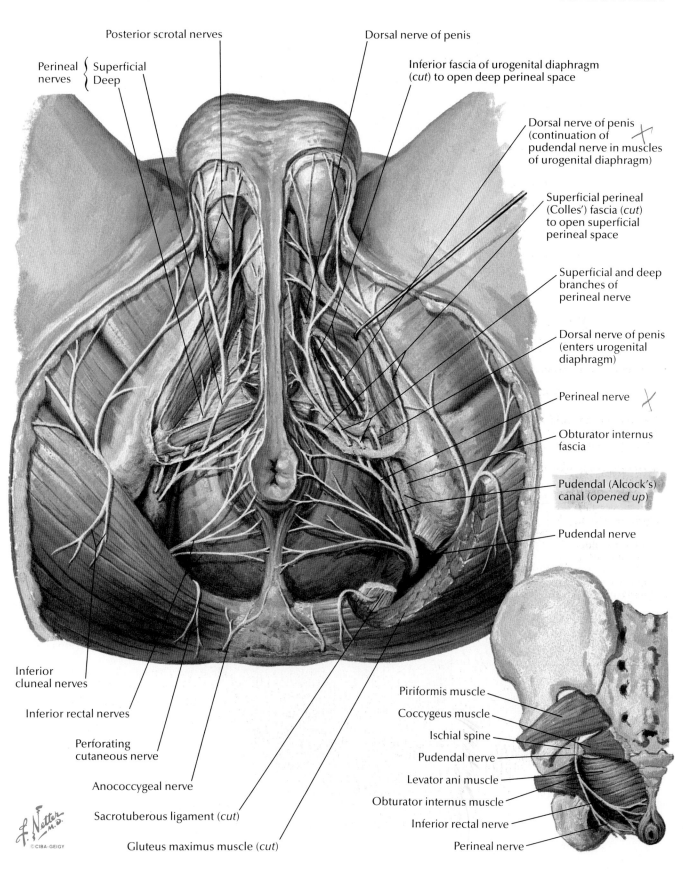

Posterior scrotal nerves

Dorsal nerve of penis

Perineal nerves { Superficial / Deep }

Inferior fascia of urogenital diaphragm (*cut*) to open deep perineal space

Dorsal nerve of penis (continuation of pudendal nerve in muscles of urogenital diaphragm)

Superficial perineal (Colles') fascia (*cut*) to open superficial perineal space

Superficial and deep branches of perineal nerve

Dorsal nerve of penis (enters urogenital diaphragm)

Perineal nerve

Obturator internus fascia

Pudendal (Alcock's) canal (*opened up*)

Pudendal nerve

Inferior cluneal nerves

Inferior rectal nerves

Perforating cutaneous nerve

Anococcygeal nerve

Sacrotuberous ligament (*cut*)

Gluteus maximus muscle (*cut*)

Piriformis muscle

Coccygeus muscle

Ischial spine

Pudendal nerve

Levator ani muscle

Obturator internus muscle

Inferior rectal nerve

Perineal nerve

Nerves of Pelvic Viscera: Female

SEE ALSO PLATES 152, 304

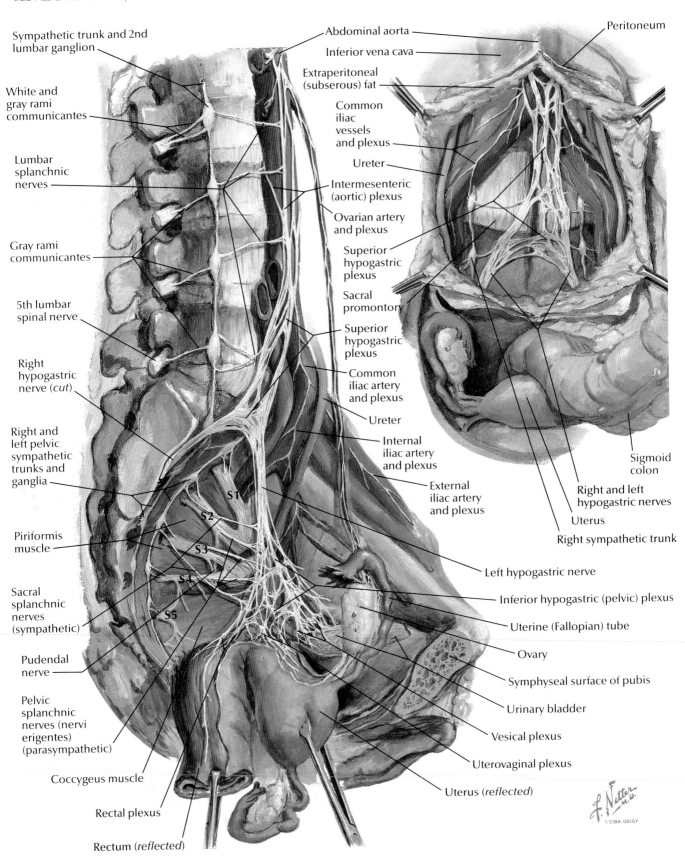

Sympathetic trunk and 2nd lumbar ganglion

White and gray rami communicantes

Lumbar splanchnic nerves

Gray rami communicantes

5th lumbar spinal nerve

Right hypogastric nerve (cut)

Right and left pelvic sympathetic trunks and ganglia

Piriformis muscle

Sacral splanchnic nerves (sympathetic)

Pudendal nerve

Pelvic splanchnic nerves (nervi erigentes) (parasympathetic)

Coccygeus muscle

Rectal plexus

Rectum (reflected)

Abdominal aorta

Inferior vena cava

Extraperitoneal (subserous) fat

Common iliac vessels and plexus

Ureter

Intermesenteric (aortic) plexus

Ovarian artery and plexus

Superior hypogastric plexus

Sacral promontory

Superior hypogastric plexus

Common iliac artery and plexus

Ureter

Internal iliac artery and plexus

External iliac artery and plexus

Peritoneum

Sigmoid colon

Right and left hypogastric nerves

Uterus

Right sympathetic trunk

Left hypogastric nerve

Inferior hypogastric (pelvic) plexus

Uterine (Fallopian) tube

Ovary

Symphyseal surface of pubis

Urinary bladder

Vesical plexus

Uterovaginal plexus

Uterus (reflected)

S1
S2
S3
S4
S5

PLATE 387

PELVIS AND PERINEUM

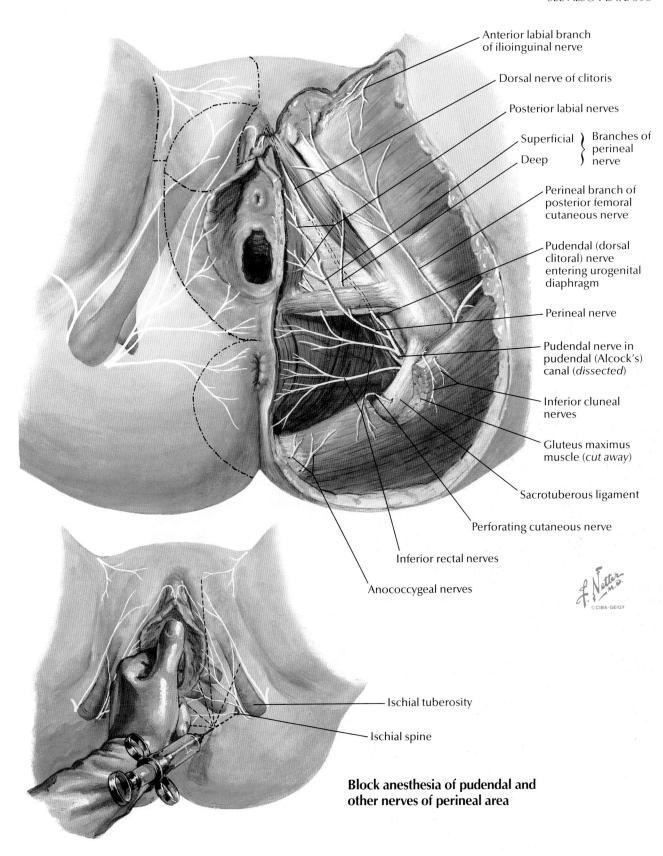

Anterior labial branch
of ilioinguinal nerve

Dorsal nerve of clitoris

Posterior labial nerves

Superficial } Branches of
perineal
Deep } nerve

Perineal branch of
posterior femoral
cutaneous nerve

Pudendal (dorsal
clitoral) nerve
entering urogenital
diaphragm

Perineal nerve

Pudendal nerve in
pudendal (Alcock's)
canal (*dissected*)

Inferior cluneal
nerves

Gluteus maximus
muscle (*cut away*)

Sacrotuberous ligament

Perforating cutaneous nerve

Inferior rectal nerves

Anococcygeal nerves

Ischial tuberosity

Ischial spine

**Block anesthesia of pudendal and
other nerves of perineal area**

Neuropathways in Parturition

SEE ALSO PLATE 152

Thoracic splanchnic nerves
- Greater
- Lesser
- Least

Celiac ganglion

Aorticorenal ganglion

Superior mesenteric ganglion

Intermesenteric (aortic) plexus

Lumbar splanchnic nerves

Iliohypogastric nerve (L1)

Ilioinguinal nerve (L1)

Vesical plexus

Dorsal nerve of clitoris

Posterior labial nerves

7th thoracic nerve (ventral ramus)

Sympathetic trunk and ganglia

11th thoracic nerve (ventral ramus)

Rami communicantes

Subcostal nerve (T12)

Inferior mesenteric ganglion

Intermesenteric (aortic) plexus

Superior hypogastric plexus

1st sacral nerve (ventral ramus)

Hypogastric nerves

Pelvic splanchnic nerves

Inferior hypogastric (pelvic) plexus

Uterovaginal plexus

Pudendal nerve (S2, 3, 4)

Inferior rectal nerve

——— Sensory fibers from uterine body and fundus accompany sympathetic fibers via pelvic plexus to T11, 12 (L1?)

——— Motor fibers to uterine body and fundus (sympathetic)

•••••• Sensory fibers from cervix and upper vagina accompany pelvic splanchnic nerves (parasympathetic) to S2, 3, 4

•••••• Motor fibers to lower uterine segment, cervix and upper vagina (parasympathetic)

– – – – Sensory fibers from lower vagina and perineum accompany somatic fibers via pudendal nerve to S2, 3, 4

– – – – Motor fibers to lower vagina and perineum via pudendal nerve (somatic)

PLATE 389

PELVIS AND PERINEUM

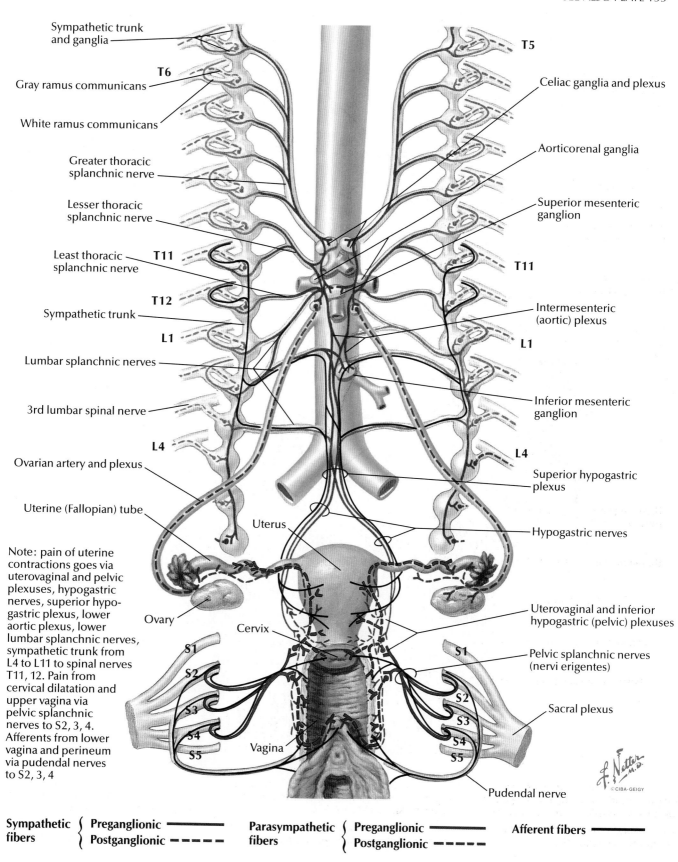

Sympathetic trunk and ganglia

T5

T6

Gray ramus communicans

White ramus communicans

Celiac ganglia and plexus

Greater thoracic splanchnic nerve

Aorticorenal ganglia

Lesser thoracic splanchnic nerve

Superior mesenteric ganglion

Least thoracic splanchnic nerve

T11

T11

T12

Sympathetic trunk

Intermesenteric (aortic) plexus

L1

L1

Lumbar splanchnic nerves

Inferior mesenteric ganglion

3rd lumbar spinal nerve

L4

L4

Ovarian artery and plexus

Superior hypogastric plexus

Uterine (Fallopian) tube

Uterus

Hypogastric nerves

Note: pain of uterine contractions goes via uterovaginal and pelvic plexuses, hypogastric nerves, superior hypo-gastric plexus, lower aortic plexus, lower lumbar splanchnic nerves, sympathetic trunk from L4 to L11 to spinal nerves T11, 12. Pain from cervical dilatation and upper vagina via pelvic splanchnic nerves to S2, 3, 4. Afferents from lower vagina and perineum via pudendal nerves to S2, 3, 4

Ovary

Cervix

Uterovaginal and inferior hypogastric (pelvic) plexuses

S1

S1

S2

S2

S3

S3

Pelvic splanchnic nerves (nervi erigentes)

Sacral plexus

S4

S4

Vagina

S5

S5

Pudendal nerve

Sympathetic fibers	Preganglionic ———	Parasympathetic fibers	Preganglionic ———	Afferent fibers ———
	Postganglionic ----		Postganglionic ----	

Innervation of Male Reproductive Organs: Schema

SEE ALSO PLATE 153

Sympathetic trunk and ganglia

Greater thoracic splanchnic nerve (T5–9)

Gray ramus communicans

White ramus communicans

Lesser thoracic splanchnic nerve

Least thoracic splanchnic nerve

Upper lumbar splanchnic nerves

Gray ramus communicans

Testicular artery and plexus

Ductus deferens and plexus

Pelvic splanchnic nerves (nervi erigentes)

Sacral plexus

Pudendal nerve

Inferior hypogastric (pelvic) plexus

Vesical plexus

Prostatic plexus

Greater and lesser cavernous nerves

T10

T11

T12

L1

L2

L3

L4

S1

S2

S3

S4

S5

Celiac ganglia

Superior mesenteric ganglion

Left aorticorenal ganglion

Renal ganglion

Intermesenteric (aortic) plexus

Inferior mesenteric ganglion

Testicular artery and plexus

Superior hypogastric plexus

Hypogastric nerves

Ductus deferens and plexus

Pelvic splanchnic nerves (nervi erigentes)

Sacral plexus

Pudendal nerve

Dorsal nerves of penis

Epididymis

Testis

S1

S2

S3

S4

S5

| Sympathetic fibers | Preganglionic —————
Postganglionic - - - - - | Parasympathetic fibers | Preganglionic —————
Postganglionic - - - - - | Afferent fibers ————— |

PLATE 391

PELVIS AND PERINEUM

Innervation of Urinary Bladder and Lower Ureter: Schema

SEE ALSO PLATE 153

Spinal ganglia

Dorsal root

Ventral root

White } Rami
Gray } communicantes

Renal ganglion

Celiac ganglia

Superior mesenteric ganglion

Aorticorenal ganglion

Renal artery and plexus

Intermesenteric (aortic) plexus

Inferior mesenteric ganglion

Superior hypogastric plexus

Hypogastric nerves

Inferior hypogastric (pelvic) plexus

Urinary bladder

1st and 2nd lumbar splanchnic nerves

Lumbar part of spinal cord

2nd lumbar spinal nerve

Sacral part of spinal cord

Ureter

Sacral splanchnic nerves from sacral sympathetic trunk to inferior hypogastric (pelvic) plexus

Sympathetic trunk

Ascending fibers

Descending fibers

Gray rami communicantes

S2

S3

S4

Pudendal nerve

Vesical plexus

Sacral plexus

Prostatic plexus

Pelvic splanchnic nerves (nervi erigentes)

Sphincter muscle of membranous urethra between fascial layers of urogenital diaphragm

Bulbospongiosus muscle

Sympathetic fibers { Preganglionic ———— Postganglionic – – – –

Parasympathetic fibers { Preganglionic ———— Postganglionic – – – –

Somatic efferent fibers ————
Afferent fibers ————

Homologues of External Genitalia

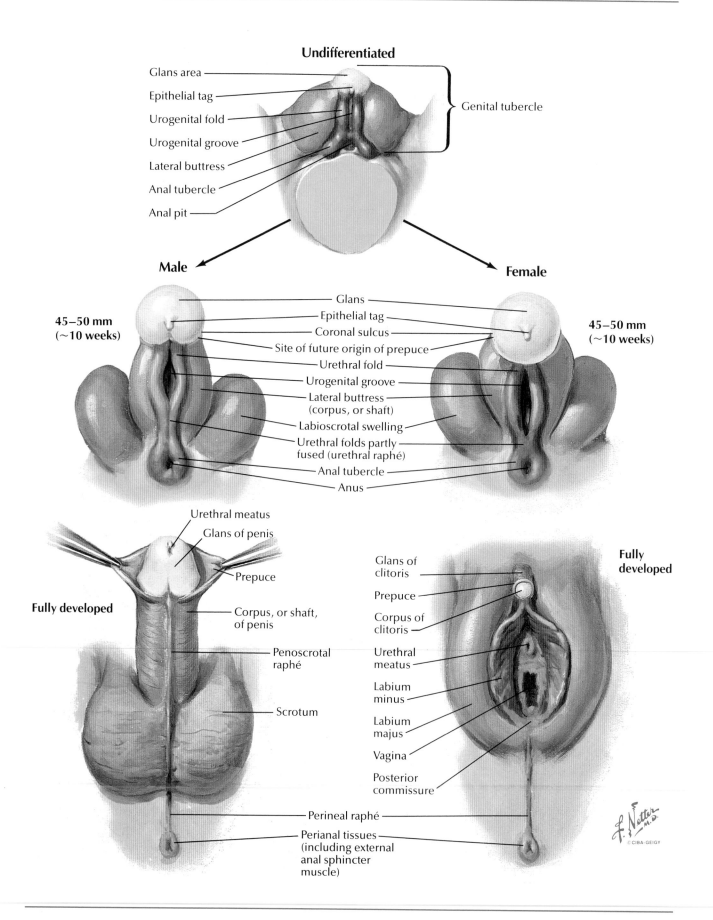

Undifferentiated

Glans area

Epithelial tag

Urogenital fold

Urogenital groove

Lateral buttress

Anal tubercle

Anal pit

Genital tubercle

Male

Female

45–50 mm
(~10 weeks)

45–50 mm
(~10 weeks)

Glans

Epithelial tag

Coronal sulcus

Site of future origin of prepuce

Urethral fold

Urogenital groove

Lateral buttress
(corpus, or shaft)

Labioscrotal swelling

Urethral folds partly
fused (urethral raphé)

Anal tubercle

Anus

Urethral meatus

Glans of penis

Prepuce

Fully developed

Corpus, or shaft,
of penis

Penoscrotal
raphé

Scrotum

**Fully
developed**

Glans of
clitoris

Prepuce

Corpus of
clitoris

Urethral
meatus

Labium
minus

Labium
majus

Vagina

Posterior
commissure

Perineal raphé

Perianal tissues
(including external
anal sphincter
muscle)

PLATE 393

PELVIS AND PERINEUM

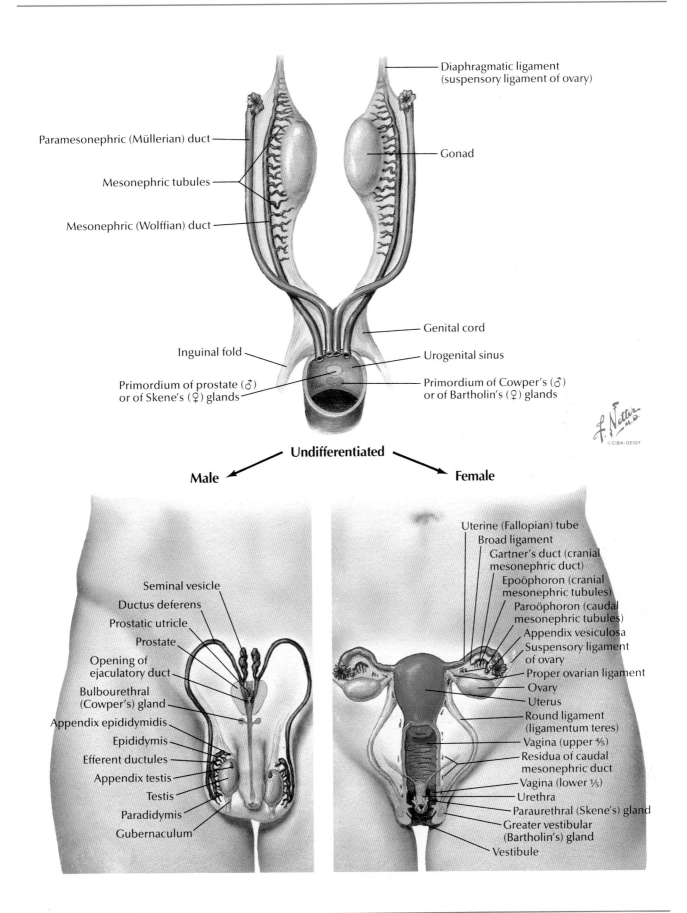

Diaphragmatic ligament (suspensory ligament of ovary)

Paramesonephric (Müllerian) duct

Mesonephric tubules

Mesonephric (Wolffian) duct

Gonad

Genital cord

Inguinal fold

Urogenital sinus

Primordium of prostate (♂) or of Skene's (♀) glands

Primordium of Cowper's (♂) or of Bartholin's (♀) glands

Undifferentiated

Male

Female

Seminal vesicle

Ductus deferens

Prostatic utricle

Prostate

Opening of ejaculatory duct

Bulbourethral (Cowper's) gland

Appendix epididymidis

Epididymis

Efferent ductules

Appendix testis

Testis

Paradidymis

Gubernaculum

Uterine (Fallopian) tube

Broad ligament

Gartner's duct (cranial mesonephric duct)

Epoöphoron (cranial mesonephric tubules)

Paroöphoron (caudal mesonephric tubules)

Appendix vesiculosa

Suspensory ligament of ovary

Proper ovarian ligament

Ovary

Uterus

Round ligament (ligamentum teres)

Vagina (upper ⅘)

Residua of caudal mesonephric duct

Vagina (lower ⅕)

Urethra

Paraurethral (Skene's) gland

Greater vestibular (Bartholin's) gland

Vestibule

Section VI

UPPER LIMB

Right clavicle

Superior surface

Acromial extremity

Posterior

Anterior

Sternal extremity

Inferior surface

Acromial extremity

Anterior

Impression for costoclavicular ligament (costal tubercle)

Trapezoid line

Posterior

Sternal extremity

Conoid tubercle

Groove for subclavius muscle

Trapezius muscle

Superior surface

Muscle origins
Muscle insertions
Ligament attachments

Posterior

Sternocleidomastoid muscle

Deltoid muscle

Anterior

Deltoid muscle

Pectoralis major muscle

Inferior surface

Pectoralis major muscle

Anterior

Costoclavicular ligament

Coracoclavicular ligament

Trapezoid ligament

Posterior

Conoid ligament

Subclavius muscle

Sternohyoid muscle

Sternoclavicular joint

Anterior sternoclavicular ligament

Interclavicular ligament

Articular disc

Clavicle

Joint cavity

Subclavius muscle

Costoclavicular ligament

1st rib

Sternocostal synchondrosis

Costal cartilages

Manubrium

Sternocostal synovial joint

2nd rib

Radiate sternocostal ligament

Sternal synchondrosis

Humerus and Scapula: Anterior Views

SEE ALSO PLATE 170

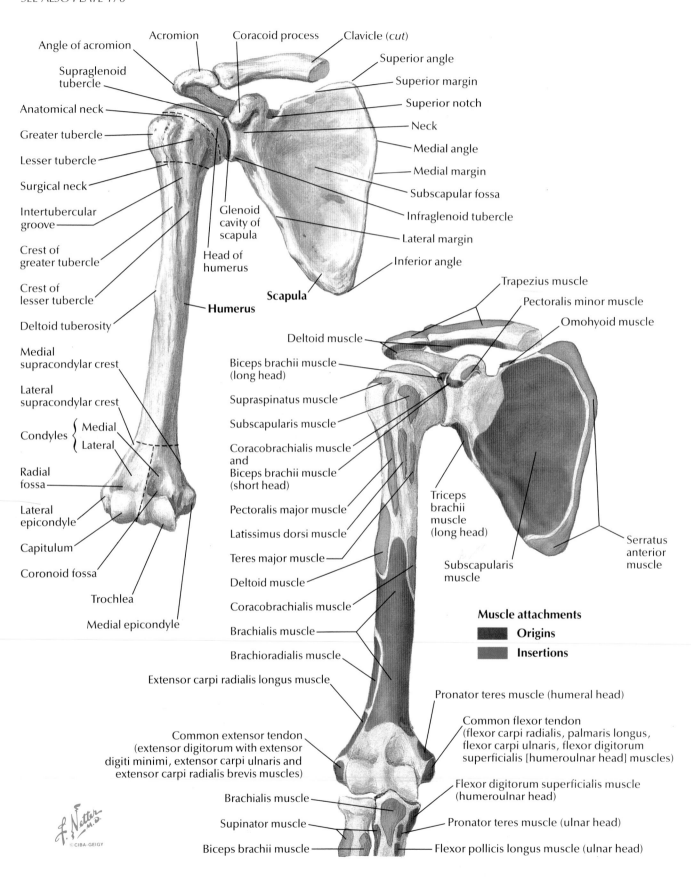

Angle of acromion

Acromion

Coracoid process

Clavicle (cut)

Superior angle

Supraglenoid tubercle

Superior margin

Superior notch

Anatomical neck

Neck

Greater tubercle

Medial angle

Lesser tubercle

Medial margin

Surgical neck

Subscapular fossa

Intertubercular groove

Infraglenoid tubercle

Crest of greater tubercle

Glenoid cavity of scapula

Lateral margin

Head of humerus

Inferior angle

Crest of lesser tubercle

Scapula

Deltoid tuberosity

Humerus

Trapezius muscle

Pectoralis minor muscle

Omohyoid muscle

Deltoid muscle

Medial supracondylar crest

Biceps brachii muscle (long head)

Lateral supracondylar crest

Supraspinatus muscle

Subscapularis muscle

Condyles { Medial
Lateral

Coracobrachialis muscle and Biceps brachii muscle (short head)

Radial fossa

Triceps brachii muscle (long head)

Pectoralis major muscle

Lateral epicondyle

Latissimus dorsi muscle

Subscapularis muscle

Capitulum

Teres major muscle

Serratus anterior muscle

Coronoid fossa

Deltoid muscle

Trochlea

Coracobrachialis muscle

Medial epicondyle

Brachialis muscle

Muscle attachments

Origins

Insertions

Brachioradialis muscle

Pronator teres muscle (humeral head)

Extensor carpi radialis longus muscle

Common flexor tendon (flexor carpi radialis, palmaris longus, flexor carpi ulnaris, flexor digitorum superficialis [humeroulnar head] muscles)

Common extensor tendon (extensor digitorum with extensor digiti minimi, extensor carpi ulnaris and extensor carpi radialis brevis muscles)

Flexor digitorum superficialis muscle (humeroulnar head)

Brachialis muscle

Pronator teres muscle (ulnar head)

Supinator muscle

Biceps brachii muscle

Flexor pollicis longus muscle (ulnar head)

PLATE 396

UPPER LIMB

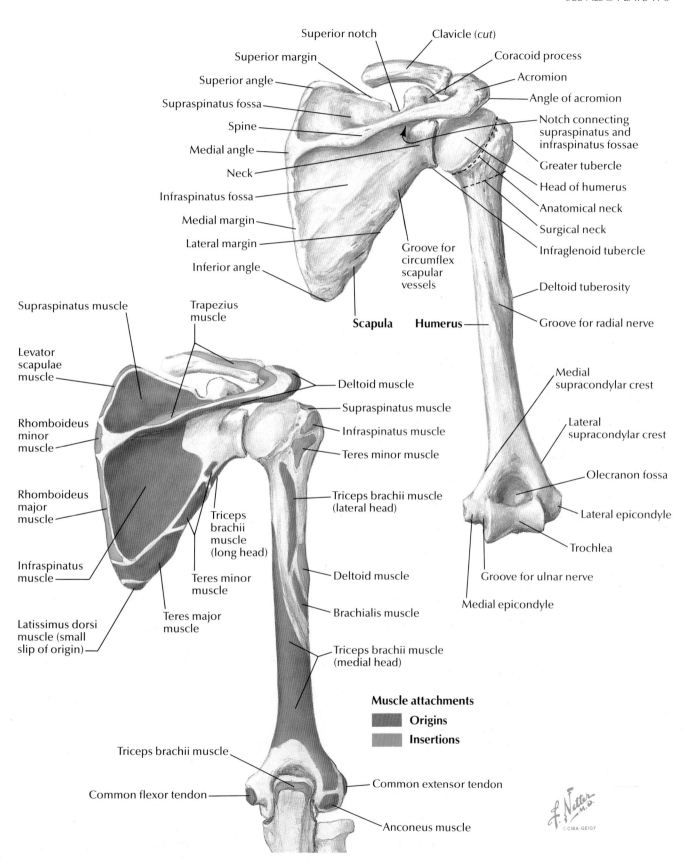

Superior notch

Clavicle (*cut*)

Superior margin

Coracoid process

Superior angle

Acromion

Supraspinatus fossa

Angle of acromion

Spine

Notch connecting supraspinatus and infraspinatus fossae

Medial angle

Greater tubercle

Neck

Head of humerus

Infraspinatus fossa

Anatomical neck

Medial margin

Surgical neck

Lateral margin

Infraglenoid tubercle

Inferior angle

Groove for circumflex scapular vessels

Deltoid tuberosity

Scapula   **Humerus**

Groove for radial nerve

Supraspinatus muscle

Trapezius muscle

Levator scapulae muscle

Deltoid muscle

Medial supracondylar crest

Rhomboideus minor muscle

Supraspinatus muscle

Lateral supracondylar crest

Infraspinatus muscle

Olecranon fossa

Teres minor muscle

Rhomboideus major muscle

Triceps brachii muscle (lateral head)

Lateral epicondyle

Triceps brachii muscle (long head)

Infraspinatus muscle

Trochlea

Teres minor muscle

Deltoid muscle

Groove for ulnar nerve

Latissimus dorsi muscle (small slip of origin)

Teres major muscle

Brachialis muscle

Medial epicondyle

Triceps brachii muscle (medial head)

Muscle attachments

■ **Origins**

■ **Insertions**

Triceps brachii muscle

Common flexor tendon

Common extensor tendon

Anconeus muscle

Glenohumeral Joint

Anterior view

Acromion

Coracoacromial ligament

Supraspinatus tendon (*cut*)

Coracohumeral ligament

Greater tubercle and Lesser tubercle of humerus

Transverse ligament of humerus

Intertubercular synovial sheath (communicates with synovial cavity)

Subscapularis tendon (*cut*)

Biceps brachii tendon (long head)

Capsular ligaments

Clavicle

Trapezoid ligament

Conoid ligament

Coraco-clavicular ligament

Superior transverse scapular ligament and scapular notch

Coracoid process

Openings of subscapular bursa to shoulder joint

Broken line indicates position of subscapular bursa

Anterior view

Deltoid muscle (*reflected*)

Capsular ligament

Supraspinatus muscle

Subdeltoid bursa with extension under acromion and coracoacromial ligament

Subscapularis muscle

Coracoacromial ligament

Acromion

Supraspinatus tendon (joined to capsule)

Subdeltoid bursa

Infraspinatus tendon (joined to capsule)

Glenoid cavity (cartilage)

Teres minor tendon (joined to capsule)

Synovial membrane (*cut edge*)

Openings of subscapular bursa

Coracoid process

Coracohumeral ligament

Biceps brachii tendon (long head)

Superior glenohumeral ligament

Subscapularis tendon (joined to capsule)

Middle glenohumeral ligament

Inferior glenohumeral ligament

Joint opened: lateral view

Subdeltoid bursa

Supraspinatus tendon

Capsular ligament

Synovial membrane

Acromion

Glenoid labrum

Deltoid muscle

Glenoid cavity of scapula

Axillary recess

Coronal section through joint

PLATE 398

UPPER LIMB

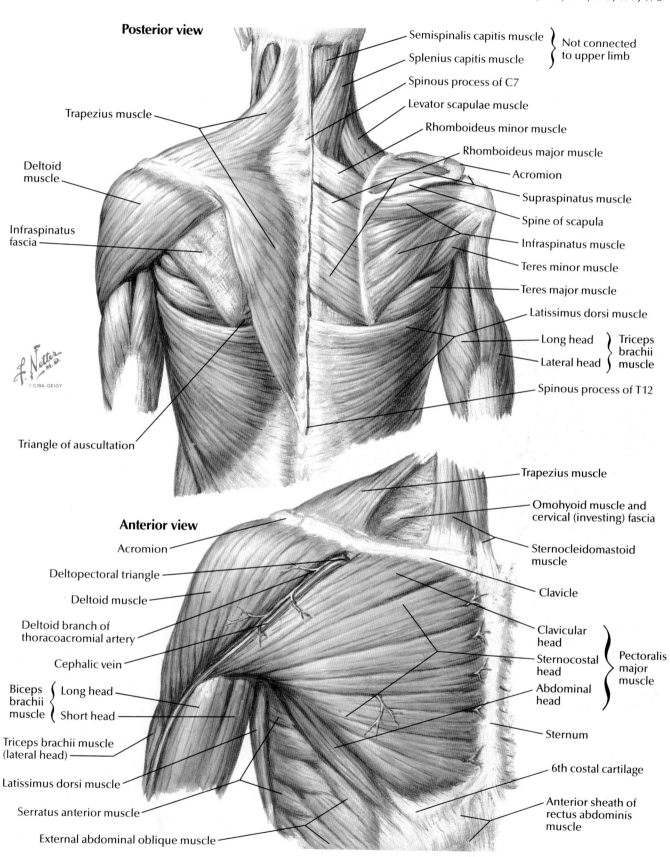

Posterior view

Semispinalis capitis muscle ⎫ Not connected
Splenius capitis muscle ⎭ to upper limb
Spinous process of C7
Levator scapulae muscle
Rhomboideus minor muscle
Rhomboideus major muscle
Acromion
Supraspinatus muscle
Spine of scapula
Infraspinatus muscle
Teres minor muscle
Teres major muscle
Latissimus dorsi muscle
Long head ⎫ Triceps
Lateral head ⎭ brachii muscle
Spinous process of T12

Trapezius muscle
Deltoid muscle
Infraspinatus fascia
Triangle of auscultation

Trapezius muscle
Omohyoid muscle and cervical (investing) fascia
Sternocleidomastoid muscle
Clavicle
Clavicular head ⎫
Sternocostal head ⎬ Pectoralis major muscle
Abdominal head ⎭
Sternum
6th costal cartilage
Anterior sheath of rectus abdominis muscle

Anterior view

Acromion
Deltopectoral triangle
Deltoid muscle
Deltoid branch of thoracoacromial artery
Cephalic vein
Biceps brachii muscle ⎰ Long head
⎱ Short head
Triceps brachii muscle (lateral head)
Latissimus dorsi muscle
Serratus anterior muscle
External abdominal oblique muscle

Muscles of Rotator Cuff

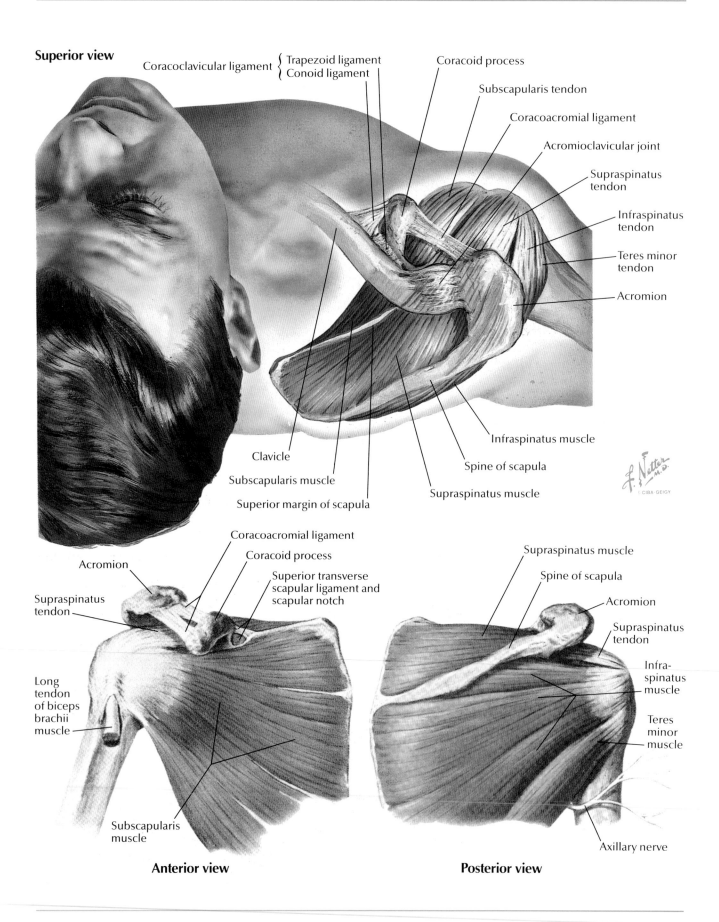

Superior view

Coracoclavicular ligament { Trapezoid ligament / Conoid ligament

Coracoid process

Subscapularis tendon

Coracoacromial ligament

Acromioclavicular joint

Supraspinatus tendon

Infraspinatus tendon

Teres minor tendon

Acromion

Infraspinatus muscle

Spine of scapula

Supraspinatus muscle

Clavicle

Subscapularis muscle

Superior margin of scapula

Acromion

Supraspinatus tendon

Coracoacromial ligament

Coracoid process

Superior transverse scapular ligament and scapular notch

Supraspinatus muscle

Spine of scapula

Acromion

Supraspinatus tendon

Infra-spinatus muscle

Teres minor muscle

Long tendon of biceps brachii muscle

Subscapularis muscle

Axillary nerve

Anterior view

Posterior view

PLATE 400

UPPER LIMB

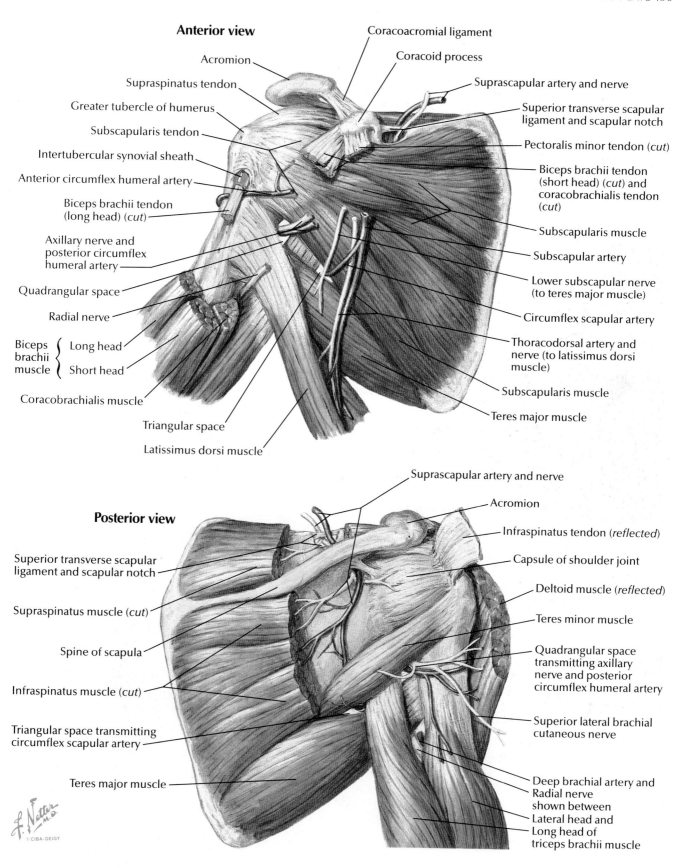

Anterior view

Coracoacromial ligament

Coracoid process

Acromion

Suprascapular artery and nerve

Suprapinatus tendon

Greater tubercle of humerus

Superior transverse scapular ligament and scapular notch

Subscapularis tendon

Pectoralis minor tendon (*cut*)

Intertubercular synovial sheath

Biceps brachii tendon (short head) (*cut*) and coracobrachialis tendon (*cut*)

Anterior circumflex humeral artery

Biceps brachii tendon (long head) (*cut*)

Subscapularis muscle

Axillary nerve and posterior circumflex humeral artery

Subscapular artery

Quadrangular space

Lower subscapular nerve (to teres major muscle)

Radial nerve

Circumflex scapular artery

Biceps brachii muscle { Long head / Short head }

Thoracodorsal artery and nerve (to latissimus dorsi muscle)

Coracobrachialis muscle

Subscapularis muscle

Triangular space

Teres major muscle

Latissimus dorsi muscle

Posterior view

Suprascapular artery and nerve

Acromion

Infraspinatus tendon (*reflected*)

Superior transverse scapular ligament and scapular notch

Capsule of shoulder joint

Supraspinatus muscle (*cut*)

Deltoid muscle (*reflected*)

Spine of scapula

Teres minor muscle

Quadrangular space transmitting axillary nerve and posterior circumflex humeral artery

Infraspinatus muscle (*cut*)

Triangular space transmitting circumflex scapular artery

Superior lateral brachial cutaneous nerve

Teres major muscle

Deep brachial artery and Radial nerve shown between Lateral head and Long head of triceps brachii muscle

Axillary Artery and Anastomoses Around Scapula

SEE ALSO PLATES 28, 409

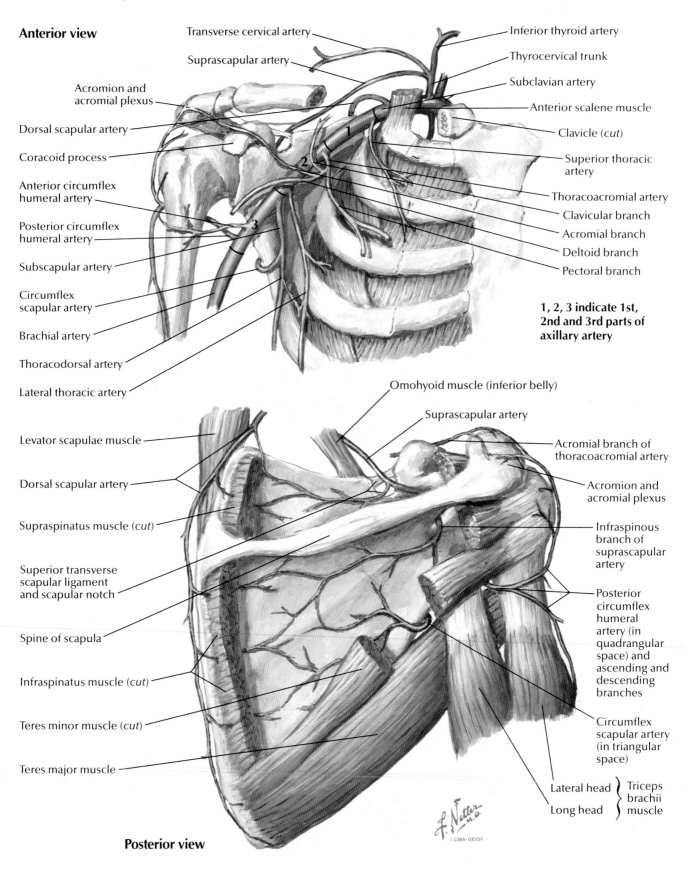

Anterior view

Transverse cervical artery

Suprascapular artery

Acromion and acromial plexus

Dorsal scapular artery

Coracoid process

Anterior circumflex humeral artery

Posterior circumflex humeral artery

Subscapular artery

Circumflex scapular artery

Brachial artery

Thoracodorsal artery

Lateral thoracic artery

Inferior thyroid artery

Thyrocervical trunk

Subclavian artery

Anterior scalene muscle

Clavicle (*cut*)

Superior thoracic artery

Thoracoacromial artery

Clavicular branch

Acromial branch

Deltoid branch

Pectoral branch

1, 2, 3 indicate 1st, 2nd and 3rd parts of axillary artery

Omohyoid muscle (inferior belly)

Suprascapular artery

Levator scapulae muscle

Dorsal scapular artery

Supraspinatus muscle (*cut*)

Superior transverse scapular ligament and scapular notch

Spine of scapula

Infraspinatus muscle (*cut*)

Teres minor muscle (*cut*)

Teres major muscle

Acromial branch of thoracoacromial artery

Acromion and acromial plexus

Infraspinous branch of suprascapular artery

Posterior circumflex humeral artery (in quadrangular space) and ascending and descending branches

Circumflex scapular artery (in triangular space)

Lateral head } Triceps brachii muscle

Long head }

Posterior view

PLATE 402

UPPER LIMB

Thoracoacromial artery

Coracoid process

Cephalic vein

Deltoid muscle

Pectoralis major muscle (cut)

Biceps brachii muscle
Short head
Long head

Fascia (cut edge) over coracobrachialis and biceps brachii muscles

Trapezius muscle

Omohyoid muscle invested by fascia of infrahyoid muscles

Clavicle

Fascia investing subclavius muscle*

Costocoracoid ligament*

Costoclavicular ligament

Costocoracoid membrane*

Fascia investing pectoralis minor muscle*

Suspensory ligament of axilla*

Pectoralis major muscle and pectoral fascia (2 layers)

Latissimus dorsi fascia

Serratus anterior fascia

Axillary fascia (anterior part)

*Components of clavipectoral fascia

Anterior view

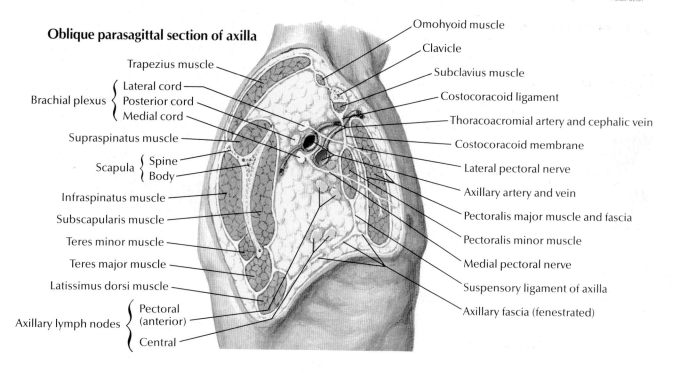

Oblique parasagittal section of axilla

Trapezius muscle

Brachial plexus
{ Lateral cord
Posterior cord
Medial cord

Supraspinatus muscle

Scapula { Spine
Body

Infraspinatus muscle

Subscapularis muscle

Teres minor muscle

Teres major muscle

Latissimus dorsi muscle

Axillary lymph nodes { Pectoral (anterior)
Central

Omohyoid muscle

Clavicle

Subclavius muscle

Costocoracoid ligament

Thoracoacromial artery and cephalic vein

Costocoracoid membrane

Lateral pectoral nerve

Axillary artery and vein

Pectoralis major muscle and fascia

Pectoralis minor muscle

Medial pectoral nerve

Suspensory ligament of axilla

Axillary fascia (fenestrated)

Axilla (Dissection): Anterior View

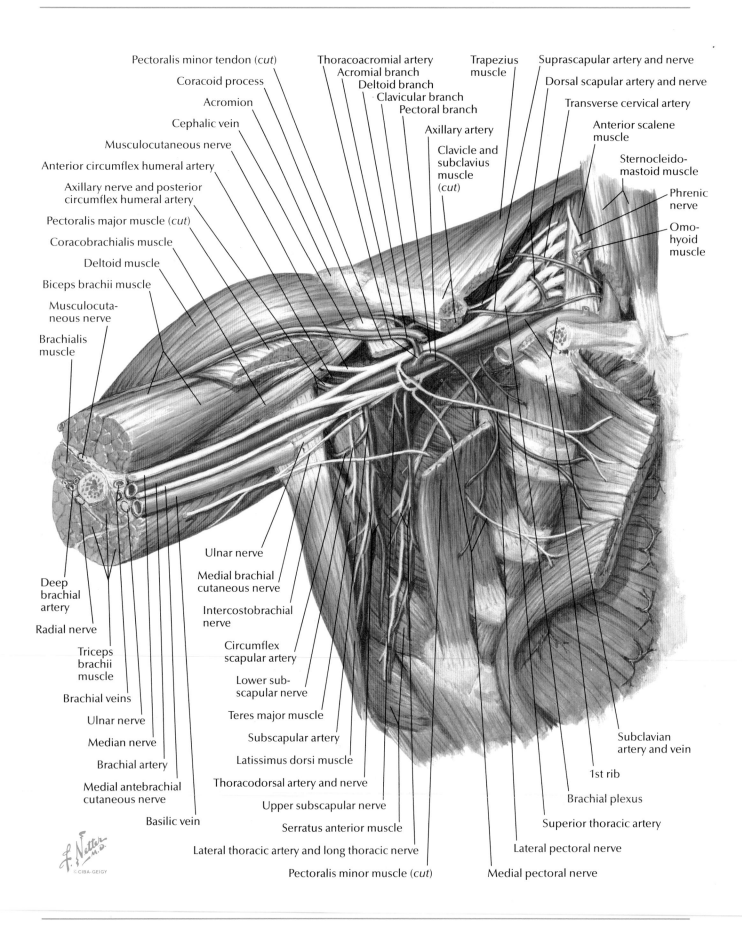

Pectoralis minor tendon (*cut*)

Coracoid process

Acromion

Cephalic vein

Musculocutaneous nerve

Anterior circumflex humeral artery

Axillary nerve and posterior circumflex humeral artery

Pectoralis major muscle (*cut*)

Coracobrachialis muscle

Deltoid muscle

Biceps brachii muscle

Musculocutaneous nerve

Brachialis muscle

Deep brachial artery

Radial nerve

Triceps brachii muscle

Brachial veins

Ulnar nerve

Median nerve

Brachial artery

Medial antebrachial cutaneous nerve

Basilic vein

Ulnar nerve

Medial brachial cutaneous nerve

Intercostobrachial nerve

Circumflex scapular artery

Lower subscapular nerve

Teres major muscle

Subscapular artery

Latissimus dorsi muscle

Thoracodorsal artery and nerve

Upper subscapular nerve

Serratus anterior muscle

Lateral thoracic artery and long thoracic nerve

Pectoralis minor muscle (*cut*)

Thoracoacromial artery
Acromial branch
Deltoid branch
Clavicular branch
Pectoral branch

Axillary artery

Clavicle and subclavius muscle (*cut*)

Trapezius muscle

Suprascapular artery and nerve

Dorsal scapular artery and nerve

Transverse cervical artery

Anterior scalene muscle

Sternocleido-mastoid muscle

Phrenic nerve

Omo-hyoid muscle

Subclavian artery and vein

1st rib

Brachial plexus

Superior thoracic artery

Lateral pectoral nerve

Medial pectoral nerve

PLATE 404

UPPER LIMB

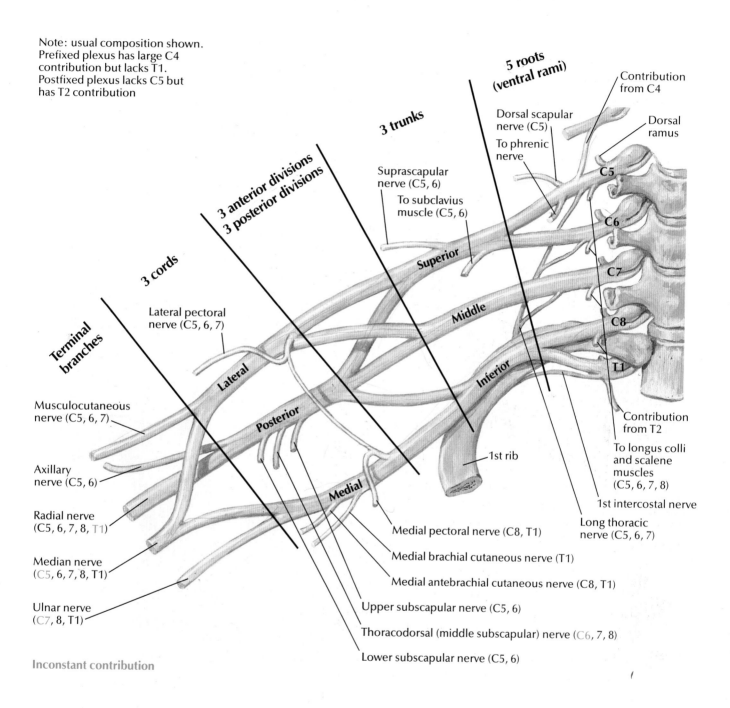

Note: usual composition shown.
Prefixed plexus has large C4
contribution but lacks T1.
Postfixed plexus lacks C5 but
has T2 contribution

**5 roots
(ventral rami)**

Contribution
from C4

3 trunks

Dorsal scapular
nerve (C5)

Dorsal
ramus

To phrenic
nerve

C5

Suprascapular
nerve (C5, 6)

To subclavius
muscle (C5, 6)

C6

**3 anterior divisions
3 posterior divisions**

C7

Superior

3 cords

Middle

C8

Lateral pectoral
nerve (C5, 6, 7)

Inferior

T1

**Terminal
branches**

Lateral

Contribution
from T2

Musculocutaneous
nerve (C5, 6, 7)

Posterior

To longus colli
and scalene
muscles
(C5, 6, 7, 8)

Axillary
nerve (C5, 6)

1st rib

1st intercostal nerve

Radial nerve
(C5, 6, 7, 8, T1)

Medial

Long thoracic
nerve (C5, 6, 7)

Median nerve
(C5, 6, 7, 8, T1)

Medial pectoral nerve (C8, T1)

Medial brachial cutaneous nerve (T1)

Ulnar nerve
(C7, 8, T1)

Medial antebrachial cutaneous nerve (C8, T1)

Upper subscapular nerve (C5, 6)

Thoracodorsal (middle subscapular) nerve (C6, 7, 8)

Lower subscapular nerve (C5, 6)

Inconstant contribution

Muscles of Arm: Anterior Views

SEE ALSO PLATE 447

Coracoacromial ligament

Subdeltoid bursa

Greater tubercle,
Lesser tubercle
of humerus

Intertubercular
synovial sheath

Deltoid muscle
(*reflected*)

Pectoralis major
muscle (*reflected*)

Anterior circumflex
humeral artery

Biceps
brachii
muscle { Long head

Short head

Brachial artery (*cut*)

Median nerve (*cut*)

Brachialis muscle

Lateral antebrachial
cutaneous nerve

Bicipital aponeurosis

Biceps brachii tendon

Brachioradialis muscle

Pronator teres muscle

Flexor carpi
radialis muscle

Acromion

Coracoid process

Pectoralis minor tendon (*cut*)

Subscapularis muscle

Musculocutaneous nerve (*cut*)

Coracobrachialis muscle

Circumflex scapular artery (*cut*)

Teres major muscle

Latissimus dorsi muscle

Biceps brachii
tendons (*cut*)
Short head
Long head

Coracobrachialis muscle

Musculocutaneous nerve

Deltoid muscle (*cut*)

Superficial layer

Brachialis muscle

Medial
intermuscular
septum

Lateral intermuscular septum

Lateral epicondyle of humerus

Lateral antebrachial cutaneous nerve

Head of radius

Biceps brachii tendon

Tuberosity of radius

Medial
epicondyle
of humerus

Tuberosity of ulna

Deep layer

PLATE 406

UPPER LIMB

SEE ALSO PLATE 450

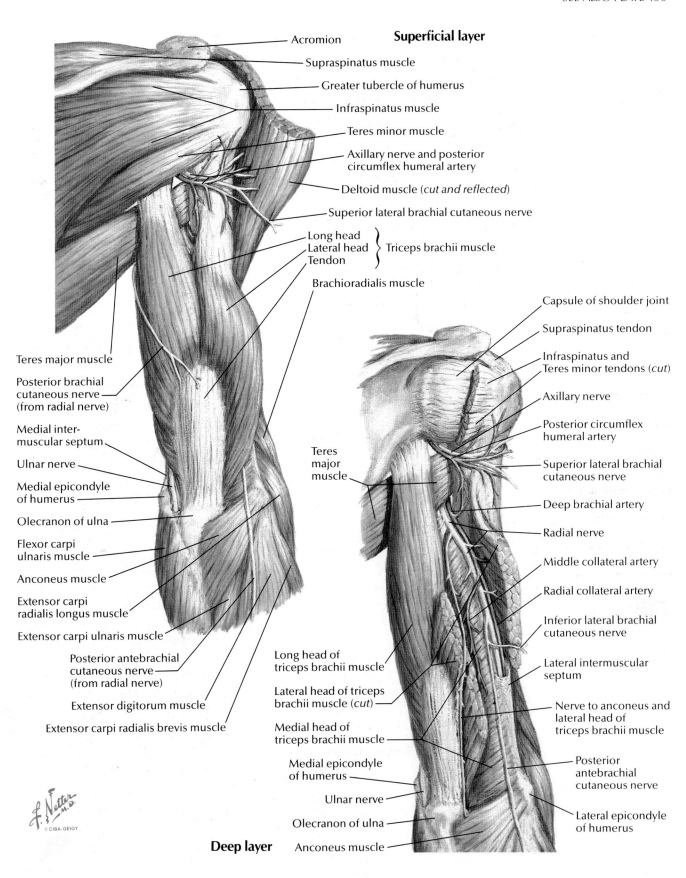

Superficial layer

Acromion

Supraspinatus muscle

Greater tubercle of humerus

Infraspinatus muscle

Teres minor muscle

Axillary nerve and posterior circumflex humeral artery

Deltoid muscle (*cut and reflected*)

Superior lateral brachial cutaneous nerve

Long head
Lateral head } Triceps brachii muscle
Tendon

Brachioradialis muscle

Capsule of shoulder joint

Supraspinatus tendon

Infraspinatus and Teres minor tendons (*cut*)

Axillary nerve

Posterior circumflex humeral artery

Superior lateral brachial cutaneous nerve

Deep brachial artery

Radial nerve

Middle collateral artery

Radial collateral artery

Inferior lateral brachial cutaneous nerve

Lateral intermuscular septum

Nerve to anconeus and lateral head of triceps brachii muscle

Posterior antebrachial cutaneous nerve

Lateral epicondyle of humerus

Teres major muscle

Posterior brachial cutaneous nerve (from radial nerve)

Medial inter-muscular septum

Ulnar nerve

Medial epicondyle of humerus

Olecranon of ulna

Flexor carpi ulnaris muscle

Anconeus muscle

Extensor carpi radialis longus muscle

Extensor carpi ulnaris muscle

Posterior antebrachial cutaneous nerve (from radial nerve)

Extensor digitorum muscle

Extensor carpi radialis brevis muscle

Teres major muscle

Long head of triceps brachii muscle

Lateral head of triceps brachii muscle (*cut*)

Medial head of triceps brachii muscle

Medial epicondyle of humerus

Ulnar nerve

Olecranon of ulna

Deep layer   Anconeus muscle

Brachial Artery In Situ

Coracoid process

Deltoid muscle

Anterior circumflex humeral artery

Humerus

Pectoralis major muscle and tendon (cut)

Biceps brachii muscle { Long head / Short head }

Coracobrachialis muscle

Brachial artery

Muscular branch

Median nerve

Muscular branch

Biceps brachii muscle

Brachialis muscle

Radial recurrent artery

Biceps brachii tendon

Radial artery

Axillary artery

Pectoralis minor muscle (cut)

Lateral cord, Medial cord of brachial plexus

Musculocutaneous nerve

Subscapularis muscle

Anterior and posterior circumflex humeral arteries

Teres major muscle

Latissimus dorsi muscle

Deep brachial artery

Medial brachial cutaneous nerve

Ulnar nerve

Medial antebrachial cutaneous nerve

Long head / Medial head } Triceps brachii muscle

Superior ulnar collateral artery

Medial intermuscular septum

Inferior ulnar collateral artery

Medial epicondyle of humerus

Bicipital aponeurosis

Pronator teres muscle

Ulnar artery

Flexor carpi radialis muscle

Brachioradialis muscle

PLATE 408

UPPER LIMB

Clavicular branch

Pectoral branch

Acromial branch

Deltoid branch

Thoracoacromial artery

Superior thoracic artery

Axillary artery

Anterior circumflex humeral artery

Lateral thoracic artery

Posterior circumflex humeral artery

Subscapular artery

Circumflex scapular artery

Brachial artery

Thoracodorsal artery

Deep brachial artery

Level of lower margin of teres major muscle is landmark for name change from axillary to brachial artery

Radial collateral artery

Middle collateral artery

Superior ulnar collateral artery

Inferior ulnar collateral artery

Radial recurrent artery

Interosseous recurrent artery

Anterior ulnar recurrent artery

Posterior interosseous artery

Posterior ulnar recurrent artery

Radial artery

Common interosseous artery

Anterior interosseous artery

Ulnar artery

Arm: Serial Cross Sections

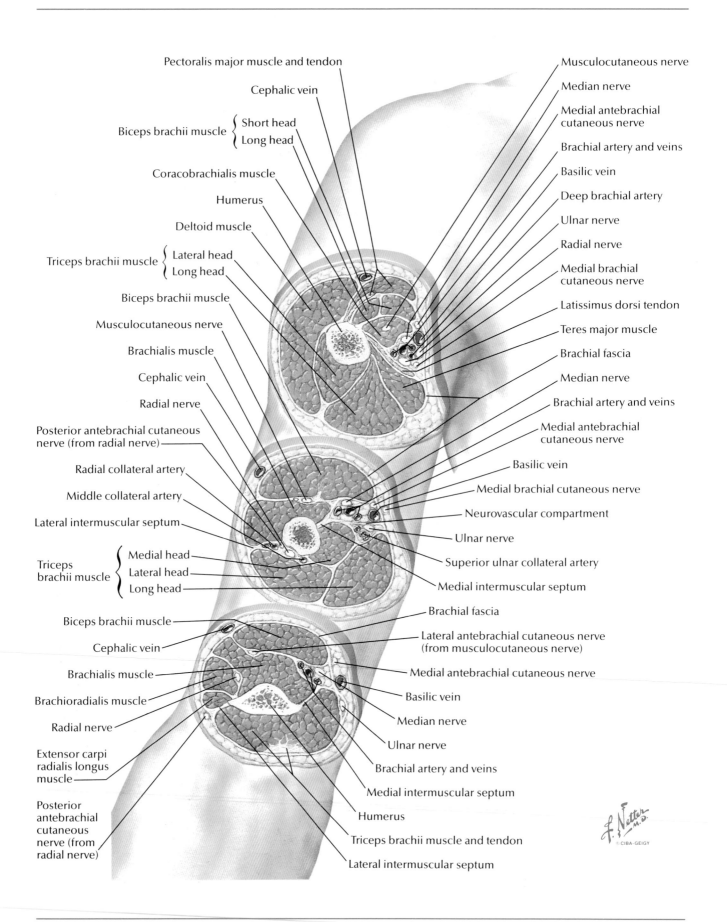

Pectoralis major muscle and tendon

Cephalic vein

Biceps brachii muscle { Short head / Long head }

Coracobrachialis muscle

Humerus

Deltoid muscle

Triceps brachii muscle { Lateral head / Long head }

Biceps brachii muscle

Musculocutaneous nerve

Brachialis muscle

Cephalic vein

Radial nerve

Posterior antebrachial cutaneous nerve (from radial nerve)

Radial collateral artery

Middle collateral artery

Lateral intermuscular septum

Triceps brachii muscle { Medial head / Lateral head / Long head }

Biceps brachii muscle

Cephalic vein

Brachialis muscle

Brachioradialis muscle

Radial nerve

Extensor carpi radialis longus muscle

Posterior antebrachial cutaneous nerve (from radial nerve)

Musculocutaneous nerve

Median nerve

Medial antebrachial cutaneous nerve

Brachial artery and veins

Basilic vein

Deep brachial artery

Ulnar nerve

Radial nerve

Medial brachial cutaneous nerve

Latissimus dorsi tendon

Teres major muscle

Brachial fascia

Median nerve

Brachial artery and veins

Medial antebrachial cutaneous nerve

Basilic vein

Medial brachial cutaneous nerve

Neurovascular compartment

Ulnar nerve

Superior ulnar collateral artery

Medial intermuscular septum

Brachial fascia

Lateral antebrachial cutaneous nerve (from musculocutaneous nerve)

Medial antebrachial cutaneous nerve

Basilic vein

Median nerve

Ulnar nerve

Brachial artery and veins

Medial intermuscular septum

Humerus

Triceps brachii muscle and tendon

Lateral intermuscular septum

PLATE 410

UPPER LIMB

Right elbow

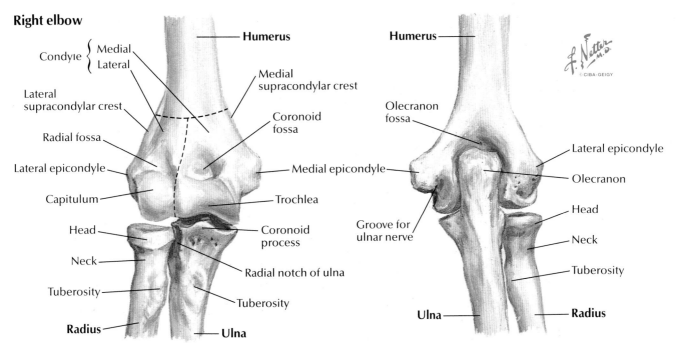

Condyle { Medial / Lateral

Lateral supracondylar crest

Radial fossa

Lateral epicondyle

Capitulum

Head

Neck

Tuberosity

Radius

Humerus

Medial supracondylar crest

Coronoid fossa

Medial epicondyle

Trochlea

Coronoid process

Radial notch of ulna

Tuberosity

Ulna

In extension: anterior view

Humerus

Olecranon fossa

Groove for ulnar nerve

Ulna

Lateral epicondyle

Olecranon

Head

Neck

Tuberosity

Radius

In extension: posterior view

Humerus

Radius

Ulna

Humerus

In extension: lateral view

In extension: medial view

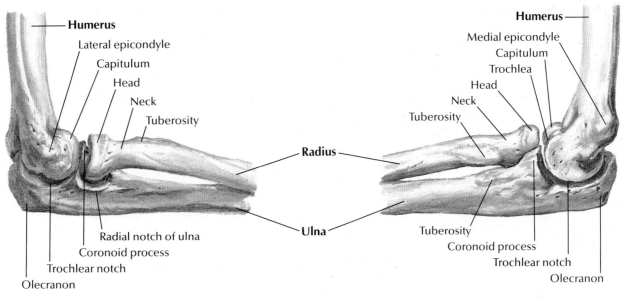

Humerus

Lateral epicondyle

Capitulum

Head

Neck

Tuberosity

Radius

Ulna

Radial notch of ulna

Coronoid process

Trochlear notch

Olecranon

In 90° flexion: lateral view

Humerus

Medial epicondyle

Capitulum

Trochlea

Head

Neck

Tuberosity

Radius

Ulna

Tuberosity

Coronoid process

Trochlear notch

Olecranon

In 90° flexion: medial view

Ligaments of Elbow

Right elbow

Anterior view

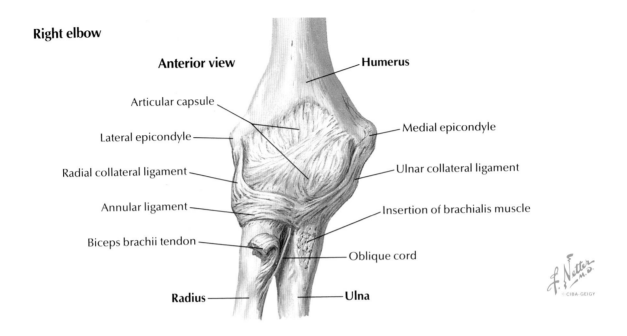

Humerus

Articular capsule

Lateral epicondyle

Radial collateral ligament

Annular ligament

Biceps brachii tendon

Medial epicondyle

Ulnar collateral ligament

Insertion of brachialis muscle

Oblique cord

Radius — — **Ulna**

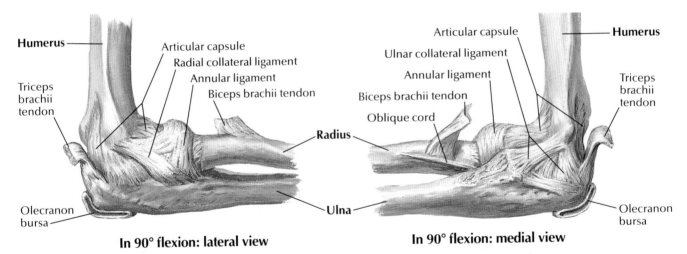

Humerus —

Triceps brachii tendon

Articular capsule
Radial collateral ligament
Annular ligament
Biceps brachii tendon

Radius

Olecranon bursa

In 90° flexion: lateral view

Articular capsule
Ulnar collateral ligament
Annular ligament
Biceps brachii tendon
Oblique cord

Radius

Ulna —

Humerus

Triceps brachii tendon

Olecranon bursa

In 90° flexion: medial view

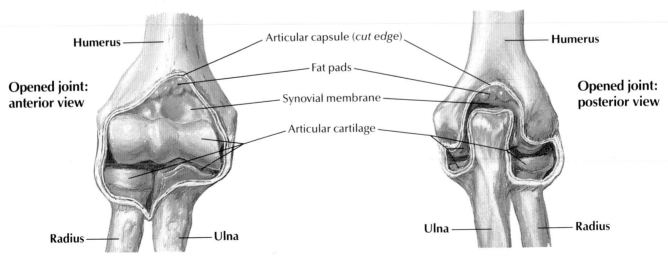

Opened joint: anterior view

Humerus —

Articular capsule (*cut edge*)

Fat pads

Synovial membrane

Articular cartilage

Humerus

Opened joint: posterior view

Radius — — **Ulna**

Ulna — — **Radius**

PLATE 412

UPPER LIMB

Right radius and ulna in supination: anterior view

Olecranon

Trochlear notch

Coronoid process

Head

Radial notch of ulna

Neck

Tuberosity of ulna

Tuberosity of radius

Oblique cord

Radius

Ulna

Anterior surface

Anterior surface

Anterior margin

Anterior margin

Interosseous margin

Interosseous margin

Interosseous membrane

Right radius and ulna in pronation: anterior view

Coronoid process

Oblique cord

Tuberosity of ulna

Radius

Ulna

Lateral surface

Posterior margin

Posterior surface

Interosseous membrane

Groove for extensor pollicis longus muscle

Groove for extensor digitorum and extensor indicis muscles

Dorsal tubercle

Groove for extensor carpi radialis longus and brevis muscles

Area for extensor pollicis brevis and abductor pollicis longus muscles

Styloid process

Styloid process

Styloid process

Styloid process

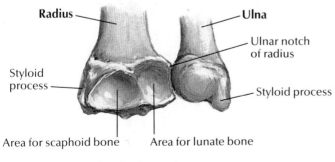

Radius

Ulna

Ulnar notch of radius

Styloid process

Styloid process

Area for scaphoid bone

Area for lunate bone

Carpal articular surface

Coronal section of radius demonstrates how thickness of cortical bone of shaft diminishes to thin layer over cancellous bone at distal end

Right forearm: anterior view

Supination

Pronation

Lateral epicondyle

Medial epicondyle

Medial epicondyle

Lateral epicondyle

Supinator

Pronator teres

Ulna

Radius

Radius

Ulna

Pronator quadratus

PLATE 414

UPPER LIMB

Individual Muscles of Forearm: Extensors of Wrist and Digits

Note: anconeus muscle not shown because it is extensor of elbow

Medial epicondyle

Olecranon

Lateral epicondyle

Common extensor tendon

Ulna

Extensors of wrist

Extensor carpi radialis longus

Extensor carpi radialis brevis

Extensor carpi ulnaris

Extensors of digits (except thumb)

Extensor digitorum

Extensor digiti minimi

Extensor indicis

Extensors of thumb

Abductor pollicis longus

Extensor pollicis brevis

Extensor pollicis longus

Extensor indicis tendon

Medial epicondyle

Olecranon

Lateral epicondyle

Common extensor tendon

Extensor digitorum and extensor digiti minimi (*cut away*)

Interosseous membrane

Radius

Ulna

Extensor digitorum and extensor digiti minimi tendons (*cut*)

Right forearm: posterior (dorsal) views

ELBOW AND FOREARM

PLATE 415

Note: brachioradialis muscle not shown
because it is flexor of elbow

Lateral epicondyle

Medial epicondyle

Common flexor tendon

Flexor carpi radialis

Palmaris longus

Flexor carpi ulnaris

Radius

Ulna

Pisiform bone

Hamulus of hamate bone

Palmar aponeurosis (*cut*)

**Right forearm:
anterior (palmar) view**

PLATE 416

UPPER LIMB

Medial epicondyle

Lateral epicondyle

Common flexor tendon

Coronoid process

Interosseous membrane

Radius

Flexor digitorum superficialis

Flexor digitorum profundus

Flexor pollicis longus

Radius

Ulna

Medial epicondyle

Lateral epicondyle

Common flexor tendon

Coronoid process

Interosseous membrane

Radius

Radius

Ulna

Flexor digitorum superficialis tendons (*cut away*)

Right forearm: anterior (palmar) views

Muscles of Forearm (Superficial Layer): Posterior View

SEE ALSO PLATE 451

Posterior ulnar recurrent artery

Ulnar nerve

Medial epicondyle of humerus

Olecranon of ulna

Anconeus muscle

Flexor carpi ulnaris muscle

Extensor carpi ulnaris muscle

Extensor retinaculum
(compartments numbered)

Dorsal branch of ulnar nerve

Extensor carpi ulnaris tendon
Extensor digiti minimi tendon
Extensor digitorum tendons
Extensor indicis tendon

5th metacarpal bone

Triceps brachii muscle

Brachioradialis muscle

Extensor carpi radialis longus muscle

Common extensor tendon

Extensor carpi radialis brevis muscle

Extensor digitorum muscle

Extensor digiti minimi muscle

Abductor pollicis longus muscle

Extensor pollicis brevis muscle

Extensor pollicis longus tendon
Extensor carpi radialis brevis tendon
Extensor carpi radialis longus tendon

Superficial branch of radial nerve

Abductor pollicis longus tendon
Extensor pollicis brevis tendon
Extensor pollicis longus tendon

Anatomical snuffbox

6 5 4 3 2 1

PLATE 418

UPPER LIMB

Superior and inferior ulnar collateral branches of deep brachial artery

Medial intermuscular septum

Ulnar nerve

Posterior ulnar recurrent artery

Medial epicondyle of humerus

Triceps brachii tendon (*cut*)

Olecranon of ulna

Anconeus muscle

Flexor carpi ulnaris muscle

Interosseous recurrent artery

Posterior interosseous artery

Ulna

Extensor pollicis longus muscle

Extensor indicis muscle

Anterior interosseous artery (termination)

Extensor carpi ulnaris tendon (*cut*)

Extensor digiti minimi tendon (*cut*)

Extensor digitorum tendons (*cut*)

Extensor retinaculum (compartments numbered)

5th metacarpal bone

Middle collateral branch of deep brachial artery

Lateral intermuscular septum

Brachioradialis muscle

Extensor carpi radialis longus muscle

Lateral epicondyle of humerus

Common extensor tendon (*partially cut*)

Extensor carpi radialis brevis muscle

Supinator muscle

Deep branch of radial nerve

Pronator teres muscle (slip of origin)

Radius

Posterior interosseous nerve

Abductor pollicis longus muscle

Extensor pollicis brevis muscle

Extensor carpi radialis brevis tendon

Extensor carpi radialis longus tendon

Radial artery

1st metacarpal bone

2nd metacarpal bone

1st dorsal interosseous muscle

SEE ALSO PLATES 448, 449

Biceps brachii muscle

Brachial artery and median nerve

Lateral antebrachial cutaneous nerve (terminal musculocutaneous nerve)

Brachialis muscle

Biceps brachii tendon

Radial artery

Bicipital aponeurosis

Brachioradialis muscle

Extensor carpi radialis longus muscle

Extensor carpi radialis brevis muscle

Flexor pollicis longus muscle and tendon

Radial artery

Median nerve

Transverse fibers of palmar aponeurosis (palmar carpal ligament)

Thenar muscles

Palmar aponeurosis

Medial antebrachial cutaneous nerve

Ulnar nerve

Triceps brachii muscle

Medial intermuscular septum

Ulnar artery

Medial epicondyle of humerus

Common flexor tendon

Pronator teres muscle

Flexor carpi radialis muscle

Palmaris longus muscle

Flexor carpi ulnaris muscle

Flexor digitorum superficialis muscle

Superficial flexor muscles

Palmaris longus tendon

Dorsal branch of ulnar nerve

Ulnar artery and nerve

Flexor digitorum superficialis tendons

Pisiform bone

Palmar branch of median nerve

Hypothenar muscles

f. Netter M.D.
©CIBA-GEIGY

PLATE 420

UPPER LIMB

Biceps brachii muscle

Brachialis muscle

Lateral antebrachial cutaneous nerve (*cut*)
(from musculocutaneous nerve)

Radial nerve
Deep branch
Superficial branch

Biceps brachii tendon

Radial recurrent artery

Radial artery

Brachioradialis muscle

Supinator muscle

Flexor digitorum superficialis
muscle (radial head)

Pronator teres muscle (*cut*)

Flexor pollicis longus muscle

Transverse fibers of palmar
aponeurosis (palmar carpal
ligament) with palmaris longus
tendon (*cut and reflected*)

Flexor carpi radialis
tendon (*cut*)

Superficial palmar branch
of radial artery

Ulnar nerve

Median nerve

Brachial artery

Medial intermuscular septum

Pronator teres muscle (humeral head)
(*cut and reflected*)

Medial epicondyle

Flexor carpi radialis and palmaris
longus tendons (*cut*)

Anterior ulnar recurrent artery

Flexor digitorum superficialis
muscle (humeroulnar head)

Ulnar artery

Common interosseous artery

Pronator teres muscle (ulnar head) (*cut*)

Anterior interosseous artery

Flexor carpi ulnaris muscle

Flexor digitorum superficialis muscle

Ulnar artery

Ulnar nerve and dorsal branch

Median nerve

Palmar branches of median and ulnar nerves

Pisiform bone

Deep palmar branches of ulnar nerve and artery

Superficial branch of ulnar nerve

Flexor retinaculum

Muscles of Forearm (Deep Layer): Anterior View

SEE ALSO PLATES 448, 449

Brachialis muscle

Musculocutaneous nerve

Lateral antebrachial cutaneous nerve

Lateral intermuscular septum

Radial nerve

Lateral epicondyle

Biceps brachii tendon (cut)

Radial recurrent artery

Radial artery

Supinator muscle

Posterior and anterior interosseous arteries

Flexor digitorum superficialis muscle (radial head) (cut)

Pronator teres muscle (cut and reflected)

Radial artery

Flexor pollicis longus muscle and tendon (cut)

Radius

Pronator quadratus muscle

Brachioradialis tendon (cut)

Radial artery and superficial palmar branch

Flexor pollicis longus tendon (cut)

Flexor carpi radialis tendon (cut)

Abductor pollicis longus tendon

Extensor pollicis brevis tendon

1st metacarpal bone

Ulnar nerve

Median nerve

Brachial artery

Medial intermuscular septum

Pronator teres muscle (cut and reflected)

Anterior ulnar recurrent artery

Medial epicondyle of humerus

Flexor carpi radialis, palmaris longus, flexor digitorum superficialis (humeroulnar head) and flexor carpi ulnaris muscles (cut)

Posterior ulnar recurrent artery

Ulnar artery

Common interosseous artery

Pronator teres muscle (ulnar head) (cut)

Median nerve (cut)

Flexor digitorum profundus muscle

Anterior interosseous artery and nerve

Ulnar nerve and dorsal branch

Palmar carpal branches of radial and ulnar arteries

Flexor carpi ulnaris tendon (cut)

Pisiform bone

Deep palmar branches of ulnar artery and nerve

Hamulus of hamate bone

5th metacarpal bone

PLATE 422

Median antebrachial vein

Pronator teres muscle

Radial artery and superficial branch of radial nerve

Radius

Brachioradialis muscle

Cephalic vein and lateral antebrachial cutaneous nerve (from musculocutaneous nerve)

Supinator muscle

Deep branch of radial nerve

Extensor carpi radialis longus muscle

Extensor carpi radialis brevis muscle

Extensor digitorum muscle

Extensor digiti minimi muscle

Extensor carpi ulnaris muscle

Flexor carpi radialis muscle

Brachioradialis muscle

Radial artery and superficial branch of radial nerve

Flexor pollicis longus muscle

Extensor carpi radialis longus muscle and tendon

Radius

Extensor carpi radialis brevis muscle and tendon

Abductor pollicis longus muscle

Extensor digitorum muscle

Extensor digiti minimi muscle

Extensor carpi ulnaris muscle

Flexor carpi radialis tendon

Radial artery

Brachioradialis tendon

Flexor pollicis longus muscle

Abductor pollicis longus tendon

Superficial branch of radial nerve

Extensor pollicis brevis tendon

Extensor carpi radialis longus tendon

Extensor carpi radialis brevis tendon

Extensor pollicis longus tendon

Radius

Flexor digitorum superficialis muscle (radial head)

Anterior branch of medial antebrachial cutaneous nerve

Flexor pollicis longus muscle

Interosseous membrane

Flexor carpi radialis muscle

Ulnar artery and median nerve

Palmaris longus muscle

Flexor digitorum superficialis muscle (humeroulnar head)

Common interosseous artery

Ulnar nerve

Flexor carpi ulnaris muscle

Basilic vein

Flexor digitorum profundus muscle

Ulna and antebrachial fascia

Anconeus muscle

Posterior antebrachial cutaneous nerve (from radial nerve)

Palmaris longus muscle

Flexor digitorum superficialis muscle

Median nerve

Ulnar artery and nerve

Flexor carpi ulnaris muscle

Anterior interosseous artery and nerve (from median nerve)

Flexor digitorum profundus muscle

Ulna and antebrachial fascia

Interosseous membrane and extensor pollicis longus muscle

Posterior interosseous artery and nerve (from deep branch of radial nerve)

Palmaris longus tendon

Median nerve

Flexor digitorum superficialis muscle and tendons

Flexor carpi ulnaris muscle and tendon

Ulnar artery and nerve

Dorsal branch of radial nerve

Flexor digitorum profundus muscle and tendons

Antebrachial fascia

Ulna

Extensor carpi ulnaris tendon

Pronator quadratus muscle and interosseous membrane

Extensor indicis muscle and tendon

Extensor digitorum tendons

Bony Attachments of Muscles of Forearm: Anterior View

Brachioradialis muscle

Extensor carpi radialis longus muscle

Extensor carpi radialis brevis, extensor digitorum, extensor digiti minimi, extensor carpi ulnaris muscles } Common extensor tendon

Brachialis muscle

Biceps brachii muscle

Supinator muscle

Flexor digitorum superficialis muscle (radial head)

Pronator teres muscle

Flexor pollicis longus muscle

Radius

Pronator quadratus muscle

Brachioradialis muscle

Abductor pollicis longus muscle

Flexor carpi radialis muscle

Flexor pollicis longus muscle

Brachialis muscle

Pronator teres muscle (humeral head)

Common flexor tendon } Pronator teres, flexor carpi radialis, palmaris longus, flexor carpi ulnaris, flexor digitorum superficialis (humeroulnar head) muscles

Flexor digitorum superficialis muscle (humeroulnar head)

Pronator teres muscle (ulnar head)

Flexor digitorum profundus muscle

Ulna

Pronator quadratus muscle

Note: attachments of intrinsic muscles of hand not shown

Flexor carpi ulnaris muscle

Extensor carpi ulnaris muscle

Flexor digitorum superficialis muscle

Flexor digitorum profundus muscle

■ Origins   ■ Insertions

PLATE 424

UPPER LIMB

Note: attachments of intrinsic muscles of hand not shown

Triceps brachii muscle (medial head)

Triceps brachii tendon

Flexor carpi ulnaris muscle (humeral origin via common flexor tendon)

Anconeus muscle

Flexor carpi ulnaris muscle (ulnar origin)

Biceps brachii muscle

Supinator muscle

Flexor digitorum profundus muscle

Abductor pollicis longus muscle

Extensor carpi ulnaris muscle (ulnar origin)

Pronator teres muscle

Extensor pollicis longus muscle

Extensor pollicis brevis muscle

Extensor indicis muscle

Ulna

Radius

Extensor carpi radialis longus muscle

Brachioradialis muscle

Extensor carpi radialis brevis muscle

Abductor pollicis longus muscle

Extensor carpi ulnaris muscle

Extensor pollicis brevis muscle

Extensor digitorum muscle (central bands)

Extensor digiti minimi muscle

Extensor pollicis longus muscle

Extensor indicis muscle

Extensor digitorum communis muscle (lateral bands)

■ Origins   ■ Insertions

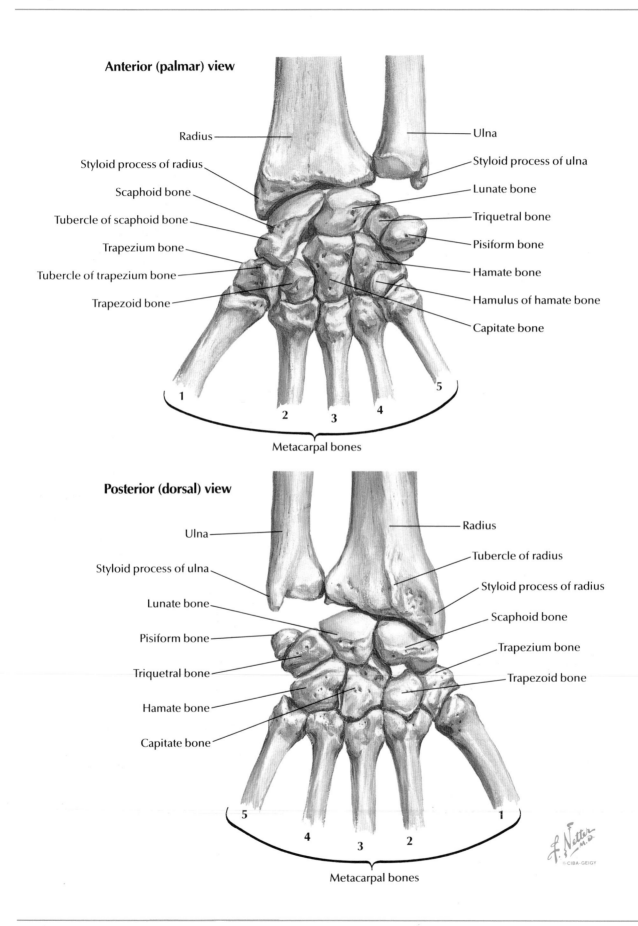

Anterior (palmar) view

Radius

Styloid process of radius

Scaphoid bone

Tubercle of scaphoid bone

Trapezium bone

Tubercle of trapezium bone

Trapezoid bone

Ulna

Styloid process of ulna

Lunate bone

Triquetral bone

Pisiform bone

Hamate bone

Hamulus of hamate bone

Capitate bone

1 2 3 4 5

Metacarpal bones

Posterior (dorsal) view

Ulna

Styloid process of ulna

Lunate bone

Pisiform bone

Triquetral bone

Hamate bone

Capitate bone

Radius

Tubercle of radius

Styloid process of radius

Scaphoid bone

Trapezium bone

Trapezoid bone

5 4 3 2 1

Metacarpal bones

PLATE 426

UPPER LIMB

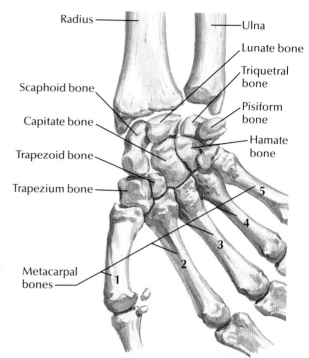

Position of carpal bones with hand in abduction: anterior (palmar) view

Position of carpal bones with hand in adduction: anterior (palmar) view

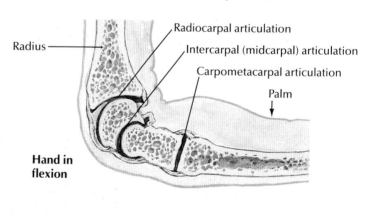

Hand in flexion

Hand in anatomical position

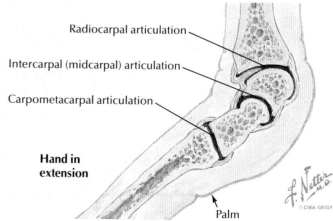

Hand in extension

Sagittal sections through wrist and middle finger

Ligaments of Wrist

Carpal tunnel: palmar view

Radius

Palmaris longus tendon

Palmar carpal ligament (thickening of deep antebrachial fascia) (*cut and reflected*)

Radial artery and superficial palmar branch

Flexor carpi radialis tendon

Flexor pollicis longus tendon

Median nerve

Palmar aponeurosis

Tubercle of scaphoid bone

Tubercle of trapezium bone

Flexor retinaculum

Ulna

Interosseous membrane

Ulnar artery and nerve

Flexor carpi ulnaris tendon

Flexor digitorum profundus tendons

Flexor digitorum superficialis tendons

Pisiform bone

Deep palmar branches of ulnar artery and nerve

Hamulus of hamate bone

1 2 3 4 5

Metacarpal bones

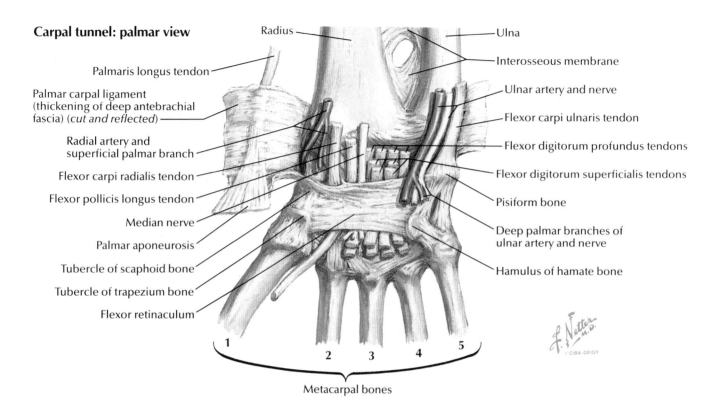

Flexor retinaculum removed: palmar view

Radius

Interosseous membrane

Superficial capsular tissue (*cut away*)

Palmar radiocarpal ligament { Radioscapholunate part / Radiotriquetral part / Radiocapitate part

Space (of Poirier)

Radial collateral ligament

Tubercle of scaphoid bone

Tubercle of trapezium bone

Capitate bone

Capitotriquetral ligament (part of radiate capitate ligament)

Palmar carpometacarpal ligaments

Ulna

Palmar radioulnar ligament

Area of articular disc

Ulnolunate part } Palmar ulno-
Ulnotriquetral part } carpal ligament

Ulnar collateral ligament

Flexor carpi ulnaris tendon (*cut*)

Triquetral bone

Pisiform bone

Lunate bone (covered by ligament)

Pisohamate ligament

Pisometacarpal ligament

Hamulus of hamate bone

Palmar metacarpal ligaments

1 2 3 4 5

Metacarpal bones

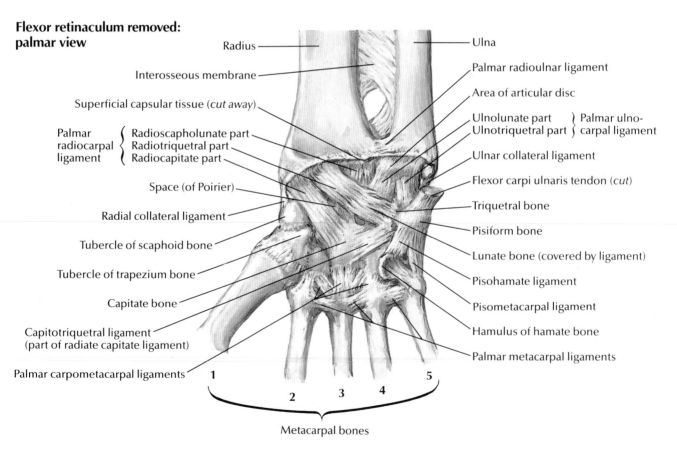

PLATE 428

UPPER LIMB

Posterior (dorsal) view

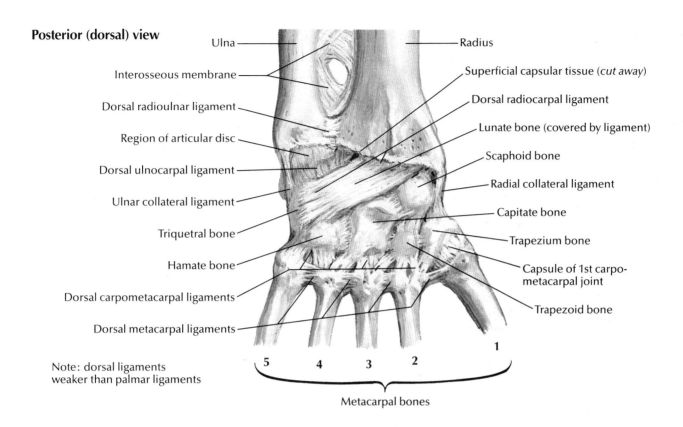

Ulna

Interosseous membrane

Dorsal radioulnar ligament

Region of articular disc

Dorsal ulnocarpal ligament

Ulnar collateral ligament

Triquetral bone

Hamate bone

Dorsal carpometacarpal ligaments

Dorsal metacarpal ligaments

Note: dorsal ligaments
weaker than palmar ligaments

Radius

Superficial capsular tissue (*cut away*)

Dorsal radiocarpal ligament

Lunate bone (covered by ligament)

Scaphoid bone

Radial collateral ligament

Capitate bone

Trapezium bone

Capsule of 1st carpo-
metacarpal joint

Trapezoid bone

5 4 3 2 1

Metacarpal bones

Coronal section: dorsal view

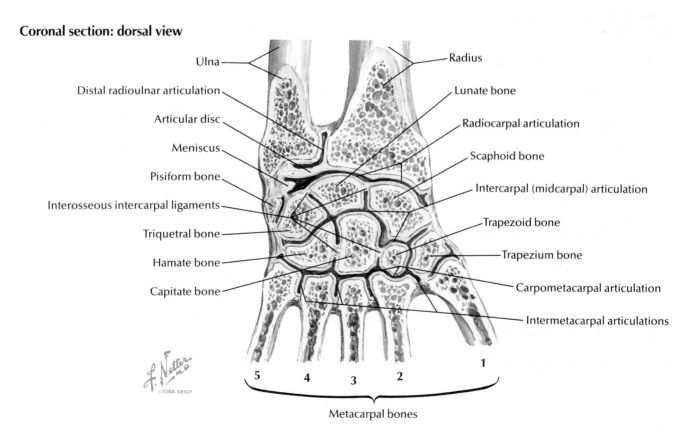

Ulna

Distal radioulnar articulation

Articular disc

Meniscus

Pisiform bone

Interosseous intercarpal ligaments

Triquetral bone

Hamate bone

Capitate bone

Radius

Lunate bone

Radiocarpal articulation

Scaphoid bone

Intercarpal (midcarpal) articulation

Trapezoid bone

Trapezium bone

Carpometacarpal articulation

Intermetacarpal articulations

5 4 3 2 1

Metacarpal bones

Bones of Wrist and Hand

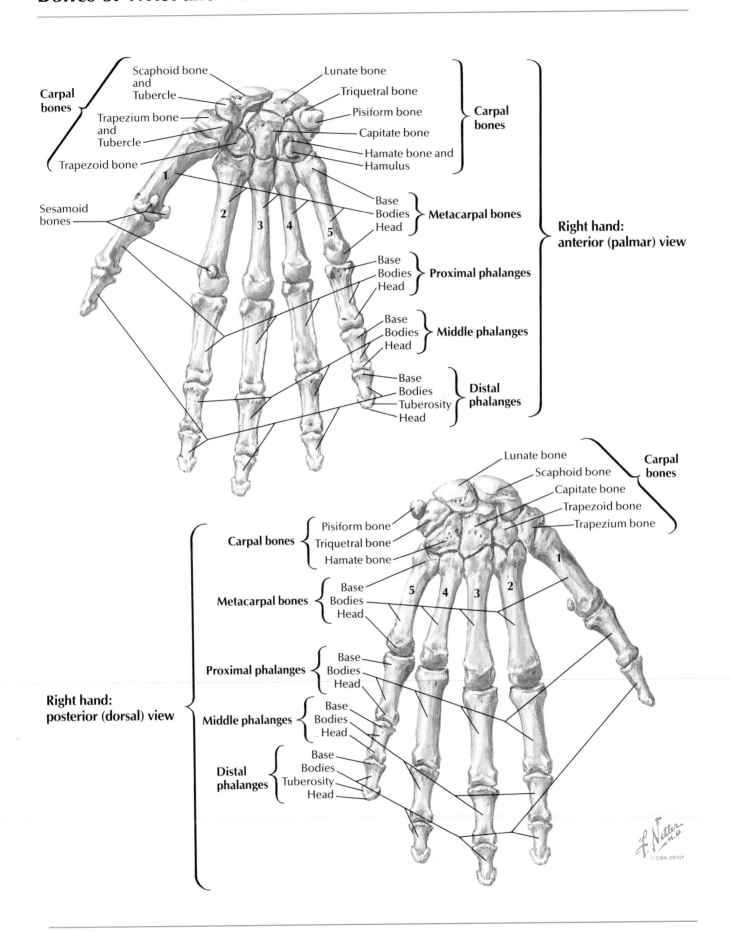

Carpal bones
- Scaphoid bone and Tubercle
- Trapezium bone and Tubercle
- Trapezoid bone

Sesamoid bones

Lunate bone
Triquetral bone
Pisiform bone
Capitate bone
Hamate bone and Hamulus

Carpal bones

1
2
3
4
5

Base
Bodies
Head — Metacarpal bones

Base
Bodies
Head — Proximal phalanges

Base
Bodies
Head — Middle phalanges

Base
Bodies
Tuberosity
Head — Distal phalanges

Right hand: anterior (palmar) view

Lunate bone
Scaphoid bone
Capitate bone
Trapezoid bone
Trapezium bone

Carpal bones

Pisiform bone
Triquetral bone
Hamate bone

Carpal bones

1
2
3
4
5

Metacarpal bones
Base
Bodies
Head

Proximal phalanges
Base
Bodies
Head

Middle phalanges
Base
Bodies
Head

Distal phalanges
Base
Bodies
Tuberosity
Head

Right hand: posterior (dorsal) view

PLATE 430

UPPER LIMB

Metacarpophalangeal and Interphalangeal Ligaments

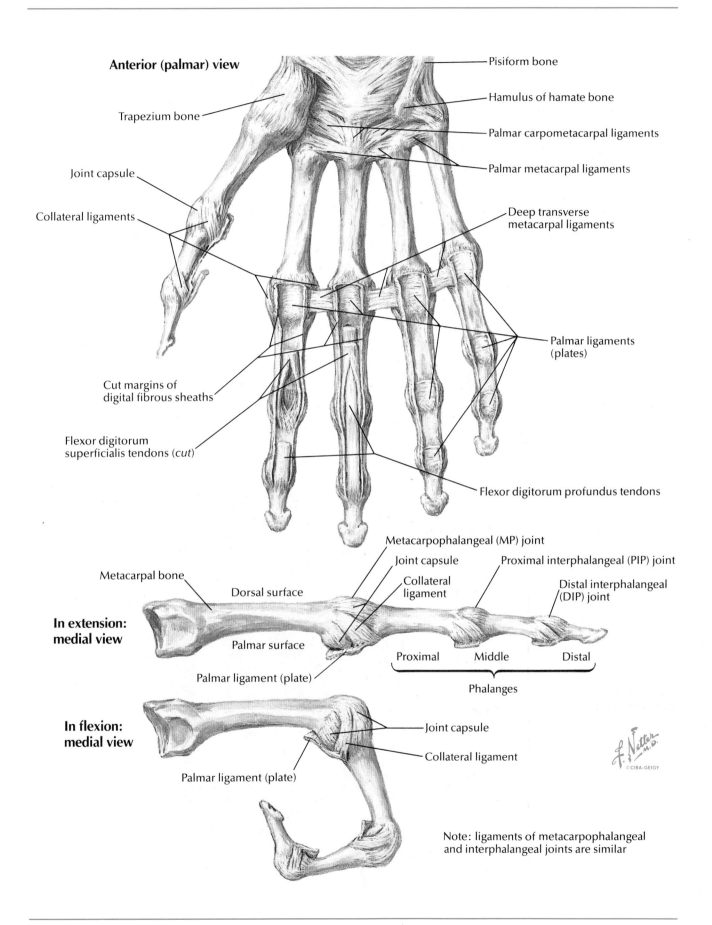

Anterior (palmar) view

Pisiform bone

Hamulus of hamate bone

Palmar carpometacarpal ligaments

Palmar metacarpal ligaments

Trapezium bone

Deep transverse metacarpal ligaments

Joint capsule

Collateral ligaments

Palmar ligaments (plates)

Cut margins of digital fibrous sheaths

Flexor digitorum superficialis tendons (*cut*)

Flexor digitorum profundus tendons

Metacarpophalangeal (MP) joint

Joint capsule

Proximal interphalangeal (PIP) joint

Collateral ligament

Distal interphalangeal (DIP) joint

Metacarpal bone

Dorsal surface

In extension: medial view

Palmar surface

Proximal   Middle   Distal

Palmar ligament (plate)

Phalanges

In flexion: medial view

Joint capsule

Collateral ligament

Palmar ligament (plate)

Note: ligaments of metacarpophalangeal and interphalangeal joints are similar

Wrist and Hand: Superficial Palmar Dissections

Palmaris longus tendon

Branch of superficial radial nerve to skin of lateral thenar area

Palmar carpal ligament (thickening of deep antebrachial fascia)

Palmar branch of median nerve

Thenar muscles

Motor branch of median nerve to thenar muscles

Minute fasciculi attaches palmar aponeurosis to dermis

Palmar branch of ulnar nerve

Pisiform bone

Deep palmar branches of ulnar artery and nerve

Superficial branch of ulnar nerve

Ulnar artery

Palmaris brevis muscle

Hypothenar muscles

Palmar aponeurosis

Anterior (palmar) views

Palmaris brevis muscle (*reflected*)

Palmar digital nerves from superficial branch of ulnar nerve to 5th and medial half of 4th fingers

Palmar aponeurosis

Transverse fasciculi

Palmar digital arteries and nerves

Superficial metacarpal ligaments

PLATE 432

UPPER LIMB

Radial artery and venae comitantes

Flexor carpi radialis tendon

Radial bursa (containing flexor pollicis longus tendon)

Median nerve

Palmaris longus tendon and palmar carpal ligament

Flexor retinaculum

Thenar muscles

Proper palmar digital nerves of thumb

Synovial sheath of flexor pollicis longus tendon (radial bursa)

Probe in 1st lumbrical muscle sheath

Common palmar digital artery

Proper palmar digital arteries

Septa from palmar aponeurosis forming canals

Palmar aponeurosis (reflected)

Ulnar artery with venae comitantes and ulnar nerve

Flexor carpi ulnaris tendon

Ulnar bursa containing superficialis and profundus flexor tendons

Pisiform bone

Deep palmar branches of ulnar artery and nerve

Superficial branch of ulnar nerve

Palmar digital nerves to 5th finger and medial half of 4th finger

Median nerve

Ulnar bursa

Superficial palmar arterial and venous arches

2nd, 3rd and 4th lumbrical muscles (in sheaths)

Synovial flexor tendon sheaths

Anterior (palmar) views

Proper palmar digital nerves of thumb

Fascia over adductor pollicis muscle

1st dorsal interosseous muscle

Probe in dorsal extension of thenar space deep to adductor pollicis muscle

Thenar space (deep to flexor tendons and 1st lumbrical muscle)

Septum separating thenar from midpalmar space

Common palmar digital artery

Proper palmar digital arteries and nerves

Annular and cruciate ligaments of fibrous sheath over synovial flexor tendon sheaths

Superficial palmar branch of radial artery and branch of median nerve to thenar muscles

Ulnar artery and nerve

Common palmar digital branches of median nerve

Hypothenar muscles

Ulnar bursa

5th finger synovial sheath

Probe in midpalmar space

Midpalmar space (deep to flexor tendons and lumbrical muscles)

Insertion of superficial flexor tendon

Insertion of deep flexor tendon

Flexor Tendons, Arteries and Nerves at Wrist

Median duo { Palmaris longus tendon
Median nerve

Radial trio { Radial artery
Flexor carpi radialis tendon
Flexor pollicis longus tendon in radial bursa

Palmar carpal ligament (*reflected*)
Synovial tendon sheath
Flexor retinaculum
Trapezium bone
1st metacarpal bone
Opponens pollicis muscle
Abductor pollicis brevis muscle (*reflected*)
Flexor pollicis brevis muscle (*reflected*)
Adductor pollicis muscle

Flexor digitorum superficialis tendons and flexor digitorum profundus tendons } Two tendon quartets
Ulnar bursa

Ulnar artery
Ulnar nerve
Flexor carpi ulnaris tendon } Ulnar trio

Pisiform bone
Abductor digiti minimi muscle
Flexor digiti minimi brevis muscle
Opponens digiti minimi muscle
Superficial palmar arterial arch
Lumbrical muscles

Schematic cross section proximal to flexor retinaculum

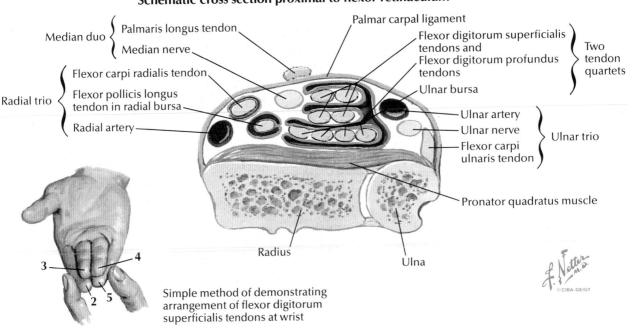

Median duo { Palmaris longus tendon
Median nerve

Radial trio { Flexor carpi radialis tendon
Flexor pollicis longus tendon in radial bursa
Radial artery

Palmar carpal ligament
Flexor digitorum superficialis tendons and Flexor digitorum profundus tendons } Two tendon quartets
Ulnar bursa

Ulnar artery
Ulnar nerve
Flexor carpi ulnaris tendon } Ulnar trio

Pronator quadratus muscle

Radius
Ulna

3 4
2 5

Simple method of demonstrating arrangement of flexor digitorum superficialis tendons at wrist

PLATE 434

UPPER LIMB

Pronator quadratus muscle

Flexor carpi radialis tendon

Flexor pollicis longus tendon in radial bursa

Flexor retinaculum (*reflected*)

Flexor digitorum profundus tendons

Flexor pollicis longus tendon in radial bursa

Fascia over adductor pollicis muscle

Ulnar bursa

Flexor digitorum superficialis tendons

Ulnar bursa (*opened*)

Lumbrical muscles in sheaths

Thenar space
(deep to flexor tendon
and 1st lumbrical muscle)

Digital synovial sheath

Lumbrical muscles in sheaths
(*cut and reflected*)

Annular and cruciate ligaments
of digital fibrous sheath (over
digital synovial sheath)

Midpalmar space
(deep to flexor tendons
and lumbrical muscles)

Digital fibrous and synovial
sheaths (*opened*)

Flexor digitorum superficialis
tendon

Flexor digitorum profundus
tendon

Dorsal subcutaneous space

Fascia of dorsum of hand

Dorsal subaponeurotic space

Dorsal interosseous fascia

Hypothenar muscles

Flexor tendons
to 5th digit
in ulnar bursa

Lumbrical muscle
in its sheath

Palmar digital artery and nerve

Palmar aponeurosis

Extensor tendons

Dorsal interosseous muscles

Palmar interosseous muscles

Palmar interosseous fascia

Adductor pollicis muscle

Extensor pollicis
longus tendon

Flexor pollicis
longus tendon
in radial bursa

Midpalmar space

Septa forming canals

Thenar space

Septum between midpalmar and thenar spaces

Profundus and superficialis flexor tendons to 3rd digit

Lumbrical Muscles and Bursae, Spaces and Sheaths: Schema

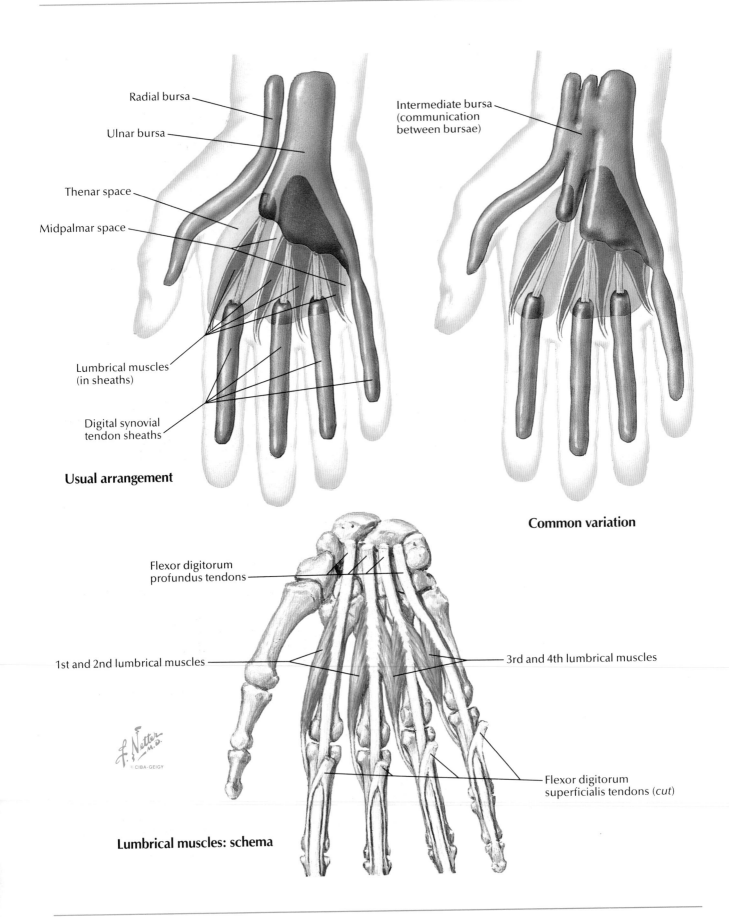

Radial bursa

Ulnar bursa

Thenar space

Midpalmar space

Intermediate bursa
(communication
between bursae)

Lumbrical muscles
(in sheaths)

Digital synovial
tendon sheaths

Usual arrangement

Common variation

Flexor digitorum
profundus tendons

1st and 2nd lumbrical muscles

3rd and 4th lumbrical muscles

Flexor digitorum
superficialis tendons (*cut*)

Lumbrical muscles: schema

PLATE 436

UPPER LIMB

Posterior (dorsal) view

Insertion of central band of extensor tendon to base of middle phalanx

Triangular aponeurosis

Slips of long extensor tendon to lateral bands

Dorsal expansion (hood)

Long extensor tendon

Interosseous muscles

Metacarpal bone

Insertion of extensor tendon to base of distal phalanx

Lateral bands

Interosseous tendon slip to lateral band

Lumbrical muscle

Part of interosseous tendon passes to base of proximal phalanx and joint capsule

Finger in extension: lateral view

Insertion of extensor tendon to base of middle phalanx

Insertion of extensor tendon to base of distal phalanx

Lateral band

Central band

Dorsal expansion (hood)

Long extensor tendon

Metacarpal bone

Collateral ligaments

Vinculum breve

Vincula longa

Flexor digitorum profundus tendon

Flexor digitorum superficialis tendon

Interosseous muscles

Lumbrical muscle

Finger in flexion: lateral view

Collateral ligament

Extensor tendon

Insertion of small deep slip of extensor tendon to proximal phalanx and joint capsule

Attachment of interosseous muscle to base of proximal phalanx and joint capsule

Interosseous muscles

Lumbrical muscle

Insertion of lumbrical muscle to extensor tendon

Palmar ligament (plate)

Flexor digitorum superficialis tendon (cut)

Collateral ligaments

Flexor digitorum profundus tendon (cut)

Palmar ligament (plate)

Note: black arrows indicate pull of long extensor tendon; red arrows indicate pull of interosseous and lumbrical muscles

WRIST AND HAND

PLATE 437

Intrinsic Muscles of Hand

Radial artery and palmar carpal branch

Radius

Superficial palmar branch of radial artery

Flexor retinaculum (*reflected*)

Opponens pollicis muscle

Branches of median nerve to thenar muscles and to 1st and 2nd lumbrical muscles

Abductor pollicis brevis muscle (*cut*)

Flexor pollicis brevis muscle

Adductor pollicis muscle

1st dorsal interosseous muscle

Branches from deep branch of ulnar nerve to 3rd and 4th lumbrical muscles and to all interosseous muscles

Lumbrical muscles (*reflected*)

Pronator quadratus muscle

Ulnar nerve

Ulnar artery and palmar carpal branch

Flexor carpi ulnaris tendon

Pisiform bone

Palmar carpal arterial arch

Median nerve

Abductor digiti minimi muscle (*cut*)

Deep palmar branches of ulnar artery and nerve

Flexor digiti minimi brevis muscle (*cut*)

Opponens digiti minimi muscle

Deep palmar arterial arch

Palmar metacarpal arteries

Common palmar digital arteries

Deep transverse metacarpal ligaments

Anterior (palmar) view

Ulna

Radius

Ulna

Radius

Radial artery

Abductor pollicis brevis muscle

Dorsal interosseous muscles

Abductor digiti minimi muscle

Posterior (dorsal) view

Palmar interosseous muscles

Deep transverse metacarpal ligaments

Anterior (palmar) view

Tendinous slips to hoods of extensor digitorum muscles

Note: arrows indicate action of muscles

PLATE 438

UPPER LIMB

Radial artery

Median nerve and palmar branch

Superficial palmar branch of radial artery

Abductor pollicis brevis muscle (cut)

Opponens pollicis muscle

Flexor pollicis brevis muscle

Motor branch of median nerve to thenar muscles

Proper digital nerves and arteries to thumb

Adductor pollicis muscle

Branches of median nerve to 1st and 2nd lumbrical muscles

Flexor tendons, synovial and fibrous sheaths

Ulnar artery and nerve

Palmar carpal ligament

Flexor retinaculum

Deep palmar branches of ulnar artery and nerve

Superficial branch of ulnar nerve

Ulnar bursa

Superficial palmar arterial arch

Common palmar digital nerves and arteries

Anastomosis between branches of median and ulnar nerves

Proper palmar digital nerves and arteries

Branches of proper palmar digital nerves and arteries to dorsum of middle and distal phalanges

Radial artery

Median nerve

Superficial palmar branch of radial artery

Deep palmar arterial arch

Princeps pollicis artery

Proper digital arteries and nerves of thumb

Distal limit of superficial palmar arch

Radialis indicis artery

Palmar metacarpal arteries

Common palmar digital arteries

Proper palmar digital arteries

Proper palmar digital nerves from median nerve

Ulnar artery and nerve

Palmar carpal branches of radial and ulnar arteries

Pisiform bone

Deep palmar branches of ulnar artery and nerve

Branches to hypothenar muscles

Superficial branch of ulnar nerve

Hamulus of hamate bone

Deep palmar branch of ulnar nerve to 3rd and 4th lumbrical, all interosseous, adductor pollicis and deep head of flexor pollicis brevis muscles

Anastomosis between median and ulnar nerves

Proper palmar digital nerves from ulnar nerve

Wrist and Hand: Superficial Radial Dissection

Lateral (radial) view

Extensor retinaculum

Dorsal carpal branch of radial artery

Extensor carpi radialis brevis tendon

Extensor carpi radialis longus tendon

Radial artery

Ist dorsal interosseous muscle

Fascia (*cut*)

Superficial branch of radial nerve

Medial branch

Lateral branch

Dorsal digital branches of radial nerve

Scaphoid bone

Radial artery in anatomical snuffbox

Trapezium bone

Insertion of abductor pollicis longus tendon

1st metacarpal bone

Insertion of extensor pollicis brevis tendon

Insertion of extensor pollicis longus tendon

PLATE 440

UPPER LIMB

Posterior (dorsal) view

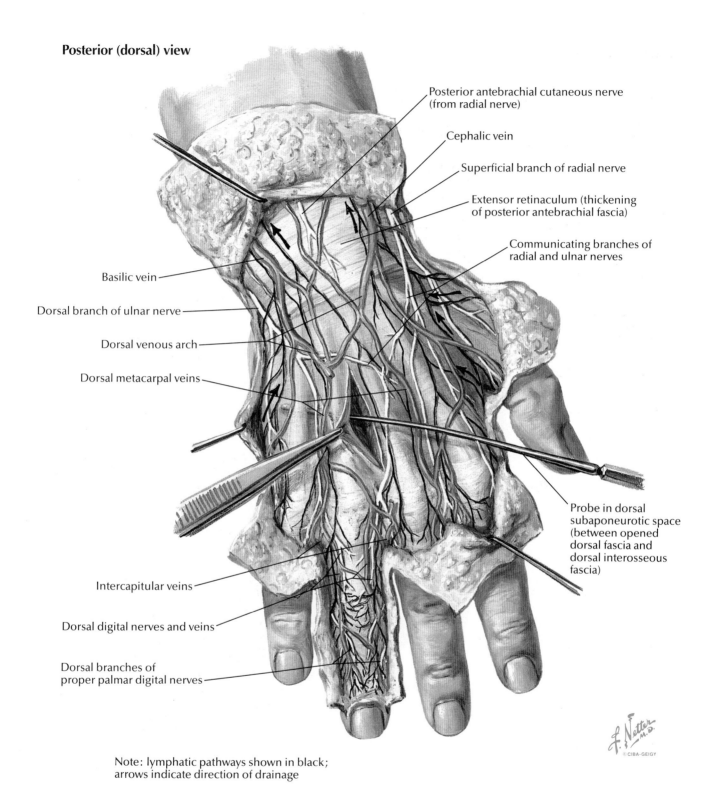

Posterior antebrachial cutaneous nerve
(from radial nerve)

Cephalic vein

Superficial branch of radial nerve

Extensor retinaculum (thickening
of posterior antebrachial fascia)

Communicating branches of
radial and ulnar nerves

Basilic vein

Dorsal branch of ulnar nerve

Dorsal venous arch

Dorsal metacarpal veins

Probe in dorsal
subaponeurotic space
(between opened
dorsal fascia and
dorsal interosseous
fascia)

Intercapitular veins

Dorsal digital nerves and veins

Dorsal branches of
proper palmar digital nerves

Note: lymphatic pathways shown in black;
arrows indicate direction of drainage

Wrist and Hand: Deep Dorsal Dissection

Medial antebrachial cutaneous nerve

Posterior antebrachial cutaneous branch of radial nerve

Extensor retinaculum

Dorsal branch of ulnar nerve

Dorsal carpal branch of ulnar artery

Extensor carpi ulnaris tendon

Dorsal carpal arterial arch

Dorsal metacarpal arteries

Dorsal digital branches of dorsal branch of ulnar nerve

Dorsal branches of proper palmar digital branches of ulnar nerve and of proper palmar digital arteries to dorsum of middle and distal phalanges of 5th and ulnar half of 4th fingers

Lateral antebrachial cutaneous nerve (terminal part of musculocutaneous nerve)

Superficial branch of radial nerve

Extensor digitorum, extensor digiti minimi and extensor indicis tendons (cut)

Radial artery in anatomical snuffbox

Abductor pollicis longus tendon
Extensor pollicis brevis tendon
Extensor pollicis longus tendon
Extensor carpi radialis longus tendon
Extensor carpi radialis brevis tendon

Dorsal digital arteries

Dorsal digital branches of superficial branch of radial nerve to 1st, 2nd, 3rd and radial half of 4th fingers

Posterior (dorsal) view

Dorsal branches of proper palmar digital branches of median nerve and of proper palmar digital arteries to dorsum of middle and distal phalanges of 2nd, 3rd and radial half of 5th fingers

PLATE 442

UPPER LIMB

Posterior (dorsal) view

Extensor carpi ulnaris – **Compartment 6**

Extensor digiti minimi – **Compartment 5**

Extensor digitorum } **Compartment 4**
Extensor indicis }

Extensor pollicis longus – **Compartment 3**

Extensor carpi radialis brevis } **Compartment 2**
Extensor carpi radialis longus }

Abductor pollicis longus } **Compartment 1**
Extensor pollicis brevis }

Radial artery in anatomical snuffbox

Dorsal interosseous muscles

Extensor retinaculum

Abductor digiti minimi muscle

Intertendinous connections

Transverse fibers of dorsal expansions (hoods)

Cross section at proximal wrist

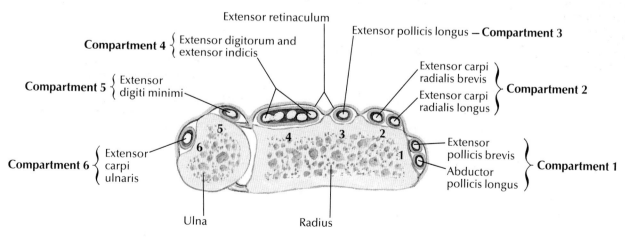

Extensor retinaculum

Compartment 4 { Extensor digitorum and extensor indicis

Extensor pollicis longus – **Compartment 3**

Extensor carpi radialis brevis }
Extensor carpi radialis longus } **Compartment 2**

Compartment 5 { Extensor digiti minimi

Compartment 6 { Extensor carpi ulnaris

Extensor pollicis brevis }
Abductor pollicis longus } **Compartment 1**

Ulna

Radius

Fingers

Sagittal section

Epiphysis

Nail matrix

Nail root

Cuticle (eponychium)

Lunula

Nail bed

Nail body

Distal phalanx

Nerves Arteries Septa

Distal anterior closed space (pulp)

Synovial membrane

Articular cartilage

Middle phalanx

Extensor digitorum tendon

Flexor digitorum superficialis tendon

Fibrous digital sheath

Synovial sheath of flexor tendons

Flexor digitorum profundus tendon

Palmar ligament (plate)

Joint cavity

Cross section through distal phalanx

Subungual space

Minute arteries

Fine nerves

Nail body

Nail bed

Distal phalanx

Fibrous septa and areolar tissue in anterior closed space (pulp)

Dorsal branches of proper palmar digital arteries and nerves to dorsum of middle and terminal phalanges

Dorsal digital artery and nerve

Arteries and nerves

Nutrient branches to metaphysis

Nutrient branch to epiphysis

Proper palmar digital artery and nerve

Proper palmar digital artery to neighboring digit

PLATE 444

UPPER LIMB

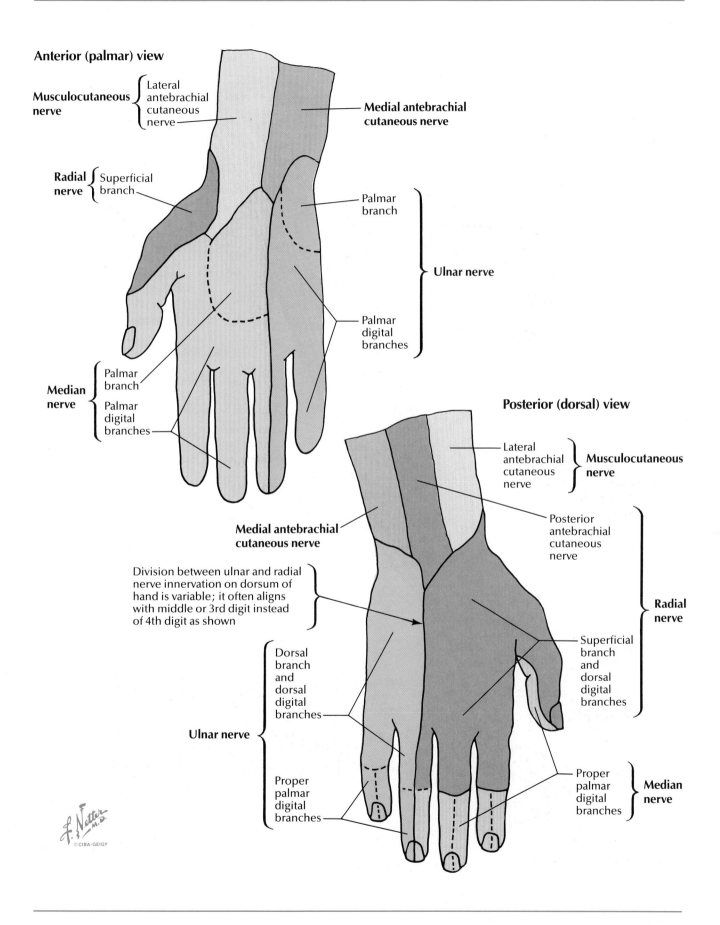

Anterior (palmar) view

Musculocutaneous nerve { Lateral antebrachial cutaneous nerve

Medial antebrachial cutaneous nerve

Radial nerve { Superficial branch

Palmar branch

Ulnar nerve

Palmar digital branches

Median nerve { Palmar branch / Palmar digital branches

Posterior (dorsal) view

Lateral antebrachial cutaneous nerve } **Musculocutaneous nerve**

Medial antebrachial cutaneous nerve

Posterior antebrachial cutaneous nerve

Division between ulnar and radial nerve innervation on dorsum of hand is variable; it often aligns with middle or 3rd digit instead of 4th digit as shown

Radial nerve

Dorsal branch and dorsal digital branches

Superficial branch and dorsal digital branches

Ulnar nerve

Proper palmar digital branches

Proper palmar digital branches } **Median nerve**

Arteries and Nerves of Upper Limb

Anterior view

Deltoid muscle

Coracobrachialis muscle

Biceps brachii muscle
- Short head (*cut*)
- Long head (*cut*)

Musculocutaneous nerve

Brachialis muscle

Biceps brachii muscle (*cut*) and tendon

Lateral antebrachial cutaneous nerve (from musculocutaneous nerve)

Radial nerve
- Deep branch
- Superficial branch

Brachioradialis muscle

Supinator muscle

Radial artery

Pronator teres muscle (*partially cut*)

Median nerve

Flexor pollicis longus muscle

Flexor carpi radialis tendon (*cut*)

Flexor retinaculum

Superficial branch of radial nerve

Motor branch of median nerve to thenar muscles

Common palmar digital branches of median nerve

Proper palmar digital branches of median nerve

Intercostobrachial nerve

Medial brachial cutaneous nerve

Radial nerve

Ulnar nerve

Medial antebrachial cutaneous nerve

Median nerve

Brachial artery

Bicipital aponeurosis

Humeral head (*cut*)
Ulnar head
} Pronator teres muscle

Flexor carpi radialis muscle (*cut*)

Humeroulnar head
Radial head
} Flexor digitorum superficialis muscle (*cut*)

Flexor digitorum profundus muscle

Flexor carpi ulnaris muscle

Ulnar artery and nerve

Dorsal branch of ulnar nerve

Flexor digitorum superficialis tendons (*cut*)

Deep palmar branches of ulnar artery and nerve

Superficial branch of ulnar nerve

Superficial palmar arterial arch (*cut*)

Common palmar digital branch of ulnar nerve

Anastomosis between branches of median and ulnar nerves

Proper palmar digital branches of ulnar nerve

PLATE 446

UPPER LIMB

Anterior view

Note: only muscles innervated by musculocutaneous nerve shown

Musculocutaneous nerve (C5, 6, 7)

Coracobrachialis muscle

Biceps brachii muscle (*reflected*)

Brachialis muscle

Articular branch

Lateral antebrachial cutaneous nerve

Anterior branch

Posterior branch

Medial
Posterior } Cords of brachial plexus
Lateral

Medial brachial cutaneous nerve

Medial antebrachial cutaneous nerve

Ulnar nerve

Median nerve

Radial nerve

Axillary nerve

Cutaneous innervation

Anterior (palmar) view

Posterior (dorsal) view

Median Nerve

Anterior view

Note: only muscles innervated by median nerve shown

Musculocutaneous nerve

Median nerve (C 5, 6, 7, 8, T1)
Inconstant contribution

Pronator teres muscle (humeral head)

Articular branch

Flexor carpi radialis muscle

Palmaris longus muscle

Pronator teres muscle (ulnar head)

Flexor digitorum superficialis muscle (turned up)

Flexor digitorum profundus muscle (lateral part supplied by anterior interosseous nerve; medial part supplied by ulnar nerve)

Anterior interosseous nerve

Flexor pollicis longus muscle

Pronator quadratus muscle

Palmar branch of median nerve

Thenar muscles
{
Abductor pollicis brevis
Opponens pollicis
Flexor pollicis brevis (superficial head; deep head often supplied by ulnar nerve)
}

1st and 2nd lumbrical muscles

Dorsal branches to dorsum of middle and distal phalanges

Medial
Posterior } Cords of brachial plexus
Lateral

Medial brachial cutaneous nerve

Medial antebrachial cutaneous nerve

Axillary nerve

Radial nerve

Ulnar nerve

F. Netter M.D.
© CIBA-GEIGY

Cutaneous innervation

Palmar view

Anastomotic branch to ulnar nerve

Common palmar digital nerves

Proper palmar digital nerves

Posterior (dorsal) view

PLATE 448

UPPER LIMB

Anterior view

Note: only muscles innervated by ulnar nerve shown

Ulnar nerve (C7, 8, T1) (no branches above elbow)

Inconstant contribution

Cutaneous innervation

Medial epicondyle

Articular branch (behind condyle)

Flexor digitorum profundus muscle (medial part only; lateral part supplied by anterior interosseous branch of median nerve)

Palmar view

Posterior (dorsal) view

Flexor carpi ulnaris muscle (*drawn aside*)

Dorsal branch of ulnar nerve

Palmar branch

Flexor pollicis brevis muscle (deep head only; superficial head and other thenar muscles supplied by median nerve)

Superficial branch

Deep branch

Palmaris brevis

Abductor digiti minimi

Adductor pollicis muscle

Flexor digiti minimi brevis

Opponens digiti minimi

Hypothenar muscles

Common palmar digital nerve

Anastomotic branch to median nerve

Palmar and dorsal interosseous muscles

3rd and 4th lumbrical muscles (*turned down*)

Proper palmar digital nerves (dorsal digital nerves are from dorsal branch)

Dorsal branches to dorsum of middle and distal phalanges

F. Netter M.D.
©CIBA-GEIGY

Radial Nerve in Arm and Nerves of Posterior Shoulder

Posterior view

Dorsal scapular nerve (C5)

Supraspinatus muscle

Suprascapular nerve (C5, 6)

Levator scapulae muscle (supplied also by branches from C5 and C6)

Deltoid muscle

Teres minor muscle

Axillary nerve (C5, 6)

Superior lateral brachial cutaneous nerve

Rhomboideus minor muscle

Radial nerve (C5, 6, 7, 8, T1)

Inconstant contribution

Rhomboideus major muscle

Inferior lateral brachial cutaneous nerve

Posterior antebrachial cutaneous nerve

Infraspinatus muscle

Teres major muscle

Lateral intermuscular septum

Lower subscapular nerve (C5, 6)

Posterior brachial cutaneous nerve (branch of radial nerve in axilla)

Brachialis muscle (lateral part; remainder of muscle supplied by musculocutaneous nerve)

Triceps brachii muscle { Long head / Lateral head / Medial head

Brachioradialis muscle

Triceps brachii tendon

Medial epicondyle

Extensor carpi radialis longus muscle

Olecranon

Anconeus muscle

Extensor carpi radialis brevis muscle

Extensor digitorum muscle

Extensor carpi ulnaris muscle

PLATE 450

UPPER LIMB

Radial nerve (C5, 6, 7, 8, T1)   Inconstant contribution

Superficial (terminal) branch

Deep (terminal) branch

Posterior view

Lateral epicondyle

Anconeus muscle

Brachioradialis muscle

Extensor carpi radialis longus muscle

Supinator muscle

Extensor carpi radialis brevis muscle

Extensor carpi ulnaris muscle

Extensor digitorum muscle and
extensor digiti minimi muscle

Extensor-supinator
group of muscles

Extensor indicis muscle

Extensor pollicis longus muscle

Abductor pollicis longus muscle

Extensor pollicis brevis muscle

Posterior interosseous nerve
(deep branch of radial nerve distal to muscular branches)

Superficial branch of radial nerve

From axillary nerve

Superior
lateral brachial
cutaneous nerve

Inferior
lateral brachial
cutaneous nerve

Posterior brachial
cutaneous nerve

From radial nerve

Posterior antebrachial
cutaneous nerve

Superficial branch of
radial nerve and dorsal
digital branches

Dorsal digital nerves

**Cutaneous innervation from
radial and axillary nerves**

Cutaneous Nerves and Superficial Veins of Shoulder and Arm

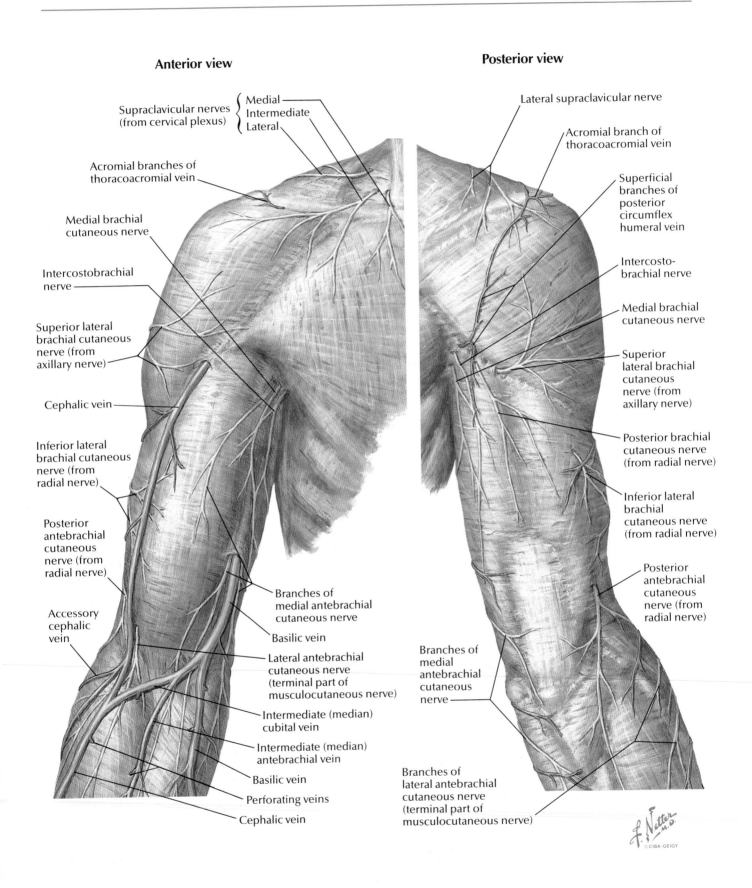

Anterior view

Supraclavicular nerves (from cervical plexus) { Medial / Intermediate / Lateral

Acromial branches of thoracoacromial vein

Medial brachial cutaneous nerve

Intercostobrachial nerve

Superior lateral brachial cutaneous nerve (from axillary nerve)

Cephalic vein

Inferior lateral brachial cutaneous nerve (from radial nerve)

Posterior antebrachial cutaneous nerve (from radial nerve)

Accessory cephalic vein

Branches of medial antebrachial cutaneous nerve

Basilic vein

Lateral antebrachial cutaneous nerve (terminal part of musculocutaneous nerve)

Intermediate (median) cubital vein

Intermediate (median) antebrachial vein

Basilic vein

Perforating veins

Cephalic vein

Posterior view

Lateral supraclavicular nerve

Acromial branch of thoracoacromial vein

Superficial branches of posterior circumflex humeral vein

Intercosto-brachial nerve

Medial brachial cutaneous nerve

Superior lateral brachial cutaneous nerve (from axillary nerve)

Posterior brachial cutaneous nerve (from radial nerve)

Inferior lateral brachial cutaneous nerve (from radial nerve)

Posterior antebrachial cutaneous nerve (from radial nerve)

Branches of medial antebrachial cutaneous nerve

Branches of lateral antebrachial cutaneous nerve (terminal part of musculocutaneous nerve)

PLATE 452

UPPER LIMB

Cutaneous Nerves and Superficial Veins of Forearm

Anterior (palmar) view

Cephalic vein

Posterior antebrachial cutaneous nerve (from radial nerve)

Lateral antebrachial cutaneous nerve (from musculo-cutaneous nerve)

Accessory cephalic vein

Intermediate (median) cephalic vein

Cephalic vein

Intermediate (median) antebrachial vein

Note: in 70% of cases an intermediate cubital vein (tributary to basilic vein) replaces intermediate cephalic and intermediate basilic veins (see plate 452)

Superficial branch of radial nerve

Palmar branch of median nerve

Intercapitular veins

Basilic vein

Anterior branch and Posterior branch of medial antebrachial cutaneous nerve

Intermediate (median) basilic vein

Bicipital aponeurosis

Basilic vein

Perforating veins

Palmar branch of ulnar nerve

Dorsal branch of ulnar nerve

Palmar carpal ligament

Palmar aponeurosis

Superficial transverse metacarpal ligament

Proper palmar digital nerves and palmar digital veins

Posterior (dorsal) view

Posterior branch of medial antebrachial cutaneous nerve

Basilic vein

Dorsal branch of ulnar nerve

Dorsal metacarpal veins

Intercapitular veins

Posterior antebrachial cutaneous nerve (from radial nerve)

Accessory cephalic vein

Posterior branch of lateral antebrachial cutaneous nerve (from musculocu-taneous nerve)

Cephalic vein

Superficial branch of radial nerve

Dorsal venous arch

Dorsal digital nerves and veins

Cutaneous Innervation of Upper Limb

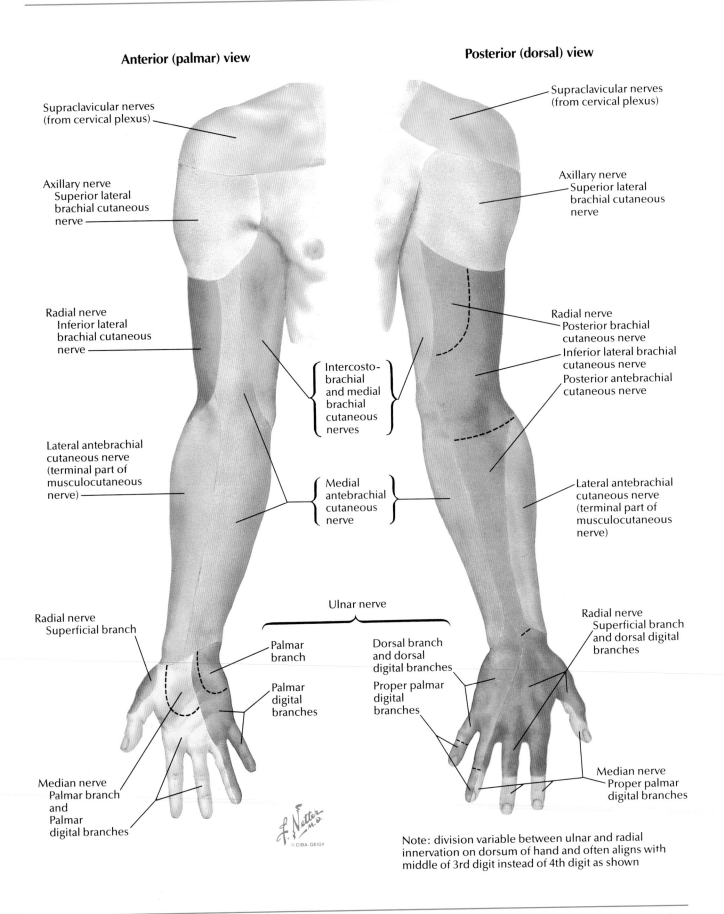

Anterior (palmar) view

Supraclavicular nerves
(from cervical plexus)

Axillary nerve
Superior lateral
brachial cutaneous
nerve

Radial nerve
Inferior lateral
brachial cutaneous
nerve

Lateral antebrachial
cutaneous nerve
(terminal part of
musculocutaneous
nerve)

Intercosto-
brachial
and medial
brachial
cutaneous
nerves

Medial
antebrachial
cutaneous
nerve

Radial nerve
Superficial branch

Ulnar nerve

Palmar
branch

Palmar
digital
branches

Median nerve
Palmar branch
and
Palmar
digital branches

Posterior (dorsal) view

Supraclavicular nerves
(from cervical plexus)

Axillary nerve
Superior lateral
brachial cutaneous
nerve

Radial nerve
Posterior brachial
cutaneous nerve
Inferior lateral brachial
cutaneous nerve
Posterior antebrachial
cutaneous nerve

Lateral antebrachial
cutaneous nerve
(terminal part of
musculocutaneous
nerve)

Radial nerve
Superficial branch
and dorsal digital
branches

Dorsal branch
and dorsal
digital branches

Proper palmar
digital
branches

Median nerve
Proper palmar
digital branches

Note: division variable between ulnar and radial
innervation on dorsum of hand and often aligns with
middle of 3rd digit instead of 4th digit as shown

F. Netter M.D.
© CIBA-GEIGY

PLATE 454

UPPER LIMB

Note: schematic demarcation of dermatomes
shown as distinct segments. There is actually
considerable overlap between adjacent dermatomes

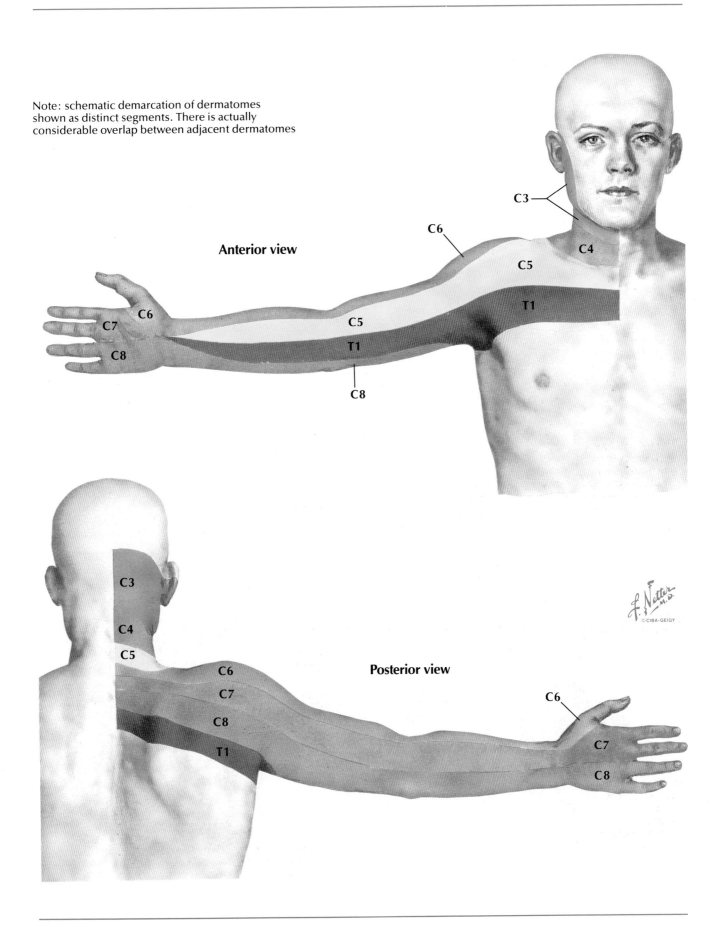

Anterior view

C3

C6

C4

C5

T1

C5

C6

C7

T1

C8

C8

C3

C4

C5

C6

C7

C8

T1

Posterior view

C6

C7

C8

SEE ALSO PLATES 169, 441

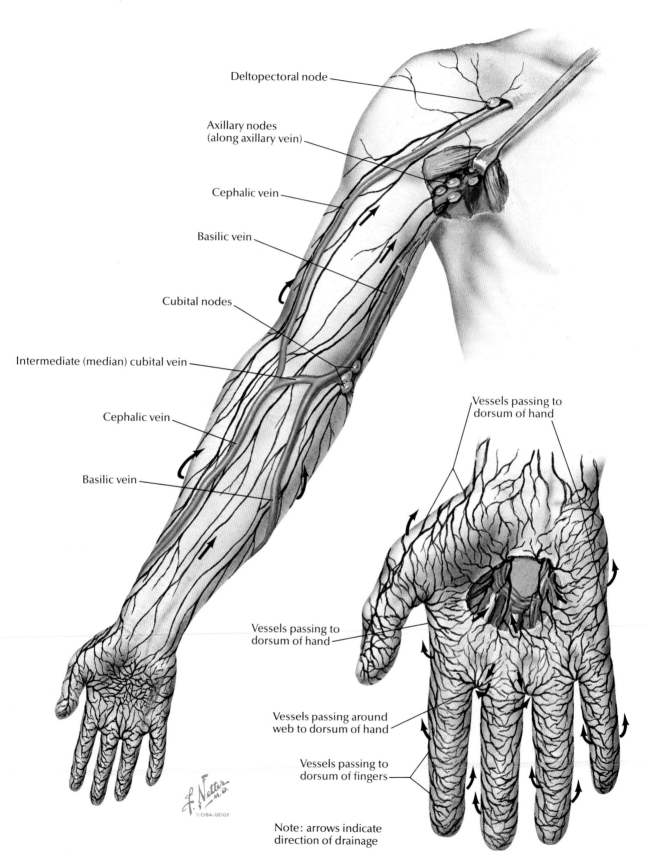

Deltopectoral node

Axillary nodes
(along axillary vein)

Cephalic vein

Basilic vein

Cubital nodes

Intermediate (median) cubital vein

Cephalic vein

Basilic vein

Vessels passing to
dorsum of hand

Vessels passing to
dorsum of hand

Vessels passing around
web to dorsum of hand

Vessels passing to
dorsum of fingers

Note: arrows indicate
direction of drainage

PLATE 456

UPPER LIMB

Section VII

LOWER LIMB

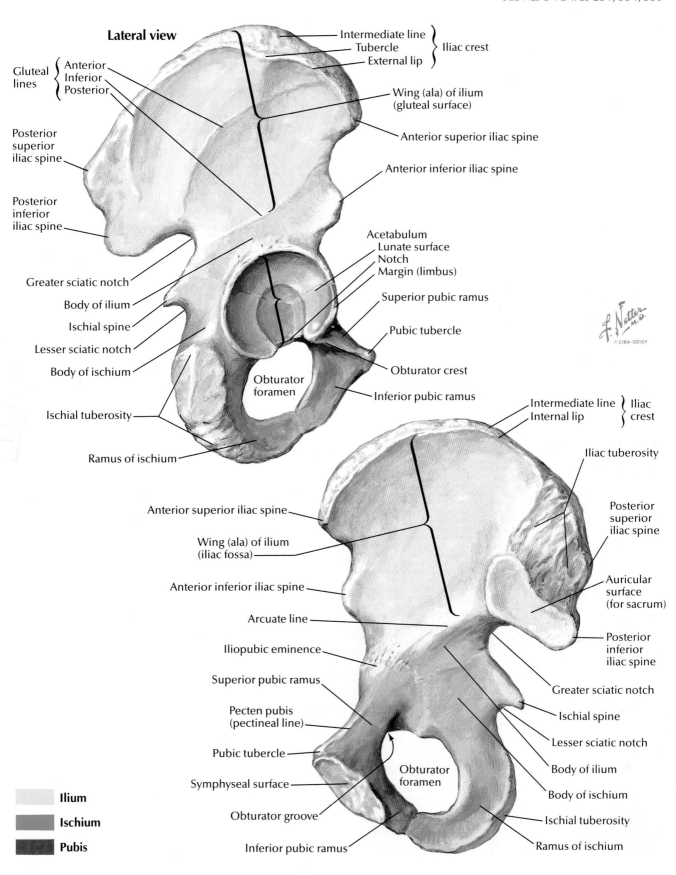

Lateral view

Gluteal lines { Anterior / Inferior / Posterior

Intermediate line
Tubercle } Iliac crest
External lip

Wing (ala) of ilium (gluteal surface)

Anterior superior iliac spine

Anterior inferior iliac spine

Posterior superior iliac spine

Posterior inferior iliac spine

Acetabulum
Lunate surface
Notch
Margin (limbus)

Superior pubic ramus

Pubic tubercle

Greater sciatic notch

Body of ilium

Ischial spine

Lesser sciatic notch

Body of ischium

Obturator crest

Inferior pubic ramus

Obturator foramen

Ischial tuberosity

Ramus of ischium

Intermediate line
Internal lip } Iliac crest

Iliac tuberosity

Posterior superior iliac spine

Anterior superior iliac spine

Wing (ala) of ilium (iliac fossa)

Anterior inferior iliac spine

Arcuate line

Iliopubic eminence

Superior pubic ramus

Pecten pubis (pectineal line)

Pubic tubercle

Symphyseal surface

Auricular surface (for sacrum)

Posterior inferior iliac spine

Greater sciatic notch

Ischial spine

Lesser sciatic notch

Body of ilium

Body of ischium

Ischial tuberosity

Obturator groove

Obturator foramen

Inferior pubic ramus

Ramus of ischium

Ilium

Ischium

Pubis

Hip Joint

Anterior view

Anterior superior iliac spine

Anterior inferior iliac spine

Greater trochanter

Intertrochanteric line

Lesser trochanter

Iliofemoral ligament (Y ligament of Bigelow)

Iliopectineal bursa (over gap in ligaments)

Pubofemoral ligament

Obturator crest

Superior pubic ramus

Posterior view

Iliofemoral ligament

Ischiofemoral ligament

Zona orbicularis

Greater trochanter

Ischial spine

Ischial tuberosity

Protrusion of synovial sac

Intertrochanteric crest

Lesser trochanter

Joint opened: lateral view

Lunate surface of acetabulum

Articular cartilage

Greater trochanter

Head of femur

Neck of femur

Intertrochanteric line

Round ligament (ligamentum capitis femoris) (cut)

Lesser trochanter

Ischial tuberosity

Anterior superior iliac spine

Anterior inferior iliac spine

Iliopubic eminence

Acetabular labrum (fibrocartilaginous)

Fat in acetabular fossa (covered by synovial membrane)

Obturator artery

Anterior branch

Posterior branch

Acetabular artery

Obturator membrane

Transverse acetabular ligament

PLATE 458

LOWER LIMB

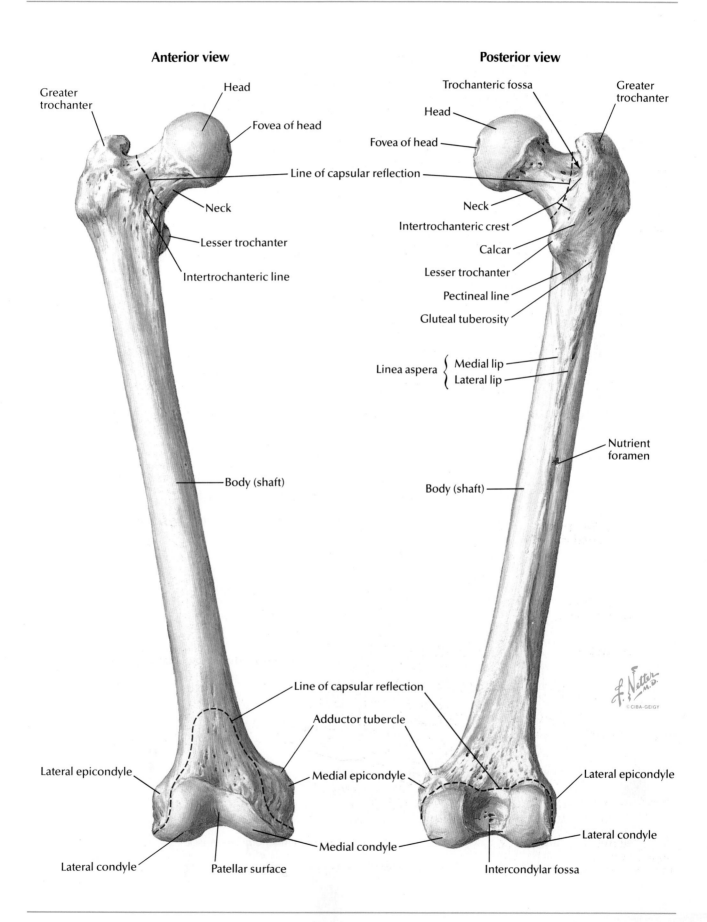

Anterior view

Greater trochanter

Head

Fovea of head

Line of capsular reflection

Neck

Lesser trochanter

Intertrochanteric line

Body (shaft)

Line of capsular reflection

Adductor tubercle

Medial epicondyle

Lateral epicondyle

Medial condyle

Lateral condyle

Patellar surface

Posterior view

Trochanteric fossa

Greater trochanter

Head

Fovea of head

Neck

Intertrochanteric crest

Calcar

Lesser trochanter

Pectineal line

Gluteal tuberosity

Linea aspera { Medial lip / Lateral lip

Nutrient foramen

Body (shaft)

Lateral epicondyle

Lateral condyle

Intercondylar fossa

Bony Attachments of Muscles of Hip and Thigh: Anterior View

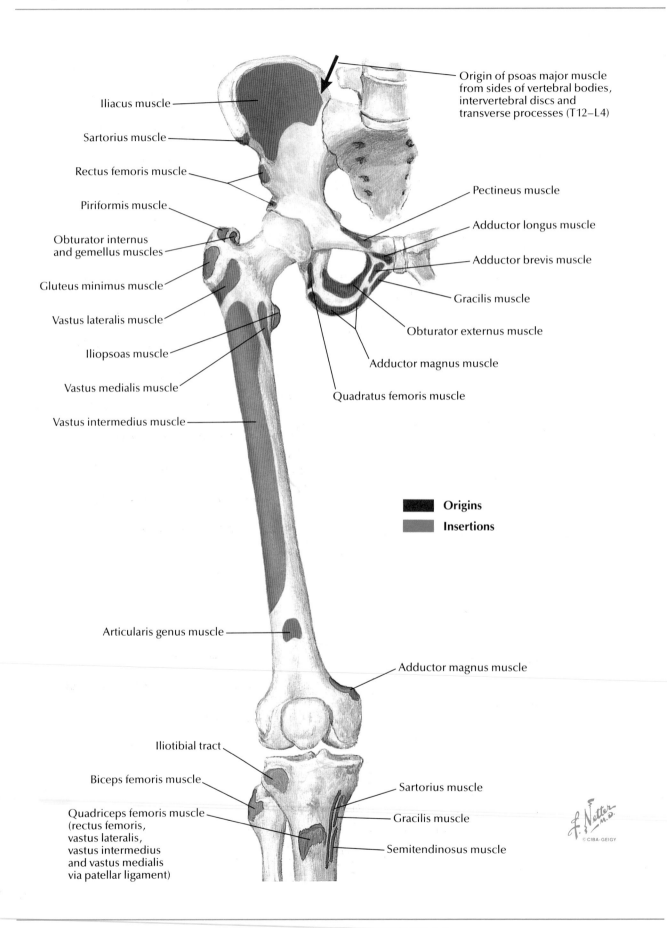

Iliacus muscle

Sartorius muscle

Rectus femoris muscle

Piriformis muscle

Obturator internus and gemellus muscles

Gluteus minimus muscle

Vastus lateralis muscle

Iliopsoas muscle

Vastus medialis muscle

Vastus intermedius muscle

Origin of psoas major muscle from sides of vertebral bodies, intervertebral discs and transverse processes (T12–L4)

Pectineus muscle

Adductor longus muscle

Adductor brevis muscle

Gracilis muscle

Obturator externus muscle

Adductor magnus muscle

Quadratus femoris muscle

■ Origins

■ Insertions

Articularis genus muscle

Adductor magnus muscle

Iliotibial tract

Biceps femoris muscle

Quadriceps femoris muscle (rectus femoris, vastus lateralis, vastus intermedius and vastus medialis via patellar ligament)

Sartorius muscle

Gracilis muscle

Semitendinosus muscle

PLATE 460

LOWER LIMB

Gluteus medius muscle

Gluteus minimus muscle

Tensor fasciae latae muscle

Sartorius muscle

Rectus femoris muscle

Obturator externus muscle

Gluteus medius muscle

Quadratus femoris muscle

Iliopsoas muscle

Gluteus maximus muscle

Vastus lateralis muscle

Adductor magnus muscle

Adductor brevis muscle

Vastus intermedius muscle

Biceps femoris muscle (short head)

Adductor magnus muscle

Vastus lateralis muscle

Plantaris muscle

Gastrocnemius muscle (lateral head)

Popliteus muscle

Gluteus maximus muscle

Superior gemellus muscle

Inferior gemellus muscle

Quadratus femoris muscle

Obturator internus muscle

Adductor magnus muscle

Biceps femoris (long head)
and semitendinosus muscles

Semimembranosus muscle

Pectineus muscle

Vastus medialis muscle

Adductor longus muscle

Adductor magnus muscle

Gastrocnemius muscle (medial head)

Semimembranosus muscle

Popliteus muscle

■ **Origins**
■ **Insertions**

Muscles of Thigh: Anterior Views

Anterior superior iliac spine

Iliacus muscle

Psoas major muscle

Gluteus medius muscle

Inguinal ligament

Pubic tubercle

Iliopsoas muscle

Tensor fasciae latae muscle

Pectineus muscle

Tensor fasciae latae muscle (origin)

Rectus femoris muscle (origin)

Greater trochanter

Iliopsoas muscle (cut)

Adductor longus muscle

Gracilis muscle

Sartorius muscle

Rectus femoris muscle

Vastus lateralis muscle

Vastus intermedius muscle

Vastus medialis muscle

Iliotibial tract

Rectus femoris tendon

Lateral patellar retinaculum

Patella

Medial patellar retinaculum

Patellar ligament

Sartorius tendon
Gracilis tendon
Semitendinosus tendon

Pes anserinus

Tibial tuberosity

Anterior superior iliac spine

Sartorius muscle (origin)

Anterior inferior iliac spine

Ligaments of hip joint

Pectineus muscle

Iliotibial tract (cut)

Rectus femoris tendon (cut)

Patella

Lateral patellar retinaculum

Medial patellar retinaculum

Head of fibula

Patellar ligament

Tibial tuberosity

Sartorius tendon

PLATE 462

LOWER LIMB

Deep dissection

Anterior superior iliac spine

Anterior inferior iliac spine

Ligaments of hip joint

Greater trochanter of femur

Iliopsoas muscle (*cut*)

Pectineus muscle
(*cut and reflected*)

Adductor brevis muscle
(*cut and reflected*)

Vastus intermedius muscle

Adductor longus muscle
(*cut and reflected*)

Femoral artery and vein
passes through hiatus
of adductor magnus muscle

Vastus medialis muscle (*cut*)

Rectus femoris tendon (*cut*)

Vastus lateralis muscle (*cut*)

Lateral epicondyle of femur

Patella

Lateral patellar retinaculum

Fibular collateral ligament

Head of fibula

Patellar ligament

Tibial tuberosity

Pectineus muscle (*cut and reflected*)

Superior ramus of pubis

Adductor longus muscle (*cut and reflected*)

Adductor brevis muscle (*cut*)

Pubic tubercle

Gracilis muscle (*cut*)

Obturator externus muscle

Quadratus femoris muscle

Adductor minimus part of
Adductor magnus muscle

Openings for perforating branches
of deep femoral artery

Medial epicondyle of femur
(adductor tubercle)

Gracilis muscle (*cut*)

Tibial collateral ligament

Medial patellar retinaculum

Sartorius tendon (*cut*)

Gracilis tendon

Semitendinosus tendon

Muscles of Hip and Thigh: Lateral View

Iliac crest

External abdominal oblique muscle

Fascia (gluteal aponeurosis) over gluteus medius muscle

Anterior superior iliac spine

Gluteus maximus muscle

Sartorius muscle

Tensor fasciae latae muscle

Rectus femoris muscle

Vastus lateralis muscle

Iliotibial tract

Biceps femoris muscle { Long head

Short head

Lateral epicondyle of tibia and Gerdy's tubercle

Semimembranosus muscle

Lateral patellar retinaculum

Fibular collateral ligament

Patella

Plantaris muscle

Extensor digitorum longus muscle

Gastrocnemius muscle (lateral head)

Patellar ligament

Head of fibula

Peroneus longus muscle

Tibialis anterior muscle

PLATE 464

LOWER LIMB

FOR PIRIFORMIS AND OBTURATOR INTERNUS SEE ALSO PLATES 337, 338; FOR OBTURATOR EXTERNUS SEE PLATE 463

Superficial dissection

Deeper dissection

Iliac crest

Fascia (gluteal aponeurosis) over
Gluteus medius muscle

Gluteus minimus muscle

Gluteus maximus muscle

Piriformis muscle

Sciatic nerve

Sacrospinous ligament

Superior gemellus muscle

Obturator internus muscle

Inferior gemellus muscle

Sacrotuberous ligament

Quadratus femoris muscle

Ischial tuberosity

Greater trochanter

Semitendinosus muscle

Biceps femoris muscle (long head)

Adductor minimus part of
Adductor magnus muscle

Semimembranosus muscle

Iliotibial tract

Gracilis muscle

Biceps femoris muscle
Short head
Long head

Semimembranosus muscle

Semitendinosus muscle

Popliteal vessels and tibial nerve

Common peroneal nerve

Plantaris muscle

Gastrocnemius muscle
Medial head
Lateral head

Sartorius muscle

Popliteus muscle

Soleus muscle

Plantaris tendon (*cut*)

Psoas and Iliacus Muscles

SEE ALSO PLATE 246

Quadratus lumborum muscle

12th rib

Transversus abdominis muscle (*cut*)

Iliohypogastric nerve

Ilioinguinal nerve

Psoas minor muscle

Psoas major muscle

Genitofemoral nerve

Lateral femoral cutaneous nerve

Iliacus muscle

Femoral nerve

Superior pubic ramus

Greater trochanter of femur

Iliopsoas muscle passes backward to insertion on lesser trochanter

Body (shaft) of femur

Origin of psoas major muscle from vertebral bodies, transverse processes and intervertebral discs (T12–L4) and origin of psoas minor muscle from vertebral bodies (T12, L1)

Lumbar plexus

Lumbosacral trunk

Iliac crest

Anterior superior iliac spine

Iliopectineal bursa

Iliofemoral ligament of hip joint (Y ligament of Bigelow)

Abductors (Gluteus medius and minimus muscles)

Adductors

Note: arrows indicate direction of action of iliopsoas muscle

PLATE 466

Intercostal nerve (T11)

Subcostal nerve (T12)

Iliohypogastric nerve (T12, L1)

Ilioinguinal nerve (L1)

To psoas major and psoas minor muscles

Genitofemoral nerve (L1, 2)

Lateral femoral cutaneous nerve (L2, 3)

Genital branch and Femoral branch of genitofemoral nerve

To psoas major and iliacus muscles

Anterior branches and Lateral branches of subcostal and iliohypogastric nerves

Lumbosacral trunk

To quadratus femoris and inferior gemellus muscles (L4, 5, S1)

To obturator internus and superior gemellus muscles (L5, S1, 2)

Superior gluteal nerve (L4, 5, S1)

To piriformis muscle (S1, 2)

Obturator nerve (L2, 3, 4)

Accessory obturator nerve (L3, 4) (inconstant)

Inferior gluteal nerve (L5, S1, 2)

Femoral nerve (L2, 3, 4)

Sciatic nerve

Posterior femoral cutaneous nerve (S1, 2, 3)

Pudendal nerve (S2, 3, 4)

Sciatic nerve {
Common peroneal nerve (L4, 5, S1, 2)

Tibial nerve (L4, 5, S1, 2, 3)

Rami communicantes

Anterior division
Posterior division

T12

Sympathetic trunk

L1

L2

Lumbar plexus

L3

L4

L5

S1

Sacral plexus

S2

S3

S4

S5
Co

Coccygeal plexus

Pelvic splanchnic nerves (nervi erigentes)

Perforating cutaneous nerve (S2, 3)

To levator ani and coccygeus muscles (S3, 4)

Perineal branch of 4th sacral nerve

Anococcygeal nerves

Obturator nerve

Inferior rectal nerve

Dorsal nerve of penis (clitoris)

Posterior femoral cutaneous nerve

Perineal nerve and Posterior scrotal (labial) branches

Lumbar Plexus

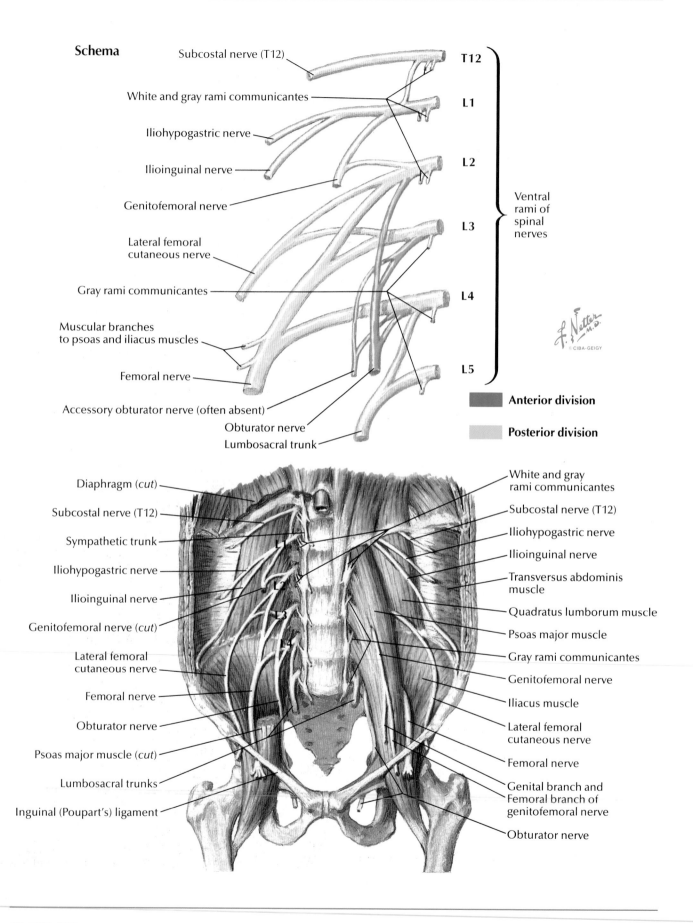

Schema

Subcostal nerve (T12)

White and gray rami communicantes

Iliohypogastric nerve

Ilioinguinal nerve

Genitofemoral nerve

Lateral femoral cutaneous nerve

Gray rami communicantes

Muscular branches to psoas and iliacus muscles

Femoral nerve

Accessory obturator nerve (often absent)

Obturator nerve

Lumbosacral trunk

T12

L1

L2

L3

L4

L5

Ventral rami of spinal nerves

Anterior division

Posterior division

Diaphragm (cut)

Subcostal nerve (T12)

Sympathetic trunk

Iliohypogastric nerve

Ilioinguinal nerve

Genitofemoral nerve (cut)

Lateral femoral cutaneous nerve

Femoral nerve

Obturator nerve

Psoas major muscle (cut)

Lumbosacral trunks

Inguinal (Poupart's) ligament

White and gray rami communicantes

Subcostal nerve (T12)

Iliohypogastric nerve

Ilioinguinal nerve

Transversus abdominis muscle

Quadratus lumborum muscle

Psoas major muscle

Gray rami communicantes

Genitofemoral nerve

Iliacus muscle

Lateral femoral cutaneous nerve

Femoral nerve

Genital branch and Femoral branch of genitofemoral nerve

Obturator nerve

PLATE 468

LOWER LIMB

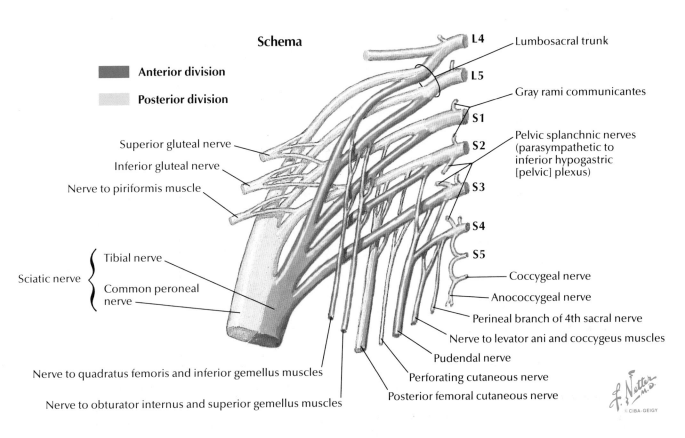

Schema

■ **Anterior division**

☐ **Posterior division**

L4 — Lumbosacral trunk

L5

Gray rami communicantes

S1

S2 — Pelvic splanchnic nerves (parasympathetic to inferior hypogastric [pelvic] plexus)

Superior gluteal nerve

Inferior gluteal nerve

Nerve to piriformis muscle

S3

S4

S5

Tibial nerve

Sciatic nerve {

Common peroneal nerve

Coccygeal nerve

Anococcygeal nerve

Perineal branch of 4th sacral nerve

Nerve to levator ani and coccygeus muscles

Pudendal nerve

Nerve to quadratus femoris and inferior gemellus muscles

Perforating cutaneous nerve

Posterior femoral cutaneous nerve

Nerve to obturator internus and superior gemellus muscles

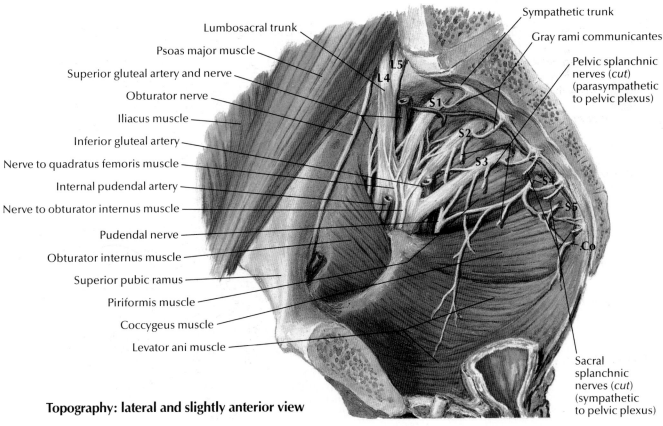

Lumbosacral trunk

Psoas major muscle

Superior gluteal artery and nerve

Obturator nerve

Iliacus muscle

Inferior gluteal artery

Nerve to quadratus femoris muscle

Internal pudendal artery

Nerve to obturator internus muscle

Pudendal nerve

Obturator internus muscle

Superior pubic ramus

Piriformis muscle

Coccygeus muscle

Levator ani muscle

Sympathetic trunk

Gray rami communicantes

Pelvic splanchnic nerves (cut) (parasympathetic to pelvic plexus)

L5

L4

S1

S2

S3

S4

S5

Co

Sacral splanchnic nerves (cut) (sympathetic to pelvic plexus)

Topography: lateral and slightly anterior view

Arteries and Nerves of Thigh: Anterior Views

SEE ALSO PLATE 506

Superficial dissections

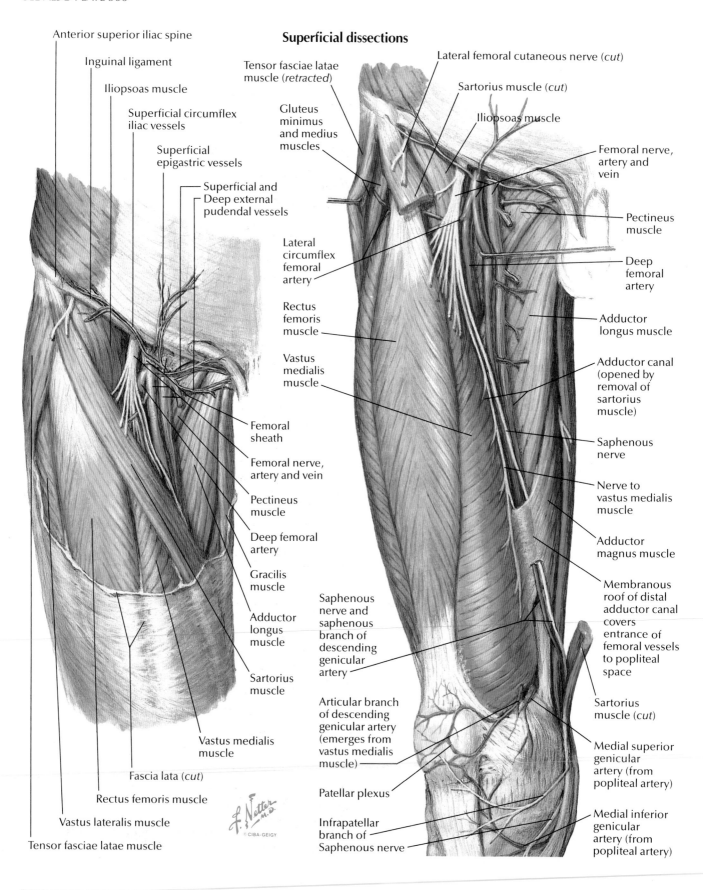

Anterior superior iliac spine

Inguinal ligament

Iliopsoas muscle

Superficial circumflex iliac vessels

Superficial epigastric vessels

Superficial and Deep external pudendal vessels

Tensor fasciae latae muscle (*retracted*)

Gluteus minimus and medius muscles

Lateral circumflex femoral artery

Rectus femoris muscle

Vastus medialis muscle

Femoral sheath

Femoral nerve, artery and vein

Pectineus muscle

Deep femoral artery

Gracilis muscle

Adductor longus muscle

Sartorius muscle

Vastus medialis muscle

Fascia lata (*cut*)

Rectus femoris muscle

Vastus lateralis muscle

Tensor fasciae latae muscle

Saphenous nerve and saphenous branch of descending genicular artery

Articular branch of descending genicular artery (emerges from vastus medialis muscle)

Patellar plexus

Infrapatellar branch of Saphenous nerve

Lateral femoral cutaneous nerve (*cut*)

Sartorius muscle (*cut*)

Iliopsoas muscle

Femoral nerve, artery and vein

Pectineus muscle

Deep femoral artery

Adductor longus muscle

Adductor canal (opened by removal of sartorius muscle)

Saphenous nerve

Nerve to vastus medialis muscle

Adductor magnus muscle

Membranous roof of distal adductor canal covers entrance of femoral vessels to popliteal space

Sartorius muscle (*cut*)

Medial superior genicular artery (from popliteal artery)

Medial inferior genicular artery (from popliteal artery)

F. Netter m.d.

©CIBA-GEIGY

PLATE 470

LOWER LIMB

Deep dissection

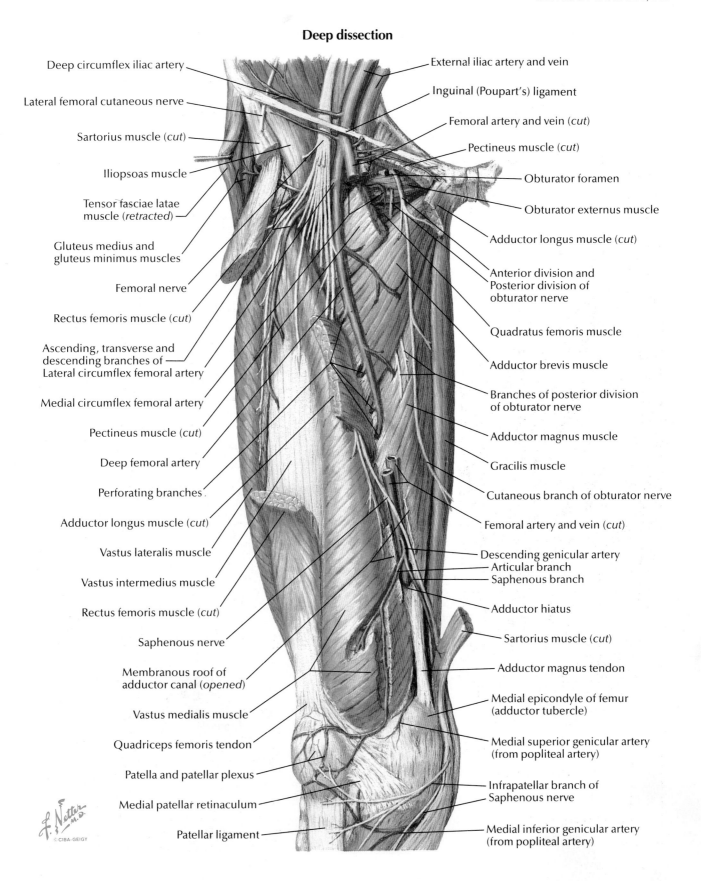

Deep circumflex iliac artery

Lateral femoral cutaneous nerve

Sartorius muscle (*cut*)

Iliopsoas muscle

Tensor fasciae latae muscle (*retracted*)

Gluteus medius and gluteus minimus muscles

Femoral nerve

Rectus femoris muscle (*cut*)

Ascending, transverse and descending branches of Lateral circumflex femoral artery

Medial circumflex femoral artery

Pectineus muscle (*cut*)

Deep femoral artery

Perforating branches

Adductor longus muscle (*cut*)

Vastus lateralis muscle

Vastus intermedius muscle

Rectus femoris muscle (*cut*)

Saphenous nerve

Membranous roof of adductor canal (*opened*)

Vastus medialis muscle

Quadriceps femoris tendon

Patella and patellar plexus

Medial patellar retinaculum

Patellar ligament

External iliac artery and vein

Inguinal (Poupart's) ligament

Femoral artery and vein (*cut*)

Pectineus muscle (*cut*)

Obturator foramen

Obturator externus muscle

Adductor longus muscle (*cut*)

Anterior division and Posterior division of obturator nerve

Quadratus femoris muscle

Adductor brevis muscle

Branches of posterior division of obturator nerve

Adductor magnus muscle

Gracilis muscle

Cutaneous branch of obturator nerve

Femoral artery and vein (*cut*)

Descending genicular artery
Articular branch
Saphenous branch

Adductor hiatus

Sartorius muscle (*cut*)

Adductor magnus tendon

Medial epicondyle of femur (adductor tubercle)

Medial superior genicular artery (from popliteal artery)

Infrapatellar branch of Saphenous nerve

Medial inferior genicular artery (from popliteal artery)

Deep dissection

Superior cluneal nerves

Gluteus maximus muscle (*cut*)

Middle cluneal nerves

Inferior gluteal artery and nerve

Pudendal nerve

Nerve to obturator internus and superior gemellus muscles

Posterior femoral cutaneous nerve

Sacrotuberous ligament

Ischial tuberosity

Inferior cluneal nerves (*cut*)

Adductor magnus muscle

Gracilis muscle

Sciatic nerve

Muscular branches of sciatic nerve

Semitendinosus muscle (*retracted*)

Semimembranosus muscle

Sciatic nerve

Articular branch

Adductor hiatus

Popliteal vein and artery

Medial superior genicular artery

Adductor tubercle (medial epicondyle of femur)

Tibial nerve

Gastrocnemius muscle (medial head)

Medial sural cutaneous nerve

Lesser saphenous vein

Iliac crest

Fascia (gluteal aponeurosis) and gluteus medius muscle (*cut*)

Superior gluteal artery and nerve

Gluteus minimus muscle

Tensor fasciae latae muscle

Piriformis muscle

Gluteus medius muscle (*cut*)

Superior gemellus muscle

Greater trochanter of femur

Obturator internus muscle

Inferior gemellus muscle

Gluteus maximus muscle (*cut*)

Quadratus femoris muscle

Medial circumflex femoral artery

Vastus lateralis muscle and iliotibial tract

Adductor minimus part of adductor magnus muscle

1st perforating artery (from deep femoral artery)

Adductor magnus muscle

2nd and 3rd perforating arteries (from deep femoral artery)

4th perforating artery (termination of deep femoral artery)

Long head (*retracted*) ⎫ Biceps femoris
Short head ⎬ muscle

Lateral superior genicular artery

Common peroneal nerve

Plantaris muscle

Gastrocnemius muscle (lateral head)

Lateral sural cutaneous nerve

PLATE 472

LOWER LIMB

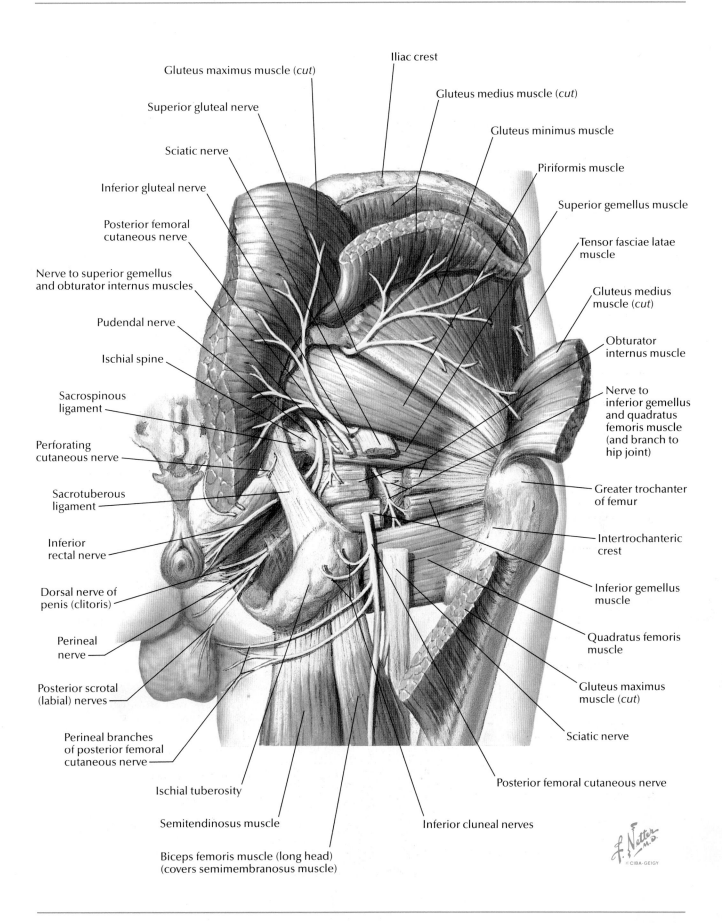

Gluteus maximus muscle (*cut*)

Iliac crest

Superior gluteal nerve

Gluteus medius muscle (*cut*)

Sciatic nerve

Gluteus minimus muscle

Inferior gluteal nerve

Piriformis muscle

Posterior femoral cutaneous nerve

Superior gemellus muscle

Nerve to superior gemellus and obturator internus muscles

Tensor fasciae latae muscle

Pudendal nerve

Gluteus medius muscle (*cut*)

Ischial spine

Obturator internus muscle

Sacrospinous ligament

Nerve to inferior gemellus and quadratus femoris muscle (and branch to hip joint)

Perforating cutaneous nerve

Greater trochanter of femur

Sacrotuberous ligament

Intertrochanteric crest

Inferior rectal nerve

Inferior gemellus muscle

Dorsal nerve of penis (clitoris)

Quadratus femoris muscle

Perineal nerve

Gluteus maximus muscle (*cut*)

Posterior scrotal (labial) nerves

Sciatic nerve

Perineal branches of posterior femoral cutaneous nerve

Posterior femoral cutaneous nerve

Ischial tuberosity

Semitendinosus muscle

Inferior cluneal nerves

Biceps femoris muscle (long head) (covers semimembranosus muscle)

Arteries of Femoral Head and Neck

SEE ALSO PLATE 481

Anterior view

Retinacular arteries (subsynovial) { Superior / Anterior / Inferior }

Anastomosis between medial and lateral circumflex femoral arteries

Iliofemoral (Y) ligament and joint capsule

Ascending, Transverse, Descending branches of Lateral circumflex femoral artery

Foveolar artery (*often minute*)

Iliopsoas tendon

Medial circumflex femoral artery

Deep femoral artery

Nutrient artery of femur

Posterior view

Retinacular arteries (subsynovial) { Superior / Posterior / Inferior }

Anastomosis

Ischiofemoral ligament and joint capsule

Medial circumflex femoral artery

Lateral circumflex femoral artery

Nutrient artery of femur

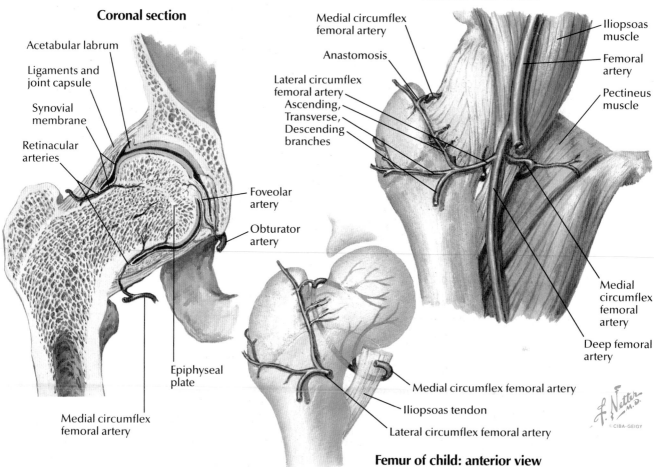

Coronal section

Acetabular labrum

Ligaments and joint capsule

Synovial membrane

Retinacular arteries

Medial circumflex femoral artery

Foveolar artery

Obturator artery

Epiphyseal plate

Anterior view in situ

Medial circumflex femoral artery

Anastomosis

Lateral circumflex femoral artery
Ascending, Transverse, Descending branches

Iliopsoas muscle

Femoral artery

Pectineus muscle

Medial circumflex femoral artery

Deep femoral artery

Medial circumflex femoral artery

Iliopsoas tendon

Lateral circumflex femoral artery

Femur of child: anterior view

PLATE 474

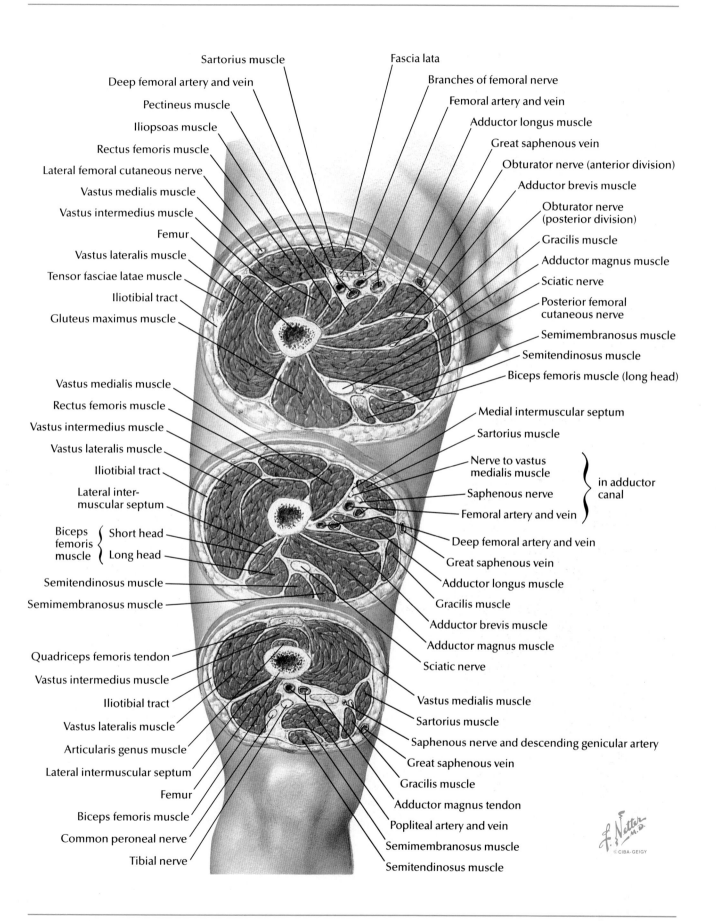

Sartorius muscle

Deep femoral artery and vein

Pectineus muscle

Iliopsoas muscle

Rectus femoris muscle

Lateral femoral cutaneous nerve

Vastus medialis muscle

Vastus intermedius muscle

Femur

Vastus lateralis muscle

Tensor fasciae latae muscle

Iliotibial tract

Gluteus maximus muscle

Fascia lata

Branches of femoral nerve

Femoral artery and vein

Adductor longus muscle

Great saphenous vein

Obturator nerve (anterior division)

Adductor brevis muscle

Obturator nerve (posterior division)

Gracilis muscle

Adductor magnus muscle

Sciatic nerve

Posterior femoral cutaneous nerve

Semimembranosus muscle

Semitendinosus muscle

Biceps femoris muscle (long head)

Vastus medialis muscle

Rectus femoris muscle

Vastus intermedius muscle

Vastus lateralis muscle

Iliotibial tract

Lateral intermuscular septum

Biceps femoris muscle { Short head / Long head }

Semitendinosus muscle

Semimembranosus muscle

Medial intermuscular septum

Sartorius muscle

Nerve to vastus medialis muscle

Saphenous nerve

Femoral artery and vein

} in adductor canal

Deep femoral artery and vein

Great saphenous vein

Adductor longus muscle

Gracilis muscle

Adductor brevis muscle

Adductor magnus muscle

Sciatic nerve

Quadriceps femoris tendon

Vastus intermedius muscle

Iliotibial tract

Vastus lateralis muscle

Articularis genus muscle

Lateral intermuscular septum

Femur

Biceps femoris muscle

Common peroneal nerve

Tibial nerve

Vastus medialis muscle

Sartorius muscle

Saphenous nerve and descending genicular artery

Great saphenous vein

Gracilis muscle

Adductor magnus tendon

Popliteal artery and vein

Semimembranosus muscle

Semitendinosus muscle

Knee: Lateral and Medial Views

Lateral view

Iliotibial tract

Biceps femoris muscle { Long head / Short head

Bursa under iliotibial tract

Fibular collateral ligament and bursa under it

Plantaris muscle

Biceps femoris tendon and bursa under it

Common peroneal nerve

Head of fibula

Gastrocnemius muscle

Soleus muscle

Peroneus longus muscle

Vastus lateralis muscle

Quadriceps femoris tendon

Patella

Lateral patellar retinaculum

Joint capsule

Patellar ligament

Tuberosity of tibia

Tibialis anterior muscle

Medial view

Vastus medialis muscle

Quadriceps femoris tendon

Adductor tubercle (medial epicondyle of femur)

Patella

Medial patellar retinaculum

Joint capsule

Patellar ligament

Tuberosity of tibia

Sartorius muscle

Gracilis muscle

Semitendinosus muscle

Semimembranosus muscle

Adductor magnus tendon

Parallel fibers } Tibial collateral ligament
Oblique fibers }

Bursa under semimembranosus muscle

Anserine bursa under Semitendinosus, Gracilis and Sartorius tendons } Pes anserinus

Gastrocnemius muscle

Soleus muscle

PLATE 476

LOWER LIMB

Right knee in extension

Vastus intermedius muscle

Vastus lateralis muscle

Iliotibial tract

Lateral patellar retinaculum

Lateral condyle of femur

Fibular collateral ligament and bursa

Biceps femoris tendon and bursa

Broken line indicates bursa under iliotibial tract

Insertion of iliotibial tract to Gerdy's tubercle and oblique line of tibia

Common peroneal nerve

Head of fibula

Peroneus longus muscle

Extensor digitorum longus muscle

Tibialis anterior muscle

Femur

Articularis genus muscle

Vastus medialis muscle

Quadriceps femoris tendon

Patella

Medial condyle of femur

Medial patellar retinaculum

Tibial collateral ligament

Semitendinosus, Gracilis and Sartorius tendons } Pes anserinus

Anserine bursa

Medial condyle of tibia

Patellar ligament

Tuberosity of tibia

Gastrocnemius muscle

Joint opened, knee slightly in flexion

Femur

Articularis genus muscle

Synovial membrane (*cut edge*)

Lateral condyle of femur

Origin of popliteus tendon (*covered by synovial membrane*)

Subpopliteal recess

Lateral meniscus

Fibular collateral ligament

Head of fibula

Patella (articular surface)

Vastus lateralis muscle (*reflected*)

Suprapatellar synovial bursa

Cruciate ligaments (*covered by synovial membrane*)

Medial condyle of femur

Infrapatellar synovial fold

Medial meniscus

Alar folds

Infrapatellar fat pads (*under synovial membrane*)

Suprapatellar synovial bursa (*roof reflected*)

Vastus medialis muscle (*reflected*)

KNEE

PLATE 477

Inferior view

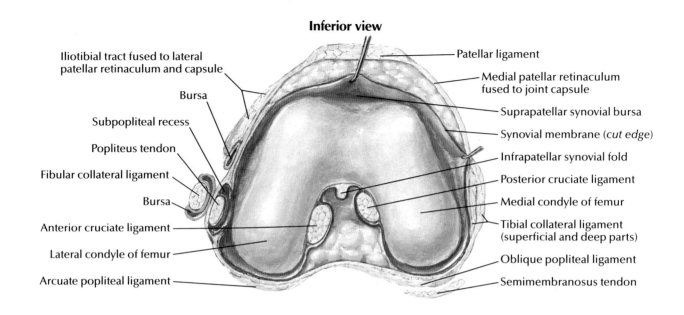

Iliotibial tract fused to lateral patellar retinaculum and capsule

Bursa

Subpopliteal recess

Popliteus tendon

Fibular collateral ligament

Bursa

Anterior cruciate ligament

Lateral condyle of femur

Arcuate popliteal ligament

Patellar ligament

Medial patellar retinaculum fused to joint capsule

Suprapatellar synovial bursa

Synovial membrane (*cut edge*)

Infrapatellar synovial fold

Posterior cruciate ligament

Medial condyle of femur

Tibial collateral ligament (superficial and deep parts)

Oblique popliteal ligament

Semimembranosus tendon

Superior view

Posterior meniscofemoral ligament

Arcuate popliteal ligament

Fibular collateral ligament

Bursa

Popliteus tendon

Subpopliteal recess

Lateral meniscus

Superior articular surface of tibia (lateral facet)

Iliotibial tract fused to capsule

Infrapatellar fat body

Semimembranosus tendon

Oblique popliteal ligament

Posterior cruciate ligament

Tibial collateral ligament (deep part bound to medial meniscus)

Medial meniscus

Superior articular surface of tibia (medial facet)

Synovial membrane

Joint capsule

Anterior cruciate ligament

Patellar ligament

Superior view: ligaments and cartilage removed

Attachment of posterior cruciate ligament

Attachment of synovial membrane

Superior articular surface of tibia (lateral facet)

Attachments of horns of lateral meniscus

Attachment of anterior cruciate ligament

Intercondylar eminence

Attachment of synovial membrane

Superior articular surface of tibia (medial facet)

Attachments of horns of medial meniscus

Tibial tuberosity

PLATE 478

LOWER LIMB

Right knee in flexion: anterior view

Anterior cruciate ligament

Lateral condyle of femur (articular surface)

Popliteus tendon

Fibular collateral ligament

Lateral meniscus

Transverse ligament of knee

Head of fibula

Gerdy's tubercle

Posterior cruciate ligament

Medial condyle of femur (articular surface)

Medial meniscus

Tibial collateral ligament

Medial condyle of tibia

Tuberosity of tibia

Right knee in extension: posterior view

Adductor tubercle (medial epicondyle of femur)

Medial condyle of femur (articular surface)

Medial meniscus

Tibial collateral ligament

Medial condyle of tibia

Posterior cruciate ligament

Anterior cruciate ligament

Posterior meniscofemoral ligament

Lateral condyle of femur (articular surface)

Popliteus tendon

Fibular collateral ligament

Lateral meniscus

Head of fibula

Knee: Posterior and Sagittal Views

Right knee: posterior view

Adductor magnus tendon

Medial head of gastrocnemius muscle and bursa beneath it

Tibial collateral ligament

Semimembranosus tendon

Oblique popliteal ligament (tendinous expansion of semimembranosus muscle)

Bursa under tendon (*broken line*)

Popliteus muscle

Femur

Attachment of joint capsule

Plantaris muscle

Lateral head of gastrocnemius muscle and bursa beneath it

Fibular collateral ligament and bursa beneath it

Biceps femoris tendon and bursa beneath it

Arcuate popliteal ligament (edge of capsule that arches over popliteus muscle)

Head of fibula

Posterior ligament of head of fibula

Attachment of joint capsule

Interosseous membrane

Tibia

Femur

Articularis genus muscle

Quadriceps femoris tendon

Suprapatellar fat body

Suprapatellar synovial bursa

Patella

Subcutaneous prepatellar bursa

Articular cavity

Infrapatellar fat body

Patellar ligament

Synovial membrane

Subcutaneous infrapatellar bursa

Deep (subtendinous) infrapatellar bursa

Lateral meniscus

Tuberosity of tibia

Bursa under lateral head of gastrocnemius muscle

Synovial membrane

Articular cartilages

Tibia

Parasagittal section (lateral to midline)

PLATE 480

LOWER LIMB

Deep circumflex iliac artery

Superficial circumflex iliac artery

Femoral artery

Ascending branch,
Transverse branch,
Descending branch of
Lateral circumflex
femoral artery

Deep femoral artery

Perforating branches

Femoral artery passes
through adductor hiatus

Lateral superior genicular artery

Patellar plexus

Lateral inferior genicular artery
(*partially in phantom*)

Posterior tibial recurrent artery
(*phantom*)

Circumflex fibular artery

Anterior tibial artery

Interosseous membrane

External iliac artery

Inferior epigastric artery

Superficial epigastric artery

Superficial external pudendal artery

Obturator artery

Deep external pudendal artery

Medial circumflex femoral artery

Femoral artery

Muscular branches

Descending genicular artery
Articular branch
Saphenous branch

Medial superior genicular artery

Popliteal artery (*phantom*)

Middle genicular artery (*phantom*)

Medial inferior genicular artery
(*partially in phantom*)

Anterior recurrent tibial artery

Posterior tibial artery (*phantom*)

Peroneal artery (*phantom*)

Tibia and Fibula

Anterior view

Posterior view

Intercondylar eminence

Lateral
intercondylar
tubercle

Medial
intercondylar
tubercle

Anterior
intercondylar area

Lateral condyle

Apex,
Head,
Neck
of
fibula

Medial
condyle

Gerdy's tubercle
(insertion of
iliotibial tract)

Oblique line

Tuberosity

Lateral
surface

Lateral surface

Anterior border

Anterior
border

Interosseous
border

Interosseous
border

Medial surface

Medial
surface

Medial border

Fibula

Tibia

Lateral
malleolus

Medial
malleolus

Malleolar
articular surface

Inferior
articular
surface

Malleolar
articular surface

Intercondylar eminence

Medial
intercondylar
tubercle

Lateral
intercondylar
tubercle

Posterior
intercondylar
area

Superior
articular surfaces
(medial and
lateral facets)

Lateral condyle

Apex,
Head,
Neck
of
fibula

Groove for
insertion of
semimembranosus
tendon

Soleal line

Nutrient
foramen

Interosseous
border

Posterior
surface

Posterior
surface

Medial crest

Medial border

Lateral surface

Tibia

Fibula

Posterior
border

Groove for
tibialis posterior
and flexor digitorum
longus tendons

Medial
malleolus

Fibular notch

Lateral
malleolus

Fossa of
lateral
malleolus

Malleolar
articular surface

Inferior
articular
surface

PLATE 482

LOWER LIMB

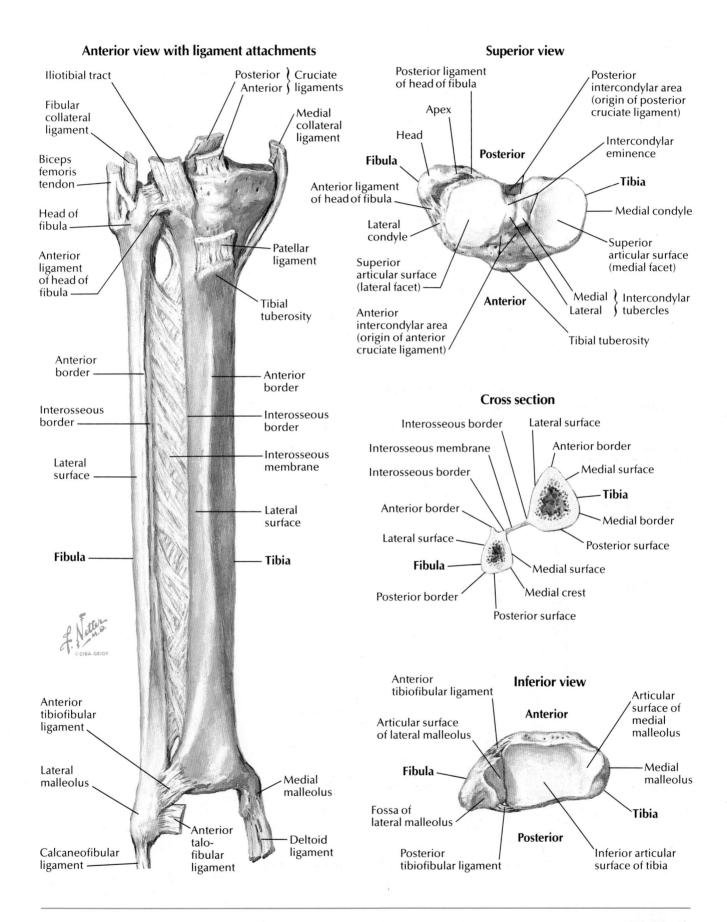

Anterior view with ligament attachments

Iliotibial tract

Posterior ⎫ Cruciate
Anterior ⎬ ligaments

Medial collateral ligament

Fibular collateral ligament

Biceps femoris tendon

Head of fibula

Anterior ligament of head of fibula

Patellar ligament

Tibial tuberosity

Anterior border

Interosseous border

Lateral surface

Fibula

Anterior border

Interosseous border

Interosseous membrane

Lateral surface

Tibia

Anterior tibiofibular ligament

Lateral malleolus

Calcaneofibular ligament

Anterior talo-fibular ligament

Medial malleolus

Deltoid ligament

Superior view

Posterior ligament of head of fibula

Apex

Head

Fibula

Anterior ligament of head of fibula

Lateral condyle

Superior articular surface (lateral facet)

Anterior intercondylar area (origin of anterior cruciate ligament)

Posterior

Posterior intercondylar area (origin of posterior cruciate ligament)

Intercondylar eminence

Tibia

Medial condyle

Superior articular surface (medial facet)

Medial ⎫ Intercondylar
Lateral ⎬ tubercles

Tibial tuberosity

Anterior

Cross section

Interosseous border

Interosseous membrane

Interosseous border

Anterior border

Lateral surface

Fibula

Posterior border

Lateral surface

Anterior border

Medial surface

Tibia

Medial border

Posterior surface

Medial surface

Medial crest

Posterior surface

Inferior view

Anterior tibiofibular ligament

Anterior

Articular surface of lateral malleolus

Fibula

Fossa of lateral malleolus

Posterior tibiofibular ligament

Posterior

Articular surface of medial malleolus

Medial malleolus

Tibia

Inferior articular surface of tibia

Bony Attachments of Muscles of Leg

Anterior view

Iliotibial tract

Biceps femoris muscle

Peroneus longus muscle

Extensor digitorum longus muscle

Extensor hallucis longus muscle

Peroneus brevis muscle

Peroneus tertius muscle

Peroneus brevis muscle

Peroneus tertius muscle

Extensor digitorum longus muscle

Extensor hallucis longus muscle

Sartorius muscle

Gracilis muscle

Semitendinosus muscle

Quadriceps femoris muscle via patellar ligament

Tibialis anterior muscle

Origins

Insertions

Note: attachments of intrinsic muscles of foot not shown

Posterior view

Plantaris muscle

Gastrocnemius muscle (medial head)

Gastrocnemius muscle (lateral head)

Popliteus muscle

Semimembranosus muscle

Popliteus muscle

Soleus muscle

Tibialis posterior muscle

Flexor digitorum longus muscle

Flexor hallucis longus muscle

Peroneus brevis muscle

Plantaris muscle

Soleus and gastrocnemius muscles via calcaneal (Achilles) tendon

Tibialis posterior muscle

Tibialis anterior muscle

Peroneus longus muscle

Flexor hallucis longus muscle

Flexor digitorum longus muscle

f. Netter M.D.

© CIBA-GEIGY

PLATE 484

LOWER LIMB

Muscles of Leg (Superficial Dissection): Posterior View

Semitendinosus muscle

Semimembranosus muscle

Gracilis muscle

Popliteal artery and vein

Sartorius muscle

Medial superior genicular artery

Gastrocnemius muscle (medial head)

Nerve to soleus muscle

Lesser saphenous vein

Gastrocnemius muscle

Soleus muscle

Plantaris tendon

Flexor digitorum longus tendon

Tibialis posterior tendon

Posterior tibial artery and vein

Tibial nerve

Medial malleolus

Flexor hallucis longus tendon

Flexor retinaculum

Calcaneal branch of
posterior tibial artery

Iliotibial tract

Biceps femoris muscle

Tibial nerve

Common peroneal nerve

Lateral superior genicular artery

Plantaris muscle

Gastrocnemius muscle (lateral head)

Lateral sural cutaneous nerve (cut)

Medial sural cutaneous nerve (cut)

Soleus muscle

Peroneus longus tendon

Peroneus brevis tendon

Calcaneal (Achilles) tendon

Lateral malleolus

Superior peroneal retinaculum

Peroneal artery

Calcaneal branches of peroneal artery

Tuberosity of calcaneus

Adductor magnus tendon

Popliteal artery and vein

Medial superior genicular artery

Gastrocnemius muscle (medial head) (cut)

Tibial collateral ligament

Semimembranosus tendon (cut)

Medial inferior genicular artery

Popliteus muscle

Tendinous arch of Soleus muscle

Plantaris tendon

Gastrocnemius muscle (cut)

Soleus muscle inserting into calcaneal (Achilles) tendon

Flexor digitorum longus tendon

Tibialis posterior tendon

Posterior tibial artery and vein

Tibial nerve

Medial malleolus

Flexor hallucis longus tendon

Flexor retinaculum

Calcaneal (Achilles) tendon

Calcaneal branch of posterior tibial artery

Tibial nerve

Common peroneal nerve (cut)

Lateral superior genicular artery

Lateral and medial sural cutaneous nerves (cut)

Gastrocnemius muscle (lateral head) (cut)

Fibular collateral ligament

Biceps femoris tendon (cut)

Plantaris muscle

Lateral inferior genicular artery

Head of fibula

Common peroneal nerve (cut)

Nerve to soleus muscle

Peroneus longus muscle

Soleus muscle

Peroneus longus tendon

Peroneus brevis tendon

Lateral malleolus

Superior peroneal retinaculum

Peroneal artery

Calcaneal branches of peroneal artery

Tuberosity of calcaneus

PLATE 486

LOWER LIMB

Muscles of Leg (Deep Dissection): Posterior View

Medial superior genicular artery

Gastrocnemius muscle (medial head) (*cut*)

Sural (muscular) branches

Popliteal artery and tibial nerve

Tibial collateral ligament

Semimembranosus tendon (*cut*)

Medial inferior genicular artery

Popliteus muscle

Posterior tibial recurrent artery

Tendinous arch of soleus muscle

Posterior tibial artery

Flexor digitorum longus muscle

Tibial nerve

Tibialis posterior muscle

Calcaneal (Achilles) tendon (*cut*)

Flexor digitorum longus tendon

Tibialis posterior tendon

Medial malleolus and posterior medial malleolar branch of posterior tibial artery

Flexor retinaculum

Medial calcaneal branches of posterior tibial artery and tibial nerve

Tibialis posterior tendon

Medial plantar artery and nerve

Lateral plantar artery and nerve

Flexor hallucis longus tendon

1st metatarsal bone

Lateral superior genicular artery

Plantaris muscle (*cut*)

Gastrocnemius muscle (lateral head) (*cut*)

Fibular collateral ligament

Biceps femoris tendon (*cut*)

Lateral inferior genicular artery

Head of fibula

Common peroneal nerve

Soleus muscle (*cut and reflected*)

Anterior tibial artery

Peroneal artery

Flexor hallucis longus muscle (*retracted*)

Peroneal artery

Interosseous membrane

Perforating branch } of peroneal
Communicating branch } artery

Peroneus longus tendon

Peroneus brevis tendon

Lateral malleolus and posterior lateral malleolar branch of peroneal artery

Superior peroneal retinaculum

Lateral calcaneal branch of peroneal artery

Lateral calcaneal branch of sural nerve

Inferior peroneal retinaculum

Peroneus brevis tendon

Peroneus longus tendon

Flexor digitorum longus tendon

5th metatarsal bone

LEG

PLATE 487

Muscles of Leg (Superficial Dissection): Anterior View

SEE ALSO PLATE 510

Vastus lateralis muscle

Quadriceps femoris tendon

Iliotibial tract

Lateral superior genicular artery

Lateral patellar retinaculum

Biceps femoris tendon

Lateral inferior genicular artery

Common peroneal nerve

Head of fibula

Peroneus longus muscle

Tibialis anterior muscle

Superficial peroneal nerve (*cut*)

Peroneus brevis muscle

Extensor digitorum longus muscle

Fibula

Superior extensor retinaculum

Lateral malleolus

Inferior extensor retinaculum

Extensor digitorum longus tendons

Peroneus tertius tendon

Extensor digitorum brevis tendons

Dorsal digital nerves

Vastus medialis muscle

Patella

Medial superior genicular artery

Tibial collateral ligament

Medial patellar retinaculum

Medial inferior genicular artery

Infrapatellar branch (*cut*) of Saphenous nerve (*cut*)

Joint capsule

Patellar ligament

Insertion of sartorius muscle

Tibial tuberosity

Tibia

Gastrocnemius muscle

Soleus muscle

Extensor hallucis longus muscle

Medial malleolus

Tibialis anterior tendon

Medial branch of deep peroneal nerve

Extensor hallucis longus tendon

Extensor hallucis brevis tendon

Dorsal digital branches of deep peroneal nerve

PLATE 488

LOWER LIMB

Muscles of Leg (Deep Dissection): Anterior View

SEE ALSO PLATE 510

Lateral superior genicular artery

Fibular collateral ligament

Lateral patellar retinaculum

Iliotibial tract (*cut*)

Biceps femoris tendon (*cut*)

Lateral inferior genicular artery

Common peroneal nerve

Head of fibula

Peroneus longus muscle (*cut*)

Anterior tibial artery

Extensor digitorum longus muscle (*cut*)

Superficial peroneal nerve

Deep peroneal nerve

Peroneus longus muscle

Extensor digitorum longus muscle

Peroneus brevis muscle and tendon

Peroneus longus tendon

Perforating branch of peroneal artery

Anterior lateral malleolar artery

Lateral malleolus and arterial plexus

Lateral tarsal artery and lateral branch of deep peroneal nerve

Extensor digitorum brevis and extensor hallucis brevis muscles (*cut*)

Peroneus brevis tendon

Posterior perforating branches from deep plantar arch

Extensor digitorum longus tendons (*cut*)

Extensor digitorum brevis tendons (*cut*)

Dorsal digital arteries

Branches of proper plantar digital arteries and nerves

Medial superior genicular artery

Quadriceps femoris tendon

Tibial collateral ligament

Medial patellar retinaculum

Infrapatellar branch of saphenous nerve (*cut*)

Medial inferior genicular artery

Saphenous nerve (*cut*)

Patellar ligament

Insertion of sartorius tendon

Anterior tibial recurrent artery and recurrent branch of deep peroneal nerve

Interosseous membrane

Tibialis anterior muscle (*cut*)

Gastrocnemius muscle

Soleus muscle

Tibia

Superficial peroneal nerve (*cut*)

Extensor hallucis longus muscle and tendon (*cut*)

Interosseous membrane

Anterior medial malleolar artery

Medial malleolus and arterial plexus

Dorsalis pedis artery

Tibialis anterior tendon

Medial tarsal artery

Medial branch of deep peroneal nerve

Arcuate artery

Deep plantar artery

Dorsal metatarsal arteries

Extensor hallucis longus tendon (*cut*)

Extensor hallucis brevis tendon (*cut*)

Dorsal digital branches of deep peroneal nerve

F. Netter
© CIBA-GEIGY

Biceps femoris muscle { Long head

Short head

Tendon

Fibular collateral ligament

Common peroneal nerve

Lateral inferior genicular artery

Head of fibula

Gastrocnemius muscle

Soleus muscle

Peroneus longus muscle and tendon

Peroneus brevis muscle and tendon

Fibula

Lateral malleolus

Calcaneal (Achilles) tendon

Subtendinous bursa

Superior peroneal retinaculum

Inferior peroneal retinaculum

Peroneus longus tendon passing to sole of foot

Vastus lateralis muscle

Iliotibial tract

Lateral superior genicular artery

Quadriceps femoris tendon

Patella

Lateral patellar retinaculum

Lateral condyle of tibia

Patellar ligament

Tuberosity of tibia

Tibialis anterior muscle

Extensor digitorum longus muscle

Superficial peroneal nerve (cut)

Extensor digitorum longus tendon

Extensor hallucis longus muscle and tendon

Superior extensor retinaculum

Inferior extensor retinaculum

Extensor digitorum brevis muscle

Extensor hallucis longus tendon

Extensor digitorum longus tendons

Peroneus brevis tendon

Peroneus tertius tendon

5th metatarsal bone

PLATE 490

LOWER LIMB

Leg: Cross Sections and Fascial Compartments

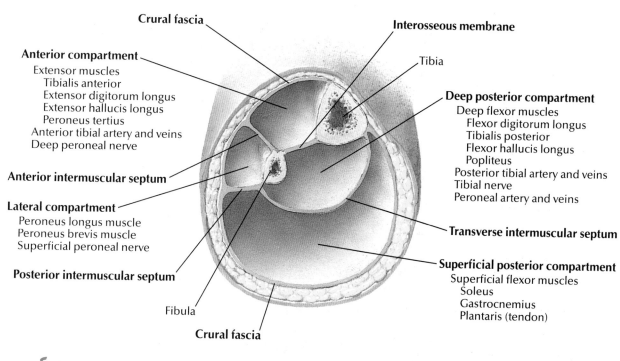

Crural fascia

Interosseous membrane

Tibia

Anterior compartment
Extensor muscles
Tibialis anterior
Extensor digitorum longus
Extensor hallucis longus
Peroneus tertius
Anterior tibial artery and veins
Deep peroneal nerve

Anterior intermuscular septum

Lateral compartment
Peroneus longus muscle
Peroneus brevis muscle
Superficial peroneal nerve

Posterior intermuscular septum

Fibula

Crural fascia

Deep posterior compartment
Deep flexor muscles
Flexor digitorum longus
Tibialis posterior
Flexor hallucis longus
Popliteus
Posterior tibial artery and veins
Tibial nerve
Peroneal artery and veins

Transverse intermuscular septum

Superficial posterior compartment
Superficial flexor muscles
Soleus
Gastrocnemius
Plantaris (tendon)

Cross section just above middle of left leg

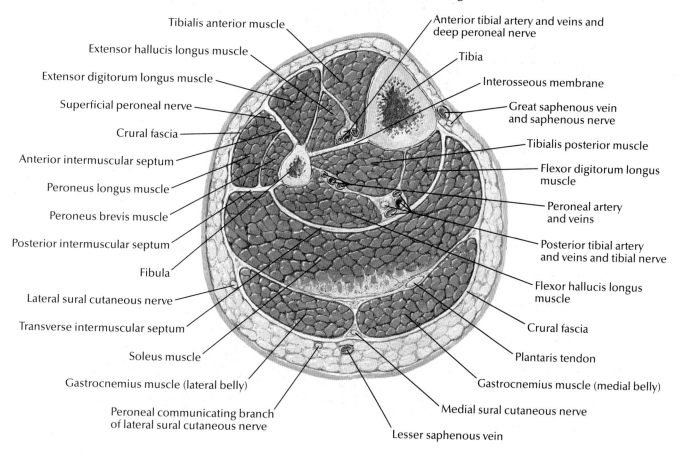

Tibialis anterior muscle

Extensor hallucis longus muscle

Extensor digitorum longus muscle

Superficial peroneal nerve

Crural fascia

Anterior intermuscular septum

Peroneus longus muscle

Peroneus brevis muscle

Posterior intermuscular septum

Fibula

Lateral sural cutaneous nerve

Transverse intermuscular septum

Soleus muscle

Gastrocnemius muscle (lateral belly)

Peroneal communicating branch
of lateral sural cutaneous nerve

Anterior tibial artery and veins and
deep peroneal nerve

Tibia

Interosseous membrane

Great saphenous vein
and saphenous nerve

Tibialis posterior muscle

Flexor digitorum longus
muscle

Peroneal artery
and veins

Posterior tibial artery
and veins and tibial nerve

Flexor hallucis longus
muscle

Crural fascia

Plantaris tendon

Gastrocnemius muscle (medial belly)

Medial sural cutaneous nerve

Lesser saphenous vein

Bones of Foot

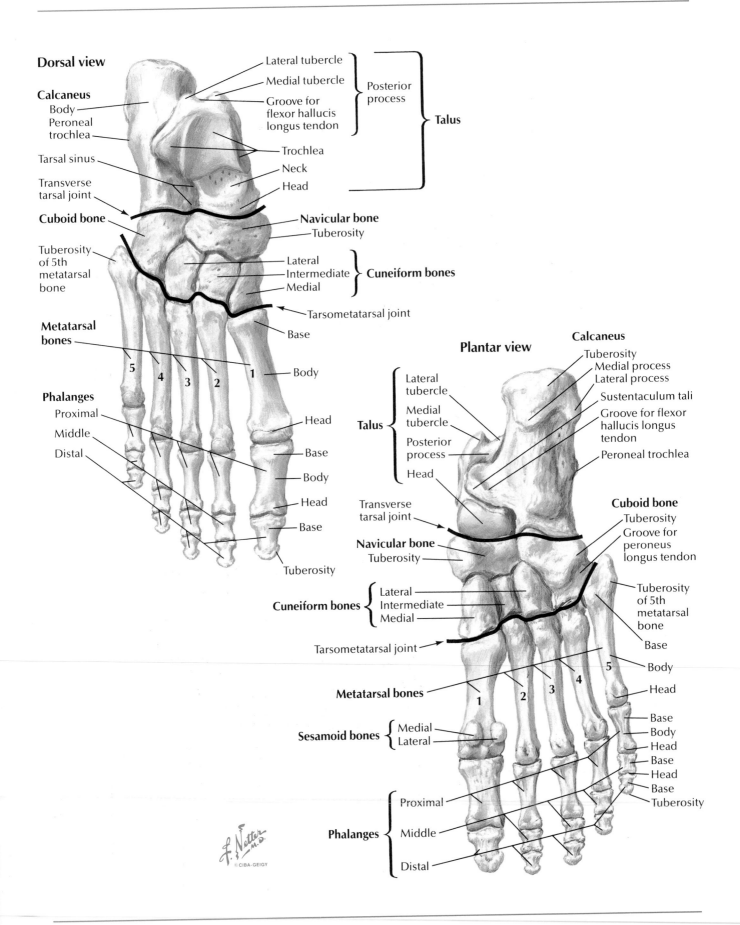

Dorsal view

Calcaneus
- Body
- Peroneal trochlea

Tarsal sinus

Transverse tarsal joint

Cuboid bone

Tuberosity of 5th metatarsal bone

Metatarsal bones

Phalanges
- Proximal
- Middle
- Distal

Lateral tubercle
Medial tubercle
Groove for flexor hallucis longus tendon } Posterior process

Trochlea
Neck
Head

Navicular bone
- Tuberosity

Lateral
Intermediate
Medial } Cuneiform bones

Tarsometatarsal joint

Base

Talus

5 4 3 2 1 — Body

Head
Base
Body
Head
Base
Tuberosity

Plantar view

Calcaneus
- Tuberosity
- Medial process
- Lateral process

Sustentaculum tali

Groove for flexor hallucis longus tendon

Peroneal trochlea

Lateral tubercle
Medial tubercle
Posterior process
Head } Talus

Transverse tarsal joint

Navicular bone
- Tuberosity

Cuneiform bones { Lateral
Intermediate
Medial

Tarsometatarsal joint

Metatarsal bones

Sesamoid bones { Medial
Lateral

Cuboid bone
- Tuberosity
- Groove for peroneus longus tendon

Tuberosity of 5th metatarsal bone

Base

1 2 3 4 5 — Body

Head
Base
Body
Head
Base
Head
Base
Tuberosity

Phalanges { Proximal
Middle
Distal

f. Netter
M.D.
© CIBA-GEIGY

PLATE 492

LOWER LIMB

Lateral view

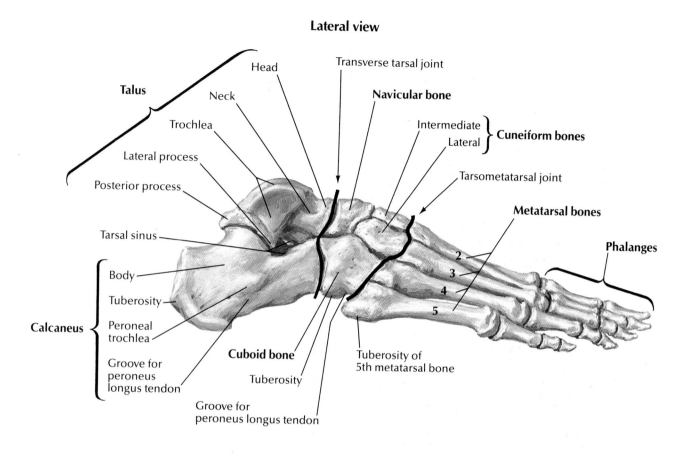

Talus
- Head
- Neck
- Trochlea
- Lateral process
- Posterior process

Transverse tarsal joint

Navicular bone

Intermediate } **Cuneiform bones**
Lateral

Tarsometatarsal joint

Metatarsal bones

Phalanges

2
3
4
5

Tarsal sinus

Calcaneus
- Body
- Tuberosity
- Peroneal trochlea
- Groove for peroneus longus tendon

Cuboid bone

Tuberosity

Groove for peroneus longus tendon

Tuberosity of 5th metatarsal bone

Medial view

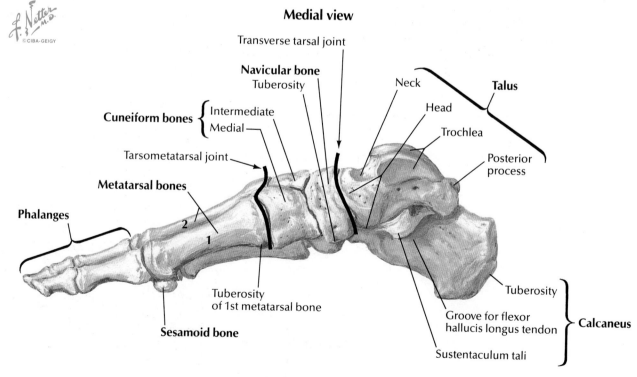

Transverse tarsal joint

Navicular bone
Tuberosity

Neck
Head
Trochlea

Talus

Posterior process

Cuneiform bones {
Intermediate
Medial

Tarsometatarsal joint

Metatarsal bones

Phalanges

2
1

Tuberosity of 1st metatarsal bone

Sesamoid bone

Groove for flexor hallucis longus tendon

Sustentaculum tali

Tuberosity

Calcaneus

Calcaneus

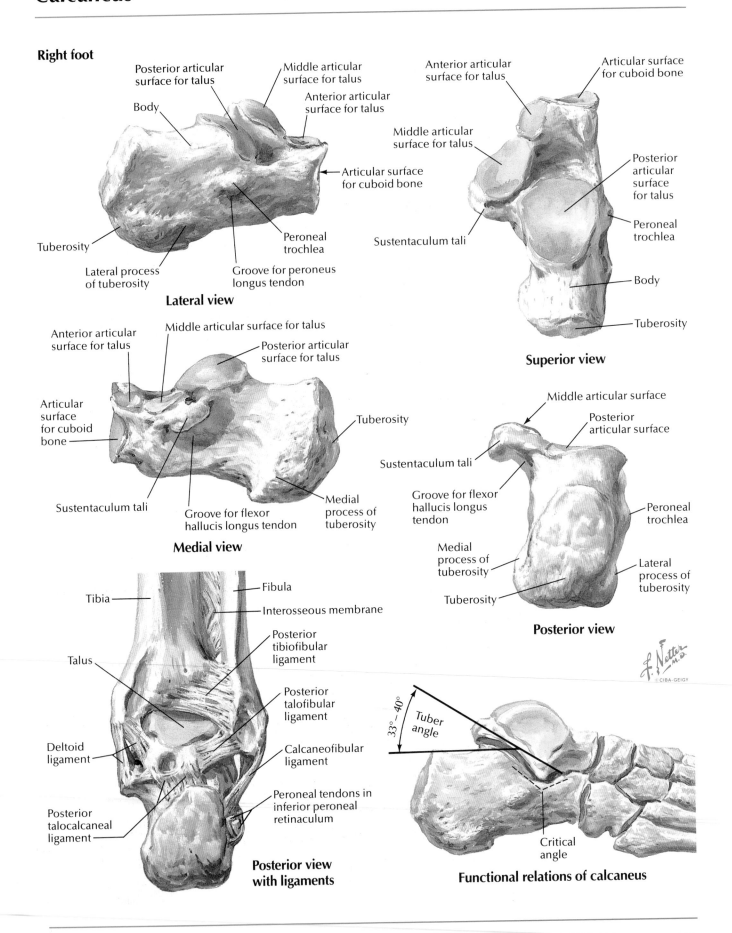

Right foot

Lateral view

Posterior articular surface for talus
Middle articular surface for talus
Body
Anterior articular surface for talus
Articular surface for cuboid bone
Tuberosity
Peroneal trochlea
Lateral process of tuberosity
Groove for peroneus longus tendon

Superior view

Anterior articular surface for talus
Articular surface for cuboid bone
Middle articular surface for talus
Posterior articular surface for talus
Sustentaculum tali
Peroneal trochlea
Body
Tuberosity

Medial view

Anterior articular surface for talus
Middle articular surface for talus
Posterior articular surface for talus
Articular surface for cuboid bone
Tuberosity
Sustentaculum tali
Groove for flexor hallucis longus tendon
Medial process of tuberosity

Posterior view

Middle articular surface
Posterior articular surface
Sustentaculum tali
Groove for flexor hallucis longus tendon
Medial process of tuberosity
Tuberosity
Peroneal trochlea
Lateral process of tuberosity

Posterior view with ligaments

Tibia
Fibula
Interosseous membrane
Posterior tibiofibular ligament
Talus
Posterior talofibular ligament
Calcaneofibular ligament
Deltoid ligament
Peroneal tendons in inferior peroneal retinaculum
Posterior talocalcaneal ligament

Functional relations of calcaneus

33° – 40°
Tuber angle
Critical angle

PLATE 494

LOWER LIMB

Right foot: lateral view

Tibia

Fibula

Posterior talofibular ligament
Calcaneofibular ligament
Anterior talofibular ligament
} Components of lateral collateral ligament

Anterior and Posterior tibiofibular ligaments

Interosseous talocalcaneal ligament
Dorsal talonavicular ligament
Calcaneonavicular part
Calcaneocuboid part
} of bifurcate ligament

Superior peroneal retinaculum

Calcaneal (Achilles) tendon (*cut*)

Dorsal cuboideonavicular ligament
Dorsal cuneonavicular ligaments
Dorsal intercuneiform ligaments
Dorsal tarsometatarsal ligaments

Inferior peroneal retinaculum

Lateral talocalcaneal ligament

Long plantar ligament

Peroneus longus tendon

Peroneus brevis tendon

Dorsal calcaneocuboid ligament

Cuboid bone

Dorsal cuneocuboid ligament

Dorsal metatarsal ligaments

Right foot: medial view

Tibia

Deltoid ligament {
Posterior tibiotalar ligament
Tibiocalcaneal ligament
Tibionavicular ligament
Anterior tibiotalar ligament

Medial talocalcaneal ligament

Posterior process of talus

Posterior talocalcaneal ligament

Dorsal talonavicular ligament

Navicular bone

Dorsal cuneonavicular ligaments

Medial cuneiform bone

Dorsal intercuneiform ligament

Dorsal tarsometatarsal ligaments

1st metatarsal bone

Tuberosity

Calcaneal (Achilles) tendon (*cut*)

Sustentaculum tali

Tibialis anterior tendon

Tibialis posterior tendon

Plantar calcaneonavicular (spring) ligament

Long plantar ligament

Ligaments and Tendons of Foot: Plantar View

Flexor digitorum longus tendon to 2nd toe (*cut*)

Flexor digitorum brevis tendon to 2nd toe (*cut*)

4th distal phalanx

4th middle phalanx

Deep transverse metatarsal ligaments

5th proximal phalanx

4th lumbrical tendon (*cut*)

Abductor digiti minimi and flexor digiti minimi brevis tendons (*cut*)

Plantar ligaments (plates)

Interosseous muscles (*cut*)

5th metatarsal bone

Plantar metatarsal ligaments

Tuberosity of 5th metatarsal bone

Peroneus brevis tendon

Cuboid bone

Peroneus longus tendon

Tuberosity of cuboid bone

Long plantar ligament

Plantar calcaneocuboid (short plantar) ligament

Calcaneus

Medial process and Lateral process of Tuberosity of calcaneus

1st distal phalanx

Interphalangeal (IP) joint

Flexor hallucis longus tendon (*cut*)

1st proximal phalanx

Metatarsophalangeal (MP) joint

Sesamoid bones

Abductor hallucis and medial head of flexor hallucis brevis tendons (*cut*)

Adductor hallucis and lateral head of flexor hallucis brevis tendons (*cut*)

1st metatarsal bone

Plantar tarsometatarsal ligaments

Medial cuneiform bone

Tibialis anterior tendon (*cut*)

Plantar cuneonavicular ligament

Plantar cuboideonavicular ligament

Tuberosity of navicular bone

Plantar calcaneonavicular (spring) ligament

Tibialis posterior tendon

Flexor digitorum longus tendon (*cut*)

Sustentaculum tali

Flexor hallucis longus tendon (cut)

Posterior process of talus (medial and lateral tubercles)

Phalanges

Distal Middle Proximal

Articular capsule

Metatarsal bone

Capsules and ligaments of metatarsophalangeal and interphalangeal joints: lateral view

Collateral ligaments

Plantar ligament (plate)

PLATE 496

LOWER LIMB

Lateral view

Soleus muscle

Peroneus longus muscle

Peroneus brevis muscle

Calcaneal (Achilles) tendon

Common sheath of peroneus longus and brevis tendons

Subcutaneous calcaneal bursa

Subtendinous calcaneal bursa

Superior and Inferior peroneal retinacula

Calcaneus

Extensor digitorum brevis muscle

Abductor digiti minimi muscle

Extensor digitorum longus muscle

Superior extensor retinaculum

Sheath of tibialis anterior tendon

Lateral malleolus and subcutaneous bursa

Inferior extensor retinaculum

Sheath of extensor digitorum longus and peroneus tertius tendons

Sheath of extensor hallucis longus tendon

Peroneus longus tendon

Peroneus brevis tendon

Peroneus tertius tendon

Tuberosity of 5th metatarsal bone

Medial view

Tibialis anterior tendon and sheath

Tibia

Sheath of tibialis posterior tendon

Superior extensor retinaculum

Medial malleolus and subcutaneous bursa

Inferior extensor retinaculum

Tibialis posterior tendon and sheath

Tibialis anterior tendon and sheath

Sheath of extensor hallucis longus tendon

1st metatarsal bone

Sheath of flexor hallucis longus tendon

Medial plantar nerve

Sheath of flexor digitorum longus tendon

Calcaneal (Achilles) tendon

Sheath of flexor digitorum longus tendon

Posterior tibial artery and tibial nerve

Sheath of flexor hallucis longus tendon

Subcutaneous and Subtendinous calcaneal bursae

Flexor retinaculum

Calcaneus

Abductor hallucis muscle (cut)

Plantar aponeurosis (cut)

Flexor digitorum brevis muscle (cut)

F. Netter *M.D.*
©CIBA-GEIGY

Muscles of Dorsum of Foot: Superficial Dissection

Superficial peroneal nerve (*cut*)

Peroneus brevis muscle

Peroneus longus tendon

Extensor digitorum longus muscle and tendon

Superior extensor retinaculum

Fibula

Perforating branch of peroneal artery

Lateral malleolus and anterior lateral malleolar artery

Inferior extensor retinaculum

Lateral tarsal artery and lateral branch of deep peroneal nerve

Peroneus brevis tendon

Peroneus tertius tendon

Tuberosity of 5th metatarsal bone

Extensor digitorum brevis and extensor hallucis brevis muscles

Extensor digitorum longus tendons

Lateral dorsal cutaneous nerve (continuation of sural nerve) (*cut*)

Dorsal metatarsal arteries

Dorsal digital arteries

Dorsal branches of proper plantar digital arteries and nerves

Tibialis anterior tendon

Anterior tibial artery and deep peroneal nerve

Tibia

Extensor hallucis longus tendon

Synovial sheath of extensor digitorum tendons

Medial malleolus

Synovial sheath of tibialis anterior tendon

Synovial sheath of extensor hallucis longus tendon

Anterior medial malleolar artery

Dorsalis pedis artery and medial branch of deep peroneal nerve

Medial tarsal artery

Arcuate artery

Deep plantar artery passing between heads of 1st dorsal interosseous muscle to join deep plantar arch

Extensor hallucis longus tendon

Extensor expansions

Dorsal digital branches of deep peroneal nerve

Dorsal digital branches of superficial peroneal nerve

PLATE 498

LOWER LIMB

Superficial peroneal nerve (*cut*)

Peroneus longus tendon

Peroneus brevis muscle and tendon

Extensor digitorum longus muscle and tendon

Fibula

Perforating branch of peroneal artery

Anterior lateral malleolar artery

Lateral malleolus

Lateral branch of deep peroneal nerve and lateral tarsal artery

Peroneus longus tendon (*cut*)

Extensor digitorum brevis and extensor hallucis brevis muscles (*cut*)

Peroneus brevis tendon (*cut*)

Peroneus tertius tendon (*cut*)

Abductor digiti minimi muscle

Dorsal metatarsal arteries

Metatarsal bones

Dorsal interosseous muscles

Lateral dorsal cutaneous nerve (continuation of sural nerve) (*cut*)

Anterior perforating branches from plantar metatarsal arteries

Dorsal digital arteries

Dorsal branches of proper plantar digital arteries and nerves

Soleus muscle

Tibialis anterior muscle and tendon

Tibia

Anterior tibial artery and deep peroneal nerve

Extensor hallucis longus muscle and tendon

Anterior medial malleolar artery

Medial malleolus

Dorsalis pedis artery

Medial branch of deep peroneal artery

Medial tarsal arteries

Tuberosity of navicular bone

Arcuate artery

Posterior perforating branches from deep plantar arch

Deep plantar artery to deep plantar arch

Abductor hallucis muscle

Extensor hallucis longus tendon

Extensor hallucis brevis tendon (*cut*)

Extensor digitorum brevis tendons (*cut*)

Extensor digitorum longus tendons (*cut*)

Extensor expansions

Dorsal digital branches of deep peroneal nerve

Dorsal digital branches of superficial peroneal nerve

Sole of Foot: Superficial Dissection

Superficial transverse metatarsal ligaments

Proper plantar digital arteries and nerves

Transverse fasciculi

Digital slips of plantar aponeurosis

Medial plantar fascia

Lateral plantar fascia

Cutaneous branches of lateral plantar artery and nerve

Cutaneous branches of medial plantar artery and nerve

Plantar aponeurosis

Lateral band of plantar aponeurosis (calcaneometatarsal ligament)

Medial calcaneal branches of tibial nerve and posterior tibial artery

Tuberosity of calcaneus with overlying fat pad (*partially cut away*)

PLATE 500

LOWER LIMB

Proper plantar digital branches
of lateral plantar nerve

Proper plantar digital branches of medial
plantar nerve

Proper plantar digital arteries

Common plantar digital arteries
from plantar metatarsal arteries

Lumbrical muscles

Digital branch of
medial plantar artery

Fibrous sheaths
of flexor tendons

Lateral head
and
Medial head
of flexor hallucis
brevis muscle

Flexor digitorum longus tendons
(overlying flexor digitorum
brevis tendons)

Flexor hallucis longus tendon

Plantar metatarsal branch of
lateral plantar artery

Abductor hallucis muscle
and tendon

Flexor digiti minimi brevis muscle

Flexor digitorum brevis muscle

Abductor digiti minimi muscle

Plantar aponeurosis (cut)

Medial process
and
Lateral process
of
Tuberosity
of calcaneus

Medial calcaneal branches of tibial
nerve and posterior tibial artery

Proper plantar digital branches
of medial plantar nerve

Proper plantar digital branches
of lateral plantar nerve

Flexor digiti minimi
brevis muscle

Superficial branch
and
Deep branch
of lateral
plantar nerve

Lateral plantar nerve and artery

Quadratus plantae muscle

Abductor digiti minimi muscle (cut)

Nerve to abductor digiti minimi muscle
(from tibial nerve)

Flexor digitorum brevis muscle
and plantar aponeurosis (cut)

Lateral calcaneal nerve and artery
(from sural nerve and peroneal artery)

Flexor digitorum longus tendons

Flexor digitorum brevis tendons

Fibrous sheaths (opened)

Sesamoid bones

Common plantar digital
nerves and arteries

Lumbrical muscles

Lateral head
and
Medial head of
flexor hallucis brevis muscle

Flexor hallucis longus tendon

Abductor hallucis tendon
and muscle (cut)

Flexor digitorum longus tendon

Medial plantar artery and nerve

Tibialis posterior tendon

Flexor hallucis longus tendon

Posterior tibial artery and
tibial nerve (dividing)

Flexor retinaculum

Abductor hallucis muscle (cut)

Medial calcaneal artery and nerve

Tuberosity of calcaneus

PLATE 502

LOWER LIMB

Proper plantar digital branches of medial plantar nerve

Proper plantar digital branches of lateral plantar nerve

Proper plantar digital branch of medial plantar artery

Anterior perforating arteries to dorsal metatarsal arteries

Tendons of lumbrical muscles (*cut*)

Sesamoid bones

Flexor digitorum longus tendons

Transverse head and Oblique head of adductor hallucis muscle

Flexor digitorum brevis tendons (*cut*)

Medial head and Lateral head of flexor hallucis brevis muscle

Flexor digiti minimi brevis muscle

Flexor hallucis longus tendon (*cut*)

Plantar metatarsal arteries

Abductor hallucis muscle (*cut*)

Plantar interosseous muscles

Flexor digitorum longus tendon (*cut*)

Superficial branch of lateral plantar nerve

Tibialis posterior tendon

Deep plantar arterial arch and deep branches of lateral plantar nerve

Medial plantar artery and nerve

Tuberosity of 5th metatarsal bone

Flexor hallucis longus tendon

Peroneus brevis tendon

Flexor retinaculum

Peroneus longus tendon and fibrous sheath

Abductor hallucis muscle (*cut*)

Quadratus plantae muscle (*cut and slightly retracted*)

Flexor digitorum brevis muscle and plantar aponeurosis (*cut*)

Lateral plantar artery and nerve

Abductor digiti minimi muscle (*cut*)

Medial calcaneal artery and nerve

Lateral calcaneal artery and nerve

Tuberosity of calcaneus

Interosseous Muscles and Deep Arteries of Foot

Dorsal view

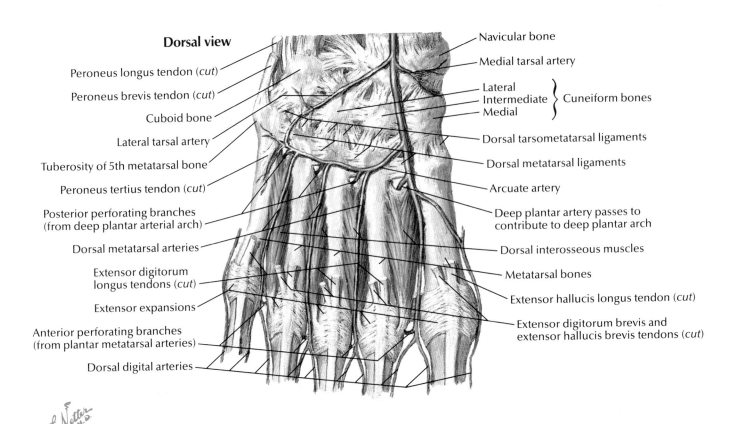

Peroneus longus tendon (*cut*)

Peroneus brevis tendon (*cut*)

Cuboid bone

Lateral tarsal artery

Tuberosity of 5th metatarsal bone

Peroneus tertius tendon (*cut*)

Posterior perforating branches
(from deep plantar arterial arch)

Dorsal metatarsal arteries

Extensor digitorum
longus tendons (*cut*)

Extensor expansions

Anterior perforating branches
(from plantar metatarsal arteries)

Dorsal digital arteries

Navicular bone

Medial tarsal artery

Lateral
Intermediate } Cuneiform bones
Medial

Dorsal tarsometatarsal ligaments

Dorsal metatarsal ligaments

Arcuate artery

Deep plantar artery passes to
contribute to deep plantar arch

Dorsal interosseous muscles

Metatarsal bones

Extensor hallucis longus tendon (*cut*)

Extensor digitorum brevis and
extensor hallucis brevis tendons (*cut*)

Plantar view

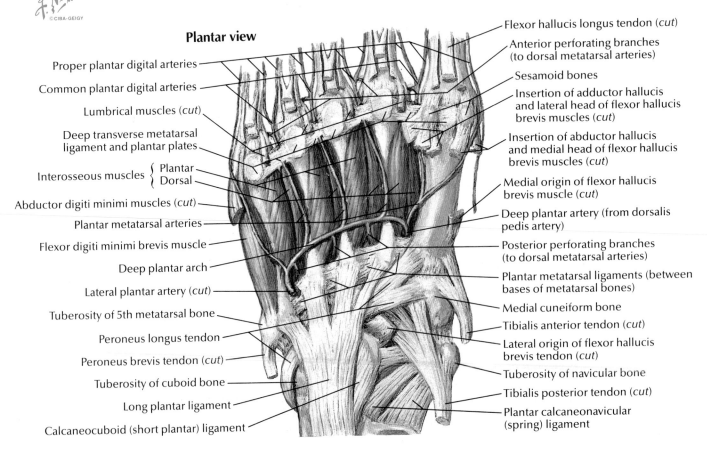

Proper plantar digital arteries

Common plantar digital arteries

Lumbrical muscles (*cut*)

Deep transverse metatarsal
ligament and plantar plates

Interosseous muscles { Plantar
Dorsal

Abductor digiti minimi muscles (*cut*)

Plantar metatarsal arteries

Flexor digiti minimi brevis muscle

Deep plantar arch

Lateral plantar artery (*cut*)

Tuberosity of 5th metatarsal bone

Peroneus longus tendon

Peroneus brevis tendon (*cut*)

Tuberosity of cuboid bone

Long plantar ligament

Calcaneocuboid (short plantar) ligament

Flexor hallucis longus tendon (*cut*)

Anterior perforating branches
(to dorsal metatarsal arteries)

Sesamoid bones

Insertion of adductor hallucis
and lateral head of flexor hallucis
brevis muscles (*cut*)

Insertion of abductor hallucis
and medial head of flexor hallucis
brevis muscles (*cut*)

Medial origin of flexor hallucis
brevis muscle (*cut*)

Deep plantar artery (from dorsalis
pedis artery)

Posterior perforating branches
(to dorsal metatarsal arteries)

Plantar metatarsal ligaments (between
bases of metatarsal bones)

Medial cuneiform bone

Tibialis anterior tendon (*cut*)

Lateral origin of flexor hallucis
brevis tendon (*cut*)

Tuberosity of navicular bone

Tibialis posterior tendon (*cut*)

Plantar calcaneonavicular
(spring) ligament

PLATE 504

LOWER LIMB

Dorsal view

Cuboid bone

Tuberosity of 5th metatarsal bone

Dorsal interosseous muscles (bipennate)

5th metatarsal bone

5th proximal phalanx

5th middle phalanx

5th distal phalanx

Navicular bone

Lateral
Intermediate } Cuneiform bones
Medial

1st metatarsal bone

1st proximal phalanx

1st distal phalanx

Plantar view

5th distal phalanx

5th middle phalanx

5th proximal phalanx

Plantar interosseous muscles (unipennate)

5th metatarsal bone

Tuberosity of 5th metatarsal bone

Cuboid bone

1st distal phalanx

1st proximal phalanx

Sesamoid bones

1st metatarsal bone

Lateral
Intermediate } Cuneiform bones
Medial

Navicular bone

Femoral Nerve and Lateral Femoral Cutaneous Nerve

Lateral femoral cutaneous nerve (L2, 3)

Femoral nerve (L2, 3, 4)

Obturator nerve

Iliacus muscle

Psoas major muscle (lower part)

Articular branch

Sartorius muscle
(cut and reflected)

Pectineus muscle

Rectus femoris
muscle (cut
and reflected)

Quadriceps
femoris
muscle

Vastus
intermedius muscle

Vastus
medialis muscle

Vastus
lateralis muscle

Articularis genus muscle

T12

L1

L2

L3

L4

Lumbar plexus

Lumbosacral trunk

Lateral femoral
cutaneous nerve

Anterior cutaneous
branches of
femoral nerve

Sartorius muscle
(cut and reflected)

Saphenous nerve

Infrapatellar branch
of saphenous nerve

Medial crural cutaneous
branches of saphenous nerve

Cutaneous
innervation

Note: only muscles
innervated by femoral
nerve shown

PLATE 506

LOWER LIMB

Iliohypogastric nerve

Ilioinguinal nerve

Genitofemoral nerve

Lateral femoral cutaneous nerve

Femoral nerve

Obturator nerve (L2, 3, 4)

Posterior branch

Articular branch

Anterior branch

Posterior branch

Cutaneous branch

Articular branch to knee joint

Hiatus of adductor canal

L1

L2

L3

L4

Lumbar plexus

Lumbosacral trunk

Obturator externus muscle

Adductor brevis muscle

Adductor longus muscle (*cut*)

Adductor magnus muscle (ischiocondylar part supplied by sciatic nerve)

Gracilis muscle

Cutaneous innervation

Note: only muscles innervated by obturator nerve shown

Sciatic Nerve and Posterior Femoral Cutaneous Nerve

Posterior femoral cutaneous nerve (S1, 2, 3)

Inferior cluneal nerves

Perineal branches

Tibial segment of sciatic nerve

Long head (*cut*) of biceps femoris muscle

Adductor magnus muscle (also partially supplied by obturator nerve)

Semitendinosus muscle

Semimembranosus muscle

Tibial nerve

Articular branch

Plantaris muscle

Medial sural cutaneous nerve

Gastrocnemius muscle

Sural nerve

Soleus muscle

Tibial nerve

Medial calcaneal branches

Medial and lateral plantar nerves

Greater sciatic foramen

Sciatic nerve (L4, 5, S1, 2, 3)

Common peroneal segment of sciatic nerve

Short head of biceps femoris muscle

Long head (*cut*) of biceps femoris muscle

Common peroneal nerve

Articular branch

Lateral sural cutaneous nerve

Peroneal communicating branch

Lateral calcaneal branches

Lateral dorsal cutaneous nerve

Cutaneous innervation

Posterior femoral cutaneous nerve

Common peroneal nerve via lateral sural cutaneous nerve

Medial sural cutaneous nerve

Superficial peroneal nerve

Sural nerve

Tibial nerve via medial calcaneal branches

From sciatic nerve

PLATE 508

LOWER LIMB

**Tibial nerve
(L4, 5, S1, 2, 3)**

Medial sural
cutaneous nerve (*cut*)

Articular branches

Plantaris muscle

Gastrocnemius
muscle (*cut*)

Nerve to popliteus muscle

Popliteus muscle

Interosseous crural nerve

Soleus muscle (*cut*)

Flexor digitorum
longus muscle

Tibialis posterior muscle

Flexor hallucis
longus muscle

Sural nerve (*cut*)

Lateral calcaneal branch

Medial
calcaneal branch

Flexor retinaculum (*cut*)

Lateral dorsal
cutaneous nerve

Common peroneal nerve

Articular branch

Lateral sural cutaneous nerve (*cut*)

From
tibial nerve
{
Medial calcaneal
branches
(S1, 2)

Medial
plantar nerve
(L4, 5)

Lateral
plantar nerve
(S1, 2)
}

Saphenous nerve
(L3, 4)

Sural nerve
(S1, 2) via
lateral calcaneal
and lateral dorsal
cutaneous
branches

Cutaneous innervation of sole

Flexor
retinaculum
(*cut*)

**Tibial
nerve**

Medial
calcaneal
branch

**Medial plantar
nerve**

Flexor digitorum
brevis muscle
and nerve

Abductor hallucis
muscle and nerve

Flexor hallucis
brevis muscle
and nerve

1st lumbrical
muscle and
nerve

Common
plantar
digital
nerves

Proper
plantar
digital
nerves

Lateral calcaneal
branch of sural nerve

**Lateral plantar
nerve**

Nerve to abductor
digiti minimi muscle

Quadratus plantae
muscle and nerve

Abductor digiti
minimi muscle

Deep branch to
interosseous
muscles,
2nd, 3rd and 4th
lumbrical muscles
and
Adductor hallucis
muscle

**Superficial
branch** to
4th interosseous
muscle
and
Flexor digiti minimi
brevis muscle

Common and
Proper plantar
digital nerves

Note: articular branches not shown

Common Peroneal Nerve

Common peroneal nerve (*phantom*)

Biceps femoris tendon

Common peroneal nerve (L4, 5, S1, 2)

Head of fibula

Peroneus longus muscle (*cut*)

Superficial peroneal nerve

Branches of lateral sural cutaneous nerve

Peroneus longus muscle

Peroneus brevis muscle

Medial dorsal cutaneous nerve

Intermediate dorsal cutaneous nerve

Inferior extensor retinaculum (*partially cut*)

Lateral dorsal cutaneous nerve (branch of sural nerve)

Dorsal digital nerves

Lateral sural cutaneous nerve (*phantom*)

Articular branches

Recurrent articular nerve

Extensor digitorum longus muscle (*cut*)

Deep peroneal nerve

Tibialis anterior muscle

Extensor digitorum longus muscle

Extensor hallucis longus muscle

Lateral branch of deep peroneal nerve to
Extensor hallucis brevis and
Extensor digitorum brevis muscles

Medial branch of deep peroneal nerve

Cutaneous innervation

Lateral sural cutaneous nerve

Superficial peroneal nerve

Deep peroneal nerve

Sural nerve via lateral dorsal cutaneous branch

PLATE 510

LOWER LIMB

Autonomous sensory zones

Anterior view

Posterior view

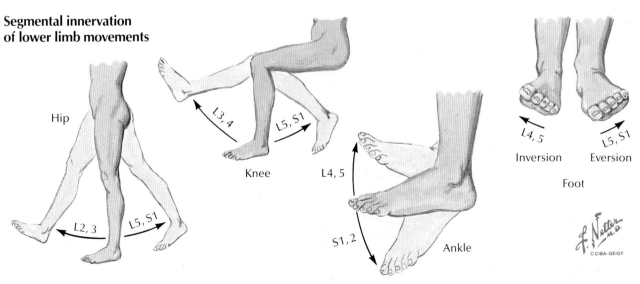

Segmental innervation of lower limb movements

Hip

Knee

Ankle

Inversion Eversion

Foot

Superficial Nerves and Veins of Lower Limb: Anterior View

Lateral cutaneous branch of subcostal nerve

Inguinal (Poupart's) ligament

Superficial circumflex iliac vein

Femoral branches of genitofemoral nerve

Lateral femoral cutaneous nerve

Fossa ovalis (saphenous opening)

Fascia lata

Anterior femoral cutaneous nerves (from femoral nerve)

Patellar nerve plexus

Branches of lateral sural cutaneous nerve (from common peroneal nerve)

Crural fascia

Superficial peroneal nerve

Medial dorsal cutaneous branch

Intermediate dorsal cutaneous branch

Lesser saphenous vein and lateral dorsal cutaneous nerve (from sural nerve)

Lateral dorsal digital nerve and vein of 5th toe

Dorsal metatarsal veins

Dorsal digital nerves and veins

Superficial epigastric vein

Ilioinguinal nerve (scrotal branch)

Genital branch of genitofemoral nerve

Femoral vein

Superficial external pudendal vein

Accessory saphenous vein

Great saphenous vein

Cutaneous branches of obturator nerve

Infrapatellar branch of saphenous nerve

Saphenous nerve (terminal branch of femoral nerve)

Great saphenous vein

Dorsal digital nerves

Dorsal venous arch

Dorsal digital nerve and vein of medial side of great toe

Dorsal digital branch of deep peroneal nerve

PLATE 512

LOWER LIMB

Superficial Nerves and Veins of Lower Limb: Posterior View

Lateral cutaneous branch of iliohypogastric nerve

Iliac crest

Superior cluneal nerves (from dorsal rami of L1, 2, 3)

Inferior cluneal nerves (from posterior femoral cutaneous nerve)

Branches of lateral femoral cutaneous nerve

Middle cluneal nerves (from dorsal rami of S1, 2, 3)

Perforating cutaneous nerve (from dorsal rami of S1, 2, 3)

Branches of posterior femoral cutaneous nerve

Accessory saphenous vein

Branch of anterior femoral cutaneous nerve

Cutaneous branch of obturator nerve

Terminal branches of posterior femoral cutaneous nerve

Great saphenous vein

Lateral sural cutaneous nerve (from common peroneal nerve)

Lesser saphenous vein

Peroneal communicating nerve

Branches of saphenous nerve

Medial sural cutaneous nerve (from tibial nerve)

Sural nerve

Lateral calcaneal branches of sural nerve

Medial calcaneal branches of tibial nerve

Lateral dorsal cutaneous nerve (continuation of sural nerve)

Plantar cutaneous branches of medial plantar nerve

Plantar cutaneous branches of lateral plantar nerve

NEUROVASCULATURE

PLATE 513

Lymph Vessels and Nodes of Lower Limb

SEE ALSO PLATES 382, 383

Superficial inguinal lymph nodes

Cribriform fascia over fossa ovalis

Superficial inguinal lymph nodes

Great saphenous vein

Fascia lata

Superficial lymph vessels

Crural fascia

Great saphenous vein

Popliteal vein

Popliteal lymph nodes

Lesser saphenous vein

External iliac lymph nodes

Femoral nerve

Inguinal (Poupart's) ligament

Ductus (vas) deferens

Femoral sheath

Femoral canal (*opened*)

Femoral artery and vein

Great saphenous vein

Femoral ring

Lacunar (Gimbernat's) ligament

Deep inguinal lymph nodes

PLATE 514

LOWER LIMB

REFERENCES

Plate 52

Braus H. Anatomie des Menschen. Berlin, Verlag von Julius Springer, 1924

Plate 85

Nishida S. The Structure of the Eye. New York, Elsevier North-Holland, 1982

Plate 150

Keegan JJ. J. Neurosurg 1947;4:115

Plate 158

Turnbull IM. Blood supply of the spinal cord. In Vinken PJ, Bruyn GW (eds). Handbook of Clinical Neurology, XII. Amsterdam, North-Holland, 1972, pp 478–491

Plates 188, 189

Jackson CL, Huber JF. Correlated applied anatomy of the bronchial tree and lungs with a system of nomenclature. Dis Chest 1943;9:319–326

Plate 191

Ikeda S, Ono Y, Miyazawa S, et al. Flexible bronchofiberscope. Otolaryngology (Tokyo) 1970;42:855–861

Plate 265

DiDio LJA. Anatomo-Fisiologia do Piloro ileo-ceco-colica no homem, Actas das Primeiras Jornadas Interuniversitarías Argentinas de Gastroenterologia, Rosario, 1954

———. Dados anatomicos sobre o "piloro" ileo-ceco-colico. (Com observacao direta in vivo de "papila" ileo-ceco-colica.) (English summary). Thesis, Fac Med, Univ de São Paulo, 1952

Plate 273

Healey JE Jr, Schroy. Anatomy of the biliary duct within the human liver; analysis of the prevailing pattern of branchings and the major variations of the biliary ducts. Arch Surg 1953;66:599

———, Sörensen. The intrahepatic distribution of the hepatic artery in man. J Int Coll Surg 1953;20:133

Plates 274, 275

Elias H. Liver morphology. Biol Rev 1955;30:263

———. Origin and early development of the liver in various vertebrates. Act Hepat 1955;3:1

———. Morphology of the liver. In "Liver Injury," Trans 11th Conference. New York, Macy Foundation, 1953

———. A re-examination of the structure of the mammalian liver; the hepatic lobule and its relation to the vascular and biliary system. Am J Anat 1949;85:379

———. A re-examination of the structure of the mammalian liver; parenchymal architecture. Am J Anat 1949;84:311

Plates 288, 289

Michels NA. Blood Supply and Anatomy of the Upper Abdominal Organs, With a Descriptive Atlas. Philadelphia, JB Lippincott, 1955

Plate 312

Thomas MD. In The Ciba Collection of Medical Illustrations, Vol 3, Part II. Summit NJ, CIBA, p 78

Plate 378

Flocks RH, Kerr HD, Elkins HB, et al. Treatment of carcinoma of the prostate by interstitial radiation with radio-active gold (Au198): A preliminary report. J Urol 1952;68(2):510–522

Plate 455

Keegan JJ, Garrett FD. The segmental distribution of the cutaneous nerves in the limbs of man. Anat Rec 1948;102:409–437

Plate 511

Keegan JJ. J Bone Joint Surg 1944;26:238

Last RJ. Innervation of the limbs. J Bone Joint Surg 1949;31(B):452

Index

References are to plate numbers; numbers in bold refer to primary sources. In most cases, structures are listed under singular nouns

A

Abdomen
arteries of 238, 247—see also arteries of individual organs
bones of 231
cross sections of 331, 332
lymph nodes of 249, 299–301, 325—see also lymph nodes of individual organs
muscles of 232–237, 246
nerves of 240, 241, 250—see also nerves of individual organs
veins of 239, 248—see also veins of individual organs
viscera of—see individual organs
Acetabulum 334, 457
Achilles—see Tendon, Achilles; calcaneal
Acinus 192
Acromion 22, 170, 174, 178, **396**–402, 404, 406, 407
Action of
extrinsic eye muscles 79
infrahyoid muscles 24
intrinsic laryngeal muscles 73
jaws 11
suprahyoid muscles 24
wrist 427
Adam's apple—see Prominence, laryngeal
Adamkiewicz—see Artery, of Adamkiewicz
Adenohypophysis 133, 140
Adenoid—see Tonsil, pharyngeal
Adhesion, interthalamic 100, 102, 105, 109, 139
Aditus of larynx 57, 60, 223
Adrenergic neurons 154
Agger nasi 32, 33
Air cell—see Cell (air)
Ala of
central cerebellar lobule 107
ilium 231, 334, 339, 457
sacrum 145
vomer 5
Albini—see Nodule, Albini's
Alveolus of
lung 192, 193
pancreas 279

Alveus of hippocampus 106
Ampulla
of ductus deferens 362
of duodenum 262, 276
hepatopancreatic 278
of inner ear 87
labyrinthine 90, 118
of lactiferous duct 167
of semicircular duct 90, 118
of uterine tube 350
of Vater—see Ampulla, of duodenum
of vestibule 91
Anastomosis
between
carotid and vertebral arteries 131
cervical and occipital arteries 28
circumflex femoral arteries 474
external and internal carotid arteries 80, 131
intercostal and lumbar arteries 218, 238
median and ulnar nerves 446, 448, 449
pancreatic arteries 284–286
pubic branches of obturator and inferior epigastric arteries 344
subclavian and carotid arteries 131
subclavian and vertebral arteries 131
at elbow 409
paravertebral 158
portacaval 297
prevertebral 158
scapular 402
Angiogram, coronary—see Arteriogram of coronary arteries
Angle
anterior chamber, of eye 82, 83, 86
iridocorneal—see Angle, anterior chamber, of eye
of Louis—see Joint, sternomanubrial
of mandible 9, 10, 60
of mastoid 6
of rib 170, 171
scapular 396, 397
of sternum 170
subpubic 336
Ankle
bones of 482, 483, 492–494
ligaments of 495
lymph nodes of 514
Annulus fibrosus of
heart 210, 213
intervertebral disc 144
Anoderm 369
Anomaly of
cervical ribs 173

Anomaly *cont.*
right inferior laryngeal nerve 74
right subclavian artery 74
Ansa
cervicalis 26, **27**, 29, 65, 68, 122, 123
hypoglossi—see Ansa cervicalis
subclavia 124, 198, 214, 215, 228
Anteflexion of uterus 352
Antihelix of external ear 88
Antitragus of external ear 88
Antrum
mastoid 89
pyloric 258
tympanic 89
Anus 341, 354, 358, 360, 371, 373, 393
Aorta
abdominal 165, 181, 217, 220, 246, **247**, 253, 256, 257, 261, 279, 282, 284, 290, 310, 313, 315, 316, 318, 324, 328, 329, 331–333, 343, 344, 348, 373, 375–378, 387
arch of 30, 68, 69, 74, 131, 184, 195, 196, 199–203, 208, 209, 213, 217, 219, **220**, 221, 225
ascending 131, 194, 203, 208, 211, 212
descending 131, 180, 194, 196, 219, 220, 225, 230
thoracic 156, 158, 179, 217, 219, 221, **225**
Aperture—see also Opening
lateral, of 4th ventricle 102, 103, 139
median, of 4th ventricle 102, 103, 109, 139
Apex of
bladder 342
fibula 482, 483
heart 201, 202
lung 184, 185, 187
sacrum 145
tongue 52
Aponeurosis
bicipital 406, 408, 420, 446, 453
external abdominal oblique 232–235, 240, 242, 244, 331, 332
gluteal 316, 464, 465, 472
internal abdominal oblique 234, 235, 240, 332
palatine 46, 59
palmar 416, 420, 421, 428, 432, 433, 435, 453
pharyngeal 59, 61, 223
plantar 497, 500–503
of scalp 17, 20, 21, 164—see also Galea aponeurotica
transversus abdominis 161, 162, 165, 235, 237, 238, 316, 328, 332

Bone *cont.*
  talus 492–494
  tarsal—see Bone, of foot
  temporal 1–3, 5, 6, 8, 9
  of thigh 475, 458
  of thorax 170, 171
  tibia—see Tibia
  trapezium 426, 427, 430, 431, 434, 440
  trapezoid 426, 427, 429, 430
  triquetral 426–430
  vertebra—see Vertebra
  vomer—see Vomer
  of wrist 426, 427, 430
  zygomatic 1, 2, 5, 8, 76
Bowel—see Colon
Bowman—see Capsule, Bowman's
Boyden—see Sphincter, of common bile duct
Brachium of
  inferior colliculus 105, 108
  superior colliculus 105, 108
Brain 96, 99, 109
Brainstem 108, 110, 111
Bregma 4
Brim, pelvic 145, 349—see also Linea, terminalis of pelvis
Bronchiole 192, 193
Bronchus
  anteromedial basal 191
  cardiac (left lung) 191
  eparterial 187, 190, 191, 194, 195, 220
  extrapulmonary 190
  intermediate 191, 195
  intrapulmonary 190, 192
  lingular 190, 191
  lobar 191
  lower lobe 187, 190, 191, 194
  main **190**, 191, 194–196, 198, 218–222, 230
  middle lobe 190, 191, 194
  nomenclature of 191
  2nd order 191—see also Bronchus, lobar
  3rd order 191—see also Bronchus, segmental
  4th order 191
  primary 190, 195, 196, 198—see also Bronchus, main
  segmental 192
  subsegmental 192
  superior division 190, 191
  upper lobe 187, 190, 191, 194, 195
    right—see also Bronchus, eparterial
Brunner—see Gland, duodenal
Buck—see Fascia, Buck's
Bulb
  of corpus spongiosum 360
  duodenal 259, 262
  olfactory 101, 113
  of penis 347, 360–363
  urethral 347, 361, 362
  vestibular 349, 355–357, 379
Bulla, ethmoidal 32, 33
Bundle
  atrioventricular 213
  Bachmann's 213

Bundle *cont.*
  of His 213
  interatrial conduction—see Bundle, Bachmann's
  of Kent (accessory atrioventricular) 213
  oval 151
Burns—see Space, of Burns
Bursa
  anserine 476, 477
  of biceps femoris tendon 476, 477, 480
  of fibular collateral ligament 476–478, 480
  of gastrocnemius muscle 480
  iliopectineal 458, 466
  of iliotibial tract 476–478
  olecranon 412
  omental 256, 331, 333—see also Sac, lesser peritoneal
  radial 433–436
  of semimembranosus muscle 476, 480
  subcutaneous
    calcaneal 497
    infrapatellar 480
    lateral malleolar 497
    medial malleolar 497
    prepatellar 480
  subdeltoid 398, 406
  subscapular 398
  subtendinous
    calcaneal 490, 497
    infrapatellar 480
    suprapatellar 477, 478, 480
  ulnar 433–436, 439

C

Calcaneus 492–**494**, 496, 497
Calcar avis 105, 106
Calot—see Lymph node, of Calot; Triangle, cystic
Calvaria 4, 96
Calyx of kidney 317
Camper—see Fascia, Camper's
Canal
  adductor 470, 471, 475
  Alcock's 287, 296, 368, 373, 374, 377, 379, 380, 386, 388
  anal 341, 368, 369
  carotid 5, 93
  central, of spinal cord 102, 103, 109
  cervical, of uterus 350
  condylar 5, 7
  dental root 51
  facial 118
  femoral 244, 514
  gastric 259
  of Hering 274, 275—see also Ductule, bile
  Hunter—see Canal, adductor
  hyaloid, of eye 82
  hypoglossal 3, 5, 7, 16, 122
  incisive 3, 32–37
  infraorbital 40

Canal *cont.*
  inguinal 244
  mandibular 54
  nasofrontal 33
  nasolacrimal 33
  obturator 236, 334, 337, 339, 345, 346, 348, 377
  optic 1, 3, 7, 78
  pudendal 287, 296, 368, 373, 374, 377, 379, 380, 386, 388
  pyloric 258
  sacral 145
  of Schlemm 82–84, 86
  semicircular 90–92
  spinal—see Canal, vertebral
  vertebral 13, 143, 144
Canaliculus
  bile 275
  lacrimal 77
  mastoid 5
  tympanic 5
Cap of duodenum 259, 262
Capillary
  intrapulmonary 193
  subpleural 193
Capitate—see Bone, capitate
Capitulum of
  humerus 396, 411
  mandible—see Caput of mandible
Capsule—see also Ligament; Joint
  atlantoaxial 14, 15
  atlantooccipital 14, 15
  of basal ganglia
    external 104
    internal 102, 104, 134
  Bowman's 321
  glomerular 321
  of kidney 317, 321, 322, 328
  lens 82, 83, 85
  of liver 273
  of suprarenal gland 329
  temporomandibular 11
  Tenon's 78, 82
  of vertebral joint, lateral 14, 15
  zygapophyseal 14, 15, 146
Caput of mandible 2, 10
Carpal—see Bone, carpal
Cartilage
  alar 31, 33, 34
  arytenoid 59, 71, 72
  of auditory tube 46, 49, 59, 61, 93
  corniculate 59, 71
  costal 170, 171, 180, 184, 231, 241
  cricoid 9, 23, 24, 57, 59, 62, 68, **71**, 72, 184, 190, 195, 221–223
  laryngeal 71
  nasal
    lateral 31, 33, 34
    septal 31, 34
  thyroid 9, 23, 24, 26, 57, 59, 62, 68, **71**, 72, 184, 190, 195, 221–223
  tracheal 190
Caruncle
  hymenal 354

Fovea
  caudal—see Fovea, inferior, of 4th
    ventricle
  centralis, in macula lutea 82, 86
  of head of femur 459
  inferior, of 4th ventricle 109
  superior, of 4th ventricle 109
Foveola, granular 4, 94, 96
Frenulum of
  clitoris 354
  lip 45
  penis 360
  tongue 45, 55
  vermiform appendix 265
Fundus of
  gallbladder 270, 276
  stomach 221, 224, 258
  urinary bladder 342, 347
  uterus 341, 343, 348, 350
Funiculus, lateral 109

G

Galea aponeurotica 17, 20, 21, 96, 164
Galen—see Vein, of Galen
Gallaudet—see Fascia, Gallaudet's
Gallbladder 120, 153, 184, 252, 255, 258,
  269–271, **276**, 277, 284, 331
Ganglion
  aorticorenal 152, 153, 250, **304**, 306–310,
    326, **327**, 330, 384, 385, 389–392
  basal 102, 104, 134
  celiac 120, 152–154, 228, 250, **304**,
    305–**310**, 311, 313, 314, 326, 330,
    331, 384, 385, 389–392
  cervical sympathetic
    inferior—see Ganglion, cervico-
      thoracic; stellate
    middle 65, 124, 152, 154, 214, 215, 228
    superior 28, 39, 54, 119, 122, **124,
      125**–128, 152, 154, 199, 214, 215, 228
  cervicothoracic 124, 152, 198, 215, 228
  ciliary 40, 81, 115, 116, 125, **126**, 152, 153
  of cochlea, spiral 91, 118
  geniculate 39, 41, 110, 117–119, 125, 129
  of glossopharyngeal nerve
    inferior 119, 128, 129
    jugular—see Ganglion, of glosso-
      pharyngeal nerve, superior
    petrosal 129—see also Ganglion,
      of glossopharyngeal nerve,
      inferior
    superior 119
  intermediate—see Ganglion, of
    sympathetic trunk, vertebral
  lumbar sympathetic 156, 216, 304, 326,
    327, **384, 385,** 387, 389–391
  mesenteric
    inferior 152–154, 304, **309**, 310, 326,
      384, 385, 389–392
    superior 120, 152–154, 250, 304,
      306–**308, 309**–311, 314, 326, 327,
      330, 384, 385, 389–392

Ganglion *cont.*
  nodose 129—see also Ganglion, of
    vagus nerve, inferior
  otic 11, 41, 49, 116, 117, 119, 125, 127, **128**,
    129, 152, 153
  petrosal 129—see also Ganglion, of
    glossopharyngeal nerve, inferior
  phrenic 306, 313
  pterygopalatine 37–40, 56, 65, 115–117,
    119, 125, **127**, 129, 152, 153
  renal 326, 327, 330, 391, 392
  sacral sympathetic 154, 304
  semilunar 40, 41, 81, 129—see also
    Ganglion, trigeminal
  spinal **155**, 156, 166, 179, 241, 307, 310,
    311, 313, 314, 327, 392
  stellate 124, 152, 198, 214, 215, 228
  submandibular 41, 53, 55, 65, 116, 117,
    125, **127**, 152, 153
  of sympathetic trunk
    cervical
      inferior—see Ganglion,
        cervicothoracic; stellate
      middle 65, 124, 152, 154, 214, 215,
        228
      superior 28, 39, 54, 119, 122, **124,
        125**–128, 152, 154, 199, 214, 215,
        228
    lumbar 156, 216, 304, 326, 327, **384,
      385,** 387, 389–391
    sacral 154, 304
    thoracic 126, 152, 156, 179, 198, 214,
      215, **228**, 230, 307, 311, 390, 391
    vertebral 124, 152, 214, 215, 228
  thoracic sympathetic 126, 152, 156, 179,
    198, 214, 215, **228**, 230, 307, 311,
    390, 391
  trigeminal **40**, 41, 81, 93, 98, 110, 111, 116,
    125–129
  of vagus nerve
    caudal—see Ganglion, of vagus
      nerve, inferior
    inferior 120–122, 129, 228
    jugular—see Ganglion, of vagus
      nerve, superior
    nodose 129—see also Ganglion,
      of vagus nerve, inferior
    rostral—see Ganglion, of vagus
      nerve, superior
    superior 120, 121, 228
  vertebral sympathetic 124, 152, 214, 215,
    228
  vestibular 90, 118
Gartner—see Duct, Gartner's
Gasserian ganglion—see Ganglion,
  semilunar
Geniculum of facial nerve 89, 92, 111
Genitalia
  female 354, 393
  male 358–360, 365, 393
Genu of
  corpus callosum 100, 101, 104, 106, 139
  facial nerve
    external—see Ganglion, geniculate

Genu, of facial nerve *cont.*
    internal—see Geniculum of facial
      nerve
  internal capsule 104
Gerdy—see Tubercle, Gerdy's
Gimbernat—see Ligament, Gimbernat's
Gingiva 51
Glabella 1, 2
Gland
  anal 369
  areolar 167
  Bartholin's—see Gland, vestibular,
    greater
  Brunner's—see Gland, duodenal
  bulbourethral 342, 361–363, 394
  Cowper's 342, 361–363, 394
  duodenal 262
  fundic 259
  gastric 259
  intestinal 312
  lacrimal 40, 77, 78, 80, 81, 127, 153
  lingual 45, 52
  of Littré 363
  mammary 167
  Meibomian 76
  mucous, of tongue 52
  palatine 46, 57, 58
  parathyroid 69, 70
  paraurethral 394
  parotid **19**, 22, 23, 26, 54, 55, 60, 66, 119,
    128, 153, 154
    accessory 55
  pineal—see Body, pineal
  pituitary 32, 98, 100, 101, 140
  preputial 360
  prostate—see Prostate
  pyloric 259
  retromolar 46
  salivary 54, 55—see also Gland, parotid;
    sublingual; submandibular
  sebaceous 76
  serous, of Ebner 52
  Skene's 394
  Stenson's—see Gland, parotid
  sublingual 41, 45, 47, 54, 55, 117, 127,
    153
  submandibular 22, 23, 26, 27, **41**, 47, 54,
    55, 60, 63, 64, 117, 127, 153
  suprarenal 153, 154, 185, 255, 257, 261, 270,
    279, 281, 315, 317, 328, **329**–331, 364
  sweat 153, 154, 369
  tarsal 76
  thymus 200, 218, 219
  thyroid 23, 24, 26, 28, 30, 57, 64, **68**, 69,
    70, 184, 186, 195
  Tyson's 360
  urethral 357, 363
  vestibular, greater 356, 379, 394
  Wharton's—see Gland, submandibular
Glans of
  clitoris 354, 393
  penis 342, 360, 363, 393
Glisson—see Capsule, of liver
Globus pallidus 102, 104

Nerve *cont.*
  of shoulder 450–452
  of sigmoid colon 153
  of small intestine 153, 308, 310, 312
  to sphincter of pupil 115, 153
  spinal
    cervical 18, 27, 30, 65, 108, 121, 148, 149, 152, 163, 164, 166, 182, 215, 216
    lumbar 147–149, 152, 156, 163, 165, 166, 215, 216, 237, 241, 385, 390, 392
    sacral 148, 149, 152, 163, 166, 389
    thoracic 126–128, 148, 149, 152, 155, 156, 163, **166**, 178, 179, 215, 216, 237, **241**, 311—see also Nerve, intercostal
  spinosus—see Nerve, meningeal branches of mandibular
  splanchnic
    lumbar 152, 153, 304, 309, 310, 326, 327, 330, 384, 385, 387, 389–392
    pelvic 152–154, 250, 304, 310, 326, 327, 385, 387, 389–392, 467, 469
    sacral 152, 153, 309, 310, 326, 385, 387, 392, 469
    thoracic
      greater 152, 153, 180, 181, **198**, 216, 218, 219, 228, 230, 241, 246, 250, 304–311, 313, 314, 326, 330, 384, 385, 389–391
      least 152, 153, 181, 198, 216, 246, 250, 304–311, 326, 327, 330, 331, 384, 385, 389–391
      lesser 152, 153, 181, **198**, 216, 241, 246, 250, 304–311, 326, 327, 330, 331, 384, 385, 389–391
  to stapedius muscle 117
  to sternohyoid muscle 27—see also Ansa cervicalis
  to sternothyroid muscle 27—see also Ansa cervicalis
  of stomach 153, 304–307
  to stylohyoid muscle 19
  to stylopharyngeus muscle 119
  to subclavius muscle 405
  subcostal 148, 237, 240, 250, 315, 316, 384, 389, 467, 468, 512
  sublingual 41
  of sublingual gland 153
  of submandibular gland 153
  suboccipital 14, 164
  subscapular
    lower 401, 404, 405, 450
    middle 405—see also Nerve, thoracodorsal
    upper 404, 405
  superficial branch of
    lateral plantar 502, 503, 509
    radial 418, 421, 423, 432, 440–442, 445, 446, 451, 453, 454
    ulnar 421, 432, 433, 439, 446, 449
  to superior gemellus muscle 467, 469, 472, 473

Nerve *cont.*
  supraclavicular 18, 26, 27, 123, 240, 452, 454
  supraorbital 18, 31, 40, 76, 81, 116
  of suprarenal glands 153, 330
  suprascapular 401, 404, 405, 450
  supratrochlear 18, 31, 40, 76, 81, 116
  sural 508, 509, 513
    cutaneous
      dorsal lateral 498, 499, 508–510, 512, 513
      lateral 472, 485, 486, 491, 508–513
      medial 472, 485, 486, 491, 508, 509, 513
  of sweat gland 153
  sympathetic 39, 115–117, 126–128, 152–154, 199, 215, 216, 307, 310, 311, 313, 314, 327, 330, 389–392
  of teeth 40, 41
  temporal branch of facial 19, 117
  temporal branches of mandibular, deep 35, 41, 65, 116
  to tensor tympani muscle 41, 116
  to tensor veli palatini muscle 41, 65, 116
  tentorial branch of ophthalmic 40, 81, 116
  of thigh 470–472, 506–508
  thoracic, long 174, 175, 177, 240, 404, 405
  of thoracic wall 179
  thoracodorsal 401, 404, 405
  to thyrohyoid muscle 27, 29—see also Ansa cervicalis
  of thyroid gland 68
  tibial 465, 467, 469, 472, 475, 485–487, 491, 497, 502, 508, 509
  of tongue 53, 56
  tonsillar branch of glossopharyngeal 56, 58, 65, 119
  of trachea 153, 199
  of tracheobronchial tree 199
  transverse cervical 18, 26, 27, 123
  trigeminal 18, 40, 41, 56, 92, 108, 110–112, **116**, 125, 127–129, 137
  trochlear 78, 81, 98, 108–112, **115**
  tubal, of tympanic plexus 119
  tympanic 89, 117, 119, 128
  ulnar 404, 405, 407, 408, 410, 418–423, 428, 433, 434, 438, 439, 441, 445–**449**, 454
  of ureter 326, 327, 392
  of urinary bladder 153, 326, 392
  vagus 27–30, 56, 63–65, 68–70, 74, 98, 108, 110–112, 119, **120**, 121, 124, 125, 129, 152–154, 182, 195, 198–201, 214, 215, 218–220, 228, 310, 311, 327
  vestibular 87, 90, 92, 118
  vestibulocochlear 87, 90, 92, 98, 108, 110–112, **118**, 125
  Vidian 37–40, 116, 117, 119, 125, 127, 129
  of wrist 445
  zygomatic branch of
    facial 19, 117
    maxillary 40, 115, 116

Nerve *cont.*
  zygomaticofacial 18, 40, 65, 116
  zygomaticotemporal 18, 40, 65, 116
Nervi erigentes 309, 310, 326, 385, 387, 390–392, 467—see also Nerve, splanchnic, pelvic
Nervous system
  autonomic 39, 110–112, 115–117, 119, 120, **124**–128, 152–154, **198**, 199, 215, 216, 228, **304**–314, 326, 327, 330, 384, 385, 387, 389–392
  parasympathetic 39, 115–117, 119, 120, 126–128, 152–154, 199, 215, 307, 310, 311, 313, 314, 327, 389–392
  sympathetic 39, 115–117, 126–128, 152–154, 199, 215, 216, 307, 310, 311, 313, 314, 327, 330, 389–392
Nervus
  intermedius 56, 98, 108, 112, 117, 118, 129
  spinosus—see Nerve, meningeal branches of mandibular
Neurohypophysis 133, 140
Nipple of breast 167, 184
Node
  atrioventricular (AV) 213
  lymph—see Lymph node
  sinoatrial (SA) 204, 213
Nodule
  Albini's 211
  Arantii 211
  of cerebellum 107, 137
  fibrous, of mitral valve 211
  lymph—see Lymph nodule
  of semilunar valve 211
Nodulus of cerebellum 109
Nomenclature of bronchi 191
Nose
  concha of 32–34
  external 31
  lateral wall of 32, 33
  medial wall of 34
  septum of 34
Notch
  of acetabulum 334, 457
  angular, of stomach 258
  anterior cerebellar 107
  cardiac, of
    lung 184, 186, 187
    stomach 224, 258
  cerebellar 107
  fibular 482
  greater sciatic 231, 457
  inferior vertebral 143, 144
  interarytenoid 60, 75
  intertragic 88
  ischiatic—see Notch, sciatic
  jugular 23, 170, 184
  lesser sciatic 231, 457
  pancreatic 279
  posterior cerebellar 107
  preoccipital 99
  radial, of ulna 411, 413
  scapular 170, 396–398, 400–402
  sciatic 231, 457